I0057284

Diagnostic Pathology: Beyond the Basics

Diagnostic Pathology: Beyond the Basics

Edited by Terence Glover

hayle
medical

New York

Hayle Medical,
750 Third Avenue, 9th Floor,
New York, NY 10017, USA

Visit us on the World Wide Web at:
www.haylemedical.com

© Hayle Medical, 2019

This book contains information obtained from authentic and highly regarded sources. Copyright for all individual chapters remain with the respective authors as indicated. All chapters are published with permission under the Creative Commons Attribution License or equivalent. A wide variety of references are listed. Permission and sources are indicated; for detailed attributions, please refer to the permissions page and list of contributors. Reasonable efforts have been made to publish reliable data and information, but the authors, editors and publisher cannot assume any responsibility for the validity of all materials or the consequences of their use.

ISBN: 978-1-63241-729-9

Trademark Notice: Registered trademark of products or corporate names are used only for explanation and identification without intent to infringe.

Cataloging-in-Publication Data

   Diagnostic pathology : beyond the basics / edited by Terence Glover.
      p. cm.
   Includes bibliographical references and index.
   ISBN 978-1-63241-729-9
   1. Diagnosis, Laboratory. 2. Diagnosis. 3. Pathology. I. Glover, Terence.
RB37 .D53 2019
616.075--dc23

Table of Contents

Preface

The field of diagnostic pathology is concerned with the causal study of diseases. It addresses primarily four components of a disease- its cause, pathogenesis, morphological changes and clinical manifestations. The study of disease involves a study of varied disease markers using techniques that are specific to organs and tissue types. The fields of anatomical and clinical pathology are intrinsic to diagnostic pathology. Anatomical pathology involves a gross, chemical, immunologic and molecular examination of tissues, organs and whole bodies. It includes cytopathology, dermatopathology, neuropathology, renal pathology, etc. Clinical pathology employs various visual and microscopic tests to analyze the biophysical properties of tissue samples involving cultures and automated analyzers. Immunopathology, hematopathology and radiation pathology fall within the domain of clinical pathology. The aim of this book is to present researches that have transformed this discipline and aided its advancement. It covers in detail some existing theories and innovative practices of diagnostic pathology. It aims to equip students and experts with the advanced topics and upcoming concepts in this field.

After months of intensive research and writing, this book is the end result of all who devoted their time and efforts in the initiation and progress of this book. It will surely be a source of reference in enhancing the required knowledge of the new developments in the area. During the course of developing this book, certain measures such as accuracy, authenticity and research focused analytical studies were given preference in order to produce a comprehensive book in the area of study.

This book would not have been possible without the efforts of the authors and the publisher. I extend my sincere thanks to them. Secondly, I express my gratitude to my family and well-wishers. And most importantly, I thank my students for constantly expressing their willingness and curiosity in enhancing their knowledge in the field, which encourages me to take up further research projects for the advancement of the area.

Editor

GATA3 is a sensitive marker for primary genital extramammary paget disease: an immunohistochemical study of 72 cases with comparison to gross cystic disease fluid protein 15

Ming Zhao[1†], Lixin Zhou[2†], Li Sun[2], Yan Song[3], Yunquan Guo[4], Xun Zhang[3], Feng Zhao[4], Peng Wang[5], Junqiu Yue[6], Dongfeng Niu[2], Zhongwu Li[2], Xiaozheng Huang[2], Qiang Kang[2], Lin Jia[2], Jinping Lai[7] and Dengfeng Cao[8*]

Abstract

Background: GATA-binding protein 3 (GATA3) has been identified as a sensitive marker for breast carcinoma but its sensitivity in primary genital extramammary Paget diseases (EMPDs) has not been well studied.

Methods: Here we investigated immunohistochemical expression of GATA3 in 72 primary genital EMPDs (35 from female, 37 from male; 45 with intraepithelial disease only, 26 with both intraepithelial disease and invasive adenocarcinoma including 14 also metastasis, 1 with metastatic adenocarcinoma only for study). We also compared GATA3 to gross cystic disease fluid protein 15 (GCDFP15) for their sensitivity.

Results: Positive GATA3 staining was seen in all 71 (100%) intraepithelial diseases, 25/26 (96%; female 10/10, male 15/16) invasive adenocarcinomas and 14/15 (93%; female 3/3, male 11/12) metastatic adenocarcinomas, respectively. Positive GCDFP15 staining was seen in 46/71 (65%; female 28/34 or 82%, male 18/37 or 49%) intraepithelial diseases, 20/26 (77%; female 9/10, male 11/16) invasive adenocarcinomas, and 12/15 (80%; female 2/3, male 10/12) metastatic adenocarcinomas, respectively (GATA3 versus GCDFP15: $p < 0.01$ for both intraepithelial disease and invasive adenocarcinoma, $p = 0.28$ for metastatic adenocarcinoma). In positive-stained cases, GATA3 stained more tumor cells than GCDFP15 (79% versus 25% for intraepithelial disease, 71% vs 34% for invasive adenocarcinoma, 73% vs 50% for metastatic adenocarcinoma, $p < 0.01$ for all 3 components).

Conclusions: Our findings indicate that GATA3 is a very sensitive marker for primary genital EMPDs and is more sensitive than GCDFP15.

Keywords: GATA3, GCDFP15, Extramammary Paget disease, Immunohistochemical marker

* Correspondence: dcao@path.wustl.edu
†Equal contributors
[8]Department of Pathology and Immunology, Washington University School of Medicine, 660 S South Euclid Avenue Campus Box 8118, Saint Louis, MO 63110, USA
Full list of author information is available at the end of the article

Background

Paget disease (PD) is a distinct intraepidermal adenocarcinoma with a pagetoid growth pattern. PDs are classified as mammary and extramammary subtypes according to their locations and their relationship to breast [1, 2]. Mammary PDs account for 90% of the PDs occurring on the skin of nipple/areola complex and most of them represent tumor spread to the epidermis from an underlying invasive ductal carcinoma (53–60%) or ductal carcinoma in situ (24–43%). Compared to breast PD, primary extramammary PDs (EMPDs) are relatively uncommon and their histogenesis is less clear [1, 2].

Primary EMPDS are found in areas rich in apocrine glands. The most common site of primary EMPDs is vulva followed by perianal skin, scrotum and penis, and axilla etc. [1–6]. In women, more than 80% of primary EMPDs are in the vulva [1–4, 6]. In men, approximately half of EMPDs are in the penoscrotal region [4–8]. Most primary EMPDs are intraepithelial at their initial presentation (type Ia disease) but some have both intraepithelial disease and invasive adenocarcinoma i.e. invasive EMPDs [1–11]. The invasive adenocarcinomas seen in primary EMPDs include those arising from intraepithelial EMPD (type Ib disease) and those giving rise to the intraepithelial disease (type Ic disease, underlying adenocarcinoma with subsequent epidermal involvement i.e. Paget disease as manifestation of an underlying adenocarcinoma) [3]. Among patients with invasive EMPDs (type Ib and type Ic), 20% to 40% had lymph node metastasis [4–7, 9, 11]. Up to 17% to 50% patients with invasive EMPDs also develop concurrent or subsequent distant metastasis [4, 5, 7, 9–12].

Primary EMPDs should be distinguished from secondary EMPDs given their different treatment and prognosis [3]. Secondary EMPD is usually the result of intraepithelial spread from a visceral carcinoma located elsewhere, with the gastrointestinal tract (colorectum) or urogenital tract (urinary bladder, prostate) being the most 2 common sources [1–3, 9, 13–17]. EMPDs may also pose some diagnostic challenges in metastatic sites as they morphologically may mimic other tumors such as urothelial carcinoma and breast carcinoma. This diagnostic challenge is further complicated by the fact that patients with EMPDs have an increased risk of developing secondary primary tumors in which breast carcinoma, colorectal adenocarcinoma and urothelial carcinoma are among the most common ones [4–6, 9, 14–17].

Given the overlapping morphologic features between primary EMPDs and secondary ones, and between metastatic EMPDs and their mimics in metastatic sites, immunohistochemical markers are often needed to facilitate the correct diagnosis. Several immunohistochemical markers, including cytokeratin 7, carcinoembryonic antigen, androgen receptor and c-erbB2 (HER2), have been used for diagnosing primary EMPDs, however, their specificity is relatively low [18–20] and therefore limited their diagnostic utility in metastatic setting. Gross cystic duct fluid protein 15 (GCDFP15, also known as BRST-2) shows relatively high specificity for EMPDs but its sensitivity was only 60% to 85% and in many cases the staining was focal [21–26]. Primary EMPD is analogous to breast Paget disease. Recently a transcription factor GATA-binding protein 3 (GATA3) has been identified as a very sensitive marker for breast carcinoma, both in both primary and metastatic sites [27–31]. GATA3 was also reported to be highly expressed in apocrine glands and adnexal tumors [30]. Apocrine gland has been proposed as the origin of primary EPMDs according to one theory [1, 2, 21]. These findings suggest that GATA3 might be a sensitive marker for primary EMPDs. In the literature, there was only one recent report of GATA3 in 11 vulvar primary EMPDs [32].

In this study, using immunohistochemical staining we investigated the expression of GATA3 in a large series of 72 primary EMPDs (45 with intraepithelial disease only, 26 with both intraepithelial disease and invasive adenocarcinoma including 14 also with lymph node metastasis, 1 with metastatic adenocarcinoma only for study) in male and female genital regions to explore the potential diagnostic utility of GATA3 in these tumors. We also compared GATA3 to GCDFP15 in these tumors for their sensitivity.

Methods

Materials

The surgical pathology archives of the authors' hospitals were searched for primary EMPDs in male and female genital regions. A total of 72 surgically resected cases with confirmed diagnosis of primary EMPDs in the genital region were included for this study: 35 from female and 37 from male patients. All 35 female cases were from vulva, including 24 with intraepithelial disease only (type Ia disease), 10 with both intraepithelial disease and invasive adenocarcinoma (5 type Ib, 5 type Ic, 2/5 type Ic cases with metastatic adenocarcinoma in nodes) and 1 with only metastatic node disease for study (history of primary vulvar EMPD). No breast tissue or mammary-like gland was present in the adjacent vulva tissue in any of these female cases. The 37 male cases included 3 from penis, 1 from perineum, and 33 from the scrotum. Twenty-one (21 or 57%) male cases were intraepithelial diseases, 16 (43%) cases had both intraepithelial disease and invasive adenocarcinoma (14 type Ib, 2 type Ic; 12/16 also with nodal metastasis including 11/14 type Ib and 1/2 type Ic).

Immunohistochemical staining

One to two formalin-fixed, paraffin-embedded full tissue blocks from each case were retrieved to generate 4 um unstained slides for immunohistochemical staining on a Ventana Benchmark-XT automated stainer using the Ventana ultraView DAB detection kit. The antibody to GATA3 is a mouse monoclonal antibody (clone L50–823, prediluted, Biocare, Concord, CA 94520). The antibody to GCDFP15 was a rabbit monoclonal antibody (clone EP95, prediluted, Rocklin, CA 95677). The automatic immunohistochemical reaction was performed with Ventana Cell Conditioning Solution 1 (CC1) at pH 6.0. The primary antibody (antibody to GATA3, antibody to GCDFP15) was incubated at 37 degrees for 24 min. Positive control (breast ductal carcinoma as positive control) and negative control (incubation with secondary antibody only) were included for each run of immunostains. Only nuclear staining was considered positive for GATA3. The staining pattern for GCDFP15 is cytoplasmic. The percentage of tumor cells labeled was semi-quantitatively scored as 0 (<1% tumor cell staining), 1+ (1–25%), 2+ (26–50%), 3+ (51–75%), and 4+ (76–100%).

Statistical analysis

The Fisher exact test was used to compare the staining pattern for GATA3 with GCDFP15, and paired t-test was used to compare the mean percentage of tumor cells stained with GATA3 with GCDFP15 in the intraepithelial component, invasive component and metastatic components of EMPDs. A P-value of <0.05 was considered statistically significant.

Results

Expression of GATA3 and GCDFP15 in female primary extramammary Paget diseases

Among the 35 vulvar EMPDs, 24 had intraepithelial disease only, 10 had both intraepithelial disease and invasive adenocarcinoma (2 also had regional lymph node metastasis) and 1 had only the metastatic adenocarcinoma in one lymph node for study (history of vulvar primary EMPD). Among the 10 cases with both intraepithelial disease and invasive adenocarcinoma, 5 were type Ib and 5 were type Ic diseases (4 apocrine carcinomas and 1 eccrine carcinoma). The staining results of GATA3 and GCDFP15 for each component of vulvar extra-mammary diseases are summarized in Table 1.

All 34 intraepithelial disease components showed positive GATA3 staining (34/34, 100%), including 1+ in 2 (6%), 2+ in 1 (3%), 3+ in 3 (9%) and 4+ in 28 (82%), with almost all cases demonstrating moderate to strong nuclear staining (Fig. 1). The invasive adenocarcinoma showed positive GATA3 staining in all 10 cases (2+ in 2, 4+ in 8) (Figs. 2, 3). All 3 metastatic adenocarcinomas from vulvar EMPDs showed 4+ GATA3 staining (Fig. 2).

Positive GCDFP15 staining was seen in 28 of 34 (82%) intraepithelial disease components (1+ in 12/28, 2+ in 4/28, 3+ in 4/28, 4+ in 8/28) and 9 of 10 (90%) invasive adenocarcinomas (1+ in 3/10, 3+ in 1/10, and 4+ in 5/10; 5/5 type Ib disease, 4/5 type Ic disease) (Table 1, Figs. 2, 3). The only invasive adenocarcinoma that was negative for GCDFP 15 staining was the eccrine carcinoma (type Ic disease). Two of the 3 (66%) metastatic adenocarcinomas showed positive GCDFP15 staining (1+, 4+) (Fig. 2).

Expression of GATA3 and GCDFP15 in male primary extramammary Paget diseases

Among the 37 cases of male extra-mammary Paget diseases, 33 were from the scrotum, 3 from the penis and 1 from the perineum. Twenty-one (57%) had intraepithelial disease only. The remaining 16 cases (16/37 or 43%) had both intraepithelial disease and invasive adenocarcinoma (14 type Ib, 2 type Ic) including 12 (12/16, 80%)

Table 1 Immunohistochemical staining results of GATA3 and GCDFP15 in primary vulvar extramammary Paget diseases

Disease Component	GATA3 staining[a]						GCDFP15 staining[a]						P value
	0	1+	2+	3+	4+	Total	0	1+	2+	3+	4+	Total	
Intraepithelial disease (N = 34)	0	2 (6%)	1 (3%)	3 (9%)	28 (82%)	34 (100%)	6 (8%)	12 (35%)	4 (12%)	4 (12%)	8 (24%)	28 (82%)	0.0004[#]
Type Ia (N = 24)		1		3	20		4	8	4	3	5		
Type Ib (N = 5)			1		4		1	3			1		
Type Ic (N = 5)		1			4		1	1		1	2		
Invasive adenocarcinoma (N = 10)	0	0	2 (20%)	0	8 (80%)	10 (10%)	1 (10%)	3 (30%)	0	1 (10%)	5 (50%)	9 (90%)	0.1035[#]
type Ib (N = 5)					5			1		1	3		
type Ic (N = 5)			2		3		1	2			2		
Metastatic adenocarcinoma (N = 3)	0	0	0	0	3 (100%)	3 (100%)	1 (33%)	1 (33%)	0	0	1 (33%)	2 (67%)	not applicable

[a]The staining is semi-quantitatively as follows: 0: <1% tumor cell staining; 1+: 1–25% tumor cells staining; 2+: 26–50% tumor cells staining; 3+: 51–75% tumor cells staining; 4+: 76–100% tumor cells staining. *NA* non-applicable due to small number

[#]p value refers to comparison of staining patterns (0,1+,2+,3+,4+) not percentage of total positives

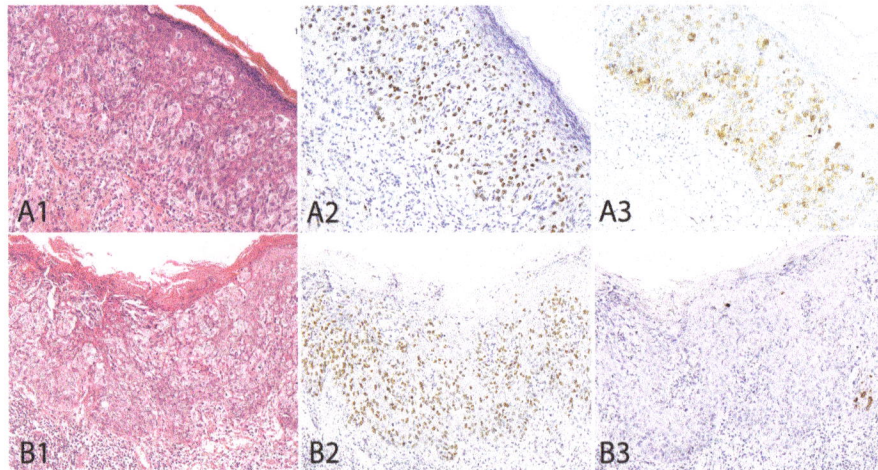

Fig. 1 Immunohistochemical staining of GATA3 and GCDFP15 in primary extramammary Paget diseases in the genital region: all intraepithelial diseases in both genders (A1, vulva; B1, scrotum) were positive for GATA3 (A2, B2). Most of intraepithelial diseases (50% male, 82% female) were also positive for GCDFP15 (A3, B3). GCDFP15 staining is often focal (B3)

with lymph node metastases. The staining results of GATA3 and GCDFP15 for each component of male extra-mammary diseases are summarized in Table 2.

Positive GATA3 staining was seen in all 37 intraepithelial disease components (100%), including 1+ in 4 (11%), 2+ in 2 (6%), 3+ in 2 (6%), and 4+ in 29 (78%) (Fig. 1). The invasive adenocarcinomas showed positive GATA3 staining in 15/16 (94%) cases including 1+ in 2 (12%), 2+ in 2 (12%), 3+ in 1 (6%) and 4+ in 10 (63%) (Fig. 2). The invasive adenocarcinoma in type Ib disease was positive for GATA3 in 13/14 cases (93%). The underlying invasive adenocarcinomas in 2 type Ic EMPDs were both positive for GATA3 (2+, 4+). Positive GATA3 staining was seen in 11/12 (92%) metastatic adenocarcinomas, including 1+ in 1 (8%), 2+ in 1 (8%), 3 + in 1 (8%) and 4+ in 8 cases (67%) (Fig. 2).

Positive GCDFP15 staining was seen in 18 of 37 (51%) intraepithelial disease components including 1+ in 12 (32%), 2+ in 4 (11%), and 4+ in 2 (6%) (Fig. 1). The invasive adenocarcinomas showed positive GCDFP15 staining in 11 of 16 (69%) cases including 1+ in 6 (38%), 2+ in 1 (6%) and 4+ in 4 (25%). The invasive adenocarcinoma in Type Ib disease was positive for GCDFP15 in 9/ 14 (64%, 1+ in 5/9, 4+ in 4/9) cases. The 2 invasive adenocarcinomas in type IC EMPDs showed positive GCDFP15 staining in both (1+, 2+). Positive GCDFP15 was seen in 10 of 12 (83%) metastatic adenocarcinomas (1+ in 3/12, 2+ in 2/12, 3+ in 1/12, 4+ in 4/12) (Fig. 2).

Comparison of GATA3 to GCDFP15 in primary genital extramammary Paget diseases

Among the 71 intraepithelial diseases (34 from female, 37 from male), all (100%) showed GATA3 staining whereas only 46 of them (46/71 or 65%, female 28/34 or

82%, male 18/37 or 51%) showed positive GCDFP15 staining ($p < 0.0001$). Among the invasive adenocarcinomas, positive GATA3 and GCDFP15 staining was seen in 25/26 (96%) and 18/26 (69%) cases, respectively ($p = 0.01$). Among the 15 metastatic adenocarcinomas, 14 (93%) showed positive GATA3 staining and 12 (80%) showed positive GCDFP15 staining ($p = 0.2825$).

Among the cases with positive immunohistochemical staining, the mean percentage of positively stained tumor cells in the intraepithelial diseases was 79% (female 83%, male 76%) for GATA3 and it was 25% (female 35%, male 10%) for GCDFP15 ($p < 0.001$). As far as the invasive adenocarcinomas were concerned, the mean percentage of tumor cells positive for GATA3 and GCDFP15 was 71% (female 76%, male 68%) and 34% (female 42%, male 34%), respectively ($p < 0.001$). The mean percentage of GATA3-positive metastatic adenocarcinoma cells was 73% (female 90%, male 68%) and it was 50% for GCDFP15 (female 65%, male 48%) ($p < 0.01$).

Expression of GATA3 in normal epidermal cells

Positive GATA3 staining was seen in some normal epidermal cells in 22/34 (65%) female and 22/37 (60%) cases, respectively, mainly in the spinous layer (typically focal but occasionally diffuse) with occasionally in the basal layer. Among the GATA3 positive cases, the GATA3 staining intensity in the normal epidermal cells was weaker than that in PD in 16/22 (73%) female and 17/22 (77%) cases, respectively. Similar GATA3 staining intensity was seen in the normal epidermal cells and in the intraepithelial PD cells in 6 of 22 (27%) female and 5 of 22 (23%) male cases, respectively. The intraepithelial PD cells typically have larger nuclei than normal epidermal cells. However, in 2 cases in each gender, the

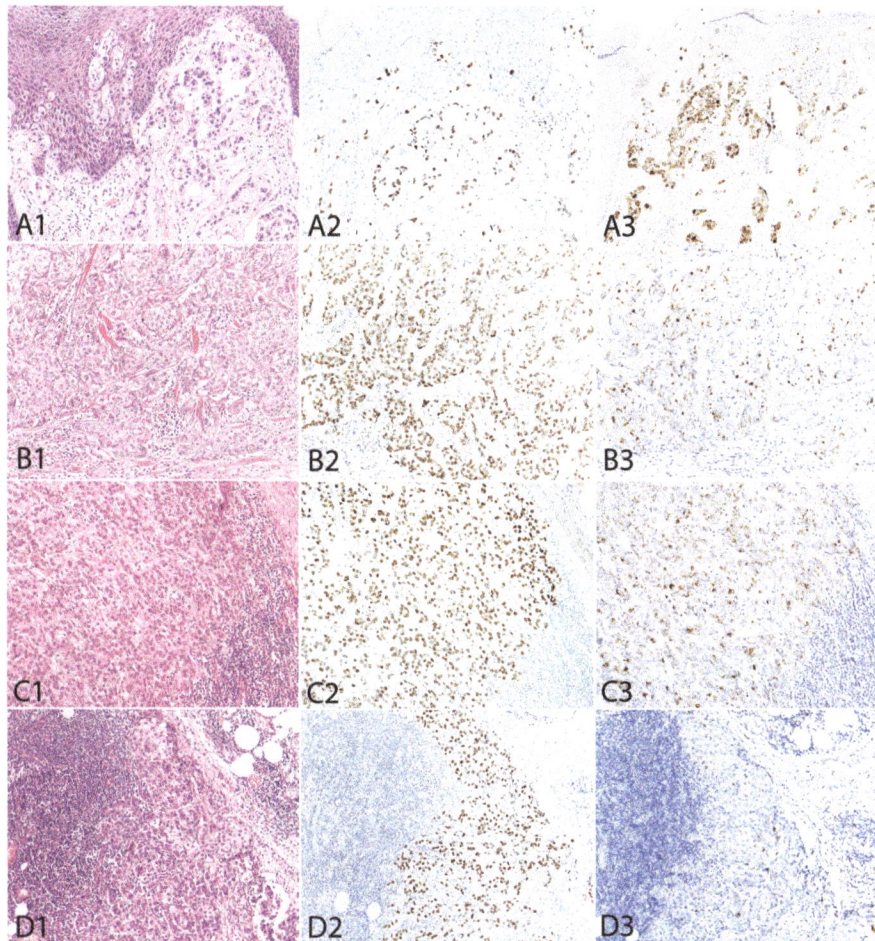

Fig. 2 The invasive adenocarcinoma in type Ib disease (primary extramammary Paget disease with invasive adenocarcinoma) (A1: vulva, with intracytoplasmic mucin; B1: scrotum) showed positive GATA3 staining in all but one cases (A2, B2) (A2 also with intraepithelial disease). Most of such invasive adenocarcinomas were also positive for GCDFP15 staining (A3, B3). All 3 metastatic adenocarcinomas from vulvar (C1) and 11 of 12 metastatic adenocarcinomas from penoscrotal (D1) extramammary Paget diseases were positive for GATA3 (C2, D2) and most of them were also positive for GCDFP15 (C3, D3). GATA3 stains more tumor cells than GCDFP15 in some cases (D2, D3)

intraepithelial PD cells focally have small nuclei and in these areas it is difficult to distinguish the intraepithelial PD cells from normal epidermal cells just based on immunohistochemical staining. Their distinction relies on the growth pattern.

Discussion

In this study, we investigated the immunohistochemical expression of GATA3 in a large series of 72 primary EMPDs in male and female genital regions. We found that GATA3 was highly expressed in the primary genital EMPDs. The high sensitivity of GATA3 is not only present in the intraepithelial disease (100%) but also in the invasive adenocarcinomas (96%) and metastatic adenocarcinomas (93%). These results indicate that GATA3 is a very sensitive marker for primary EMPDs in the genital regions.

GATA3 is a zinc-finger transcription factor involved in embryogenesis, cell proliferation and differentiation in multiple human tissues and organs, including breast, genitourinary system, parathyroid, skin, central nervous and hematopoietic systems [33–36]. In 2007, Higgins et al. found that GATA3 was a sensitive diagnostic marker for urothelial carcinoma [37]. Since then, there has been growing evidence that GATA3 could serve as a relatively sensitive diagnostic marker for breast carcinomas, parathyroid tumors, trophoblastic tumors, mesonephric adenocarcinomas, paragangliomas and pheochromocytomas etc. [28–31, 38–42]. Other tumors with a less frequent expression of GATA3 include salivary gland tumors, malignant mesotheliomas, pancreatic adenocarcinomas, skin squamous cell carcinomas, skin adnexal tumors, renal oncocytomas, chromophobe renal cell carcinomas, and yolk sac tumors [28–30]. Morbeck D et al. recently reported positive GATA3 expression in all 11 vulvar primary

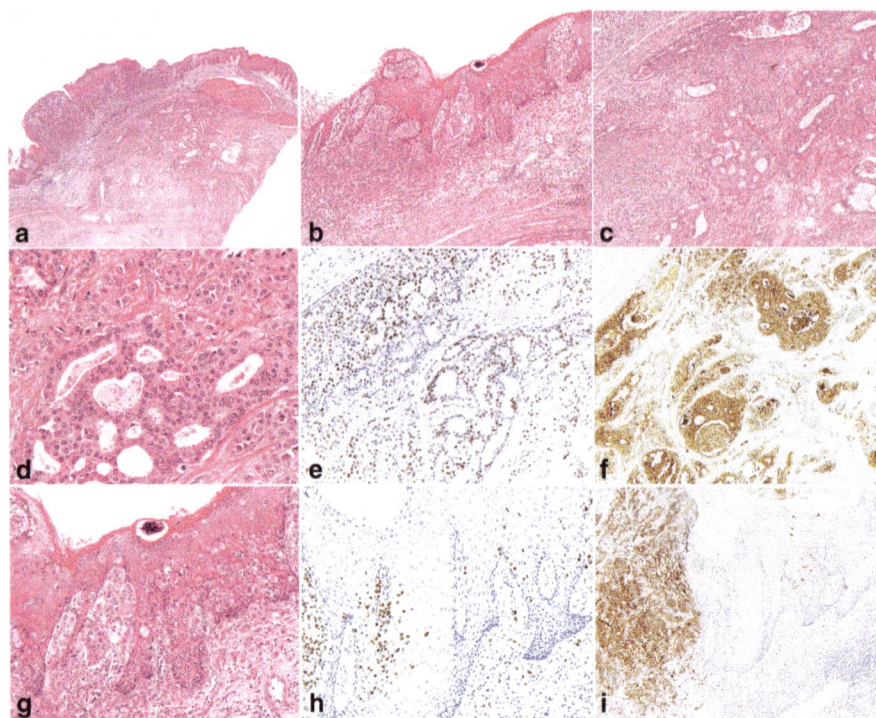

Fig. 3 Immunohistochemical staining of GATA3 and GCDFP15 in a vulvar primary extra-mammary Paget disease with an underlying apocrine adenocarcinoma (type Ic disease). The underlying apocrine adenocarcinoma formed a mass in the dermis and subcutaneous tissue but it eroded the epidermis (**a**) and grew in a pagetoid pattern within the adjacent epidermis (**b**, **g**). The underlying adenocarcinoma showed nests, solid and glandular growth patterns with some cribriform glands (**c**, **d**). Cytoplasmic apical apocrine snouts were apparent (**d**). Both the underlying invasive apocrine adenocarcinoma (**d**) and the overlying intraepithelial Paget disease (**g**) were positive for GATA3 (**e**, **h**) and GCDFP15 (**f**, **i**). Similar GATA3 findings were also observed in penoscrotal type Ic diseases

EMPDs (4 with invasive carcinoma) [32]. They did not include any metastatic adenocarcinoma from vulvar Paget disease. They did not study male genital EMPDs, either. Our findings and that of Morbeck et al. [32] add primary genital EMPDs to the list of tumors with **high** expression of GATA3. High expression of GATA3 in EMPDs has some diagnostic implications, both for primary EMPDs and their metastasis.

Distinguishing primary from secondary EMPDs is clinically critical given their different treatment and prognosis [3, 9]. Secondary EMPD in the genital region is usually the result of intraepithelial spread from a visceral carcinoma,

Table 2 Immunohistochemical staining results of GATA3 and GCDFP15 in primary male genital extramammary Paget diseases

Disease Component	GATA3 staining[a]						GCDFP15 staining[a]						P value
	0	1+	2+	3+	4+	Total	0	1+	2+	3+	4+	Total	
Intraepithelial disease (N = 37)	0	4 (11%)	2 (6%)	2 (6%)	29 (78%)	37 (100%)	19 (51%)	12 (32%)	4 (11%)	0	2 (6%)	18 (49%)	< 0.001
Type Ia (N = 21)		1			20		17	4					
Type Ib (N = 14)		3	1	2	8		1	7	4		2		
Type Ic (N = 2)			1		1		1	1					
Invasive adenocarcinoma (N = 16)	1 (6%)	2 (13%)	2 (13%)	1 (6%)	10 (63%)	15 (94%)	5 (31%)	6 (38%)	1 (6%)	0	4 (25%)	11 (69%)	0.062
type Ib (N = 14)	1	2	1	1	9		5	5			4		
type Ic (N = 2)			1		1			1	1				
Metastatic adenocarcinoma (N = 12)	1 (8%)	1 (8%)	1 (8%)	1 (8%)	8 (67%)	11 (92%)	2 (17%)	3 (25%)	2 (17%)	1 (8%)	4 (33%)	10 (83%)	0.277

[a]The staining is semi-quantitatively scored as follows: 0: < 1% tumor cell staining; 1+: 1–25% tumor cells staining; 2+: 26–50% tumor cells staining; 3+: 51–75% tumor cells staining; 4+: 76–100% tumor cells staining

with urogenital tract (urothelial carcinoma, prostate) and the gastrointestinal tract (distal colon, rectum) being the most 2 common sources [1–3, 6, 9, 12–16]. In females, secondary EMPD in vulva caused by urothelial carcinoma typically involves periurethral vulvar vestibule but it may extend to the adjacent vulvar skin and it may also become invasive [1–3, 6, 9, 12–16]. In males, both urothelial carcinoma and prostate carcinoma may involve scrotum in an intraepithelial pagetoid fashion [43–45]. Rarely urothelial carcinoma [43, 46] and prostate adenocarcinoma [43, 47, 48] may recur in the penis as a secondary EMPD. Since both primary EMPDs and urothelial carcinomas are positive for GATA3, GAT3 is not useful in distinguishing primary EMPDs from secondary EMPD caused by urothelial carcinoma and other markers should be sought for this purpose. Urothelial carcinomas are often positive for uroplakin-III, p63 and p40 whereas EMPDs have an opposite immunohistochemical profile [49–51]. GCDFP15 is often positive in primary EMPDs [20–26] but it is only rarely positive in urothelial carcinoma [43, 52]. Secondary EMPD caused by prostatic adenocarcinoma can be distinguished from primary EMPD by p501S (prostein) and GATA3. Prostatic adenocarcinoma is positive for p501S but negative for GATA3 whereas EMPD shows an opposite profile [28–30, 43, 53]. Prostatic adenocarcinoma can be rarely positive for GCDFP15 and primary EMPDs can show positive prostate specific antigen (PSA) staining in as many as 30% cases [43, 53]. Therefore, one cannot rely on PSA or GCDFP15 to distinguish primary EMPD from secondary PD caused by prostatic adenocarcinoma. Secondary EMPDs from anorectal adenocarcinomas typically extend from perianal skin to the vulva or scrotum [1–6, 9, 43, 44]. GATA3 is negative in colorectal adenocarcinoma [28–30] and therefore is useful to distinguish primary genital EMPD from secondary EMPD due to colorectal adenocarcinoma. It should be pointed out that primary EMPDs can be rarely positive for CDX2 (3%) [43]. GCDFP15 is negative in colorectal adenocarcinomas [43]. Anorectal adenocarcinoma and primary vulvar EMPDs showed overlapping profiles in CK7 and CK20 though CK7 negativity favors the former and CK20 negativity favors the latter [43]. In the genital area, rare pagetoid squamous cell carcinoma in situ can closely mimic intraepithelial EMPD [54, 55] and may be misdiagnosed as such [54]. Since some squamous cell carcinomas and normal epidermal cells are positive for GATA3 [28–30], GATA3 is not useful to distinguish primary EMPD from pagetoid squamous cell carcinoma in situ. Instead P63 should be used in this scenario (p63 negative in primary EMPD but positive in pagetoid squamous cell carcinoma in situ) [50, 51]. Lastly, melanoma in situ may closely mimic primary EMPD and rare pigmented primary

EMPD has been reported [56, 57]. Melanoma in situ was negative for GATA3 [28–30] but positive for S100, melan-A and HMB45 whereas EMPD had an opposite immunoprofile.

Although most primary EMPDs are intraepithelial, approximately 4% to 20% primary vulvar EMPDs [1–4, 9, 13, 15, 16] and 26% to 61% primary penoscrotal EMPDs were invasive at the time of presentation [5, 7, 8, 10, 58–61]. Some of these invasive adenocarcinomas arise from the intraepithelial EMPD (type Ib primary EMPDs) whereas others are underlying adenocarcinomas which showed secondary epidermotropism (type Ic primary EMPDs) [3, 6, 8, 9, 14–16]. In vulva, it is estimated that type Ic EMPDs account for at least 10–30% invasive EMPDs [1–3, 8, 9, 15, 16, 62]. Rare type Ic primary EMPD in penoscrotum has also been reported [63] and two of our cases belong to this category. Type Ic EMPDs were reported to be associated with a worse prognosis than type Ib EMPDs [3, 9] and therefore pathologists should attempt to specify the subtypes of primary invasive EMPDs (Ib versus Ic). However, it is not always feasible to distinguish them. Our findings indicate that type Ib and apocrine type Ic diseases cannot be distinguished by their GATA3 and GCDFP15 immunoprofile given their similar profile for these two markers. Type Ic EMPDs are predominantly of apocrine type, but other types of adenocarcinomas may also rarely give rise to type Ic EMPDs including eccrine sweat gland adenocarcinoma [64], Bartholin gland adenocarcinoma [65], and adenocarcinomas of mammary-like glands [66, 67] etc. One of the invasive adenocarcinomas in vulvar type Ic EMPDs in our study was an eccrine carcinoma. Cutaneous eccrine carcinomas were positive for GATA3 in 36% to 68% cases [68, 69]. The only eccrine carcinoma in our study showed 4+ GATA3 staining (>75% cells). Thus, GATA3 immunostaining cannot distinguish type Ib EMPDs from apocrine and *eccrine* type Ic primary EMPDs. Their distinction relies on morphology and other markers such as p63 and GCDFP15. Eccrine carcinomas were often positive p63 (85% to 89%) whereas primary type Ib EMPDs were not [68, 69]. Eccrine carcinomas were only rarely positive for GCDFP15 (5%) [69]. Adenocarcinoma of mammary-like gland in the vulva is rare and its diagnosis requires the presence of a transition zone between normal mammary-like glands and adenocarcinoma [66, 67, 70]. Morphologically it is similar to breast carcinoma. Both ductal type [66] and lobular-like [67] mammary-like carcinomas with Paget's disease (type Ic primary EMPD) have been reported. Although there has been no report of GATA3 in vulvar adenocarcinoma of mammary-like glands, it is conceivable that the vast majority of these tumors will be positive for GATA3 as in breast carcinoma. As expected, two thirds of vulvar mammary-like carcinomas were also positive for GCDFP15 [70]. For these reasons, rare type IC primary EMPD due to mammary-like carcinoma cannot be distinguished from type Ib EMPD or type IC EMPD due to sweat gland adenocarcinoma by GATA3 and GCDFP15 immunostaining. Primary type Ic EMPDs caused by underlying apocrine carcinomas were often negative for ER and PR. In contrast, vulvar mammary-like carcinomas were often positive for these two markers [66, 67, 70–72].

Among patients with invasive EMPDs (type Ib and Ic), some will develop metastatic disease at the time of presentation or in their subsequent disease courses. In the SEER data, 17.1% patients with invasive EMPDs have lymph node metastasis (male 16.0%, female 17.6%) and 2.5% have distant metastasis (male 3.8%, female 1.9%) at presentation [4]. In a recent Japanese study of 301 primary invasive EMPDs (both male and female), 114 (37%) had metastasis including 20% node metastasis and 17% distant metastasis (16% with both nodal and distant metastasis) [12]. Lymph nodes metastasis typically involved inguinofemoral nodes but pelvic and para-aortic nodes were also involved in some patients [9–11, 22, 58–62]. Distant metastatic sites include bone, lung, liver, lung, brain and muscle [9, 58–62]. Invasive EMPDs were morphologically similar to other types of tumors especially breast carcinoma and urothelial carcinoma, and therefore they may pose some diagnostic difficulty in metastasis, which can be further complicated by the fact that patients with primary EMPDs have an increased risk of developing other types of secondary primary tumors (overall 5–8% chance). Breast carcinoma and urothelial carcinoma are among the most common secondary tumors in these patients, and they can occur either before or after the diagnosis of primary EMPDs [6, 9, 12, 14–17, 58–60, 62]. In patients with both a primary invasive EMPD and another type of tumor (particularly urothelial and breast carcinoma), the differential diagnosis for a metastatic tumor with positive GATA3 staining should also include metastatic primary EMPDs in the list of differential diagnosis. A panel of immunohistochemical markers should be used to facilitate the correct diagnosis.

GCDFP15 was a useful marker for primary EMPDs but its sensitivity was 60% to 85% [20–26]. In this study, we showed that GATA3 is relatively more sensitive than GCDFP15 for primary EMPDs, especially in male patients. Our study is the largest series of primary EMPDs with GCDFP15 staining. It is interesting to note that GCDFP15 stains a higher percentage of primary EMPDs in female patients than male patients.

Although GATA3 is a sensitive marker for primary genital EMPDs, it should be pointed out that it is not specific for these tumors. As described above and reviewed elsewhere, several other types of tumors including urothelial carcinoma, breast carcinoma, paragangliomas/pheochromocytomas, trophoblastic tumors, and

mesonephric adenocarcinomas are often positive for GATA3 [28–31, 38–42]. In this sense, GATA3 is less specific than GCDFP15 for primary genital EMPDs. In difficult cases particularly in metastasis, both GATA3 and GCDFP15 should be used in conjunction to avoid misdiagnosis.

Lastly, high expression of GATA3 in primary EMPDs may also help shed some lights on the histogenesis of these tumors. Currently there are 3 theories: intraepidermal origin of adnexal origin such as apocrine glands, multipotent stem cells in the epidermis or infundibular stem cells from hair follicles [1, 2, 20, 73]. Positive staining for both GATA3 and GCDFP15 in primary EMPDs probably favors the first theory.

One limitation of our study is that we did not include genital secondary EMPDs. Secondary EMPDs are rare and it is difficult to collect a meaningful number of cases to do a comparison study. The two most common types of carcinomas that cause secondary EMPDs are urothelial carcinoma and colorectal carcinoma [1–3, 9, 13–17]. As discussed above, GATA3 immunoreactivity was seen in most urothelial carcinomas but not in colorectal carcinomas [28–30, 37].

Conclusions

In summary, we investigated immunohistochemical expression of GATA3 in a large series of 72 primary EMPDs in the male and female genital regions. Our findings show that GATA3 is a very sensitive marker for genital primary EMPDs and is more sensitive than GCDFP15. Although GATA3 is highly sensitive for primary EMPDs, it is not specific for these tumors. GATA3 staining cannot distinguish intraepithelial PD from pagetoid squamous cell carcinoma in situ or primary EMPD from secondary EMPD caused by urothelial carcinoma. GATA3 staining can be used to distinguish primary EMPD from pagetoid melanoma in situ and secondary EMPD caused by colorectal carcinoma. In the metastatic setting, GATA3-positive tumors should include metastatic adenocarcinoma originated from PD.

Abbreviations
EMPD: Extramammary Paget disease; GATA3: GATA-binding protein 3; GCDFP15: Gross Cystic Disease Fluid Protein 15; PD: Paget disease

Acknowledgements
None.

Funding
None.

Authors' contributions
DC conceived the research idea and designed this study along with MZ and LZ. LS, YG, FZ, PW, ND, and ZL collected samples. XH, QK and LJ performed

immunohistochemical staining. MZ, YS, and JY drafted the manuscript. XZ and JL revised the manuscript. DC revised the manuscript and finalized it. All authors read and approved the final manuscript.

Competing interests

The authors declare that they have no competing interests.

Author details

[1]Department of Pathology, Zhejiang Provincial People's Hospital, Hangzhou, China. [2]Department of Pathology, Key Laboratory of Carcinogenesis and Translational Research (Ministry of Education), Peking University Cancer Hospital (Beijing Cancer Hospital), Beijing, China. [3]Department of Pathology, Cancer Hospital of Chinese Academy of Medical Sciences, Beijing, China. [4]Department of Pathology, Xinjiang Medical University Affiliated Tumor Hospital, Urumqi, China. [5]Department of Pathology, Beijing Ditan Hospital, Beijing, China. [6]Department of Pathology, Hubei Cancer Hospital, Wuhan, China. [7]Department of Pathology, Saint Louis University School of Medicine, Saint Louis, MO, USA. [8]Department of Pathology and Immunology, Washington University School of Medicine, 660 S South Euclid Avenue Campus Box 8118, Saint Louis, MO 63110, USA.

References

1. Lloyd J, Flanagan AM. Mammary and extramammary Paget's disease. J Clin Pathol. 2000;53:742–9.
2. Kanitakis J. Mammary and extramammary Paget's disease. J Eur Acad Dermatol Venereol. 2007;21:581–90.
3. Wilkinson EJ, Brown HM. Vulvar Paget disease of urothelial origin: a report of three cases and a proposed classification of vulvar Paget disease. Hum Pathol. 2002;33:549–54.
4. Karam A, Doigo O. Treatment outcomes in a large cohert of patients with invasive extramammamry Paget's disease. Gynecol Oncol. 2012;125:346–51.
5. Herrel LA, Weiss AD, Goodman M, Johnson TV, Osunkoya AO, Delman KA, et al. Extramammary Paget's disease in males: survival outcomes in 495 patients. Ann Surg Oncol. 2015;22:1625–30.
6. Van der Zwan JM, Siesling S, Blokx WA, Blokx WA, Pierie JP, Capocaccia R. Invasive extramammary Paget's disease and the risk for secondary tumours. Eur J Surg Oncol. 2012;38:214–21.
7. Ito Y, Igawa S, Ohishi Y, Uehara J, Yamamoto AI, Iizuka H. Prognostic indicators in 35 patients with extramammary Paget's disease. Dermatol Surg. 2012;38:1938–44.
8. Liu Y, Yuan B, Wang Y, Xue F. Clinicopathologic study of vulvar Paget's disease in China. J Low Genit Tract Dis. 2014;18:281–4.
9. Parker LP, Parker JR. Bodurka-Bevers, Deavers M, Bevers MW, Shen-Gunther J, et al. Paget's disease of the vulva: pathology, pattern of involvement, and prognosis. Gynecol Oncol. 2000;77:183–9.
10. Kang Z, Zhang Q, Zhang Q, Li X, Hu T, Xu X, et al. Clinical and pathological characteristics of extramammary Paget's disease: report of 246 Chinese male patients. Int J Clin Exp Pathol. 2015;8:13233–40.
11. Wang Z, Lu M, Dong GQ, Jiang YQ, Lin MS, Cai ZK, et al. Penile and scrotal Paget's disease: 130 Chinese patients with long-term follow-up. BJU Int. 2008;102:485–8.
12. Ohara K, Fujisawa Y, Yoshino K. A proposal for a TNM staging system for extramammary Paget disease: Retrospective analysis of 301 patients with invasive primary tumors. J Dermatol Sci. 2016;83:234–9.
13. Boradman CH, Webb MJ, Cheville JC, Lerner SE, Zincke H. Transitional cell carcinoma of the bladder mimicking recurrent paget's disease of the vulva: report of two cases, with one occurring in a myocutaneous flap. Gynecol Oncol. 2001;82:200–4.
14. van Der Linden M, Meeuwuis KA, Bulten J, Bosse T, van Poelgeest MI, de Hullu JA. Paget disease of the vulva. Crit Rev Oncol Hematol. 2016;101:60–74.
15. Chanda JJ. Extramammary Paget's disease: prognosis and relationship to internal malignancy. J Am Acad Dermatol. 1985;13:1009–14.
16. Fanning J, Lambert HC, Hale TM, Morris PC, Schuerch C. Paget's disease of the vulva: prevalence of associated vulvar adenocarcinoma, invasive Paget's disease, and recurrence after surgical excision. Am J Obstet Gynecol. 1999; 180:24–7.
17. Karam A, Dorigo O. Increased risk and pattern of secondary malignancies in patients with invasive extramammary Paget disease. Br J Dermatol. 2014; 170:661–71.
18. Ohnishi T, Watanabe S. The use of cytokeratins 7 and 20 in the diagnosis of primary and secondary extramammary Paget's disease. Br J Dermatol. 2000; 142:243–7.
19. Liegl B, Horn LC, Moinfar F. Androgen receptors are frequently expressed in mammary and extramammary Paget's disease. Mod Pathol. 2005;18:1283–8.
20. Plaza JA, Torres-Cabala C, Ivan D, Prieto CG. HER-2/neu expression in extramammary Paget disease: a clinicopathologic and immunohistochemistry study of 47 cases with and without underlying malignancy. J Cutan Pathol. 2009;36:729–33.
21. Mazoujian G, Pinkus GS, Haagensen DE Jr. Extramammary Paget's disease-evidence for an apocrine origin. An immunoperoxidase study of gross cystic disease fluid protein-15, carcinoembryonic antigen, and keratin proteins. Am J Surg Pathol. 1984;8:43–50.
22. Shu B, Shen XX, Chen P, Fang XZ, Guo YL, Kong YY. Primary invasive extramammary Paget disease on penoscrotum: a clinicopathological analysis of 41 cases. Hum Pathol. 2016;47:70–7.
23. Liegl B, Leibl S, Gogg-Kamerer M, Tessaro B, Horn LC, Moinfar F. Mammary and extramammary Paget's disease: an immunohistochemical study of 83 cases. Histopathology. 2007;50:439–47.
24. Olson DJ, Fujimura M, Swanson P, Okagaki T. Immunohistochemical features of Paget's disease of the vulva with and without adenocarcinoma. Int J Gynecol Pathol. 1991;10:285–95.
25. Kohler S, Smoller BR. Gross cystic disease fluid protein-15 reactivity in extramammary Paget's disease with and without associated internal malignancy. Am J Dermatopathol. 1996;18:118–23.
26. Goldblum JR, Hart WR. Vulvar Paget's disease: a clinicopathologic and immunohistochemical study of 19 cases. Am J Surg Pathol. 1997;21:1178–87.
27. Hoch RV, Thompson DA, Baker RJ. GATA-3 is expressed in association with estrogen receptor in breast cancer. Int J Cancer. 1999;84:122–8.
28. Liu H, Shi J, Wilkerson ML, Lin F. Immunohistochemical evaluation of GATA3 expression in tumors and normal tissues: a useful immunomarker for breast and urothelial carcinomas. Am J Clin Pathol. 2012;138:57–64.
29. Ordóñez NG. Value of GATA3 immunostaining in tumor diagnosis: a review. Adv Anat Pathol. 2013;20:352–60.
30. Miettern M, McCue PA, Sarlomo-Rikala M, Rys J, Czapiewski P, Wazny K, et al. GATA3: a multispecific but potentially useful marker in surgical pathology: a systematic analysis of 2500 epithelial and nonepithelial tumors. Am J Surg Pathol. 2014;38:13–22.
31. Asch-Kendrick R, Cimino-Methews A. The role of GATA3 in breast carcinomas: a review. Hum Pathol. 2016;48:37–47.
32. Morbeck D, Tregnago AC, Netto GB, et al. GATA3 expression in primary vulvar Paget disease: a potential pitfall leading to misdiagnosis of pagetoid urothelial intraepithelial neoplasia. Histopathology. 2016;16 [Epub ahead of print]
33. Kaufman CK, Zhou P, Pasolli HA, Rendl M, Bolotin D, Lim KC, et al. GATA-3: an unexpected regulator of cell lineage determination in skin. Genes Dev. 2003;17:2108–22.
34. Tsarovina K, Pattyn A, Stubbusch J, Müller F, van der Wees J, Schneider C, et al. Essential role of Gata transcription factors in sympathetic neuron development. Development. 2004;131:4775–86.
35. Grote D, Souabni A, Busslinger M, Bouchard M. Pax 2/8-regulated Gata 3 expression is necessary for morphogenesis and guidance of the nephric duct in the developing kidney. Development. 2006;133:53–61.
36. Asselin-Labat ML, Sutherland KD, Barker H, Thomas R, Shackleton M, Forrest NC, et al. Gata-3 is an essential regulator of mammary-gland morphogenesis and luminal-cell differentiation. Nat Cell Biol. 2007;9:201–9.
37. Higgins JP, Kaygusuz G, Wang L, Montgomery K, Mason V, Zhu SX, et al. Placental S100 (S100P) and GATA3: markers for transitional epithelium and urothelial carcinoma discovered by complementary DNA microarray. Am J Surg Pathol. 2007;31:673–80.

38. So JS, Epstein JI. GATA3 expression in paragangliomas: a pitfall potentially leading to misdiagnosis of urothelial carcinoma. Mod Pathol. 2013;26:1365–70.

39. Ordonez NG. Value of GATA3 immunostaining in the diagnosis of parathyroid tumors. Appl Immunohistochem Mol Morphol. 2014;22:756–61.

40. Banet N, Gown AM, Shih Ie M, Kay Li Q, Roden RB, Nucci MR, et al. GATA-3 expression in trophoblastic tissues: an immunohistochemical study of 445 cases, including diagnostic utility. Am J Surg Pathol. 2015;39:101–8.

41. Schwartz LE, Begum S, Westra WH, Bishop JA. GATA3 immunohistochemical expression in salivary gland neoplasms. Head Neck Pathol. 2013;7:311–5.

42. Mertens RB, de Peralta-Venturina MN, Balzer BL, Frishberg DP. GATA3 Expression in Normal Skin and in Benign and Malignant Epidermal and Cutaneous Adnexal Neoplasms. Am J Dermatopathol. 2015;37:885–91.

43. Perrotto J, Abbott JJ, Ceilley RI, Ahmed I. The role of immunohistochemistry in discriminating primary from secondary extramammary Paget disease. Am J Dermatopathol. 2010;32:137–43.

44. Hoyt BS, Cohen PR. Cutaneous scrotal metastasis: origins and clinical characteristics of visceral malignancies that metastasize to the scrotum. Int J Dermatol. 2013;52:398–403.

45. Gulavita P, Mai KT. Urothelial bladder carcinoma metastasising to the scrotum mimicking primary extra-mammary Paget's disease. Pathology. 2014;46:256–7.

46. Somers K, Iorizzo L, Scott G, Mercurio MG. Extramammary Paget disease of the penis as a manifestation of recurrent transitional cell carcinoma. Dermatol Online J. 2012;15(18):3.

47. Kiyohara T, Ito K. Epidermotropic secondary extramammary Paget's disease of the glans penis from retrograde lymphatic dissemination by transitional cell carcinoma of the bladder. J Dermatol. 2013;40:214–5.

48. Roma AA, Magi-Galluzzi C, Wood H, Fergany A, McKenney JK. Metastatic prostate adenocarcinoma to the penis presenting as pagetoid carcinoma: a phenomenon not previously reported. Am J Surg Pathol. 2015;39:724–6.

49. Brown HM, Wilkinson EJ. Uroplakin-III to distinguish primary vulvar Paget disease from Paget disease secondary to urothelial carcinoma. Hum Pathol. 2002;33:545–8.

50. Yanai H, Takahashi N, Omori M, Oda W, Yamadori I, Takada S, et al. Immunohistochemistry of p63 in primary and secondary vulvar Paget's disease. Pathol Int. 2008;58:648–51.

51. Chang J, Prieto VG, Sangueza M, Plaza JA. Diagnostic utility of p63 expression in the differential diagnosis of pagetoid squamous cell carcinoma in situ and extramammary Paget disease: a histopathologic study of 70 cases. Am J Dermatopathol. 2014;36:49–53.

52. Wick MR, Lillemoe TJ, Copland GT, Swanson PE, Manivel JC, Kiang DT. Gross cystic disease fluid protein-15 as a marker for breast cancer: immunohistochemical analysis of 690 human neoplasms and comparison with alpha-lactalbumin. Hum Pathol. 1989;20:281–7.

53. Hammer A, Hager H, Steiniche T. Prostate-specific antigen-positive extramammary Paget's disease–association with prostate cancer. APMIS. 2008;116:81–8.

54. Shaco-Levy R, Bean SM, Vollmer RT, Papalas JA, Bentley RC, Selim MA, et al. Paget disease of the vulva: a histologic study of 56 cases correlating pathologic features and disease course. Int J Gynecol Pathol. 2010;29:69–78.

55. Amin A, Griffith RC, Chaux A. Penile intraepithelial neoplasia with pagetoid features: report of an unusual variant mimicking Paget disease. Hum Pathol. 2014;45:889–92.

56. Hilliard NJ, Huang C, Andea A. Pigmented extramammary Paget's disease of the axilla mimicking melanoma: case report and review of the literature. J Cutan Pathol. 2009;36:995–1000.

57. Vincent J, Taube JM. Pigmented extramammary Paget disease of the abdomen: a potential mimicker of melanoma. Dermatol Online J. 2011;17:13.

58. Hegarty PK, Suh J, Fisher MB, Taylor J, Nguyen TH, Ivan D, et al. Penoscrotal extramammary Paget's disease: the University of Texas M. D. Anderson Cancer Center contemporary experience. J Urol. 2011;186:97–102.

59. Zhu Y, Ye DW, Yao XD, Zhang SL, Dai B, Zhang HL, et al. Clinicopathological characteristics, management and outcome of metastatic penoscrotal extramammary Paget's disease. Br J Dermatol. 2009;161:577–82.

60. Dai B, Kong YY, Chang K, Qu YY, Ye DW, Zhang SL, et al. Primary invasive carcinoma associated with penoscrotal extramammary Paget's disease: a clinicopathological analysis of 56 cases. BJU Int. 2015;115:153–60.

61. Yan D, Dai H, Jin M, Zhao Y. Clinicopathologic characteristics of extramammary Paget's disease of the scrotum associated with sweat gland adenocarcinoma-a clinical retrospective study. J Chin Med Assoc. 2011;74:179–82.

62. Preti M, Micheletti L, Massobrio M, Ansai S, Wilkinson EJ. Vulvar paget disease: one century after first reported. J Low Genit Tract Dis. 2003;7:122–35.

63. Terada T, Kamo M, Sugiura M. Apocrine carcinoma of the scrotum with extramammary Paget's disease. Int J Dermatol. 2013;52:504–6.

64. Grin A, Colgan T, Laframboise S, Shaw P, Ghazarian D. "Pagetoid" eccrine carcinoma of the vulva: report of an unusual case with review of the literature. J Low Genit Tract Dis. 2008;12:134–9.

65. Hastrup N, Andersen ES. Adenocarcinoma of Bartholin's gland associated with extramammary Paget's disease of the vulva. Acta Obstet Gynecol Scand. 1988;67:375–7.

66. Meddeb S, Rhim MS, Mestiri S, Kouira M, Bibi M, Khairi H. Mammary-like adenocarcinoma of the vulva associated to Paget's disease: a case report. Pan Afr Med J. 2014;19:188.

67. Villada G, Farooq U, Yu W, Diaz JP, Milikowski C. Extramammary Paget disease of the vulva with underlying mammary-like lobular carcinoma: a case report and review of the literature. Am J Dermatopathol. 2015;37:295–8.

68. Mentrikoski MJ, Wick MR. Immunohistochemical distinction of primary sweat gland carcinoma and metastatic breast carcinoma: can it always be accomplished reliably? Am J Clin Pathol. 2015;143:430–6.

69. Wick MR, Ockner DM, Mills SE, Ritter JH, Swanson PE. Homologous carcinomas of the breasts, skin, and salivary glands. A histologic and immunohistochemical comparison of ductal mammary carcinoma, ductal sweat gland carcinoma, and salivary duct carcinoma. Am J Clin Pathol. 1998;109:75–84.

70. Abbott JJ, Ahmed I. Adenocarcinoma of mammary-like glands of the vulva: Report of a case and review of the literature. Am J Dermatopathol. 2006;28: 127–33.

71. Baykal C, Dünder I, Turkmen IC, Ozyar E. An unusual case of mammary gland-like carcinoma of vulva: case report and review of literature. Eur J Gynaecol Oncol. 2015;36:333–4.

72. Diaz de Leon E, Carcangiu ML, Prieto VG, Prieto VG, PA MC, Burchette JL, et al. Extramammary Paget disease is characterized by the consistent lack of estrogen and progesterone receptors but frequently expresses androgen receptor. Am J Clin Pathol. 2000;113:572–5.

73. Regauer S. Extramammary Paget's disease–a proliferation of adnexal origin? Histopathology. 2006;48:723–9.

2

Cytoplasmic FOXP1 expression is correlated with ER and calpain II expression and predicts a poor outcome in breast cancer

Bao-Hua Yu[1,2], Bai-Zhou Li[3], Xiao-Yan Zhou[1,2*], Da-Ren Shi[1,2] and Wen-Tao Yang[1,2]

Abstract

Background: Nuclear forkhead box protein P1 (N-FOXP1) expression in invasive breast cancer has been documented in the literature. However, the FOXP1 expression patterns at different stages of breast cancer progression are largely unknown, and the significance of cytoplasmic FOXP1 (C-FOXP1) expression in breast cancer has not been well illustrated. The aims of this study were to investigate FOXP1 expression patterns in invasive ductal carcinoma (IDC), ductal carcinoma in situ (DCIS), atypical ductal hyperplasia (ADH) and usual ductal hyperplasia (UDH), and to analyze the clinicopathological relevance of C-FOXP1 and its prognostic value in IDC.

Methods: N-FOXP1 and C-FOXP1 expression in cases of IDC, DCIS, ADH and UDH was determined using immunohistochemistry. The correlation between C-FOXP1 expression and clinicopathological parameters as well as the overall survival (OS) and disease-free survival (DFS) rates of patients with IDC were analyzed.

Results: Exclusive N-FOXP1 expression was found in 85.0% (17/20), 40.0% (8/20), 12.2% (5/41) and 10.8% (9/83) of UDH, ADH, DCIS, and IDC cases, respectively, and exclusive C-FOXP1 expression was observed in 0% (0/20), 0% (0/20), 4.9% (2/41), and 31.3% (26/83) of the cases, respectively. Both N- and C-FOXP1 staining were observed in 15.0% (3/20), 60.0% (12/20), 82.9% (34/41) and 48.2% (40/83) of the above cases, respectively, while complete loss of FOXP1 expression was observed in only 9.6% (8/83) of IDC cases. Estrogen receptor (ER) expression in C-FOXP1-positive IDC cases (31/66, 47.0%) was significantly lower than that in C-FOXP1-negative cases (13/17, 76.5%) ($p = 0.030$). Calpain II expression was observed in 83.3% (55/66) of C-FOXP1-positive IDC cases, which was significantly higher than that in C-FOXP1-negative cases (9/17, 52.9%) ($p = 0.007$). Calpain II was significantly associated with pAKT ($p = 0.029$), pmTOR ($p = 0.011$), p4E-BP1 ($p < 0.001$) and p-p70S6K ($p = 0.003$) expression levels. The 10-year OS and DFS rates of the C-FOXP1-positive patients were 60.5% and 48.7%, respectively, both of which were lower than those of the C-FOXP1-negative patients (93.3, 75.3%). The OS curve showed a dramatic impact of C-FOXP1 status on OS ($p = 0.045$).

Conclusions: Cytoplasmic relocalization of FOXP1 protein was a frequent event in breast IDC. Calpain II might play an important role in nucleocytoplasmic trafficking of FOXP1 and the AKT pathway might be involved in this process. C-FOXP1 expression was inversely associated with ER expression and might be a predictor of poor OS in patients with IDC.

Keywords: Breast cancer, FOXP1, ER, Calpain II, AKT pathway, Immunohistochemistry, Survival

* Correspondence: xyzhou100@163.com
[1]Department of Pathology, Fudan University Shanghai Cancer Center,
Dong-an Road 270, Xuhui District, Shanghai 200032, China
[2]Department of Oncology, Shanghai Medical College, Fudan University,
Shanghai, China
Full list of author information is available at the end of the article

Background

Breast cancer is the most common female malignancy and also the second leading cause of cancer-related death among women worldwide [1]. However, its molecular pathogenesis is largely unknown, and clinically useful prognostic and predictive parameters, apart from human epidermal growth factor receptor-2 (HER2), estrogen receptor (ER), progesterone receptor (PR) and lymph node status, are still insufficient, emphasizing the need for further investigating additional prognostic biomarkers and potential targets for selective therapies.

The forkhead box protein P1 (FOXP1) gene, locating on 3p14.1, is a member of the forkhead/winged helix transcription factor family, and the FOXP1 protein is widely expressed in normal tissues [2–5]. FOXP1 protein subcellular localization varies between different tissues. A predominant nuclear FOXP1 (N-FOXP1) distribution has been identified in the kidney, thyroid, cerebellum, tonsil, blood, thymus, spleen, skin, pancreas and colon, whereas cytoplasmic FOXP1 (C-FOXP1) labeling was observed in other epithelial tissues, such as the stomach [3]. Altered FOXP1 expression is also associated with various types of tumors [6]. For example, N-FOXP1 protein is up-regulated in diffuse large B-cell lymphoma (DLBCL) and extranodal marginal zone or mucosa-associated lymphoid tissue (MALT) lymphoma [7], while loss of N-FOXP1 expression characterizes malignancy in certain solid tumors, including endometrial and prostate tumors as well as familial and sporadic breast cancer [3, 8–10]. The presence of N-FOXP1 expression is correlated with ERα and/or ERβ reactivity in invasive breast cancers [8, 11, 12]. A correlation between N-FOXP1 and ERα has also been observed in endometrial adenocarcinoma [9]. Loss of FOXP1 nuclear expression is the most striking observation, and cytoplasmic expression is noted more frequently in endometrial adenocarcinoma according to the literature. However, to date, data regarding C-FOXP1 expression in breast cancer are limited, and its clinicopathological relevance, including its correlation with ER expression, has not been well illustrated.

The oncogenic functions of FOXP1 in tumors, such as DLBCL, MALT lymphoma, and hepatocellular and renal cell carcinoma, have been well documented [4, 13, 14]. On the other hand, FOXP1 might attenuate tumorigenicity to exert a tumor-suppressive effect in other tumors, such as neuroblastoma and prostate cancer [4, 15–17]. Therefore, FOXP1 is associated with cancer patient prognosis in a context-dependent manner [4, 18]. Overall, FOXP1 positivity, with either nuclear or an unspecified distribution, is associated with favorable survival in patients with breast cancer [4, 8, 18]. Nevertheless, the prognostic value of C-FOXP1 expression in breast cancer patients has not been discussed in the literature.

The underlying mechanisms of the nucleocytoplasmic shuttling of FOXP1 in breast cancer are largely unknown. The calpains are a family of calcium-dependent cysteine proteases that function in a wide range of important cellular activities [19]. The ubiquitously expressed family members, μ-calpain (calpain I) and m-calpain (calpain II), are the most extensively studied calpains [20, 21]. Calpain II activity is subject to many forms of posttranslational control in vivo, including translocation from the cytosol to the membrane [22]. Calpains are implicated in the cleavage of several apoptosis-associated proteins, notably Bax, Bcl2, JNK and JUN, amongst others [19, 23], and are involved in the regulation of some cell cycle progression-associated proteins, such as p21, cyclin D1, and p27Kip1 [24, 25]. For example, calpains may cleave Bcl-2 and Bid and permit translocation of Bax and Bid to the mitochondria, amplifying the apoptotic signaling pathway in cancer cells [26, 27]. In addition, calpains can mediate p27Kip1 degradation, and nuclear export might be necessary for this process [24]. The PI3K/AKT/mTOR signaling pathway, including its downstream molecules p4E-BP1 and p-p70S6K, plays a crucial role in initiation and progression of breast tumorigenesis and drug resistance [28, 29]. Calpain II might promote breast cancer cell proliferation through the PI3K/AKT signaling pathway [30]. However, whether calpain II plays a role in FOXP1 regulation in breast cancer has not yet been documented.

Herein, we investigated both the cytoplasmic and nuclear expression of FOXP1 protein in cases of invasive ductal cancer (IDC) or ductal carcinoma in situ (DCIS), as well as in atypical ductal hyperplasia (ADH) and usual ductal hyperplasia (UDH) of the breast, and further analyzed the association of C-FOXP1 expression with ER, calpain II and other clinicopathological parameters in IDC, and also evaluated the prognostic value of C-FOXP1.

Methods

Patient selection and tissue microarray (TMA) construction

Altogether, 83 cases of IDC, 41 of DCIS, 20 of ADH, and 20 of UDH were retrieved from the archival files of the Department of Pathology, Fudan University Shanghai Cancer Center (Shanghai, China). The study was approved by the Institutional Review Board of Fudan University Shanghai Cancer Center (Shanghai Cancer Center Ethics Committee). H&E-stained sections for each case were independently reviewed by two of the authors (BHY and BZL) according to the criteria described in the World Health Organization classification of tumors of the breast [31].

Clinical data, including follow-up data, were available for all of the 83 IDC cases. For TMA construction, H&E-stained sections from each formalin-fixed paraffin-embedded block were first observed to define representative tumor cell-rich areas and then 2 representative 0.6 mm cores were obtained from each IDC case and inserted into a recipient paraffin block in a grid pattern using a tissue arrayer (Beecher Instruments, Silver Spring, MD, USA). Four-micrometer-thick sections were then cut from the TMA blocks for routine hematoxylin and eosin (H&E) staining and immunohistochemical procedures. The H&E-stained sections were used to verify the adequate representation of the diagnostic biopsies.

Immunohistochemical staining

Following deparaffinization and heat-mediated antigen retrieval, immunohistochemical staining was carried out using an Envision system (DAKO, Glostrup, Denmark) with primary antibodies against FOXP1 (JC12, AbD Serotec, Oxford, UK), ER (SP1, Roche Tucson, AZ, USA), calpain II (CAPN2, Sigma, St. Louis, MO, USA), HER2 (4B5, Roche Tucson), pAKT (736E11, Cell signaling, Danvers, MA, USA), pmTOR (49F9, Cell signaling), p4E-BP1 (53H11, Cell signaling) and p-p70S6K (49D7, Cell signaling). The stained sections were then counterstained with hematoxylin. Appropriate positive and negative controls were carried out simultaneously for all stains.

The immunostaining results were reviewed by 2 independent qualified pathologists. Nuclear and cytoplasmic tumor cell staining for FOXP1 protein was analyzed separately. FOXP1 nuclear expression was scored using the following system: negative = 0; weak/focal staining = 1; strong focal/wide spread moderate staining = 2; or strong/widespread staining = 3. Tumors that scored 2 or 3 were considered positive for N-FOXP1 [8]. Scoring of C-FOXP1, calpain II, pAKT, pmTOR, p4E-BP1, p-p70S6K were performed in terms of the staining intensity (intensity score: 0, none; 1, weak; 2, moderate; and 3, strong) and the proportion of positive tumor cells (proportion score: less than 5% positive cells were scored as 0; 5 to 25% as 1; 26 to 50% as 2; 51 to 75% as 3; greater than 75% as 4) according to previously described scoring methods with a slight modification [9, 32, 33]. These two scores were then multiplied to yield the final score. A final score of ≥3 was defined as positive.

The status of ER, PR and HER2 were evaluated using the scoring criteria of the American Society of Clinical Oncology (ASCO)/College of American Pathologists (CAP) guideline [34, 35]. Staining was considered positive for ER when nuclear staining was present in more than 1% of the tumor cells. Immunohistochemistry for HER2 as 3+ was defined as positive. For cases of HER2 IHC 2+, Abbott-Vysis HER2 FISH assay was employed to further confirm the status of HER2 gene amplification.

Statistical analysis

All statistical analyses were performed using the SPSS software package (SPSS version 19.0, SPSS Inc., Chicago, IL, USA). Categorical variables were compared with a χ^2 test, and measurement data were analyzed using Pearson correlation analysis. Overall survival (OS) was defined as the interval from the initial diagnosis to the time of death or the last contact. Surviving patients were censored at the last known date of contact. Disease-free survival (DFS) was determined according to the time from diagnosis to the time of recurrence or the last contact. Patient survival was estimated using the Kaplan-Meier method and was compared by means of a log-rank test. All p-values were two sided, and a p-value < 0.05 was considered statistically significant.

Results

FOXP1 protein expression patterns in UDH, ADH, DCIS, and IDC of the breast

Most UDH cases (17/20, 85%) showed uniform strong N-FOXP1 staining and the other 3 cases (15.0%) showed both N- and C-FOXP1 staining (Fig. 1). As for ADH group, 40.0% (8/20) of cases demonstrated nuclear positivity and 60.0% (12/20) showed both nuclear and cytoplasmic positivity. Nevertheless, solely cytoplasmic staining was not found in these two groups. In comparison, exclusive N-FOXP1 expression was present only in 12.2% (5/41) of DCIS cases, while both N- and C-FOXP1 expression was observed in the majority of this group

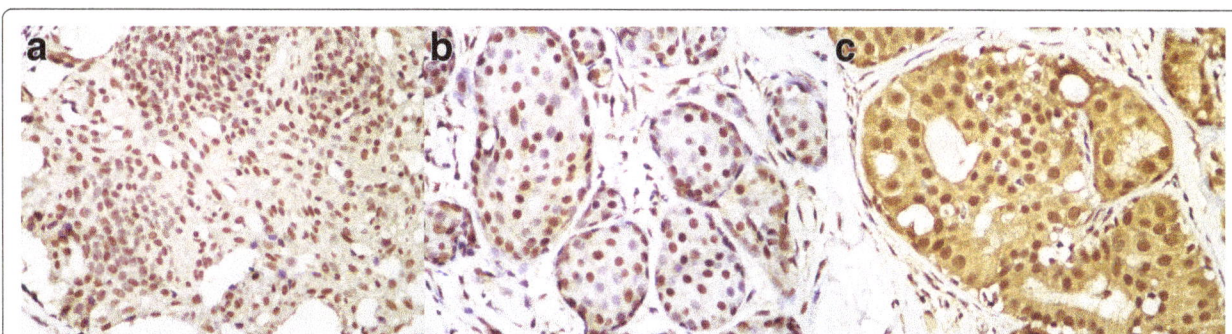

Fig. 1 Representative cases of FOXP1 expression in UDH and ADH. FOXP1 positive staining was located in the nuclei of ductal cells in UDH (**a** ×400). In ADH, FOXP1 positivity was observed in the nuclei of tumor cells (**b** ×400) or in both the nuclei and the cytoplasm (**c** ×400)

(34/41, 82.9%), and the remaining 2 cases (4.9%) revealed exclusive cytoplasmic labeling (Fig. 2). The FOXP1 expression pattern in IDC samples varied. In this group, exclusive cytoplasmic staining (26/83, 31.3%) was more frequently observed than solely nuclear staining (9/83, 10.8%), both nuclear and cytoplasmic staining accounted for 48.2% (40/83) of cases and complete loss of expression was observed in 8 cases (9.6%) (Fig. 3). Moreover, exclusive cytoplasmic FOXP1 expression was more common in IDC than that in DCIS, ADH and UDH (31.3% vs 4.9, 0 and 0%). The FOXP1 expression patterns were significantly different in UDH, ADH, DCIS and IDC ($p < 0.001$, Table 1). Even within a single case, different lesions showed diverse FOXP1 staining patterns. For example, clear nuclear and cytoplasmic staining was observed in the DCIS region, while solely nuclear staining was seen in the epithelium of adjacent benign ducts.

Correlation between C-FOXP1 expression and clinicopathological variables in breast IDC

The identified associations between C-FOXP1 expression and histopathological and clinical variables in IDC are shown in Table 2. ER staining was observed in 47.0% (31/66) of C-FOXP1-positive staining cases, which was lower than that in C-FOXP1-negative cases (13/17, 76.5%) ($p = 0.030$). Calpain II expression was found in 83.3% (55/66) of C-FOXP1 positive cases, compared

with 52.9% (9/17) of C-FOXP1-negative ones, and the difference was statistically significant ($p = 0.007$, Fig. 4). Nevertheless, there was no significant relevance between C-FOXP1 expression and patient age, tumor size, grade, tumor stage, nodal status, distant metastasis or HER2 expression (all $p > 0.05$). pAKT, pmTOR, p4E-BP1 and p-p70S6K, as key members in the AKT pathway, was expressed in 72.3% (60/83), 74.7% (62/83), 69.9% (58/83) and 73.5% (61/83) of IDC cases in the current series, respectively. Interestingly, calpain II expression was statistically associated with the expression of pAKT ($p = 0.029$), pmTOR ($p = 0.011$), p4E-BP1 ($p < 0.001$) and p-p70S6K ($p = 0.003$, Table 3).

Correlation between C-FOXP1 expression and the survival of patients with breast IDC

Among the 83 patients with breast IDC, the follow-up period ranged from 2 to 146 months (median, 67 months), and there were 32 relapses and 21 deaths. Twenty out of 66 C-FOXP1-positive patients died of disease, and 28 had relapses, whereas 1 and 4 out of 17 C-FOXP1-negative patients died or relapsed, respectively. The 10-year OS and DFS rates of the C-FOXP1-positive patients were 60.5 and 48.7%, respectively, both of which were lower than that of the C-FOXP1-negative patients (93.3, 75.3%). The OS curve showed that C-FOXP1 status had an impact on outcome ($p = 0.045$). The DFS curve suggested that

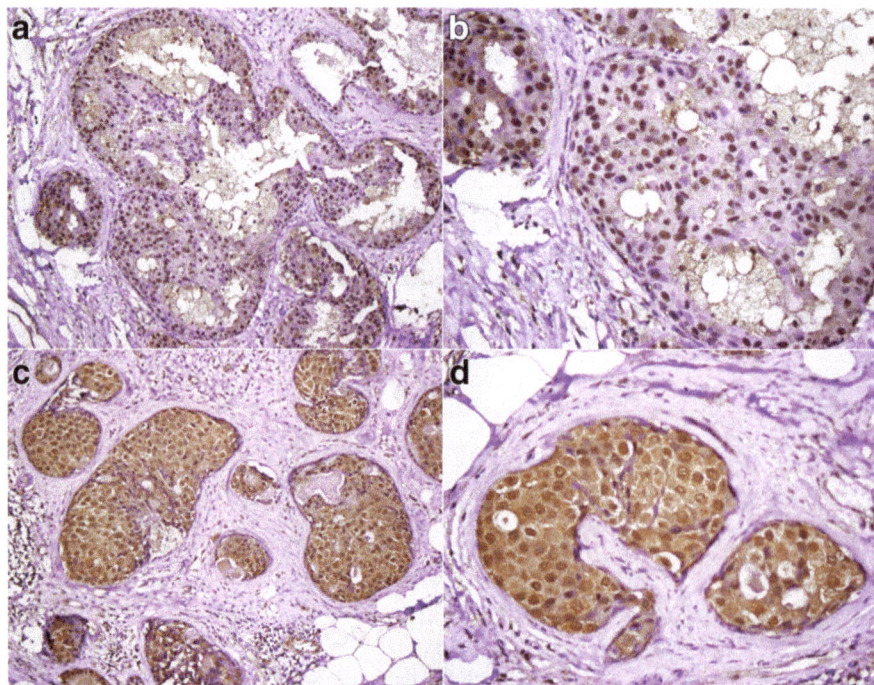

Fig. 2 FOXP1 expression patterns in DCIS. FOXP1 immunostaining was observed in the nuclei of tumor cells (**a** ×200, **b** ×400) or both the nuclei and cytoplasm (**c** ×200, **d** ×400)

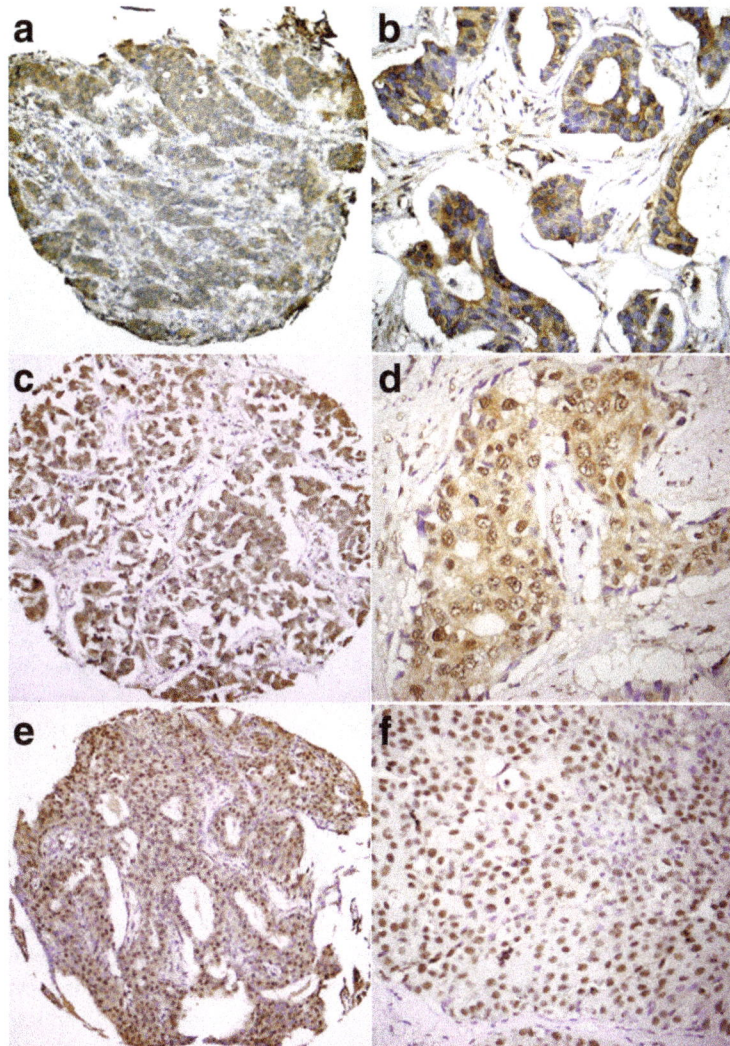

Fig. 3 FOXP1 expression patterns in IDC. The FOXP1 protein expression patterns in IDC tumor cells ranged from exclusive cytoplasmic (**a**, TMA; **b** ×400) to mixed nuclear/cytoplasmic (**c**, TMA; **d** ×400) and to exclusive nuclear (**e**, TMA; **f** ×400)

patients with C-FOXP1-negative IDCs demonstrated longer DFS than those with C-FOXP1-positive disease, but the result did not reach statistical significance ($p = 0.152$). Survival curves stratified for C-FOXP1 expression are shown in Fig. 5.

Discussion

Although N-FOXP1 expression in breast cancer has been documented in several studies, the expression patterns of FOXP1 protein at different stages of breast cancer progression, including DCIS and IDC, and in

Table 1 FOXP1 protein expression patterns in different breast lesions

Breast lesions	Total number $n = 164$	FOXP1 expression patterns			
		Exclusive nuclear expression n (%)	Both nuclear and cytoplasmic expression n (%)	Exclusive cytoplasmic expression n (%)	Complete loss of expression n (%)
UDH	20	17 (85.0)	3 (15.0)	0 (0)	0 (0)
ADH	20	8 (40.0)	12 (60.0)	0 (0)	0 (0)
DCIS	41	5 (12.2)	34 (82.9)	2 (4.9)	0 (0)
IDC	83	9 (10.8)	40 (48.2)	26 (31.3)	8 (9.6)

Table 2 The correlation between cytoplasmic FOXP1 expression and clinicopathological parameters in IDC cases

Clinicopathological parameters	Cytoplasmic FOXP1 expression		
	Positive (%) $n = 66$	Negative (%) $n = 17$	P value
ER			**0.030[a]**
Positive	31 (47.0)	13 (76.5)	
Negative	35 (53.0)	4 (23.5)	
HER2			0.443
Positive	22 (33.3)	4 (23.5)	
Negative	44 (66.7)	13 (76.5)	
Calpain II			**0.007[a]**
Positive	55 (83.3)	9 (52.9)	
Negative	11 (16.7)	8 (47.1)	
pAKT			0.863
Positive	48 (72.7)	12 (70.6)	
Negative	18 (27.3)	5 (29.4)	
pmTOR			0.093
Positive	52 (78.8)	10 (58.8)	
Negative	14 (21.2)	7 (41.2)	
p4E-BP1			0.607
Positive	47 (71.2)	11 (64.7)	
Negative	19 (28.8)	6 (35.3)	
p-p70S6K			0.363
Positive	50 (75.8)	11 (64.7)	
Negative	16 (24.2)	6 (35.3)	
Stage			0.562
Stage I	7 (10.6)	1 (5.9)	
Stage II	38 (57.6)	13 (76.5)	
Stage III	21 (31.8)	3 (17.6)	
Grade			0.325
Grade I	16 (24.2)	3 (17.6)	
Grade II	38 (57.6)	9 (52.9)	
Grade III	12 (18.2)	5 (29.4)	
Nodal status			0.090
Positive	49 (74.2)	9 (52.9)	
Negative	17 (25.8)	8 (47.1)	
Distant metastasis			0.230
Positive	26 (39.4)	4 (23.5)	
Negative	40 (60.6)	13 (76.5)	
Tumor size			0.907
≦4 cm	30 (45.5)	8 (47.1)	
> 4 cm	36 (54.5)	9 (52.9)	
Age			0.762
≦55 yrs	44 (66.7)	12 (70.6)	
> 55 yrs	22 (33.3)	5 (29.4)	

[a]Statistically significant p values are in bold

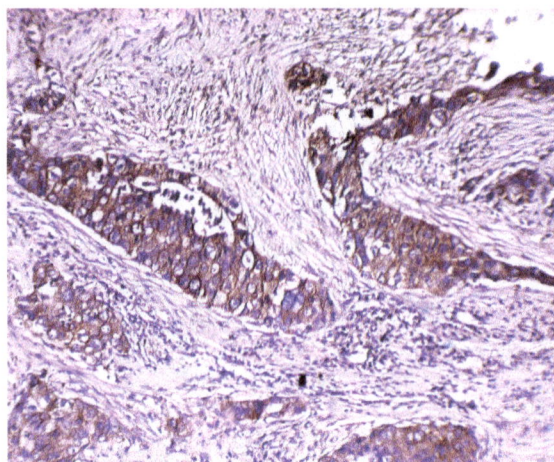

Fig. 4 Calpain II-positive staining was found in the cytoplasm of IDC tumor cells ($\times 400$)

ADH and UDH lesions, have not yet been clearly demonstrated. In the current study, heterogeneous FOXP1 expression patterns were observed in the above-mentioned cases. While FOXP1 staining was predominantly localized in the nuclei in UDH, the FOXP1 nuclear distribution gradually decreased from ADH, DCIS to IDC, and the cytoplasmic staining increased. These results were consistent with the previous reported heterogeneous expression pattern of FOXP1, in terms of the proportion of positive cells, the staining intensity, and subcellular localization [3, 36]. Our observations strongly indicated that FOXP1 expression might shift from the nucleus to the cytoplasm during breast tumorigenesis, and therefore, cytoplasmic mislocalization of FOXP1 is suggested play an important role in breast cancer progression. Similarly, subcellular localization has been suggested to play a distinct role in the pathogenesis of endometrial cancer [9]. Banham et al. also revealed that FOXP1 protein expression levels and compartmentalization varied depending on the cancer stage, although their sample sizes for each tumor were quite small [3].

Studies on the mechanisms of FOXP1 subcellular relocalization in breast cancer are very few. Calpain II has been implicated in mediating cell differentiation, necrosis, migration, and metastasis [19, 22]. Several studies, although limited, have investigated the aberrant expression and role of calpain II in breast cancer [19, 21, 25, 30, 37–40]. High calpain II expression has been established in triple-negative and basal-like IDC and calpain II might promote breast cancer cell proliferation through the AKT signaling pathway [21, 30]. Calpain-mediated cleavage of β-catenin and E-cadherin may lead to aberrant stabilization of the proteins and promote tumorigenesis in breast cancer cells [38, 39]. In addition, Ho et al. suggested that the FOXO3a subcellular location was skewed toward nuclear localization in calpain

Table 3 The correlation between calpain II expression and clinicopathological parameters in IDC cases

Clinicopathological parameters	Calpain II expression		
	Positive (%) $n = 64$	Negative (%) $n = 19$	P value
ER			0.580
Positive	35 (54.7)	9 (47.4)	
Negative	29 (45.3)	10 (52.6)	
HER2			0.597
Positive	21 (32.8)	5 (26.3)	
Negative	43 (67.2)	14 (73.7)	
pAKT			**0.029**[a]
Positive	50 (78.1)	10 (52.6)	
Negative	14 (21.9)	9 (47.4)	
pmTOR			**0.011**[a]
Positive	52 (81.3)	10 (52.6)	
Negative	12 (18.8)	9 (47.4)	
p4E-BP1			**< 0.001**[a]
Positive	52 (81.3)	6 (31.6)	
Negative	12 (18.8)	13 (68.4)	
p-p70S6K			**0.003**[a]
Positive	52 (81.3)	9 (47.4)	
Negative	12 (18.8)	10 (52.6)	
Stage			0.773
Stage I	7 (10.9)	1 (5.3)	
Stage II	37 (57.8)	14 (73.7)	
Stage III	20 (31.3)	4 (21.2)	
Grade			0.568
Grade I	16 (25.0)	3 (15.8)	
Grade II	35 (54.7)	12 (63.2)	
Grade III	13 (20.3)	4 (21.1)	
Nodal status			0.876
Positive	45 (70.3)	13 (68.4)	
Negative	19 (29.7)	6 (31.6)	
Distant metastasis			0.122
Positive	26 (40.6)	4 (21.1)	
Negative	38 (59.4)	15 (78.9)	
Tumor size			**0.013**[a]
≦4 cm	34 (53.1)	4 (21.1)	
> 4 cm	30 (46.9)	15 (78.9)	
Age			0.653
≦55 yrs	44 (68.8)	12 (63.2)	
> 55 yrs	20 (31.3)	7 (36.8)	

[a]Statistically significant p values are in bold

II-deficient cells [20]. To date, we are not aware of any literature establishing the relevance between calpain II and FOXP1 protein in breast cancer. An unexpected but

important finding in the current study was that C-FOXP1 expression was remarkably associated with calpain II in IDC. Moreover, in IDC samples in our series, calpain II was strongly correlated with the important molecules in AKT pathway, including pAKT, mTOR, p4E-BP1 and p-p70S6K. The PI3K/AKT/p70S6K signaling pathway, which has been reported to be involved in the nucleus-cytoplasm shuttling of FOXO1, another forkhead protein family member, was previously shown to participate in FOXP1 regulation in breast cancer [30, 41]. Taken together, we speculate that calpain II might play an important role in the subcellular regulation of FOXP1, and the AKT pathway might be involved in this process. Further investigations are merited to confirm this hypothesis and thoroughly explore the underlying mechanisms.

While N-FOXP1 was positively associated with ERα as well as ERβ expression in breast cancer according to the previous studies [8, 11, 12, 30, 42], the clinicopathological relevance of C-FOXP1 positivity in IDC has not been addressed until now. For the first time, we identified an inverse correlation between C-FOXP1 expression and ER expression in IDC. Our results are in line with those of a previous report by Giatromanolaki et al. concerning endometrial carcinoma [9]. They demonstrated that loss of ERα expression was a frequent event in cases with C-FOXP1 expression or loss of FOXP1 expression in endometrial carcinoma. Given that nucleus-cytoplasm shuttling might be an important event in the carcinogenesis, the interaction between ER and C-FOXP1 expression might be more clinically significant than that originally established between ER and N-FOXP1, and its biological significance should be further explored [8, 11, 30, 43, 44].

Previous studies have demonstrated that loss of FOXP1 expression is associated with a poor prognosis in primary invasive and familial breast cancer [11]. For example, both Fox et al. and Ijichi et al. indicated that FOXP1 immunoreactivity predicted better relapse-free survival but not OS in breast cancer patients [6, 8]. Moreover, FOXP1 immunoreactivity may predict a favorable prognosis for breast cancer patients treated with tamoxifen [6, 42, 44]. However, in previous studies, the FOXP1 protein was either located in the nuclei, or its subcellular location was not specified; nonetheless, cytoplasmic FOXP1 localization might play a large role in cancer cell biology because nuclear expression is characteristic of normal breast tissues [9]. Therefore, the prognostic impact of C-FOXP1 overexpression in IDC patients might be meaningful. Our results indicate for the first time that C-FOXP1 immunoreactivity is associated with an unfavorable OS and slightly inferior DFS in patients with breast IDC. Similarly, exclusive C-FOXP1 expression in early endothelial carcinoma has been linked with deep myometrial invasion and conferred a slightly worse outcome, despite an insignificant difference [9]. Hu et al.

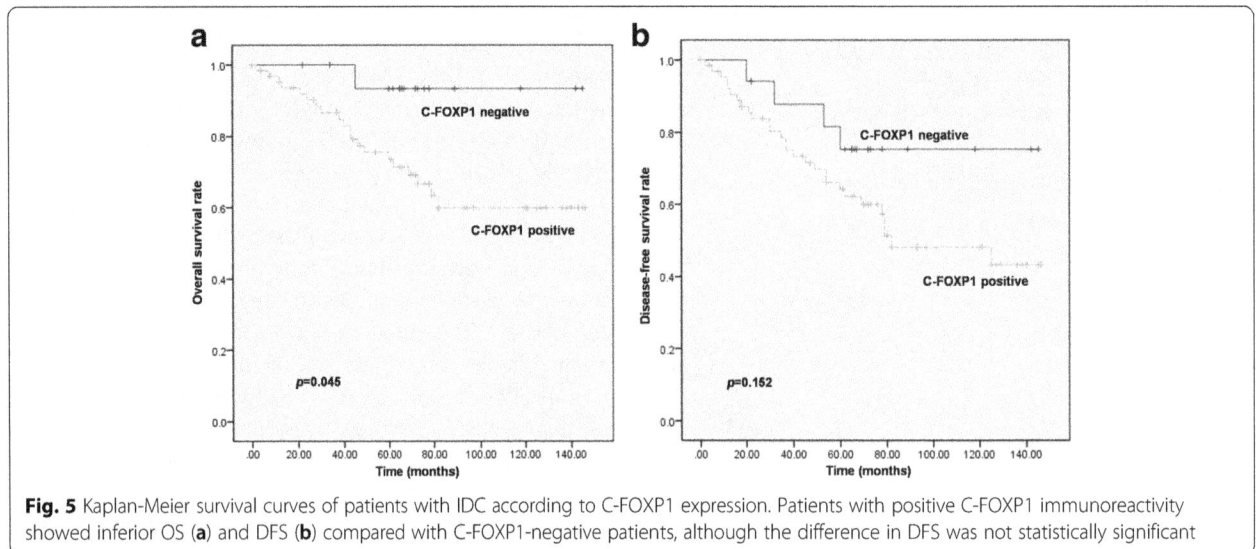

Fig. 5 Kaplan-Meier survival curves of patients with IDC according to C-FOXP1 expression. Patients with positive C-FOXP1 immunoreactivity showed inferior OS (**a**) and DFS (**b**) compared with C-FOXP1-negative patients, although the difference in DFS was not statistically significant

demonstrated that increased cytoplasmic FOXP1 expression was correlated with increased tumor grade but was not significantly associated with chemotherapy resistance and prognosis [32]. Our results provide reliable evidence regarding the prognostic importance of C-FOXP1 overexpression in breast cancer, which should be further confirmed with a much larger case series.

Conclusions

In summary, cytoplasmic relocalization of the FOXP1 protein is a frequent event in breast cancer. For the first time, we found that C-FOXP1 expression was dramatically associated with ER expression and correlated with reduced OS in patients with breast IDC. Our results indicated that C-FOXP1 might be important in both the pathogenesis and prognosis of breast cancer patients. Another noteworthy finding was that calpain II might be involved in FOXP1 trafficking from the nucleus to the cytoplasm, which might be mediated by the AKT pathway. Further investigations are needed to better understand the biological role of FOXP1 expression in breast cancer development and progression and to provide better strategies for prognosis prediction and therapeutic intervention in breast cancer.

Abbreviations
C-FOXP1: Cytoplasmic FOXP1; DCIS: Ductal carcinoma in situ; DFS: Disease-free survival; DLBCL: Diffuse large B-cell lymphoma; ER: Estrogen receptor; FOXP1: Forkhead box protein P1; HER2: Human epidermal growth factor receptor-2; IDC: Invasive ductal carcinoma; MALT: Mucosa associated lymphoid tissue; N-FOXP1: Nuclear FOXP1; OS: Overall survival; PR: Progesterone receptor; TMA: Tissue microarray

Funding
This study was supported by grants from the youth project of National Nature Science Funding of China (No. 81700195) and Shanghai Hospital Development Center Emerging Advanced Technology Joint Research Project (SHDC12014105).

Authors' contributions
BHY and XYZ conceived and designed the experiments. BHY performed the experiments. BHY and BZL reviewed the slides and analyzed the data. BHY wrote the manuscript. DRS, XYZ, WTY revised the paper and approved the final version of the manuscript. All authors read and approved the final manuscript.

Competing interests
The authors declare that they have no competing interests.

Author details
[1]Department of Pathology, Fudan University Shanghai Cancer Center, Dong-an Road 270, Xuhui District, Shanghai 200032, China. [2]Department of Oncology, Shanghai Medical College, Fudan University, Shanghai, China. [3]Department of Pathology, the Second Affiliated Hospital of Zhejiang University, 88 Jiefang Road, Hangzhou 310009, China.

References
1. Xu T, He BS, Liu XX, et al. The predictive and prognostic role of stromal tumor-infiltrating lymphocytes in HER2-positive breast cancer with trastuzumab-based treatment: a meta-analysis and systematic review. J Cancer. 2017;8:3838–48.
2. Maitra A, Wistuba II, Washington C, et al. High-resolution chromosome 3p allelotyping of breast carcinomas and precursor lesions demonstrates frequent loss of heterozygosity and a discontinuous pattern of allele loss. Am J Pathol. 2001;159:119–30.
3. Banham AH, Beasley N, Campo E, et al. The FOXP1 winged helix transcription factor is a novel candidate tumor suppressor gene on chromosome 3p. Cancer Res. 2001;61:8820–9.
4. Katoh M, Igarashi M, Fukuda H, et al. Cancer genetics and genomics of human FOX family genes. Cancer Lett. 2013;328:198–206.
5. Shu W, Yang H, Zhang L, et al. Characterization of a new subfamily of winged-helix/forkhead (fox) genes that are expressed in the lung and act as transcriptional repressors. J Biol Chem. 2001;276:27488–97.

6. Ijichi N, Ikeda K, Horie-Inoue K, Inoue S. FOXP1 and estrogen signaling in breast cancer. Vitam Horm. 2013;93:203–12.

7. Goatly A, Bacon CM, Nakamura S, et al. FOXP1 abnormalities in lymphoma: translocation breakpoint mapping reveals insights into deregulated transcriptional control. Mod Pathol. 2008;21:902–11.

8. Fox SB, Brown P, Han C, et al. Expression of the forkhead transcription factor FOXP1 is associated with estrogen receptorα and improved survival in primary human breast carcinomas. Clin Cancer Res. 2004;10:3521–7.

9. Giatromanolaki A, Koukourakis MI, Sivridis E, et al. Loss of expression and nuclear/cytoplasmic localization of the FOXP1 forkhead transcription factor are common events in early endometrial cancer: relationship with estrogen receptors and HIF-1α expression. Mod Pathol. 2006;19:9–16.

10. Banham AH, Boddy J, Launchbury R, et al. Expression of the forkhead transcription factor FOXP1 is associated both with hypoxia inducible factors (HIFs) and the androgen receptor in prostate cancer but is not directly regulated by androgens or hypoxia. Prostate. 2007;67:1091–8.

11. Bates GJ, Fox SB, Han C, et al. Expression of the forkhead transcription factor FOXP1 is associated with that of estrogen receptorb in primary invasive breast carcinomas. Breast Cancer Res Treat. 2008;111:453–9.

12. Rayoo M, Yan M, Takano EA, et al. Expression of the forkhead box transcription factor FOXP1 is associated with oestrogen receptor alpha, oestrogen receptor beta and improved survival in familial breast cancers. J Clin Pathol. 2009;62:896–902.

13. Zhang Y, Zhang S, Wang X, et al. Prognostic significance of FOXP1 as an oncogene in hepatocellular carcinoma. J Clin Pathol. 2012;65:528–33.

14. Yu B, Zhou X, Li B, et al. FOXP1 expression and its clinicopathologic significance in nodal and extranodal diffuse large B-cell lymphoma. Ann Hematol. 2011;90:701–8.

15. Koon HB, Ippolito GC, Banham AH, Tucker PW. FOXP1: a potential therapeutic target in cancer. Expert Opin Ther Targets. 2007;11:955–65.

16. Ackermann S, Kocak H, Hero B, et al. FOXP1 inhibits cell growth and attenuates tumorigenicity of neuroblastoma. BMC Cancer. 2014;14:840.

17. Takayama K, Suzuki T, Tsutsumi S, et al. Integrative analysis of FOXP1 function reveals a tumor-suppressive effect in prostate cancer. Mol Endocrinol. 2014;28:2012–24.

18. Xiao J, He B, Zou Y, et al. Prognostic value of decreased FOXP1 protein expression in various tumors: a systematic review and meta-analysis. Sci Rep. 2016;6:30437.

19. Storr SJ, Thompson N, Pu X, et al. Calpain in breast cancer: role in disease progression and treatment response. Pathobiology. 2015;82:133–41.

20. Ho WC, Pikor L, Gao Y, et al. Calpain 2 regulates Akt-FoxO-p27 (Kip1) protein signaling pathway in mammary carcinoma. J Biol Chem. 2012;287:15458–65.

21. Storr SJ, Lee KW, Woolston CM, et al. Calpain system protein expression in basal-like and triple-negative invasive breast cancer. Ann Oncol. 2012;23:2289–96.

22. Xu L, Deng X. Tobacco-specific nitrosamine 4-(methylnitrosamino)-1-(3-pyridyl)-1-butanone induces phosphorylation of mu- and m-calpain in association with increased secretion, cell migration, and invasion. J Biol Chem. 2004;279:53683–90.

23. Goll DE, Thompson VF, Li H, et al. The Calpain system. Physiol Rev. 2003;83:731–801.

24. Delmas C, Aragou N, Poussard S, et al. MAP kinase-dependent degradation of p27Kip1 by calpains in choroidal melanoma cells. J Biol Chem. 2003;278:12443–51.

25. Libertini SJ, Robinson BS, Dhillon NK, et al. Cyclin E both regulates and is regulated by calpain 2, a protease associated with metastatic breast cancer phenotype. Cancer Res. 2005;65:10700–8.

26. Gil-Parrado S, Fernández-Montalván A, Assfalg-Machleidt I. Ionomycin-activated calpain triggers apoptosis. J Biol Chem. 2002;277:27217–26.

27. Guicciardi ME, Gores GJ. Calpains can do it alone: implications for cancer therapy. Cancer Biol Ther. 2003;2:153–4.

28. Guerrero-Zotano A, Mayer IA, Arteaga CL. PI3K/AKT/mTOR: role in breast cancer progression, drug resistance, and treatment. Cancer Metastasis Rev. 2016;35:515–24.

29. Dey N, De P, Leyland-Jones B. PI3K-AKT-mTOR inhibitors in breast cancers: from tumor cell signaling to clinical trials. Pharmacol Ther. 2017;175:91–106.

30. Halacli SO, Dogan AL. FOXP1 regulation via the PI3K/Akt/p70S6K signaling pathway in breast cancer cells. Oncol Lett. 2015;9:1482–8.

31. Lakhani SR, Ellis IO, Schnitt SJ. World Health Organization classification of tumours of the breast. 4th ed. Lyon: IARC Press; 2012.

32. Hu Z, Zhu L, Gao J, et al. Expression of FOXP1 in epithelial ovarian cancer (EOC) and its correlation with chemotherapy resistance and prognosis. Tumour Biol. 2015;36:7269–75.

33. Wu N, Du Z, Zhu Y, et al. The expression and prognostic impact of the PI3K/AKT/mTOR signaling pathway in advanced esophageal squamous cell carcinoma. Technol Cancer Res Treat. 2018;17:1533033818758772. https://doi.org/10.1177/1533033818758772.

34. Hammond MEH, Hayes DF, Dowsett M, et al. American Society of Clinical Oncology/College of American Pathologists Guideline Recommendations for Immunohistochemical testing of estrogen and progesterone receptors in breast Cancer. J Clin Oncol. 2010;28:2784–95.

35. Wolff AC, Hammond ME, Hicks DG, et al. Recommendations for human epidermal growth factor receptor 2 testing in breast cancer: American Society of Clinical Oncology/College of American Pathologists clinical practice guideline update. J Clin Oncol. 2013;31:3997–4013.

36. Oskay Halacli S. FOXP1 enhances tumor cell migration by repression of NFAT1 transcriptional activity in MDA-MB-231 cell. Cell Biol Int. 2017;41:102–10.

37. Storr SJ, Zhang S, Perren T, et al. The calpain system is associated with survival of breast cancer patients with large but operable inflammatory and non-inflammatory tumours treated with neoadjuvant chemotherapy. Oncotarget. 2016;7:47927–37.

38. Rios-Doria J, Kuefer R, Ethier SP, Day ML. Cleavage of β-catenin by calpain in prostate and mammary tumor cells. Cancer Res. 2004;64:7237–40.

39. Rios-Doria J, Day KC, Kuefer R, et al. The role of calpain in the proteolytic cleavage of E-cadherin in prostate and mammary epithelial cells. J Biol Chem. 2003;278:1372–9.

40. Li CL, Yang D, Cao X, et al. Fibronectin induces epithelial-mesenchymal transition in human breast cancer MCF-7 cells via activation of calpain. Oncol Lett. 2017;13:3889–95.

41. Zhao X, Gan L, Pan H, et al. Multiple elements regulate nuclear/cytoplasmic shuttling of FOXO1: characterization of phosphorylation and 14-3-3-dependent and -independent mechanisms. Biochem J. 2004;378:839–49.

42. Shigekawa T, Ijichi N, Ikeda K, et al. FOXP1, an estrogen-inducible transcription factor, modulates cell proliferation in breast cancer cells and 5-year recurrence-free survival of patients with tamoxifen-treated breast cancer. Horm Cancer. 2011;2:286–97.

43. Kim SJ, Kim TW, Lee SY, et al. CpG methylation of the ERalpha and ERbeta genes in breast cancer. Int J Mol Med. 2004;14:289–93.

44. Ijichi N, Shigekawa T, Ikeda K, et al. Association of double-positive FOXA1 and FOXP1 immunoreactivities with favorable prognosis of tamoxifen-treated breast cancer patients. Horm Cancer. 2012;3:147–59.

3

Nucleoli cytomorphology in cutaneous melanoma cells – a new prognostic approach to an old concept

Piotr Donizy[1*], Przemyslaw Biecek[2], Agnieszka Halon[1], Adam Maciejczyk[3,4] and Rafal Matkowski[4,5]

Abstract

Background: The nucleolus is an organelle that is an ultrastructural element of the cell nucleus observed in H&E staining as a roundish body stained with eosin due to its high protein content. Changes in the nucleoli cytomorphology were one of the first histopathological characteristics of malignant tumors. The aim of this study was to assess the relationship between the cytomorphological characteristics of nucleoli and detailed clinicopathological parameters of melanoma patients. Moreover, we analyzed the correlation between cytomorphological parameters of nucleoli and immunoreactivity of selected proteins responsible for, among others, regulation of epithelial-mesenchymal transition (SPARC, N-cadherin), cell adhesion and motility (ALCAM, ADAM-10), mitotic divisions (PLK1), cellular survival (FOXP1) and the functioning of Golgi apparatus (GOLPH3, GP73).

Methods: Three characteristics of nucleoli – presence, size and number – of cancer cells were assessed in H&E-stained slides of 96 formalin-fixed paraffin-embedded primary cutaneous melanoma tissue specimens. The results were correlated with classical clinicopathological features and patient survival. Immunohistochemical analysis of the above mentioned proteins was described in details in previous studies.

Results: Higher prevalence and size of nucleoli were associated with thicker and mitogenic tumors. All three nucleolar characteristics were related to the presence of ulceration. Moreover, microsatellitosis was strongly correlated with the presence of macronucleoli and polynucleolization (presence of two or more nucleoli). Lack of immunologic response manifested as no TILs in primary tumor was associated with high prevalence of melanoma cells with distinct nucleoli. Interestingly, in nodular melanoma a higher percentage of melanoma cells with prominent nucleoli was observed. In Kaplan-Meier analysis, increased prevalence and amount, but not size of nucleoli, were connected with shorter cancer-specific and disease-free survival.

Conclusion: (1) High representation of cancer cells with distinct nucleoli, greater size and number of nucleoli per cell are characteristics of aggressive phenotype of melanoma; (2) higher prevalence and size of nucleoli are potential measures of cell kinetics that are strictly correlated with high mitotic rate; and (3) high prevalence of cancer cells with distinct nucleoli and presence of melanocytes with multiple nucleoli are features associated with unfavorable prognosis in patients with cutaneous melanoma.

Keywords: Nucleolus, Melanoma, Prognosis

* Correspondence: piotrdonizy@wp.pl
[1]Department of Pathomorphology and Oncological Cytology, Wroclaw Medical University, ul. Borowska 213, 50-556 Wroclaw, Poland
Full list of author information is available at the end of the article

The preliminary results of this study was presented during the 29th European Congress of Pathology (Amsterdam, The Netherlands; 2–6 September 2017) and the abstract was published in the congress materials [1].

Background

The nucleolus is an organelle that is an ultrastructural element of the cell nucleus observed in H&E staining as a roundish body stained with eosin due to its high protein content. In mammalian cells, nucleoli are present only in the interphase and are not observed during mitosis [2–4]. The nucleoli's main function is the synthesis of ribosomal RNA (rRNA), that is why they are referred to as the ribosome factory. Additionally, the nucleolus is a specific sequestration/storehouse of proteins which under physiological conditions serve their role in the nucleoplasm. It was shown that the Cdc14 phosphatase is sequestered in yeast cell nucleoli and released to the cytoplasm during anaphase, being the key point of cell cycle progression [5]. Other biochemical functions of the nucleoli include their role in maintaining three-dimensional organization of chromatin in the nucleus [6]. It was demonstrated that perinucleolar chromatin is enriched in Snf2h, catalytic subunit of protein complex which is involved in chromatin remodeling that is necessary for normal replication of heterochromatin of exceptionally packed structure [7]. In addition to ribosome production, the nucleolus is also involved in the biogenesis of ribonucleoprotein particles independently from the synthesis of ribosome subunits – assembly of the signal recognition particle (SRP) [8–10], modification of U2 and U6 spliceosomal small RNA [11, 12] and assembly of specific mRNPs (small nuclear ribonucleoproteins) [13].

Based on the electron microscope analysis of the ultrastructure, the nucleolus has three major components: fibrillar center (FC), dense fibrillar component (DFC) and granular component (GC) [3]. Ribosomal genes actively engaged in transcription are located dominantly in two components: FC and DFC, thus being a functionally active unit of the nucleolus that is involved in rRNA synthesis. Granular component is responsible for maturation of ribosomal subunits [14, 15].

Changes in the nucleoli cytomorphology (their entry to the cells and the evaluation of their size) were one of the first histopathological characteristics of malignant tumors, along with abnormal mitotic figures, thickened and irregular nuclear membrane and coarse chromatin [4]. Eosinophilic macronucleoli are characteristic e.g. for melanoma, serous adenocarcinoma, epithelioid sarcoma, prostatic adenocarcinoma or Hodgkin lymphoma. It must be stressed, however, that only the presence of nucleoli (micronucleoli, less often macronucleoli) is a feature of metabolically active cells. Therefore, the presence of nucleoli in the cells does not allow us to qualify the analyzed cells as malignant cancer cells – e.g. normal macrophages and hepatocytes may present with clear nucleoli which only means they are functionally active as regards protein synthesis, and not that they are undergoing cancer transformation. It must also be underlined that the cells of some clinically extremely aggressive cancers do not have prominent nucleoli (or even do not have them at all), e.g. desmoplastic small round cell tumor (DSRCT) and small cell neuroendocrine carcinoma – in our opinion it may be related with extremely high Ki67 proliferative index and high mitotic rate in the case of these two cancers, which suggests that a high percentage of cancer cell population is in the active phase of mitotic division, which excludes the presence of nucleoli within these cells.

The aim of this study was to assess the relationship between the cytomorphological characteristics of nucleoli and detailed clinicopathological parameters of melanoma patients with survival analysis. Moreover, we analyzed the correlation between cytomorphological parameters of the nucleoli and immunoreactivity of the selected proteins related, among others, with the regulation of EMT (SPARC, N-cadherin), cell adhesion and motility (ALCAM, ADAM-10), mitotic divisions (PLK1), cellular survival (FOXP1) and the functioning of Golgi apparatus (GOLPH3, GP73).

Methods

Patients

Our study group was composed of 96 cutaneous melanoma patients treated at the Lower Silesian Oncology Center in Wroclaw, Poland, diagnosed in 2005–2010. Patients were enrolled in the study based on the availability of their medical documentation and tissue material, which included paraffin blocks and histopathology slides. Comprehensive clinical data was retrieved from the archival medical records, and data concerning the diagnostic and therapeutic procedures used was sourced from the cancer outpatient clinic at the Lower Silesian Oncology Center and Lower Silesian Cancer Registry, as well as Civil Register Office. The study was reviewed and approved by the ethical committee of the Wroclaw Medical University, Wroclaw, Poland.

Records were reviewed for clinical and pathological data (age and gender, primary tumor location, tumor stratification according to AJCC (pT), presence or absence of nodal (pN) and distant (pM) metastases, information on disease recurrence and SLNB procedures (Table 1).

Histopathological parameters

Archival formalin-fixed and paraffin-embedded tumor specimens were analyzed. Specifically, all hematoxylin and eosin-stained sections of the primary tumor were

Table 1 Correlations between characteristics of nucleoli in malignant melanocytes and clinical parameters

Clinical parameters	Characteristics of nucleoli								
	Size			Presence			Number		
	Low	High	p value	Low	High	p value	Low	High	p value
Age in years (21–79)[a] mean, 57 ± 15.4; median, 58			0.463			0.883			0.480
Gender[b]									
Female	46	11	0.618	25	32	0.532	42	15	0.464
Male	29	10		20	19		32	7	
Primary tumor location[c]									
Head/neck	10	4	0.927	5	9	0.295	11	3	0.722
Extremities	33	8		20	21		30	11	
Hand/ft	2	1		0	3		3	0	
Trunk	30	8		20	18		30	8	
Primary tumor (pT)[a]									
pT1	28	6	**0.022**	21	13	**0.025**	27	7	0.233
pT2	17	0		10	7		15	2	
pT3	15	9		6	18		15	9	
pT4	15	6		8	13		17	4	
Regional lymph nodes status (pN)[b]									
No metastases (pN-)	64	17	0.735	38	43	1.000	64	17	0.326
Metastases present (pN+)	11	4		7	8		10	5	
Distant metastases (pM)[b]									
No metastases (pM-)	71	20	1.000	44	48	0.363	72	19	0.076
Metastases present (pM+)	4	1		1	4		2	3	
Sentinel lymph node biopsy status (SNLB)[b] (55 patients)									
No metastases (SNLB-)	37	8	1.000	23	22	1.000	37	8	1.000
Metastases present (SNLB+)	8	2		5	5		8	2	
Recurrence[b]									
No	64	18	1.000	39	43	0.778	63	19	1.000
Yes	11	3		6	8		11	3	

[a] p value of Wilcoxon two sample test
[b] p value of Fisher's exact test
[c] p value of chi^2 test;
Statistically significant results ($P < 0.05$) are in bold text

examined independently by two pathologists who reported data such as Breslow thickness, Clark level, histologic type, mitotic rate (number of mitotic figures per 1 mm^2), presence of ulceration, lymphangioinvasion, microsatellitosis, intensity of tumor infiltrating lymphocytes (TILs) and microscopic evidence of regression (Table 2).

Evaluation of nucleoli

Three cytomorphological parameters were introduced to characterize the nucleoli. The presence of nucleoli refers to the global/total evaluation of the presence of nucleoli in the melanoma cell nuclei using the following grouping algorithm: 0: no nucleoli in melanoma cells, 1: small number of cells with the presence of nucleoli (≤ 20% of melanoma cells in the analyzed single H&E stained specimen of the primary tumor), 2: high percentage of cells shows the presence of nucleoli (> 20% of melanoma cells in the analyzed single H&E stained specimen of primary tumor). Nucleolus size refers to the size of the analyzed nucleoli (0: no nucleoli in melanoma cell nuclei, 1: micronucleoli present (inconspicuous nucleoli), 2: macronucleoli present (prominent nucleoli). Nucleoli number refers to the number of nucleoli in melanoma cell nuclei (0: no nucleoli in melanoma cell nuclei, 1: single micro- or macronucleolus in the nucleus, 2: two or more nucleoli per one nucleus of melanoma cell) Figs. 1 and 2.

Immunohistochemistry

Immunohistochemistry on formalin-fixed paraffin embedded tissue was done as described previously [16–20].

Table 2 Correlations between characteristics of nucleoli and presence of intranuclear vacuoles in malignant melanocytes and histopathological parameters

Histopathological parameters	Characteristics of nucleoli								
	Size			Presence			Number		
	Low	High	p value	Low	High	p value	Low	High	p value
Breslow thickness[a]									
≤1 mm	28	6	**0.022**	21	13	**0.025**	27	7	0.233
1.01–2.00 mm	17	0		10	7		15	2	
2.01–4.00 mm	15	9		6	18		15	9	
>4 mm	15	6		8	13		17	4	
Clark level[a]									
II and III	55	8	**0.003**	35	28	**0.032**	48	15	0.806
IV and V	20	13		10	23		26	7	
Histologic type[b]			0.316			**0.012**			0.511
Superficial spreading melanoma (SSM)	53	11		36	28		50	14	
Nodular malignant melanoma (NMM)	20	9		9	20		21	8	
Acral-lentiginous melanoma (ALM)	2	1		0	3		3	0	
Mitotic rate[a]									
0	40	4	**0.006**	28	16	**0.004**	37	7	0.152
≥1	35	17		17	35		37	15	
Ulceration[c]									
No	46	6	**0.012**	31	21	**0.008**	45	7	**0.026**
Yes	29	15		14	30		29	15	
TILs									
No	14	3		4	13		13	4	0.585
Non-brisk	24	7	0.887	13	18	**0.038**	22	9	
Brisk	37	11		28	20		39	9	
Microsatellitosis[c]									
No	74	17	**0.008**	44	47	0.363	73	18	**0.010**
Yes	1	4		1	4		1	4	
Lymphatic invasion									
No	55	16	1.000	36	35	0.248	58	13	0.098
Yes	20	5		9	16		16	9	
Tumor regression[c]									
No	71	18	0.340	42	47	1.000	69	20	1.000
Yes	4	3		3	4		5	2	

[a] p value of Wilcoxon two sample test
[b] p value of chi² test
[c] p value of Fisher's exact test;
Statistically significant results (P < 0.05) are in bold text

Statistical analysis

Statistical analysis was performed using the R language (available online: https://www.r-project.org/). Continuous variables like the age or proportions of lymphocytes were summarized with the use of the mean, median, min and max values. As regards the analysis of correlation of individual nucleolar parameters, the following dichotomous divisions of the study group were introduced for the purposes of statistical analysis: (1) presence of nucleoli: no nucleoli in melanoma cells or small number of cells with the presence of nucleoli (≤ 20% of melanoma cells in the analyzed single H&E stained specimen of the primary tumor) versus high percentage of cells shows the presence of nucleoli (> 20% of melanoma cells in the analyzed single H&E stained specimen of primary tumor); (2) nucleolus size:

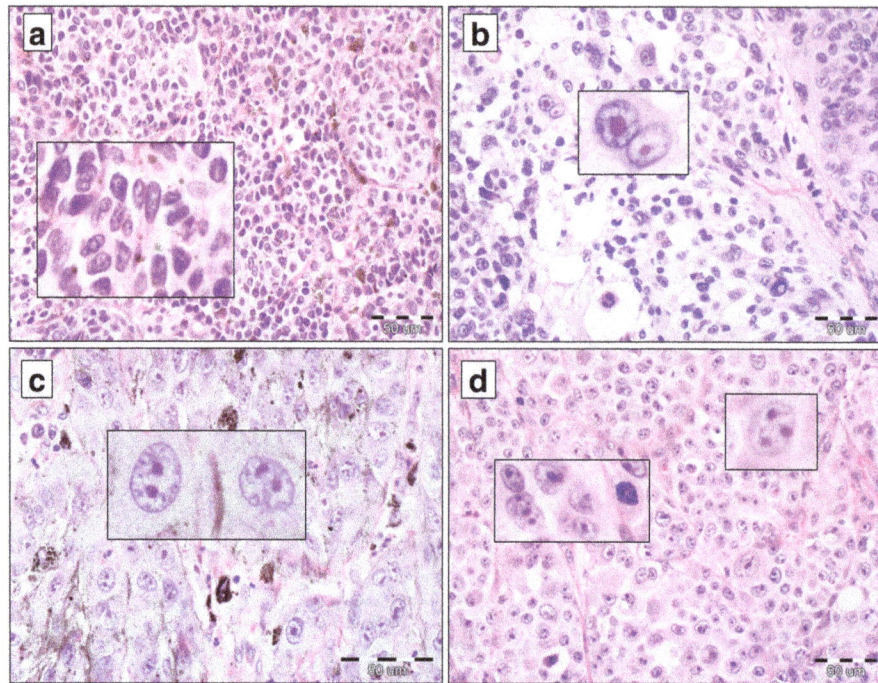

Fig. 1 Cytomorphology of nucleoli in cutaneous melanoma cells. Lack of nucleoli in neoplastic cells ((**a**), H&E staining, × 400; insert: H&E staining, × 600). Small number of melanoma cells with visible nucleoli ((**b**), H&E staining, × 400; insert: in higher magnification two cells with macro- and micronucleoli, H&E staining, × 600). High representation of cancer cells with distinct nucleoli ((**c**), H&E staining, × 600; insert: prominent binucleolization (two nucleoli per one melanoma cell), H&E staining, × 600). High percentage of melanoma cells with prominent nucleoli ((**d**), H&E staining, × 400; insert: polynucleolization of melanoma cells (three nucleoli per one melanoma cell, H&E staining, × 600)

no nucleoli in melanoma cell nuclei or micronucleoli present (inconspicuous nucleoli) versus macronucleoli present (prominent nucleoli); (3) nucleoli number: no nucleoli in melanoma cell nuclei or single micro- or macronucleolus in the nucleus versus two or more nucleoli per one nucleus of melanoma cell.

For cancer-specific overall survival (CSOS) and disease-free survival (DFS), we performed log-tests and Kaplan-Meier curves; all such analyses were conducted with the survival package for R. To assess the relation between dichotomized cytomorphological parameters of nucleoli in melanoma cells and continuous variables, the Wilcoxon two-sample test was used. The relation of cytomorphological parameters of nucleoli with binary variables was assessed by exact Fisher's exact test while the relation with other categorical variables was assessed by chi-square test. All relations were summarized by a suitable p-value, and all p-values smaller than 0.05 were considered as significant.

Results

Correlations with clinical parameters

A statistically significant correlation was shown between high percentage of melanoma cells with the presence of observable and/or clear nucleoli and higher advancement of primary tumor (pT) ($p = 0.025$). Additionally, also the size of nucleoli themselves – the presence of macronucleoli was correlated with a more advanced cancer process ($p = 0.022$). No other significant correlations were observed between cytomorphological parameters of the nucleoli and other clinical characteristics e.g. the status of regional lymph nodes or the presence of distant metastases (Table 1).

Correlations with histopathological parameters

Higher prevalence and size of nucleoli were associated with thicker primary tumor in the context of Breslow and Clark scales (p = 0.025 and p = 0.022, respectively). Moreover, these cytomorphological parameters of nucleoli were observed in primary tumor with high mitotic rate ($p = 0.004$ and $p = 0.006$, respectively). A statistically significant correlation was shown between high percentage of melanoma cells with the presence of observable nucleoli and nodular melanoma ($p = 0.012$). All three nucleolar characteristics were related to the presence of ulceration ($p = 0.008$, p = 0.012 and $p = 0.026$, respectively). Moreover, microsatellitosis was strongly correlated with the presence of macronucleoli and polynucleolization (presence of two or more nucleoli) (p = 0.008 and $p =$

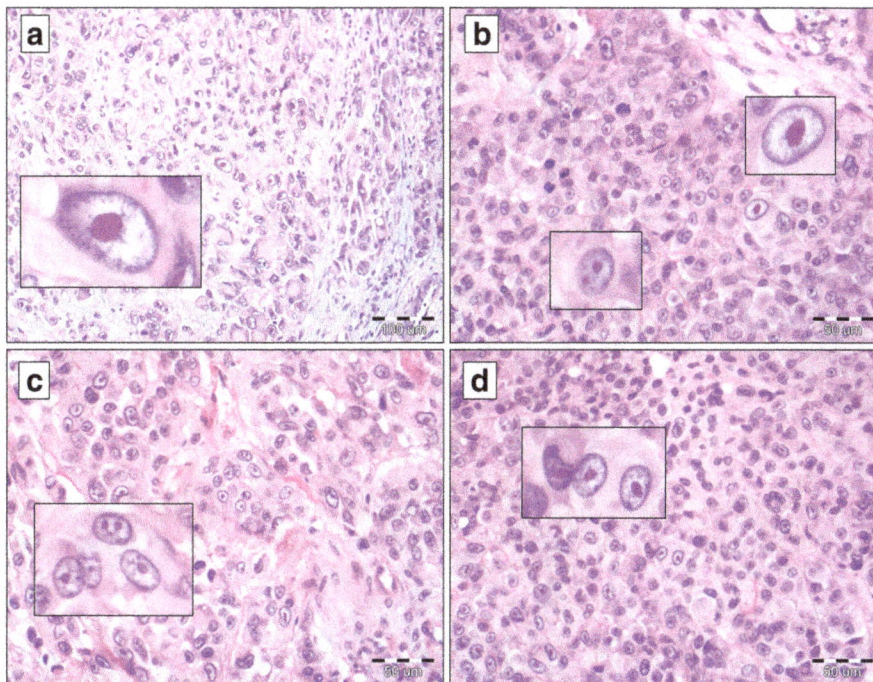

Fig. 2 Cytomorphology of nucleoli in cutaneous melanoma cells. Prominent macronucleoli in melanoma cells ((**a**), H&E staining, ×400; insert: eosinophilic roundish macronucleolus, H&E staining, ×600). Melanoma cells of high heterogeneity in the context of cytomorphological parameters of the nucleoli – cells with micronucleoli and cells with prominent macronucleoli present ((**b**), H&E staining, ×400; insert: H&E staining, ×600). High representation of cancer cells with distinct nucleoli with the feature of binucleolization ((**c**), H&E staining, ×400; insert: H&E staining, ×600; (**d**) staining, ×400; insert: eosinophilic micronucleoli, H&E staining, ×600);

0.010, respectively). Interestingly, lack of immunologic response manifested as no TILs in primary tumor was associated with high prevalence of melanoma cells with distinct nucleoli ($p = 0.038$) (Table 2).

Impact of nucleoli cytomorphology on long-term survival – Kaplan-Meier analysis

In Kaplan-Meier analysis, increased prevalence and number, but not size of nucleoli, were connected with significantly shorter disease-free and cancer-specific overall survival (Fig. 3).

Correlations between cytomorphology of nucleoli and expression parameters of selected proteins

A statistically significant correlation was demonstrated between the presence of macronucleoli and increased number of nucleoli (polynucleolization) and decreased expression of GOLPH3 protein in tumor-associated macrophages ($p = 0.034$ and $p = 0.042$, respectively). GOLPH3 immunoreactivity in melanoma cells did not show statistically significant correlations with the presence of macronucleoli and polynucleolization. No significant correlations were shown between cytomorphological parameters of the nucleoli and expression of proteins related with the regulation of EMT (SPARC, N-cadherin), cell

adhesion and motility (ALCAM, ADAM-10), regulation of mitotic divisions (PLK1) or cellular survival (FOXP1) (data not shown).

Discussion

In this study we revealed that higher prevalence and nucleolar hypertrophy were associated with thicker and mitogenic tumors. Presence of macronucleoli and polynucleolization (presence of two or more nucleoli) was strongly correlated with microsatellitosis which is postulated as an unfavorable prognostic factor in melanoma patients. All three nucleolar characteristics were related to the presence of ulceration – one of the most important histopathological bad prognostic parameter. Interestingly, lack of immunologic response manifested as no TILs in primary tumor was associated with high prevalence of melanoma cells with distinct nucleoli. Kaplan-Meier analysis confirmed that increased prevalence and number, but not size of nucleoli, were connected with shorter cancer-specific and disease-free survival.

The nucleolus that is actively engaged in transcription, and is morphologically manifested as eosinophilic, hypertrophic, prominent nucleolus (sometimes also a few nucleoli in a single cell) is strictly related with a high

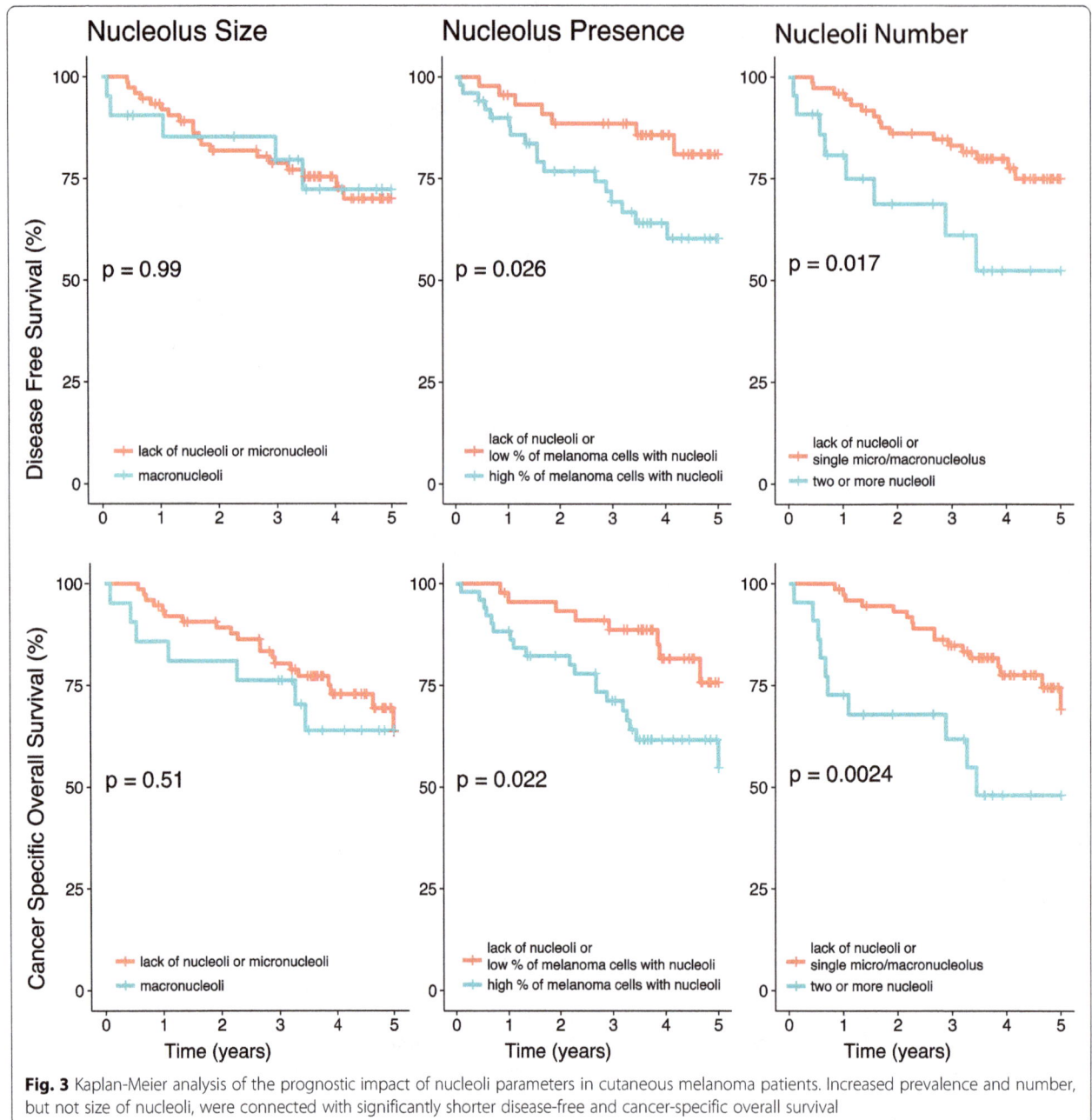

Fig. 3 Kaplan-Meier analysis of the prognostic impact of nucleoli parameters in cutaneous melanoma patients. Increased prevalence and number, but not size of nucleoli, were connected with significantly shorter disease-free and cancer-specific overall survival

translational potential of a cell and is an indicator of the cell's high demand for proteins (e.g. proto-oncogene proteins). Prominent nucleoli are specific measures of cellular kinetics, as they are a morphological equivalent of the cell preparing for mitotic division which always requires a massive number of regulatory, structural and functional proteins. We may also state that prominent nucleoli observed in a routine H&E staining are specific mirrors of extremely numerous, abnormally intensified cytobiochemical changes that occur in cancer cells. In our study we showed a statistically significant correlation between high mitotic rate and a higher prevalence and size of nucleoli, which confirms that the changes of nucleoli morphology are strictly correlated with increased proliferation potential. In other words, morphological changes of the nucleoli are basically the result of increased demand for ribosome synthesis which is a feature of cells with high proliferation potential. In our opinion, the evaluation of cytomorphology of the nuclei could be a more informative parameter than mitotic rate, since cytomorphological changes of the nucleoli occur at a much earlier stage of cancer transformation – the presence of mitotic figures in cancer melanocytes is the final stage and clue of cancer development and the nucleoli help us identify an increased proliferation potential at a much earlier stage. We should highlight the fact that the assessment of the nucleolar features is of academic interest but does not currently warrant a change in routine histopathological practice, as it does not seem to independently predict prognosis in melanoma in addition to the already well-established prognostic parameters. It could be very promising cytomorphological parameter assess only with cooperation with well-established parameters, such as: Breslow thickness, mitotic rate and ulceration. Interestingly, studies conducted by Lee et al. [21] concerning hepatocellular carcinoma showed that nucleolar hypertrophy appears to be independent of cell proliferation – most of hepatocytes in dysplastic tumors with enlarged nucleoli did not show increased cell proliferation. It may have been related with early phase of accumulation of molecular disorders in dysplastic foci that precede the development of invasive carcinoma.

In our study we observed a statistically significant correlation between the presence of macronucleoli and increased number of nucleoli (polynucleolization) and decreased expression of GOLPH3 protein in tumor-associated macrophages (TAMs). Having no factual insight into the role of GOLPH3 in TAMs, we only speculate that the reduced GOLPH3 immunoreactivity in TAMs may be associated with stable prooncogenic M2 phenotype [19]. Due to the lack of clinical and molecular data careful functional investigations are needed to explore the roles of tumor-associated macrophages in melanoma.

Studies conducted over recent several years concerning molecular biology of the nucleoli have revealed a few molecular mechanisms which might explain the processes of nucleolar hypertrophy and their increased number in cancer cells. One of them is concerned with *c-Myc* gene proto-oncogene whose translation product is necessary for cell-cycle entry [22]. Its direct effect on ribosome biogenesis was showed which involves direct enhancement of RNA polymerase and transcription activity. The main mechanism involves binding to specific consensus elements of rDNA and recruiting the selectivity factor 1 (SL1) to the rDNA promoter [3, 23, 24]. SL1 is the key factor that in cooperation with UBF (upstream binding factor) enables rDNA transcription by recruiting RNA polymerase I [25]. Additionally, c-Myc oncoprotein regulates transcription of many proteins directly involved in ribosome biogenesis such as cyclin D and E [26].

The second mechanism involves the effect of mutations in *TP53* gene which result in inactivation and accumulation of p53 protein in the nucleus. Wild-type (non-mutated) p53 binds directly to selectivity factor SL1 thus preventing the formation of SL1-UBF complex which is necessary for RNA polymerase I recruitment to the rRNA gene promoter, and finally inhibits RNA Pol I transcription [3, 27]. Mutated inactive p53 loses its function of a negative controller of rRNA transcription, significantly increasing ribosome biogenesis.

An important molecular mechanism behind a considerable increase in nucleoli volume and number in cancer cells is related with inactivation of pRB protein. Active, nonphosphorylated pRB, through binding with UBF inhibits rRNA synthesis [28, 29]. During the progression of cell cycle, phosphorylation of pRB by cyclin-dependent kinases 2 and 4 results in freeing UBF and E2Fs, which directly induces increase in rRNA transcription, morphologically manifesting as nucleolar hypertrophy and polynucleolization [30].

Prognostic importance of the nucleoli morphology was widely studied over the recent years [4]. It must be stressed, however, that most authors analyzed the presence of AgNORs and not the cytomorphology of the nucleoli assessed based on H&E staining. In line with our observations, in the vast majority of cancers the larger the size of the nucleolus (when examining AgNORs areas), the worse the prognosis of the disease [31]. A similar correlation was observed in melanoma [32]. PubMed literature research did not bring any paper that would evaluate the nucleoli morphology and its prognostic significance in melanoma based on a routine H&E staining. Our studies have showed that the evaluation of cytomorphology of the nucleoli does not need to involve special histochemical techniques – we are able to obtain reliable prognostic information from a routine H&E staining.

Conclusions

To conclude, (1) high representation of cancer cells with distinct nucleoli, greater size and number of nucleoli per cell are characteristics of aggressive phenotype of melanoma; and (2) higher prevalence and size of nucleoli are potential measures of cell kinetics that are strictly correlated with high mitotic rate.

Abbreviations
ADAM10: A disintegrin and metalloproteinase domain-containing protein 10; AgNORs: Argyrophylic nucleolar organizer regions; AJCC: American Joint Committee on Cancer; ALCAM: Activated leukocyte cell adhesion molecule; CSOS: Cancer-specific overall survival; DFC: Dense fibrillar component; DFS: Disease-free survival; DSRCT: Desmoplastic small round cell tumor; FC: Fibrillar center; FOXP1: Forkhead box P1; GC: Granular component; GOLPH3: Golgi phosphoprotein 3; GP73: Golgi protein 73; H&E: Hematoxylin and eosin; PLK1: Polo-like kinase 1; SL1: Selectivity factor 1; SNLB: Sentinel lymph node biopsy; SPARC: Secreted protein acidic and cysteine rich; SRP: Signal recognition particle; TILs: Tumor-infiltrating lymphocytes; UBF: Upstream binding factor

Acknowledgements
Not applicable.

Funding
This research was financed through a statutory subsidy by the Polish Minister of Science and Higher Education as a part of grants ST.B130.16.049 and ST.C280.17.010 (record numbers in the Simple system).

Authors' contributions

PD: study concepts and design; PD, AM, RM: data acquisition; PD, RM, AH, AM, PB: data analysis and interpretation; PB: statistical analysis; PD, RM: manuscript preparation and editing. All authors read and approved the final manuscript.

Competing interests

The authors declare that they have no competing interests.

Author details

[1]Department of Pathomorphology and Oncological Cytology, Wroclaw Medical University, ul. Borowska 213, 50-556 Wroclaw, Poland. [2]Faculty of Mathematics and Information Science, Warsaw University of Technology, Koszykowa 75, 00-662 Warsaw, Poland. [3]Department of Oncology and Clinic of Radiation Oncology, Wroclaw Medical University, pl. Hirszfelda 12, 53-413 Wroclaw, Poland. [4]Lower Silesian Oncology Centre, pl. Hirszfelda 12, 53-413 Wroclaw, Poland. [5]Department of Oncology and Division of Surgical Oncology, Wroclaw Medical University, pl. Hirszfelda 12, 53-413 Wroclaw, Poland.

References

1. Donizy P, Kaczorowski M, Biecek P, Halon A, Matkowski R. Nucleoli and nuclear pseudoinclusions in cutaneous melanoma cells - a new prognostic approach to an old concept. Virchows Arch. 2017;471suppl.1:S117.
2. Sirri V, Urcuqui-Inchima S, Roussel P, Hernandez-Verdun D. Nucleolus: the fascinating nuclear body. Histochem Cell Biol. 2008;129:13–31.
3. Montanaro L, Treré D, Derenzini M. Nucleolus, Ribosomes, and cancer. Am J Pathol. 2008;173:301–10.
4. Derenzini M, Montanaro L, Treré D. What the nucleolus says to a tumour pathologist. Histopathology. 2009;54:753–62.
5. Visintin R, Amon A. The nucleolus: the magician's hat for cell cycle tricks. Curr Opin Cell Biol. 2000;12:372–7.
6. Chubb JR, Boyle S, Perry P, Bickmore WA. Chromatin motion is constrained by association with nuclear compartments in human cells. Curr Biol. 2002;12:439–45.
7. Zhang LF, Huynh KD, Lee JT. Perinucleolar targeting of the inactive X during S phase: evidence for a role in the maintenance of silencing. Cell. 2007;129:693–706.
8. Hernandez-Verdun D. Assembly and disassembly of the nucleolus during the cell cycle. Nucleus. 2011;2:189–94.
9. Politz JC, Yarovoi S, Kilroy SM, Gowda K, Zwieb C, Pederson T. Signal recognition particle components in the nucleolus. Proc Natl Acad Sci U S A. 2000;97:55–60.
10. Leung E, Brown JD. Biogenesis of the signal recognition particle. Biochem Soc Trans. 2010;38:1093–8.
11. Ganot P, Jady BE, Bortolin ML, Darzacq X, Kiss T. Nucleolar factors direct the 2'-O-ribose methylation and pseudouridylation of U6 spliceosomal RNA. Mol Cell Biol. 1999;19:6906–17.
12. YT Y, Shu MD, Narayanan A, Terns RM, Terns MP, Steitz JA. Internal modification of U2 small nuclear (sn)RNA occurs in nucleoli of Xenopus oocytes. J Cell Biol. 2001;152:1279–88.
13. Jellbauer S, Jansen RP. A putative function of the nucleolus in the assembly or maturation of specialized messenger ribonucleoprotein complexes. RNA Biol. 2008;5:225–9.
14. Ploton D, O'Donohue MF, Cheutin T, Beorchia A, Kaplan H, Thiry M. Three-dimensional organization of rDNA and transcription. The Nucleolus. 2004: 154–69. Olson MOJ, editor. New York: Kluwer/Plenum
15. Raska I, Shaw PJ, Cmarko D. Structure and function of the nucleolus in the spotlight. Curr Opin Cell Biol. 2006;18:325–34.
16. Donizy P, Zietek M, Halon A, Leskiewicz M, Kozyra C, Matkowski R. Prognostic significance of ALCAM (CD166/MEMD) expression in cutaneous melanoma patients. Diagn Pathol. 2015;2:86.
17. Donizy P, Zietek M, Leskiewicz M, Halon A, Matkowski R. High percentage of ADAM-10 positive melanoma cells correlates with paucity of tumor-infiltrating lymphocytes but does not predict prognosis in cutaneous melanoma patients. Anal Cell Pathol (Amst). 2015;2015:975436.
18. Pieniazek M, Donizy P, Halon A, Leskiewicz M, Matkowski R. Prognostic significance of immunohistochemical epithelial-mesenchymal transition markers in skin melanoma patients. Biomark Med. 2016;10:975–85.
19. Donizy P, Kaczorowski M, Biecek P, Halon A, Szkudlarek T, Matkowski R. Golgi-related proteins GOLPH2 (GP73/GOLM1) and GOLPH3 (GOPP1/MIDAS) in cutaneous melanoma: patterns of expression and prognostic significance. Int J Mol Sci. 2016;17:E1619.
20. Kaczorowski M, Borowiec T, Donizy P, Pagacz K, Fendler W, Lipinski A, Halon A, Matkowski R. Polo-like kinase-1 immunoreactivity is associated with metastases in cutaneous melanoma. J Cutan Pathol. 2017; doi:10.1111/cup. 12985 [Epub ahead of print].
21. Lee RG, Tsamandas AC, Demetris AJ. Large cell change (liver cell dysplasia) and hepatocellular carcinoma in cirrhosis: matched case-control study, pathological analysis, and pathogenetic hypothesis. Hepatology. 1997;26:1415–22.
22. Eilers M, Picard D, Yamamoto KR, Bishop JM. Chimaeras of myc oncoprotein and steroid receptors cause hormone-dependent transformation of cells. Nature. 1989;340:66–8.
23. Arabi A, Wu S, Ridderstrale K, Bierhoff H, Shiue C, Fatyol K, Fahlen S, Hydbring P, Soderberg O, Grummt I, Larsson LG, Wright AP. C-Myc associates with ribosomal DNA and activates RNA polymerase I transcription. Nat Cell Biol. 2005;7:303–10.
24. Grandori C, Gomez-Roman N, Felton-Edkins ZA, Ngouenet C, Galloway DA, Eisenman RN, White RJ. C-Myc binds to human ribosomal DNA and stimulates transcription of rRNA genes by RNA polymerase I. Nat Cell Biol. 2005;7:311–8.
25. Grummt I. Life on a planet of its own: regulation of RNA polymerase I transcription in the nucleolus. Genes Dev. 2003;17:1691–702.
26. Voit R, Hoffmann M, Grummt I. Phosphorylation by G1-specific Cdk-cyclin complexes activates the nucleolar transcription factor UBF. EMBO J. 1999;18:1891–9.
27. Zhai W, Comai L. Repression of RNA polymerase I transcription by the tumor suppressor p53. Mol Cell Biol. 2000;20:5930–8.
28. Cavanaugh AH, Hempel WM, Taylor LJ, Rogalsky V, Todorov G, Rothblum LI. Activity of RNA polymerase I transcription factor UBF blocked by Rb gene product. Nature. 1995;374:177–80.
29. Voit R, Schafer K, Grummt I. Mechanism of repression of RNA polymerase I transcription by the retinoblastoma protein. Mol Cell Biol. 1997;17:4230–7.
30. Donjerkovic D, Scott DW. Regulation of the G1 phase of the mammalian cell cycle. Cell Res. 2000;10:1–16.
31. Pich A, Chiusa L, Margaria E. Prognostic relevance of AgNORs in tumor pathology. Micron. 2000;31:133–41.
32. Barzilai A, Goldberg I, Yulash M, Pavlotsky F, Zuckerman A, Trau H, Azizi E, Kopolovic J. Silver-stained nucleolar organizer regions (AgNORs) as a prognostic value in malignant melanoma. Am J Dermatopathol. 1998;20:473–7.

4

Tissue expression of retinoic acid receptor alpha and CRABP2 in metastatic nephroblastomas

Ana Paula Percicote[1*], Gabriel Lazaretti Mardegan[1], Elizabeth Schneider Gugelmim[2], Sergio Ossamu Ioshii[3], Ana Paula Kuczynski[4], Seigo Nagashima[5] and Lúcia de Noronha[3]

Abstract

Background: Nephroblastoma or Wilms tumor is the most frequent kidney cancer in children and accounts for 98% of kidney tumors in this age group. Despite favorable prognosis, a subgroup of these patients progresses to recurrence and death. The retinoic acid (RA) pathway plays a role in the chemoprevention and treatment of tumors due to its effects on cell differentiation and its antiproliferative, anti-oxidant, and pro-apoptotic activities. Reports describe abnormal cellular retinoic acid-binding protein 2 (CRABP2) expression in neoplasms and its correlation with prognostic factors and clinical and pathological characteristics. The aim of this study was to evaluate the immunohistochemical expression of retinoic acid receptor alpha (RARA) and CRABP2 in paraffin-embedded samples of nephroblastomas via semiquantitative and quantitative analyses and to correlate this expression with prognostic factors.

Methods: Seventy-seven cases of nephroblastomas were selected from pediatric oncology services. The respective medical records and surgical specimens were reviewed. Three representative tumor samples and one non-tumor renal tissue sample were selected for the preparation of tissue microarrays (TMA). The Allred scoring system was used for semiquantitative immunohistochemical analyses, whereas a morphometric analysis of the stained area was employed for quantitative evaluation. The nonparametric Mann-Whitney test was used for comparisons between two groups, while the nonparametric Kruskal-Wallis test was used to compare three or more groups.

Results: Immunopositivity for RARA and CRABP2 was observed in both the nucleus and cytoplasm. All histological components of the nephroblastoma (blastema, epithelium, and stroma) were positive for both markers. RARA, based on semiquantitative analyses, and CRABP2, bases on quantitative analyses, exhibited increased immunohistochemical expression in patients with metastasis, with p values of 0.0247 and 0.0128, respectively. These findings were similar to the results of the quantitative analysis of RARA expression, showing greater immunopositivity in tumor samples of patients subjected to pre-surgical chemotherapy. No significant correlation was found with the other variables studied, such as disease stage, anaplasia, risk group, histological type, nodal involvement, and clinical evolution.

Conclusions: Semiquantitative and quantitative analyses of the markers RARA and CRABP2 indicate their potential as biomarkers for tumor progression and their participation in nephroblastoma tumorigenesis.

Keywords: Nephroblastoma, Retinoic acid, CRABP2

* Correspondence: appercicote@gmail.com
[1]Federal University of Paraná, Curitiba, Brazil
Full list of author information is available at the end of the article

Background

Nephroblastoma or Wilms tumor is the most frequent kidney cancer in children and accounts for 98% of kidney tumors in this age group [1]. Nephroblastoma originates in metanephric blastema cells that histologically resemble the undifferentiated blastema, stroma, and primitive renal tubular structures of the fetal kidney [2]. The prognosis of patients with this cancer improved dramatically after the formation of cooperative groups. The development of treatment protocols resulted in global survival rates above 90% [3].

Despite this therapeutic success, prognostic factors such as lymph node metastases, anaplastic histology, bilateral disease, molecular characteristics, stage III/IV disease, tumor rupture, and renal vein and inferior vena cava thrombi are associated with relapse and reduced survival [3–5].

In a frantic search for new therapeutic targets and for a better understanding of the molecular pathways responsible for tumorigenesis and tumor progression in nephroblastoma, retinoic acid (RA) emerged as a therapeutic alternative for the treatment of this cancer. Numerous genes involved in the RA signaling pathway seem to participate in the progression and cellular differentiation of nephroblastoma [6, 7].

RA is the most active metabolite of vitamin A, and its function is essential for many biological processes, such as fetal development and the proliferation, differentiation and apoptosis of normal and tumor cells [8]. The effects of RA on the regulation of gene expression depend on intracellular RA distribution secondary to the concentration of intracellular proteins such as cellular retinoic acid-binding protein 2 (CRABP2) and to the activity on RA receptors, designated retinoic acid receptors (RARs) and retinoid X receptors (RXRs) [8–10]. Retinoic acid receptor alpha (RARA) is a ligand-dependent transcription factor that regulates target gene expression after RA binding [8]. RA can be used for the chemoprevention and treatment of tumors due to its effects on cell differentiation and its antiproliferative, anti-oxidant and pro-apoptotic activities [11, 12]. CRABPs are low-molecular-weight, intracellular proteins that act on RA-induced transcriptional activity, maintaining an adequate RA metabolism [13].

Previous studies have described changes in the RA pathway in nephroblastomas [6, 7, 14]. The overexpression of CRABP2 is related to advanced stages of this cancer, which indicates the involvement of the RA pathway in tumor progression [7, 15, 16]. CRABP2 protein expression has been observed in human fetal kidney samples during mesenchymal-epithelial transition and in the blastemal component of nephroblastoma; in the latter, the RA pathway was found to be associated with CRABP2 upregulation [2].

This study aims to evaluate the distribution of RARA and CRABP2 protein expression and positivity in nephroblastoma tissue specimens and to correlate these results with clinical and pathological prognostic factors.

Methods

Patients

We selected 77 patients diagnosed with nephroblastoma between 1994 and 2012 who were treated at pediatric oncology services of the Clinics Hospital Complex/Federal University of Paraná, Pequeno Príncipe Children's Hospital and Erasto Gaertner Hospital. This study was approved by the ethics committees of the three institutions.

Hematoxylin-eosin-stained histological slides were reviewed and classified according to the histological type and presence of anaplasia. Relevant clinical data, such as the gender of patients, age at diagnosis, initial clinical presentation, disease stage, risk group, presence of metastasis, nodal involvement, treatment received, and clinical evolution, were obtained.

Twelve tissue microarrays (TMA) containing samples representative of the tumors were constructed. For each case, three distinct tumor areas and one sample of non-tumor renal tissue were selected to construct the TMA.

Information regarding the clinical evolution, initial treatment (chemotherapy or surgery), and prognostic factors, such as disease stage, presence of metastasis, histological type, presence of anaplasia, risk group, and nodal involvement, was compiled for statistical analysis and comparison with the immunoexpression of markers in tumor samples.

Immunohistochemistry

Histological sections of 4 μm thickness were obtained for immunohistochemistry. The slides were then subjected to deparaffinization, dehydration, and rehydration. Endogenous peroxidase was blocked using methyl alcohol and hydrogen peroxide for the first blocking step and distilled water and hydrogen peroxide for the second blocking step. The next step was incubation with primary antibodies chosen for the study, including rat anti-RARA monoclonal antibody (clone 2C9-1F8; 1:800 dilution, Abcam, Cambridge, MA, USA) and rabbit anti-CRABP2 polyclonal antibody (1:50 dilution, Bioss, Woburn, MA, USA), for one hour in a humid chamber at room temperature. Secondary antibody (Advance™ HRP Dako®, Dako Corporation, Carpinteria, CA, USA) conjugated with the polymer dextran was incubated with the slides for 30 min at room temperature. For staining, the diaminobenzidine (DAB) + substrate complex (buffer for DAB dilution) was added to the slides, which were counterstained with Harris hematoxylin and subsequently dehydrated with 100% ethanol and clearing with analytical grade xylol. The stained slides were mounted in histological resin for microscopy (Entellan, Merck®). Positive and negative controls were included in all reactions [17].

Evaluation of immunoexpression

Immunohistochemical expression was evaluated through semiquantitative and quantitative analyses of both nuclear and cytoplasmic staining. For the semiquantitative analysis, the Allred scoring system was used, which consists of scores of the proportion and intensity of both nuclear and cytoplasmic staining that are summed to give the total Allred score. The proportion score was calculated as the ratio between positive cells and the total number of cells and was classified as 0 (0%), 1 (> 0–1%), 2 (≥1%–10%), 3 (> 10%–33%), 4 (> 33%–66%), and 5 (> 66%–100%). The intensity score was classified as 0 (negative), 1+ (weak), 2+ (moderate), and 3+ (strong). The total score was calculated as the sum of the proportion and intensity scores and ranged from 0 to 8 [18].

Quantitative morphometric analysis was performed using images obtained by a Zeiss Axioscan Slide Scanner (Germany) at 20× magnification, which generates digital tagged image file format (TIFF) files. After scanning, the software generated images in the photomicrograph format, which were analyzed using the image analysis software Image-Pro Plus® (Rockville, MD, USA). The immunostained area of each photomicrograph was measured, including both nuclear and cytoplasmic areas, and was expressed in square micrometers, and the mean was calculated for each case and transformed into percentage by half-magnification field (HMF) by dividing by the constant 115.226,1 μm^2 and multiplying by 100 for subsequent statistical analysis [19].

Statistical analysis

For the evaluation of the data obtained, quantitative variables were expressed as the means, medians, minimum values, maximum values, and standard deviations. Qualitative variables were expressed as frequencies and percentages. For comparisons between two groups, the non-parametric Mann-Whitney test was used for quantitative variables. Three or more groups were compared using the non-parametric Kruskal-Wallis test. The normality of the variables was evaluated by the Shapiro-Wilk test. Pearson correlation test was applied to measure the dependence of two variables. Values of $p < 0.05$ indicated statistical significance. The data were analyzed using IBM SPSS Statistics v. 20 software.

Results

Population characteristics

Of the total 77 selected patients with nephroblastoma, the mean age at diagnosis was 33.6 months (0–108 months). The main clinical findings related to diagnosis were increased abdominal girth in 40.2% ($n = 31$), abdominal mass in 37.7% ($n = 29$), abdominal pain in 11.7% ($n = 9$), fever in 10.4% ($n = 8$), vomiting in 3.9% ($n = 3$), and weight loss in 3.9% ($n = 3$) of the patients. As an initial treatment, 67.1% of the patients underwent pre-surgical chemotherapy, while 25% underwent surgery. Data regarding the initial treatment of one patient could not be retrieved. The clinical and demographic data are summarized in Table 1.

Immunohistochemical analysis

Immunopositivity for RARA and CRABP2 was observed in all three histological components of nephroblastoma (blastema, stroma, and epithelium). Cytoplasmic and nuclear positivity for CRABP2 was present in 100% and 56% of the samples, respectively. A total of 94.7% of the cases were positive for RARA in both the nucleus and cytoplasm. The total Allred score ranged from 3 to 7 for both markers, with a median of 6 for RARA and 5 for CRABP2 (Fig. 1).

The immunoexpression of RA and CRABP2 was not restricted to a specific histological type or histological

Table 1 Patients' baseline characteristics

Variable	Value
Gender (female:male)	31:46
Age (months), median	26
Metastases, n (%)	
Yes	17 (22.4)
No	59 (77.6)[a]
Histological risk group, n (%)	
High risk	9 (11.7)
Intermediate risk	68 (88.3)
Lymph nodes, n (%)	
Negative	36 (46.8)
Positive	4 (5.2)[b]
Local stage, n (%)	
I	47 (64.4)
II	13 (17.8)
III	13 (17.8)[c]
Histological classification, n (%)	
Nephroblastoma - epithelial type	10 (13.0)
Nephroblastoma - stromal type	9 (11.7)
Nephroblastoma - mixed type	37 (48.1)
Nephroblastoma - regressive type	4 (5.2)
Nephroblastoma - blastemal type	12 (15.6)
Nephroblastoma - diffuse anaplasia type	5 (6.5)
Clinical evolution, n (%)	
Disease-free	57 (74.0)
Dead	11 (14.3)[d]

[a]data could not be retrieved; [b]remaining patients did not undergo lymph node resection; [c]specimens with impaired staging; [d]patients lost to follow-up or transferred to another center during the study

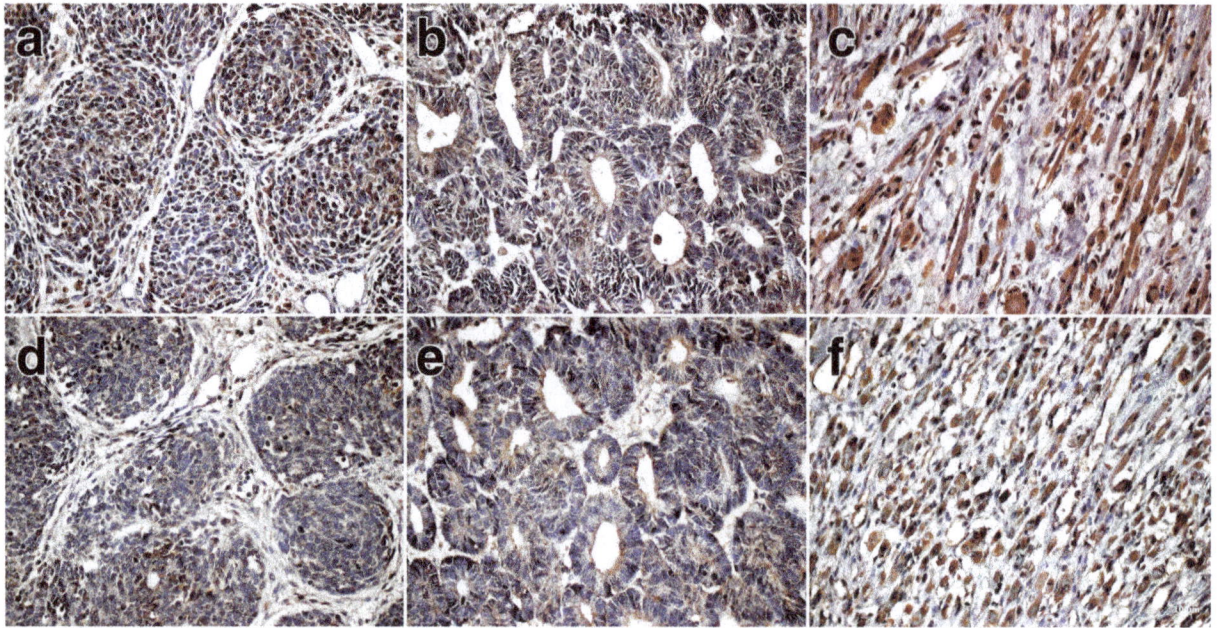

Fig. 1 Immunohistochemical expression of RARA and CRABP2 in nephroblastoma samples. RA immunoexpression: **a**, blastema; **b**, epithelium; **c**, stroma; CRABP2 immunoexpression: **d**, blastema; **e**, epithelium; **f**, stroma (40×)

Table 2 Median immunoexpression of RARA and CRABP2 in nephroblastomas based on histological subtype

Variable	Semiquantitative, median (minimum:maximum)				Quantitative analysis (%), median (minimum:maximum)			
	RARA	p value	CRABP2	p value	RARA	p value	CRABP2	p value
Metastases								
Yes	6 (4–7)	0.9428	5 (3–7)	0.0128	27.1 (17.3–33.8)	0.0247	28.7 (13.6–36.5)	0.0844
No	6 (3–7)		4 (0–7)				25.4 (4.2–40.4)	
Histological risk group								
High risk	5.5 (4–7)	0.7591	4 (3–7)	0.5615	20.0 (12.4–31.7)	0.6014	24.6 (18.9–32.3)	0.8628
Intermediate risk	6 (3–7)		5 (0–7)		24.6 (6.3–40.3)		26.2 (4.2–40.4)	
Lymph nodes								
Negative	6 (3–7)	0.3291	4.5 (0–6)	0.7087	24.6 (6.3–35.7)	0.8715	26.8	0.9197
Positive	6 (5–7)		5 (3–6)		23.2 (19.4–29.1)		25.7	
Local stage								
I	6 (3–7)	0.3425	5 (3–7)	0.8520	25.3 (6.3–40.3)	0.0525	26.2	0.4731
II	6 (5–7)		5 (0–7		20.7 (7.3–33.6)		23.4	
III	5 (4–7)		4 (3–6)		20.2 (12.4–29.1)		26.8	
Histological classification								
Nephroblastoma - epithelial type	6 (5–6)	0.8286	5 (3–7)	0.5188	27.0 (19.9–34.4)4.6	0.2300	25.9 (15.2–39.5)27.6	0.6782
Nephroblastoma - stromal type	5 (5–7)		5 (3–6)		24.3 (14.7–29.0)1		21.4 (6.2–40.4)28.4	
Nephroblastoma - mixed type	6 (3–7)		5 (3–6)		24.4 (6.3–35.6)23.6		26.9 (4.2–37.4)-7.3	
Nephroblastoma - regressive type	6 (5–7)		5 (4–6		26.4 (20.0–31.8)5		27.2(15.2–38.5)6	
Nephroblastoma - blastemal type	6 (4–7)		5 (0–5)		24.920.9 (17.3–40.3)		28.2 (15.1–37.0)27.5	
Nephroblastoma - diffuse anaplasia type	6 (4–7)		4.5 (3–7)		14.821.3 (12.4–31.8)		2.24 (20.0–28.3)4.7	
Overall nephroblastoma	6 (3–7)		5 (0–7)		24.2 (6.3–40.3)		26.3 (4.2–40.4)	
Overall non-tumor renal parenchyma	6 (5–8)		6 (4–7)		30.4 (1.4–49.7)		33.8 (0.6–52.0)	

component. Areas with rhabdomyoblastic differentiation and anaplastic nephroblastomas expressed both markers.

The results obtained by quantitative analysis of RARA and CRABP2 expression in the nephroblastoma samples showed median values of 24.2% per HMF (6.3%–40.3%) and 26.3% per HMF (4.2%–40.4%), respectively (Table 2).

The immunoexpression of RARA and CRABP2 was also observed in samples of renal parenchyma. Glomeruli and renal tubules expressed RARA and CRABP2 both in the nucleus and cytoplasm (Additional file 1: Figure S1). The median values of the total Allred score obtained for renal parenchyma samples were 6 for RARA and 5 for CRABP2 (Fig. 1).

Prognostic importance

The results obtained through quantitative and semiquantitative analyses were compared to clinical and pathological prognostic factors such as histological type, disease stage, risk group, presence of metastasis, anaplasia, clinical evolution, nodal involvement, and pre-surgical chemotherapy.

According quantitative analyses, the protein expression of RARA was increased in patients with metastasis ($p = 0.0247$) and in patients who underwent pre-surgical chemotherapy ($p = 0.0330$) (Fig. 2).

The semiquantitative analysis for CRABP2 indicated higher expression in patients with metastasis ($p = 0.0128$) (Fig. 2). This group of patients, with scores 6 and 7 in semiquantitative analysis, were mostly of intermediate risk (77.8%), without lymph node metastasis (75.0%), with histologically mixed type tumors (53.3%), with local stage I disease (66.7%) and free of disease (86.7%).

Additional evaluation did not demonstrate association between initial distant metastasis and treatment ($p = 0.1288$), local stage ($p = 0.8700$), risk group ($p = 0.9911$) or nodal involvement ($p = 0.3628$). The results were similar for the analysis between local stage and treatment ($p = 0.9034$).

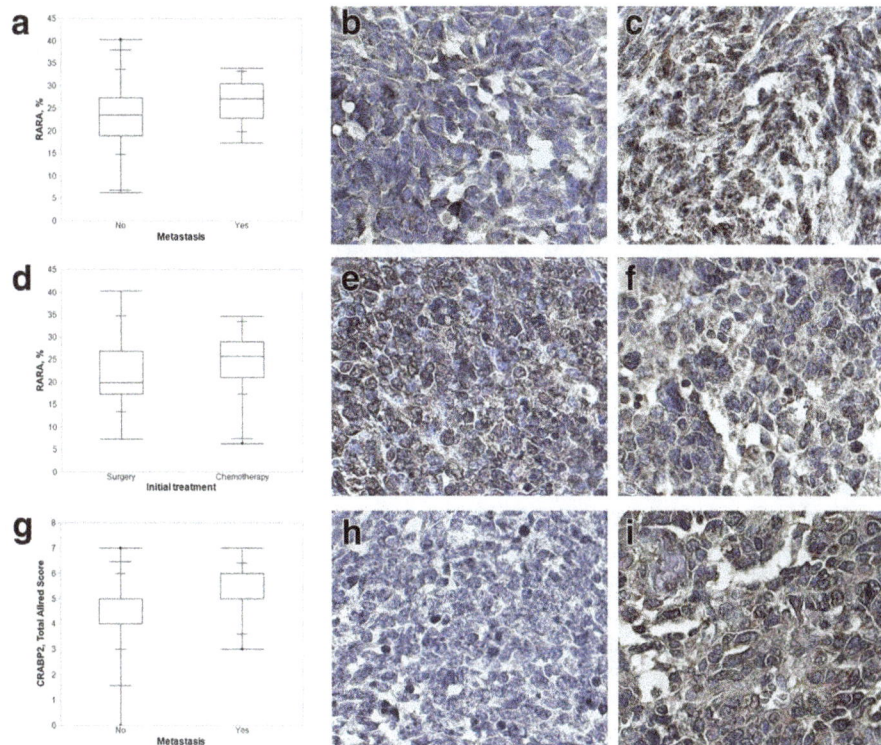

Fig. 2 a Quantitative analysis of RARA immunoexpression as a function of the presence of metastasis. The box-plot represents the results of the quantitative analysis of RARA immunoexpression according to the presence of metastasis, showing RARA immunoexpression in nephroblastomas with and without metastasis. Increased immunopositivity was observed in patients with metastasis ($p = 0.0247$). **b** and **c** Immunohistochemical expression of RARA in nephroblastomas without (**b**) and with metastasis (**c**) (63×). **d** Quantitative analysis of RARA immunoexpression as a function of the initial treatment. The box-plot represents the results of the quantitative analysis of RARA immunoexpression according to the type of initial treatment, showing RARA immunoexpression in nephroblastoma samples from patients subjected to pre-surgical chemotherapy and patients subjected to surgery as initial treatment ($p = 0.0330$). **e** and **f** Immunohistochemical expression of RARA in nephroblastoma samples from patients subjected to surgery (**e**) and pre-surgical chemotherapy (**f**) (63×). **g** Semiquantitative analysis of CRABP2 immunoexpression as a function of the presence of metastasis. The box-plot represents the results of the quantitative analysis of CRABP2 immunoexpression according to the presence of metastasis, showing CRABP2 immunoexpression in nephroblastomas with and without metastasis. Increased immunopositivity was observed in patients with metastasis ($p = 0.0128$). **h** and **i** Immunohistochemical expression of CRABP2 in nephroblastoma without (**h**) and with metastasis (**i**) (63×)

No significant correlation was found between RARA and CRABP2 immunopositivity and clinical evolution, disease stage, anaplasia, nodal involvement, risk group, or histological type ($p > 0.05$).

Discussion

The present work is the first report of the evaluation of RARA and CRABP2 immunoexpression as potential biomarkers and therapeutic targets in nephroblastomas.

The essential functions of RA in biological processes, such as differentiation, proliferation, and apoptosis, have prompted the evaluation of this protein that had not been previously studied in nephroblastomas [8]. The effects of RA depend on intracellular proteins, such as CRABP2, that maintain an adequate RA metabolism by increasing its availability and transporting it to the nucleus [10, 13, 20]. The effects of RA on gene expression are mediated by nuclear receptors, such as RARA [8]. RARA can be translocated from the cytoplasm to the nucleus after being synthesized, modified and stimulated by RA. Under physiological conditions, RARA is located in the cytoplasm and nucleus [21]. RARA gene mutations observed in promyelocytic leukemia can induce the cytoplasmic translocation of the receptor [22].

CRABP2 transports RA from the cytoplasm to the nucleus, promoting RAR ligation and RXR heterodimer formation [12]. Cytoplasmic CRABP2 functions, when coupled with RA, include transportation of RA to different cellular components and metabolization or sequestration of RA in the cytoplasm. However, knowledge about CRABP2 activity unassociated with RA is sparse [23]. Among cytoplasmic CRABP2 interactions, a connection was described with the RNA-binding protein HuR, involved in RNA stability control [24]. Upregulation of CRABP2 has been reported in the blastema of nephroblastomas during the investigation of genes related to nephrogenesis. Nuclear negativity of CRABP2 has been described in 5.31% and cytoplasmic negativity in 6.48% of blastema samples [2]. However, in the samples studied here, including three histological components of nephroblastomas (blastema, epithelium, and stroma), we observed cytoplasmic and nuclear positivity in 100% and 56% of the samples, respectively.

Gupta et al. described the overexpression of CRABP2 in nephroblastoma samples with favorable histology, with increased expression in advanced cancer stages (stage III/IV). The findings of these authors indicate the role of CRABP2 in cell migration and invasion in nephroblastomas [16]. When comparing clinical-pathological prognostic factors to values obtained in quantitative and semiquantitative analyses, we observed increased expression of RARA and CRABP2 in patients with metastasis.

Among our samples, protein expression of RARA was increased in samples from patients undergoing pre-surgical chemotherapy. Increased expression of genes in the RA pathway has been described by other authors in nephroblastoma patients treated with pre-surgical chemotherapy relative to that in patients undergoing surgery as the initial treatment [7]. This phenomenon may be associated with tissue damage and the inflammatory process caused by chemotherapy, which induce increased expression of the RA signaling pathway [25]. Both RARA and CRABP2 immunoexpression appeared to be unrelated with clinico-pathological variables, such as local stage, risk group and lymph node status.

In summary, the immunoexpression of RARA and CRABP2 was increased in samples from patients subjected to pre-surgical chemotherapy and in samples from patients with metastatic disease, respectively.

Conclusions

In conclusion, semiquantitative and quantitative analyses of the markers RARA and CRABP2 indicate these proteins as potential biomarkers of tumor progression and their participation in nephroblastoma tumorigenesis. Complementary studies are needed to better understand the mechanisms involved.

Abbreviations

CRABP2: Cellular retinoic acid-binding protein 2; DAB: Diaminobenzidine; HMF: Half-magnification field; RA: Retinoic acid; RARA: Retinoic acid receptor alpha; TIFF: Tagged image file format; TMA: Tissue microarrays

Acknowledgements

We thank the pathology services of the Clinics Hospital Complex, the Pequeno Príncipe Children's Hospital, and the Erasto Gaertner Hospital for allowing this work to be conducted and the Laboratory of Experimental Pathology of the Pontifical Catholic University of Paraná for immunohistochemical analyses and image scanning.

Funding

Immunohistochemical analyses were performed in the Laboratory of Experimental Pathology of the Pontifical Catholic University of Paraná.

Authors' contributions

APP and LN developed the project. APP selected the samples and reviewed the slides. GLM, SN and APP performed the immunohistochemical analyses. SN performed the scanning of slides and digital documentation of immunohistochemical reactions. ESG, APK and SOI provided patient data. APP performed the statistical analyses. APP and LN wrote the article. All authors have read and approved the manuscript.

Competing interests

The authors declare that they have no competing interests.

Author details

[1]Federal University of Paraná, Curitiba, Brazil. [2]Anatomic Pathology Service at the Pequeno Príncipe Hospital, Curitiba, Brazil. [3]Department of Medical Pathology, Federal University of Paraná and School of Health of the Pontifical Catholic University of Paraná, Curitiba, Brazil. [4]Oncology Service at the Pequeno Príncipe Hospital, Curitiba, Brazil. [5]School of Health of the Pontifical Catholic University of Paraná, Curitiba, Brazil.

References

1. Stiller CA, Parkin DM. Geographic and ethnic variations in the incidence of childhood cancer. Br Med Bull. 1996;52(4):682–703.
2. Maschietto M, Trapé AP, Piccoli FS, Ricca TI, Dias AAM, Coudry RA, Galante PA, Torres C, Fahhan L, Lourenço S, Grundy PE, Camargo B, Souza S, Neves EJ, Soares FA, Brentani H, Carraro DM. Temporal blastemal cell gene expression analysis in the kidney reveals new Wnt and related signaling pathway genes to be essential for Wilms' tumor onset. Cell Death Dis. 2011;2:e224.
3. Pritchard-Jones K, Moroz V, Vujanic G, Powis M, Walker J, Messahel B, Hobson R, Levitt G, Kelsey A, Mitchell C. Treatment and outcome of Wilms'tumour patients: an analysis of all cases registered in the UKW3 trial. Ann Oncol. 2012;23(9):2457–63.
4. Honeyman JN, Rich BS, Mcevoy MP, Knowles MA, Heller G, Riachy E, Kobos R, Shukla N, Wolden SL, Steinherz PG, La Quaglia MP. Factors associated with relapse and survival in Wilms tumor: a multivariate analysis. J Pediatr Surg. 2012;47(6):1228–33.
5. Dome JS, Graf N, Geller JI, Fernandez CV, Mullen EA, Spreafico F, Van Den Heuvel-Eibrink M, Pritchard-Jones K. Advances in Wilms tumor treatment and biology: progress through international collaboration. J Clin Oncol. 2015;33(27):2999–3007.
6. Zirn B, Hartmann O, Samans B, Krause M, Wittmann S, Mertens F, Graf N, Eilers M, Gessler M. Expression profiling of Wilms tumors reveals new candidate genes for different clinical parameters. Int J Cancer. 2006;118(8):1954–62.
7. Wegert J, Bausenwein S, Kneitz S, Roth S, Graf N, Geissnger E, Gessler M. Retinoic acid pathway activity in Wilms tumors and chacarecterization of biological responses in vitro. Mol Cancer. 2011;10:136.
8. Theodosiou M, Laudet V, Schubert M. From carrot to clinic: an overview of the retinoic acid signaling pathway. Cell Mol Life Sci. 2010;67(9):1423–45.
9. Passeri D, Doldo E, Tarquini C, Costanza G, Mazzaglia D, Agostinelli S, Campione E, Di Stefani A, Giunta A, Bianchi L, Orlandi A. Loss of CRABP-II characterizes human skin poorly diferrenciated squamous cell carcinomas and favors DMBA/TPA-induced carcinogenesis. J Invest Dermatol. 2016;136(6):1255–66.
10. Gupta S, Pramanik D, Mukherjee R, Campbell NR, Elumalai S, Wilde RF, Hong S, Goggins MG, Jesus-Acosta A, Laheru D, Maitra A. Molecular determinants of retinoic acid sensitivity in pancreatic cancer. Clin Cancer Res. 2012;18(1):280–9.
11. Bushue N, Wan YY. Retinoid pathway and cancer therapeutics. Adv Drug Deliv Rev. 2010;62(13):1285–98.
12. Favorskaya I, Kainov Y, Chemeris G, Komelkov A, Zborovskaya I, Tchevkina E. Expression and clinical significance of CRABP1 and CRABP2 in non-small cell lung cancer. Tumour Biol. 2014;35(10):10295–300.
13. Blomhoff R. Transport and Metabolism of vitamin a. Nutr Rev. 1994;52:S13–23.
14. Li W, Kessler P, Williams BRG. Transcript profiling of Wilms tumors reveals connections to kidney morphogenesis and expression patterns associated with anaplasia. Oncogene. 2005;24(3):457–68.
15. Zirn B, Samans B, Spangenberg C, Graf N, Eilers M, Gessler M. All-trans retinoic acid treatment of Wilms tumor cells reverses expression of genes associated with high risk and relapse in vivo. Oncogene. 2005;24(3):5246–51.
16. Gupta A, Kessler P, Rawwas J, Williams BRG. Regulation of CRABP-II expression by MycN in Wilms tumor. Exp Cell Res. 2008;314(20):3663–8.
17. Chong DC, Raboni SM, Abujamra KB, Marani DM, Nogueira MB, Tsuchiya LRV, Neto HJC, Flizikowski FBZ, Noronha L. Respiratory viruses in pediatric necropsies: an immunohistochemical study. Pediatr Dev Pathol. 2009;12(3):211–6.
18. Harvey J, Clark G, Osborne C, Allred D. Estrogen receptor status by immunohistochemistry is superior to the ligand-binding assay for predicting response to adjuvant endocrine therapy in breast cancer. J Clin Oncol. 1999;17(5):1474–81.
19. Simões MA, Pabis FC, Freitas AKE, Azevedo MLVA, Ronchi DCM. Immunoexpression of GADD45β in the myocardium of newborns experiencing perinatal hypoxia. Pathol Res Pract. 2017;213(3):222–6.
20. Noy N. Retinoid-binding proteins: mediator of retinoid action. The Biochem J. 2000;348:481–95.
21. Wang H, Yang R, Zhong L, Zhu XY, Ma PP, Yang XQ, Jiang KL, Liu BZ. Location of NLS-RARα protein in NB4 cell and nude mice. Oncol Lett. 2017;13(4):2045–52.
22. Goto E, Tomita A, Hayakawa F, Atsumi A, Kiyoi H, Naoe T. Missense mutations in PML-RARA are critical for the lack of responsiveness to arsenic trioxide treatment. Blood. 2011;118(6):1600–9.
23. Napoli JL. Biochemical pathways of retinoid transport, metabolism and signal transduction. Clin Immunol Immunopathol. 1996;80(3):S52–62.
24. Vreeland A, Yu S, Levi L, Rosseto DB, Noy N. Transcript stabilization by the RNA-binding protein HuR is regulated by cellular retinoic acid-binding protein 2. Mol Cell Biol. 2014;34(12):2135–46.
25. Liebler S, Überschär B, Kübert H, Brems S, Schnitger A, Tsukada M, Zouboulis CC, Ritz E, Wagner J. The renal retinoid system: time-dependent activation in experimental glomerulonephritis. Am J Physiol Renal Physiol. 2004;286(3):F458–65.

5

Cervical small cell carcinoma frequently presented in multiple high risk HPV infection and often associated with other type of epithelial tumors

Peifeng Li[†], Jing Ma[†], Xiumin Zhang, Yong Guo, Yixiong Liu, Xia Li, Danhui Zhao and Zhe Wang[*]

Abstract

Background: Small cell carcinoma of the uterine cervix is a rare and highly malignant tumor, and its etiopathogenesis is strongly related to high-risk HPV infections.

Methods: The clinicopathological data of 30 cases of cervical primary small cell carcinoma were retrospectively analyzed. In situ hybridization, polymerase chain reaction and reverse dot-blot hybridization were employed to detect HPV DNA in both small cell carcinoma and other coexisting epithelial tumors. Immunohistochemistry was used to detect the protein expression of p16 and p53.

Results: Amongst 30 patients with cervical primary small cell carcinoma, 15 patients simultaneously exhibited other types of epithelial tumors, including squamous cell carcinoma, adenocarcinoma, squamous cell carcinoma in situ, and adenocarcinoma in situ. Most tumor cells infected with HPV presented integrated patterns in the nuclei by in situ hybridization. HPV DNA was detected in every small cell carcinoma case (100%) by polymerase chain reaction and reverse dot blot hybridization. 27 cases (90%) harbored type 18, and 15 (50%) displayed multiple HPV18 and 16 infections. The prevalence of HPV 18 infection in small cell carcinoma was higher than in cervical squamous and glandular epithelial neoplasms ($P = 0.002$). However, similar infection rates of HPV 16 were detected in both tumors ($P = 0.383$). Both small cell carcinoma and other types of epithelial tumors exhibited strong nuclear and cytoplasmic staining for p16 in all cases. Three cases of small cell carcinoma revealed completely negative p53 immunohistochemical expression in 15 cases of composite tumors, which suggested *TP53* nonsense mutation pattern. The pure small cell carcinoma of uterine cervix had similar mutation or wild type pattern for *TP53* compared with composite tumor ($P = 0.224$).

Conclusions: Cervical small cell carcinomas are often associated with squamous or glandular epithelial tumors, which might result from multiple HPV infections, especially HPV 16 infection. Multiple HPV infections were not correlated with tumor stage, size, lymphovascular invasion, lymph node metastasis, or prognosis. Furthermore, careful observation of specimens is very important in finding little proportion of small cell carcinoma in the composite lesions, specifically in cervical biopsy specimens, in order to avoid the missed diagnosis of small cell carcinoma.

Keywords: Human papillomavirus, p16, p53, Small cell carcinoma, Uterine cervix

* Correspondence: zhwang@fmmu.edu.cn
[†]Peifeng Li and Jing Ma contributed equally to this work.
State Key Laboratory of Cancer Biology, Department of Pathology, Xijing Hospital and School of Basic Medicine, The Fourth Military Medical University, Changle West Road #169, Xi'an 710032, Shaan Xi Province, China

Background

Numerous clinical and experimental studies have demonstrated a closed etiopathogenetic relationship between the development of cervical cancers (including squamous cell carcinoma, adenocarcinoma, and small cell carcinoma) and high-risk human papillomavirus (HPV) infection [1]. It has been implicated that squamous cell carcinoma and adenocarcinoma are correlated to HPV 16 infection, whilst cervical small cell carcinoma is linked to HPV 18 [2, 3]. As an uncommon and highly malignant tumor, small cell carcinoma of uterine cervix has similar morphological features to tumors arising in the lung. The clinicopathological features of cervical small cell carcinoma and its relationship with HPV infection has been widely studied, including case series and larger retrospective population-based reports [2, 4]. Although some studies report that cervical small cell carcinoma is often associated with other cervical cancer or intraepithelial neoplasia [5], the clinicopathological features of cervical composite tumors, including small cell carcinoma, were rarely characterized. In these studies, HPV infection was detected using a variety of methods [3, 6] such as immunohistochemistry, polymerase chain reaction (PCR), in situ hybridization (ISH), reverse dot blot hybridization (RDDH), and Southern blot hybridization. The inconsistent results affected the understanding of the relationship between HPV infection and cervical small cell carcinoma. Many studies revealed the preponderant infection of HPV 18 in cervical small cell carcinoma [2], but multiple infections were rarely reported.

In this report, the clinicopathological features of 30 patients were analyzed, including 15 patients with pure cervical small cell carcinoma, and 15 cases with composite cervical tumors composed of small cell carcinoma and other types of epithelial tumors. The HPV infection in these tumors was detected by ISH and PCR-RDDH, and the expression of p16 and p53 proteins were examined using immunohistochemistry. Our results demonstrate that cervical small cell carcinoma is often associated with squamous or glandular epithelial tumors, and these tumor cells usually exhibit overexpression of p16. Small cell carcinomas and adenocarcinomas or squamous cell carcinoma in situ showed all completely negative p53 immunohistochemical expression in three of 15 composite tumors of uterine cervix. To the best of our knowledge, this is the first study to report that multiple infections of HPV 18 and 16 developed in half of cervical small cell carcinomas. Furthermore, this is the first report to make the distinction that HPV 18 infection is closely correlated to the occurrence of cervical small cell carcinoma while HPV 16 infection is involved in cervical squamous cell carcinoma or adenocarcinoma in the co-existing tumor cases. Multiple infections of HPV subtypes were not related to tumor stage, size, lymphovascular invasion, lymph node metastasis, or prognosis. In addition, our study also confirmed for the first time that

patients with composite tumors had similar HPV infection subtypes, clinicopathological features, and prognosis compared to patients with pure small cell carcinoma.

Methods

Case selection

Thirty cases of cervical primary small cell carcinoma were retrieved from the 2009–2017 surgical pathology archives of the Xijing Hospital. These included 23 hysterectomies, 1 conization, and 6 biopsies. To rule out the possibility of metastatic small cell carcinoma from the lung or other organs, the clinical data were carefully reviewed. Hematoxylin and eosin-stained slides of primary cervical neoplasm were re-examined to confirm the original diagnosis. Immunohistochemical staining for neuroendocrine markers, including Leu-19, synaptophysin, chromogranin, and neuron-specific enolase, was performed, and more than half of small cell carcinoma cells showed positive expression for two or more markers. The clinical records and follow-up of these patients were examined. This study received approval from the Ethics Committee of the Xijing Hospital.

ISH analysis

Three-micron sections containing small cell carcinoma and other types of epithelial tumors were examined for HPV DNA by ISH staining with INFORM® HPV III Family 16 and 6 Probe (Ventana Medical Systems, Inc., Tucson, AZ, USA) for high-risk HPV types (16, 18, 31, 33, 35, 39, 45, 51, 52, 56, 58, and 66) and low-risk HPV types (6 and 11), respectively. The ISH assay was performed according to the manufacturer's protocol using the Ventana BenchMark XT system (Ventana Medical Systems, Inc.). Labeling was detected with the ISH iVIEW™ Blue Plus Detection Kit (Ventana Medical Systems, Inc.). The positive and negative controls were carried out using HPV quality control slides provided by Ventana Medical Systems, Inc. The HPV signals were detected in the nuclei of tumor cells, and the signal patterns were categorized as either episomal staining pattern or punctuate staining pattern. The former presents as a homogeneous globular navy-blue to black signal in the entire nuclei of tumor cells, and the latter shows single or multiple sparsely distributed and dot-like navy-blue punctae in the nuclei of the tumor cells.

DNA extraction and HPV detection using PCR-RDDH

Eight-micron sections were prepared from formalin-fixed, paraffin-embedded (FFPE) tissues of cervical tumor samples. Tumor tissues were dissected using sterile blades from slides and were collected into 1.5 ml Eppendorf tubes. Amongst 15 specimens with composite carcinomas, small cell carcinoma and other types of epithelial tumors were successfully isolated in seven specimens. 37 samples of tumor cells were collected, including 22 cases of small cell carcinoma, 8 cases of mixed tumors, 2 cases of squamous cell carcinoma, 2 cases of adenocarcinoma, 2 cases of squamous cell carcinoma in situ, and 1 case of adenocarcinoma in situ. DNA extraction was carried out using QIAamp® DNA FFPE Tissue Kit (Cat No. 56404, QIAGEN GmbH, Hilden, Germany) following the manufacturer's guidelines. The samples were digested with proteinase K in a volume of 200 μL at 56 °C overnight, and 20 μL of DNA aliquot was obtained finally. The quality of the genomic DNA extracted was tested by agarose gel electrophoresis with ethidium bromide staining. For the PCR, 2 μL of DNA aliquot was used, and broad-spectrum HPV DNA amplification was performed using primers for GP5+/6+ (GP5+: 5'-TTTGTTACTGTGGTAGATACTAC-3', GP6 +: 5'-GAAAAATAAACTGTAAATCATATTC-3') with a total reaction volume of 50 μL. PCR amplification was performed in the following conditions: 50 °C for 15 min, 95 °C for 10 min, 94 °C for 30 s, 46 °C for 90 s, 72 °C for 30 s, 40 cycles, 72 °C for 5 min. DNA RDDH was performed with the HPV Genotyping Detection Kit (Asia Energy Biotechnology Co, Ltd., Shenzhen, China) to simultaneously identify 23 HPV subtypes, including HPV 6, 11, 16, 18, 31, 33, 35, 39, 42, 43, 45, 51, 52, 53, 56, 58, 59, 66, 68, 73, 81, 82, and 83. PCR amplification products were boiled 10 min to obtain single-stranded DNA. Samples were then added in low density gene patches with a total of 23 gene probes of different HPV subtypes and hybridization was performed at 51 °C for 3 h. The gene patches were incubated in peroxidase solution for 30 min, and then developed in color reagent (19 ml 0.1 mol/L sodium citrate, 1 ml tetramethylbenzidine, and 2 μL 30% H_2O_2) for 60 min in the dark. HPV subtypes were determined by the positive point on the HPV genotype profile on the membrane. HPV-positive and negative controls were also included in every experiment.

Immunohistochemistry

Immunohistochemistry was performed on 3 μm thick tissue sections using the Ventana BenchMark XT system (Ventana Medical Systems, Inc.). P16 (clone: 6H12) and p53 (clone: DO-7) antibodies were purchased from Maxin Corp. (Fuzhou, China) and DAKO Corp. (Carpinteria, CA), respectively. Immunohistochemical staining was conducted employing the Roche Ultraview DAB Detection Kit (Ventana Medical Systems, Inc.) following the manufacturer's instructions. The positive and negative control slices were also run simultaneously. Nuclear/cytoplasmic staining was considered positive for p16, and p53 protein showed nuclear expression. A tumor was recorded positive for p16 if more than 50% of the tumor cells showed immunoreactivity. IHC for p53 includes mutation pattern

and wild type pattern. Strong and diffuse nuclear staining or complete negative with internal control is considered to be mutation pattern, and focal and weak staining correlate with a wild type pattern of p53.

Statistics

Statistical software SPSS17.0 (SPSS, Inc., Chicago, IL, USA) was employed in this report. Pearson X^2 test or Fisher's exact test was adopted for correlation analysis of enumeration data. Wilcoxon rank sum test was used for comparison of patients' age and tumor size. $P<0.05$ was considered as a statistically significant.

Results

Clinicopathological features

Among 30 patients with cervical primary small cell carcinomas included in this study, 15 patients were diagnosed with pure cervical small cell carcinoma. In the remaining 15 cases of composite tumors, 7 cases also exhibited invasive cervical squamous cell carcinoma, 4 cases also showed cervical squamous cell carcinoma in situ, 3 cases also had cervical adenocarcinoma, and one patient also displayed cervical adenocarcinoma in situ. The age of all 30 patients at diagnosis ranged from 31 to 74 years (mean 46.4 years, median 41 years). The mean and median age of the 15 patients with cervical composite tumors was 46.4 and 45 years, respectively. 22 patients presented with abnormal vaginal bleeding or contact bleeding. Two patients showed no clinical symptoms, and the tumors were found following physical examination. Most of the tumors displayed exophytic growth with or without cervical erosion. The tumor sizes in the 24 hysterectomies and cervical conization specimens ranged from 1 to 6 cm (mean 3.0 cm, median 2.5 cm). 16 tumors (66.7%) were FIGO stage IB, 3 stage IIA, 2 stage IA, 1 stage IIB, 1 stage IIIA, and 1 stage IVB. Accurate staging information was not acquired for 6 cases of cervical biopsy specimens. 21 patients underwent radical hysterectomy with bilateral or partial adnexectomy and pelvic lymph node dissection. Two patients received radical hysterectomy with pelvic lymph node dissection, and one case underwent cervical conization owing to the superficial invasion depth of small cell carcinoma. Accurate surgical methods in 6 outpatients were not obtained in this study. 15 patients underwent postoperative chemotherapy combined with radiotherapy, and 6 patients received postoperative chemotherapy. Postoperative treatment strategies were not obtained in 9 other patients. Follow-up data of 16 cases was obtained: 7 patients died with a survival time ranging from 5 to 24 months (median survival time: 7 months). Survival time was more than two years in 4 out of 10 confirmed surviving patients, and two patients free of disease have undergone a follow-up at 67 and 88 months.

Histologically, cervical primary small cell carcinomas showed morphological features similar to those seen in the pulmonary counterpart. Densely packed small tumor cells often formed a sheet-like diffuse growth pattern. Neuroendocrine growth patterns, such as orderly tubular, trabecular, organoid, and nuclear palisading patterns, were less illustrated. Tumor cells showed round, ovoid, or spindled nuclei and scant cytoplasm. Nuclear chromatin is finely granular, and nucleoli were absent or inconspicuous. Numerous mitotic figures and extensive necrosis were commonly observed. Furthermore, squamous and glandular epithelial neoplasms were observed in 15 cases. Most squamous cell carcinomas developed in the superficial parts of small cell carcinomas (Fig. 1a). However, in two cases, the squamous cell carcinoma intermingled with the small cell carcinoma (Fig. 1b). In three cases of cervical small cell carcinoma associated with adenocarcinoma, one case illustrated mixed small cell carcinoma and adenocarcinoma (Fig. 1c), and two patients revealed adenocarcinoma present at the periphery of the small cell carcinoma (Fig. 1d). Five cases of cervical small cell carcinoma associated with carcinoma in situ all illustrated adjacent relationships between small cell carcinoma and squamous cell carcinoma in situ or adenocarcinoma in situ. Although more composite tumors were found in hysterectomy specimens than in biopsy specimens in this study, the discovery of composite lesions was not related to specimen type ($P = 0.651$). There

was no statistical difference in patients' age, FIGO stage, lymph node metastasis, lymphovascular invasion, or prognosis between pure small cell carcinoma and composite tumors (Table 1, Fig. 2). Patients with cervical composite tumors had similar prognosis to patients with pure small cell carcinoma ($P = 0.716$). The prognosis of these patients was determined by the composition of small cell carcinoma. Six cases (26.1%) had regional nodal metastasis, including 5 cases of metastatic small cell carcinoma and one case of metastatic squamous cell carcinoma. One patient displayed small cell carcinoma involving vaginal stump, and ovarian metastatic small cell carcinoma was found in another patient. In the 24 patients who underwent hysterectomies or cervical conization, lymphovascular invasion of small cell carcinoma was detected inside or within the tumor in 21 cases, of which two patients had simultaneous lymphovascular invasion of squamous cell carcinoma. Only one case presented with lymphovascular invasion of small cell carcinoma in 6 cervical biopsy specimens. Lymphovascular invasion was more likely to be found in hysterectomy or conization specimens than in biopsy specimens ($P = 0.002$).

HPV DNA detection and typing

ISH of tissue sections revealed that most specimens were positive for the INFORM HPV III Family 16 Probe in both small cell carcinomas and other types of epithelial tumors. 29 out of 30 cases of small cell carcinomas showed positive staining, including 21 cases with only one navy-blue to black puncta (Fig. 3a), 6 cases with

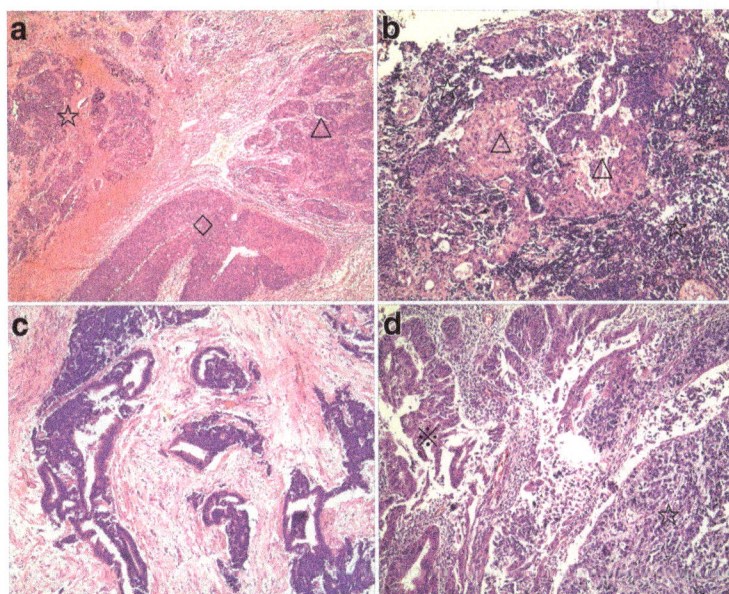

Fig. 1 Cervical small cell carcinoma associated with other types of epithelial tumors (hematoxylin-eosin staining). **a** Squamous cell carcinoma (△) and squamous cell carcinoma in situ (◇) detected in the superficial parts of small cell carcinoma (☆) (× 40). **b** Squamous cell carcinoma (△) intermingled with small cell carcinoma (☆) (× 100). **c** Small cell carcinoma (☆) mixed with adenocarcinoma (※) (× 100). **d** Adenocarcinoma (※) present at the periphery of small cell carcinoma (☆) (× 100)

Table 1 Clinicopathological features of cervical small cell carcinoma with or without other types of epithelial tumors

	Pure small cell carcinoma	Small cell carcinoma associated with other epithelial tumors	P value
Cases (n)	15	15	
Specimen type			0.651
hysterectomy or cervical conization	11	13	
biopsy	4	2	
Age (years)	46.4 (34–68)	46.4 (31–74)	0.967
Size of tumors	3.4 (2–6)	2.5 (1–4.5)	0.105
FIGO stage			0.605
I	9	9	
II	2	2	
III		1	
IV		1	
Lymph node metastasis			1.000
Yes	3	3	
No	8	9	
Lymphovascular invasion			1.000
Yes	11	11	
No	4	4	

multiple small blue puncta inside the nuclei (Fig. 3b), and 2 cases with multiple puncta-like staining to diffuse small particles (Fig. 3c). These staining signals represent viral integrative patterns in 27 cases. In some cases, the nuclear viral integrative pattern was so discrete that microscopic examination at a higher magnification (40× objective) was required to judge nuclear epithelial cell localization, which represented very low viral copy number. Two cases of small cell carcinoma showed both

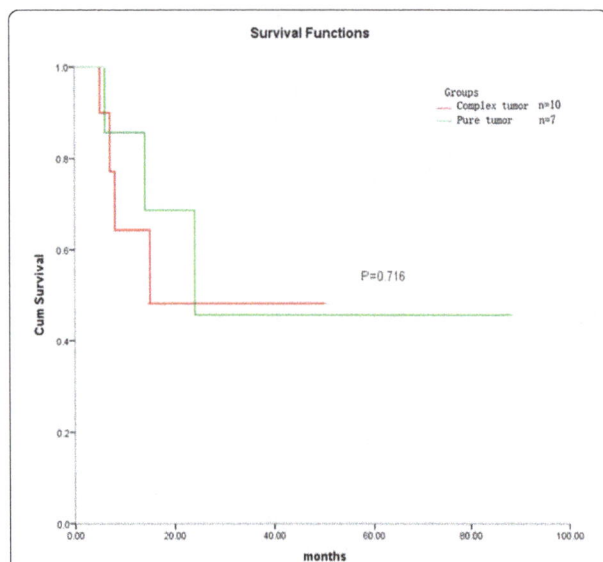

Fig. 2 Survival analysis of 17 patients with follow-up data. The patients with composite cervical tumors had similar prognosis to patients with pure small cell carcinoma

episomal and integrative staining patterns. In 7 cases of cervical squamous cell carcinoma, 5 cases illustrated punctate signals in the nuclei of tumor cells (Fig. 3d) and 2 cases displayed episomal staining patterns. Two out of four cases of squamous cell carcinoma in situ revealed episomal staining patterns (Fig. 3e), and all tumor cells of cervical adenocarcinoma and adenocarcinoma in situ illustrated punctate staining (Fig. 3f). Interestingly, one case displayed positive staining for small cell carcinoma with punctate pattern but negative for squamous cell carcinoma, and another was positive for cervical adenocarcinoma in situ with punctate staining, but negative for small cell carcinoma. The INFORM HPV III Family 6 Probe was employed to detect low-risk HPV genotypes, and no positive tumor cells were observed in both small cell carcinoma and other types of epithelial tumors.

Thirty-seven specimens of cervical small cell carcinoma and other types of epithelial tumors were tested for HPV DNA by PCR-RDDH, and all were positive (Fig. 4). The prevalence of HPV 18 and 16 was 78.4% (29/37) and 64.9% (24/37), respectively. 48.6% (18/37) of specimens demonstrated multiple infections with various HPV subtypes, and the predominant multiple infections were HPV 16 and 18 at a rate of 43.2% (16/37). The rare infection of HPV 31, 33, and 43 was detected in three cases of small cell carcinoma with multiple HPV infections. The prevalence of HPV 18 and 16 was 90.0% (27/30) and 60.0% (18/30) in the 30 cases of small cell carcinoma, respectively. Multiple infections were found in 17 cases of small cell carcinoma, among which coinfection of HPV 18 and 16 was detected in 15 cases.

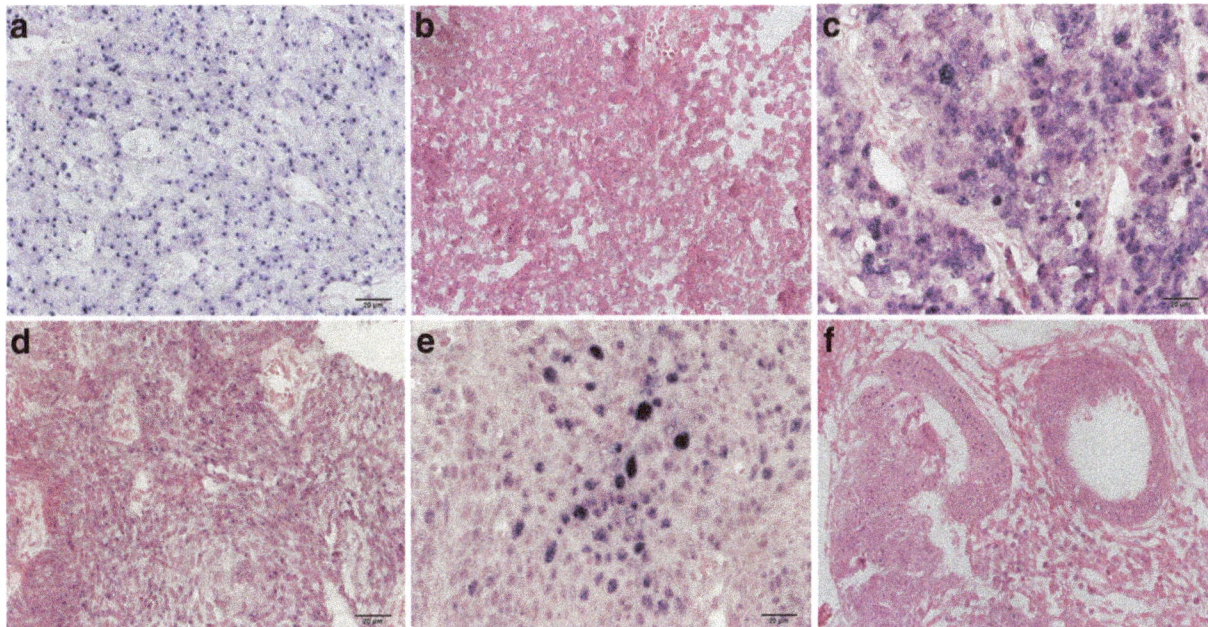

Fig. 3 HPV DNA detection using in situ hybridization (×400). **a** Small cell carcinoma illustrated punctate staining pattern with one navy-blue puncta signal in the nuclei. **b** Multiple small puncta inside the nuclei of small cell carcinoma represents low viral copy number of HPV DNA. **c** Diffuse small particles were observed in the nuclei of small cell carcinoma. **d** Squamous cell carcinoma displayed punctuate signal patterns. **e** Squamous cell carcinoma illustrated episomal staining pattern. **f** Tumor cells of adenocarcinoma positive with one navy-blue puncta

Multiple infections in composite tumors (73.3%) were more common than in pure small cell carcinoma (46.7%), but there was no statistical difference ($P = 0.136$). The infection prevalence of HPV 16 and 18 was not significantly different between the composite tumor group and the pure tumor group ($P = 0.456$ and 1.00, respectively). The HPV DNA subtypes in different tumor components were detected in seven cases of composite tumors, and the consistent HPV type was detected in two cases with single infection. Four cases showed that tumor cells of small cell carcinoma were positive for HPV both 16 and 18, while other types of epithelial tumors, including adenocarcinoma, squamous cell carcinoma, and squamous cell carcinoma in situ, only displayed HPV 16 infection. The infection rate of HPV 18 in small cell carcinoma was significantly higher than in other types of epithelial tumors ($P = 0.008$). However, similar infection rates of HPV 16 were measured in both groups ($P = 0.382$, Table 2). In addition, multiple infection with HPV subtypes was not related to tumor stage, size, lymphovascular invasion, lymph node metastasis, or prognosis ($P = 0.187$, 1.00, 1.00, 0.179, and 0.498, respectively).

Immunohistochemical expression of p16 and p53

Strong and diffuse nuclear and cytoplasmic staining for p16 protein was noted in all cases of cervical small cell carcinoma (Fig. 5a), squamous cell carcinoma (Fig. 5b), squamous cell carcinoma in situ, adenocarcinoma, and adenocarcinoma in situ. In contrast, the nonneoplastic squamous and glandular epithelia were either negative or showed focal and weak cytoplasmic positivity. Strong and diffuse nuclear staining for p53 protein was observed in one case of cervical squamous cell carcinoma (Fig. 5c) and in one case of squamous cell carcinoma in situ, which revealed *TP53* missense mutation. Scattered tumor cells illustrated weak or moderate positivity for p53 with rates ranging from 1 to 60% (Fig. 5d), which meant wild type pattern of *TP53*. Three cases of composite tumors showed negative staining both in small cell carcinoma and in adenocarcinoma or squamous cell carcinoma in situ, which suggested *TP53* nonsense mutation. The pure small cell carcinoma of uterine cervix had similar mutation or wild type pattern of *TP53* compared with composite tumor ($P = 0.224$), and there was no difference between *TP53* mutation in small cell carcinoma and those in other epithelial neoplasms of uterine cervix ($P = 0.682$).

Discussion

Small cell carcinoma of the uterine cervix is a rare and highly malignant tumor. The etiopathogenetic association between cervical small cell carcinoma and high-risk HPV infections has been well documented in some studies [1, 2, 7]. Our study extend these findings by demonstrating that all 30 cases of cervical small cell carcinomas are related to high-risk HPV types 18 and 16,

Cases	HPV16	HPV18	HPV31	HPV33	HPV43
1	■				
1△	■	■			
2	■				
2△	■				
3	■	■			
3△	■				
4	■				
4△	■				
5		■			
5△		■			
6	■	■			
6△		■			
7	■	■			
7△	■				
8*		■	■		
9*		■			
10*	■	■			
11*	■	■			
12*	■				■
13*	■	■			
14*				■	
15*		■			
16		■			
17		■			
18		■			
19	■	■			
20	■	■			
21		■			
22		■			
23	■				
24	■	■			
25		■			
26	■	■			
27	■	■			
28	■	■			
29		■			
30	■	■			

△: tumor specimens of non-small cell carcinoma
*: specimens of complex tumors
The blank areas represented negative results

Fig. 4 HPV typing using polymerase chain reaction-reverse dot blot hybridization

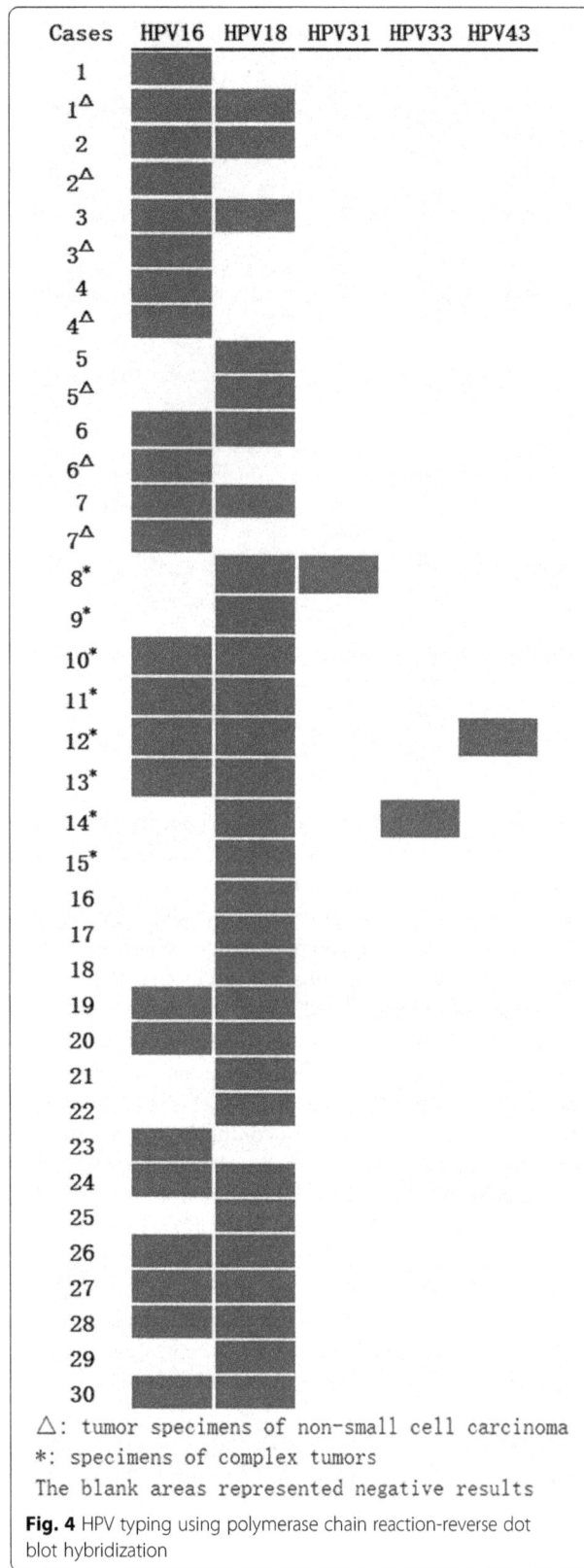

with predominant HPV 18 infection and multiple infections with HPV 18 and 16. In addition, a high frequency of cervical small cell carcinomas associated with other epithelial tumors was reported. This may be related with the common etiopathogenesis—HPV 18 and HPV 16. However, the prevalence of HPV 18 was different in cervical small cell carcinomas from squamous or glandular epithelial neoplasm.

The mean age at diagnosis for women with cervical small cell carcinoma was between 45 and 50 years [2], which is consistent with that of cervical squamous cell carcinoma. In this study, the mean age of the patients with cervical small cell carcinoma was 46.4 years. The patients had no specific clinical manifestations. Most cases presented with abnormal vaginal bleeding or contact bleeding. Exophytic growth was not different from other uterine cervical carcinomas. Of note, most of the patients in our study were in the early stage, which differs from previous studies [2, 4]. However, high rates of lymph node metastasis and poor prognosis were still observed in these stage I and II patients.

Primary small cell carcinomas of uterine cervix often coexist with squamous cell carcinomas or adenocarcinomas. Wang et al. reported that in 22 cases of primary cervical small cell carcinomas, two exhibited concordant high-grade squamous intraepithelial neoplasia and adenocarcinoma in situ [8]. In the study by Abeler et al., 12 of the 26 patients with cervical small cell carcinomas were associated with other forms of carcinoma, including squamous cell carcinoma ($n = 6$), adenocarcinoma ($n = 5$), and adenocarcinoma in situ ($n = 1$) [9]. Ishida et al. reported 10 cases of cervical small cell carcinoma, 7 of which were mixed with adenocarcinoma and/or squamous cell carcinoma, or cervical intraepithelial neoplasia [10]. Emerson et al. reported that in 19 cases of cervical small cell carcinoma, 6 cases were associated with adenocarcinoma, and three patients also had adenosquamous carcinoma, squamous cell carcinoma in situ, and adenocarcinoma [5]. In this study, 15 patients also displayed squamous or glandular epithelial neoplasms, including squamous cell carcinoma ($n = 7$), adenocarcinoma ($n = 3$), squamous cell carcinoma in situ ($n = 4$), and adenocarcinoma in situ ($n = 1$). Our results demonstrate a high frequency of cervical small cell carcinomas associated with squamous or glandular epithelial tumors. They had similar age composition and clinical manifestations as the patients of single cervical tumor. Chan et al. found that pure, rather than mixed histological pattern was a poor prognostic factor for survival [11]. However, in our study, patients of cervical small cell carcinoma with and without other types of epithelial neoplasms had similar prognosis, which was significantly worse than that of cervical squamous cell carcinoma and adenocarcinoma [12]. Therefore, the prognosis of patients with composite cervical cancer was

Table 2 HPV infection in small cell carcinoma and other types of epithelial tumors

	Small cell carcinomas	Squamous or glandular epithelial neoplasms	P value
Cases (n)	22	7	
HPV 18	19	2	0.008
HPV 16	14	6	0.382
HPV 18 + HPV 16	11	1	0.187

determined by the composition of small cell carcinoma. In addition, in the case of biopsy specimens suspected of cervical epithelial disease, careful observation should be made to avoid the omission of small cell carcinoma. In this study, more lymphovascular invasion was observed in hysterectomy and cervical conization specimens. Therefore, obtaining as many specimens as possible improves the accuracy of the diagnosis, and it will more accurately estimate the prognosis.

High-risk HPV has been implicated in the carcinogenesis of cervical small cell carcinomas [1, 7]. A meta-analysis including more than 30,000 invasive cervical cancers revealed that HPV 16 (59%), 18 (13%), 58 (5%), 33 (5%), and 45 (4%) were the most prevalent subtypes in cervical squamous cell carcinomas. HPV 18 (37%), 16 (36%), 45 (5%), 31 (2%), and 33 (2%) were the most prevalent in cervical adenocarcinomas [13]. Many studies have established that the prevalence of different high-risk HPV types in cervical small cell carcinoma ranged from 50 to 100%, and that HPV 18 may be the most prevalent type [2]. Wang et al. reported that

HPV18 and 16 were detected in 77.3 and 18.2% cases of cervical small cell carcinoma, respectively, and one case displayed HPV 18 and 16 co-infection [8]. Research by Abeler et al. demonstrated that HPV-18 is predominant in pure small cell carcinomas and in tumors with adenocarcinomatous areas, and that HPV-16 is found in pure small cell carcinomas and in tumors with areas of squamous cell differentiation [9]. In a study by Ishida et al., HPV 18 was detected in both small cell carcinomas and adenocarcinomatous components, and no other types of HPV were detected [10]. In our study, preponderant infection with HPV 18 was found in 27 of 30 cases of cervical small cell carcinoma. In the 15 cases of composite tumors, HPV 18 infection was more common in small cell carcinoma than in any other type of epithelial tumors. These findings are in line with the notion that HPV 18 infection is involved in the development of cervical small cell carcinoma and HPV 16 infection promotes the occurrence of cervical squamous cell carcinoma and adenocarcinoma.

Multiple infections were observed in more than half of the cervical small cell carcinomas in our study. Only one case of multiple infections was found in 7 cases of squamous and glandular epithelial neoplasm. Multiple infections of HPV 18 and 16, rather than pure HPV 18 infection, might play an important role in the pathogenesis of cervical small cell carcinoma. In previous studies, very few cases of multiple infections were reported [8]. One explanation for this might be found in the different detection methods or the population differences. In the research by Zhou et al., using HPV DNA detection by

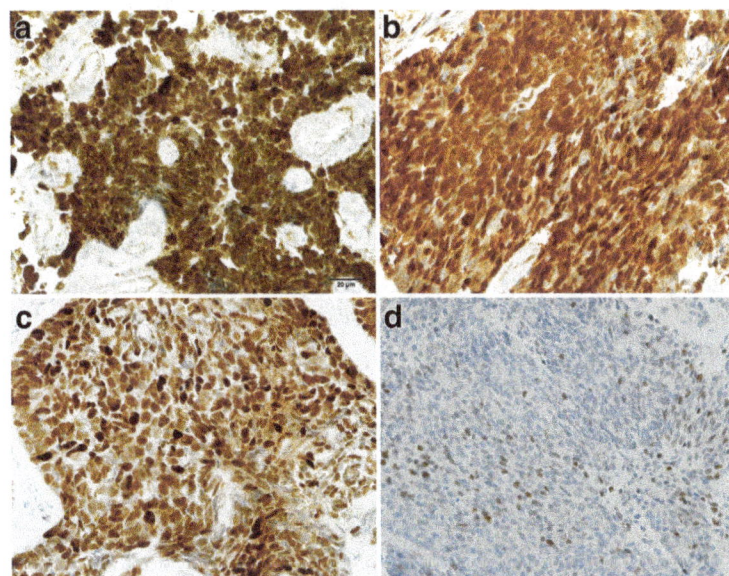

Fig. 5 Immunohistochemical expression of p16 and p53 (× 400). Strong and diffuse nuclear and cytoplasmic staining for p16 was noted in cervical small cell carcinoma (**a**) and squamous cell carcinoma (**b**). **c** Nuclear staining for p53 was observed in cervical squamous cell carcinoma, wich revealed *TP53* missense mutation. **d** Cervical small cell carcinoma illustrating scattered, weakly positive nuclear staining for p53 revealed wild type pattern of *TP53*

PCR-RDDH, multiple HPV DNA prevalence was 4.5% in 2452 women whom volunteered for cervical cancer screening in Shanghai, China [14]. A similar multiple infection prevalence rate was measured in 9012 women whom attended cervical cancer screening in Taihu River Basin, China [15]. In addition, reported HPV infection rates are closely related to the detection methods used. For example, in our study, the ISH assessment for HPV infection with low copy number was very difficult, displaying the lower sensitivity using ISH detection compared to PCR. Similar results were reported by Masumoto using ISH and direct sequencing of PCR products [16]. The prevalence of infection by multiple HPV genotypes was 20% in patients with cervical squamous cell carcinoma and adenocarcinoma [17]. One case of multiple HPV infection was confirmed in seven cases of squamous or glandular epithelial neoplasms in our study. Furthermore, the prevalence of multiple infections in small cell carcinoma was not significantly different in pure small cell carcinoma compared to the composite tumors, and multiple HPV infections did not affect the prognosis of these patients.

Overexpression of p16 has been well documented in high-risk HPV-related cervical squamous cell carcinomas and adenocarcinomas, as well as their precursor lesions [18, 19]. Many recent studies have shown that cervical small cell carcinoma also overexpressed p16 protein [20, 21]. In this study, we detected simultaneous overexpression of p16 in both small cell carcinoma and other types of epithelial tumors by immunohistochemistry. Although the overexpression of p16 was correlated with HPV18 and 16 infections in both pure tumors and composite tumors, it does not confirm that high-risk HPV infections result in the overexpression of p16. Indeed, small cell carcinoma negative for HPV DNA in the lung, colorectum, bladder, and ovaries also overexpress p16 [8, 20]. In our study, the mutation or wild type pattern of TP53 in small cell carcinoma was not significantly different between pure and composite tumors. Three patients with composite tumors showed completely negative p53 protein expression both in small cell carcinoma and in other epithelial tumors. Furthermore, two cases revealed strong and diffuse positive expression of p53 only in squamous cell carcinoma or squamous cell carcinoma in situ, while small cell carcinoma components of the same patients showed wild type pattern. These observations indicated TP53 mutation might involved in the occurrence of small cell carcinoma as in squamous cell carcinoma and adenocarcinoma of uterine cervix, but the pathogenesis of small cell carcinoma was not completely same to those of squamous cell carcinoma or adenocarcinoma.

Since only a single-center retrospective case series was studied, and limited cases were employed, this study should be repeated on a larger scale to confirm our findings. Furthermore, some patients did not complete their follow-up, thus the comprehensive and effective data were not obtained.

Conclusions

In summary, our study demonstrated that cervical small cell carcinomas closely correlate with HPV18 and HPV 16 infections. The patients of cervical small cell carcinomas with multiple infection of high-risk HPV may also promote the development of squamous or glandular epithelial neoplasms. In patients with composite cervical neoplasms, multiple infections of HPV 18 and 16 were involved in the development of cervical small cell carcinoma, while the occurrence of cervical squamous cell carcinoma or adenocarcinoma was closely related to HPV 16 infection. Multiple high-risk HPV infection was not related to tumor stage, size, lymphovascular invasion, lymph node metastasis, or prognosis in cervical small cell carcinoma. Similar HPV DNA genotypes, clinicopathological features, and prognosis were observed both in patients with pure small cell carcinomas and those with composite cervical tumors. The small cell carcinoma determined the prognosis of patients with cervical composite tumors. Because of the frequent presence of co-existing tumors, it is important to carefully examine the cervical biopsy specimens in surgical pathological examination.

Abbreviations
FIGO: International Federation of Gynecology and Obstetrics; HPV: Human papillomavirus; ISH: In Situ Hybridization; PCR: Polymerase chain reaction; RDDH: Reverse dot blot hybridization

Acknowledgements
We are grateful to the Department of Pathology, Xijing Hospital for excellent working conditions and for providing access to archival materials.

Funding
The study was funded by grants from the National Natural Science Foundation of China (81272651 and 81570180 to Zhe Wang).

Authors' contributions
ZW study design, PL, JM, XZ data acquisition, YL, DZ ISH analysis and PCR, PL, JM, XZ, YG data analysis, PL, JM, XL statistical analysis PL, JM manuscript preparation and editing. All authors read and approved the final manuscript.

Competing interests
The authors declare that they have no competing interests.

References

1. Small W Jr, Bacon MA, Bajaj A, Chuang LT, Fisher BJ, Harkenrider MM, Jhingran A, Kitchener HC, Mileshkin LR, Viswanathan AN, Gaffney DK. Cervical cancer: a global health crisis. Cancer. 2017;123: 2404–12.

2. Atienza-Amores M, Guerini-Rocco E, Soslow RA, Park KJ, Weigelt B. Small cell carcinoma of the gynecologic tract: a multifaceted spectrum of lesions. Gynecol Oncol. 2014;134:410–8.

3. Satoh T, Takei Y, Treilleux I. Gynecologic Cancer InterGroup (GCIG) consensus review for small cell carcinoma of the cervix. Int J Gynecol Cancer. 2014;24(3):S102–8.

4. Dores GM, Qubaiah O, Mody A, Ghabach B, Devesa SS. A population-based study of incidence and patient survival of small cell carcinoma in the United States, 1992-2010. BMC Cancer. 2015;15:185.

5. Emerson RE, Michael H, Wang M, Zhang S, Roth LM, Cheng L. Cervical carcinomas with neuroendocrine differentiation: a report of 28 cases with Immunohistochemical analysis and molecular genetic evidence of common clonal origin with coexisting squamous and adenocarcinomas. Int J Gynecol Pathol. 2016;35:372–84.

6. Carow K, Read C, Hafner N, Runnebaum IB, Corner A, Dürst M. A comparative study of digital PCR and real-time qPCR for the detection and quantification of HPV mRNA in sentinel lymph nodes of cervical cancer patients. BMC Res Notes. 2017;10:532.

7. Gadducci A, Carinelli S, Aletti G. Neuroendocrine tumors of the uterine cervix: a therapeutic challenge for gynecologic oncologists. Gynecol Oncol. 2017;144:637–46.

8. Wang HL, Lu DW. Detection of human papillomavirus DNA and expression of p16, Rb, and p53 proteins in small cell carcinomas of the uterine cervix. Am J Surg Pathol. 2004;28:901–8.

9. Abeler VM, Holm R, Nesland JM, Kjørstad KE. Small cell carcinoma of the cervix. A clinicopathologic study of 26 patients. Cancer. 1994;73:672–7.

10. Ishida GM, Kato N, Hayasaka T, Saito M, Kobayashi H, Katayama Y, Sasou S, Yaegashi N, Kurachi H, Motoyama T. Small cell neuroendocrine carcinomas of the uterine cervix: a histological, immunohistochemical, and molecular genetic study. Int J Gynecol Pathol. 2004;23:366–72.

11. Chan JK, Loizzi V, Burger RA, Rutgers J, Monk BJ. Prognostic factors in neuroendocrine small cell cervical carcinoma: a multivariate analysis. Cancer. 2003;97:568–74.

12. Zhou J, Wu SG, Sun JY, Tang LY, Lin HX, Li FY, Chen QH, Jin X, He ZY. Clinicopathological features of small cell carcinoma of the uterine cervix in the surveillance, epidemiology, and end results database. Oncotarget. 2017;8:40425–33.

13. Li N, Franceschi S, Howell-Jones R, Snijders PJ, Clifford G. Human papillomavirus type distribution in 30,848 invasive cervical cancers worldwide: variation by geographical region, histological type and year of publication. Int J Cancer. 2011;128:927–35.

14. Zhou XH, Shi YF, Wang LJ, Liu M, Li F. Distribution characteristics of human papillomavirus infection: a study based on data from physical examination. Asian Pac J Cancer Prev. 2017;18:1875–9.

15. Lu JF, Shen GR, Li Q. Genotype distribution characteristics of multiple human papillomavirus in women from the Taihu River basin, on the coast of eastern China. BMC Infect Dis. 2017;17:226.

16. Masumoto N, Fujii T, Ishikawa M, Saito M, Iwata T, Fukuchi T, Susumu N, Mukai M, Kubushiro K, Tsukazaki K, Nozawa S. P16 overexpression and human papillomavirus infection in small cell carcinoma of the uterine cervix. Hum Pathol. 2003;34:778–83.

17. Mazarico E, Gomez-Roig MD, Minano J, Cortes L, Gonzalez-Bosquet E. Relationship of human papilloma virus multiple genotype infection with patient's age and type of cervical lesion. Eur J Gynaecol Oncol. 2014;35: 378–81.

18. Ahmad A, Raish M, Shahid M. Batra S4, Batra V5, Husain S. The synergic effect of HPV infection and epigenetic anomaly of the p16 gene in the development of cervical cancer. Cancer Biomark. 2017;19: 375–81.

19. Togami S, Sasajima Y, Kasamatsu T, Oda-Otomo R, Okada S, Ishikawa M, Ikeda S, Kato T, Tsuda H. Immunophenotype and human papillomavirus status of serous adenocarcinoma of the uterine cervix. Pathol Oncol Res. 2015;21:487–94.

20. Carlson JW, Nucci MR, Brodsky J, Crum CP, Hirsch MS. Biomarker-assisted diagnosis of ovarian, cervical and pulmonary small cell carcinomas: the role of TTF-1, WT-1 and HPV analysis. Histopathology. 2007;51:305–12.

21. Horn LC, Hauptmann S, Leo C. pRb, p16, and cyclin D1 in small cell carcinoma of the uterine cervix. Int J Gynecol Pathol. 2007;26:269.

Gene expression profiling in uveal melanoma: technical reliability and correlation of molecular class with pathologic characteristics

Kristen M. Plasseraud[1], Jeff K. Wilkinson[2], Kristen M. Oelschlager[2], Trisha M. Poteet[2], Robert W. Cook[1], John F. Stone[2] and Federico A. Monzon[1*]

Abstract

Background: A 15-gene expression profile test has been clinically validated and is widely utilized in newly diagnosed uveal melanoma (UM) patients to assess metastatic potential of the tumor. As most patients are treated with eye-sparing radiotherapy, there is limited tumor tissue available for testing, and technical reliability and success of prognostic testing are critical. This study assessed the analytical performance of the 15-gene expression test for UM and the correlation of molecular class with pathologic characteristics.

Methods: Inter-assay, intra-assay, inter-instrument/operator, and inter-site experiments were conducted, and concordance of the 15-gene expression profile test results and associated discriminant scores for matched tumor samples were evaluated. Technical success was determined from de-identified clinical reports from January 2010 - May 2016. Pathologic characteristics of enucleated tumors were correlated with molecular class results.

Results: Inter-assay concordance on 16 samples run on 3 consecutive days was 100%, and matched discriminant scores were strongly correlated ($R^2 = 0.9944$). Inter-assay concordance of 46 samples assayed within a one year period was 100%, with an R^2 value of 0.9747 for the discriminant scores. Intra-assay concordance of 12 samples run concurrently in duplicates was 100%; discriminant score correlation yielded an R^2 of 0.9934. Concordance between two sites assessing the same tumors was 100% with an R^2 of 0.9818 between discriminant scores. Inter-operator/ instrument concordance was 96% for Class 1/2 calls and 90% for Class 1A/1B calls, and the discriminant scores had a correlation R^2 of 0.9636. Technical success was 96.3% on 5516 samples tested since 2010. Increased largest basal diameter and thickness were significantly associated with Class 1B and Class 2 vs. Class 1A signatures.

Conclusions: These results show that the 15-gene expression profile test for UM has robust, reproducible performance characteristics. The technical success rate during clinical testing remains as high as first reported during validation. As molecular testing becomes more prevalent for supporting precision medicine efforts, high technical success and reliability are key characteristics when testing such limited and precious samples. The performance of the 15-gene expression profile test in this study should provide confidence to physicians who use the test's molecular classification to inform patient management decisions.

Keywords: Uveal melanoma, Gene expression profiling, Prognosis, Analytic validity

* Correspondence: fmonzon@castlebiosciences.com
[1]Castle Biosciences, Inc., 820 S. Friendswood Drive, Suite 201, Friendswood, TX 77546, USA
Full list of author information is available at the end of the article

Background

Uveal melanoma (UM) is a rare, intraocular cancer that affects approximately 1600 patients per year in the United States [1]. Most patients are treated with eye-sparing radiotherapy, primarily through plaque brachytherapy or proton beam radiation, while only a small proportion (~10%) will undergo enucleation. Despite the high rate of primary tumor control, ~50% of patients will develop metastatic disease, primarily to the liver, after which prognosis is poor [2]. While the clinicopathologic features assessed in AJCC staging, including tumor size, ciliary body involvement, and extraocular extension, are important factors when assessing metastatic risk, even Stage I-II patients have a 12-30% UM-related mortality rate by 10 years [3, 4]. Because of this, frequent surveillance was generally recommended to monitor all UM patients for disease spread [5, 6].

Gene expression profiles that are associated with low-risk (Class 1A), intermediate-risk (Class 1B), or high-risk (Class 2) outcomes have been shown to provide information useful for risk-tailored surveillance plans [7–9]. Because treatment of the primary tumor is highly effective with plaque radiotherapy, enucleation is not common, and the amount of tumor tissue available for molecular prognostic testing is limited. During the development of the gene expression profiling test for UM prognostication (also known as DecisionDx®-UM), focus was placed on providing patients with a test that was robust and could be run successfully and reproducibly on a very small amount of tissue obtained through a fine needle aspirate biopsy (FNAB), as well as formalin-fixed paraffin embedded (FFPE) tissue from enucleations [8–10].

Recommendations for the development of clinically useful molecular biomarkers have suggested that a biomarker test needs to demonstrate clinical validity, utility, and analytic validity, and that supporting data for each must be transparent and readily available for both physicians and patients [11]. Several widely-used genomic tests for different types of cancer have achieved high levels of evidence for each of these criteria [12–17]. The clinical validity and clinical utility of the 15-gene expression profile test for UM was reported by the Cooperative Ocular Oncology Group (COOG) [9], and the prognostic accuracy of the test has been confirmed in multiple single- and multi-center studies [18–23]. The test's impact on clinical decision-making for UM patients has also been demonstrated [23, 24]. The focus of this study was to evaluate performance metrics of the test in a CLIA-certified laboratory setting, describe the rate of technical success on both FNAB and FFPE tissue from enucleations, and report correlations with pathological variables.

Methods

Tissue acquisition and processing

All samples were acquired during routine clinical testing for risk prognostication in UM patients. For FNAB samples, UM tumor aspirates were frozen in RNase-free RNA stabilization buffer by the treating physician immediately after biopsy and shipped to the Castle Biosciences' laboratory on dry ice (Fig. 1). All samples were immediately processed with the PicoPure RNA Isolation Kit (Molecular Devices, Sunnyvale, CA). For tumors removed through enucleation, five-micron sections from FFPE tissue were used; the first of six sequential sections were stained with hematoxylin and eosin. Tumor tissue containing at least 80% tumor nuclei density was marked and manually dissected from unstained slides using a sterile scalpel and processed for RNA isolation according to the Ambion RecoverAll Total Nucleic Acid Isolation Kit (Life Technologies Corporation, Grand Island, NY). Reverse transcription of RNA into cDNA was performed using the Applied Biosystems High Capacity cDNA Reverse Transcription Kit (Life Technologies Corporation).

DecisionDx-UM gene expression profiling and molecular classification

Gene expression profiling was performed as previously described [9, 25]. From 2010 through 2014, quantitative PCR was performed on a 7900HT Fast Real-Time PCR System (Thermo Fisher Scientific), after which it was performed on the current system, a QuantStudio 12K Flex Real-Time PCR System (Applied Biosystems). Complementary cDNA was pre-amplified with 14 cycles and then diluted 20-fold with Tris-EDTA (TE). Fifty microliters of diluted, pre-amplified cDNA was mixed with 50 uL of 2X Taqman Gene Expression Master Mix and loaded in triplicate onto customized microfluidics PCR cards containing the gene-specific primers and probes for the 12 discriminating genes and endogenous control genes (Additional file 1: Table S1).

After PCR amplification, the average Ct values for each triplicate are calculated. The average Ct value for each of the 12 discriminating genes is subtracted from the geometric mean of the control genes to determine the ΔCt value for each gene. A support vector machine (SVM)-learning algorithm, trained on a training set of UM cases with known gene expression profiles and long-term outcomes, which has been locked since inception, is used to determine classification of test cases. The SVM algorithm places the UM samples within the training set into a hyperplane with n-dimensional space and maximizes the hyperplane between the Class 1 and Class 2 specimens. A discriminant score for each sample is generated, which reflects the inverse distance of the patient sample to the hyperplane separating Class 1 and 2 training set samples. The output of the algorithm is

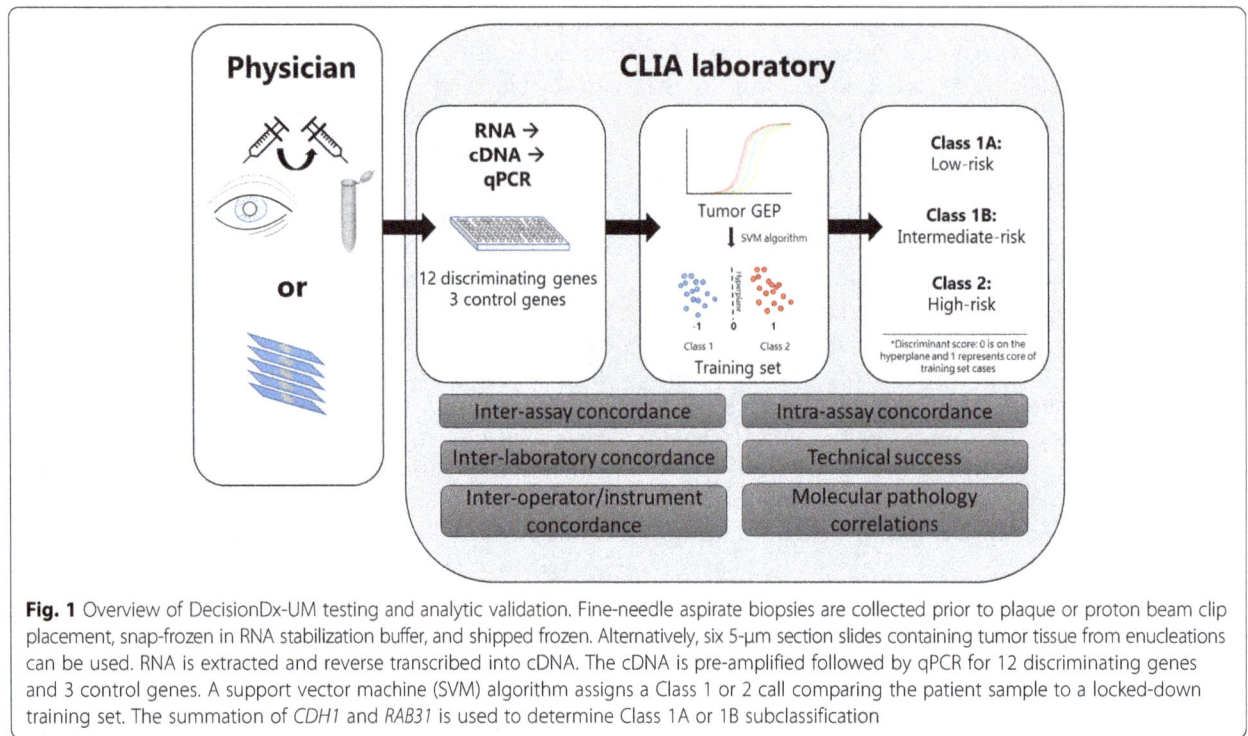

Fig. 1 Overview of DecisionDx-UM testing and analytic validation. Fine-needle aspirate biopsies are collected prior to plaque or proton beam clip placement, snap-frozen in RNA stabilization buffer, and shipped frozen. Alternatively, six 5-μm section slides containing tumor tissue from enucleations can be used. RNA is extracted and reverse transcribed into cDNA. The cDNA is pre-amplified followed by qPCR for 12 discriminating genes and 3 control genes. A support vector machine (SVM) algorithm assigns a Class 1 or 2 call comparing the patient sample to a locked-down training set. The summation of *CDH1* and *RAB31* is used to determine Class 1A or 1B subclassification

either a negative discriminant score (Class 1) or positive discriminant score (Class 2). The discriminant score can theoretically range from >0 to positive or negative infinity, however, only the absolute (positive) value of the discriminant score is reported clinically alongside the respective Class result. A discriminant score is considered reduced confidence if it is <0.1. For Class 1 cases, summation of the *RAB31* and *CDH1* ΔCt values determined whether the sample was Class 1A or Class 1B based on a mathematical threshold. Class 1B UMs have differential *RAB31/CDH1* expression relative to Class 1A tumors.

Technical reliability studies

De-identified DecisionDx-UM test results from January 2010 through May 2016 were analyzed according to tissue type, successful molecular classification, and resultant class assignment. Institutional review board submission of the technical reliability study was not required as it constitutes technical data on file only, and contains no patient-specific protected health information. As such, this analysis is exempt from the regulatory review requirements as set forth in section 46.101 (b) of 45 CFR 46 [26]. Analytic validation experiments were performed on cDNA generated from the RNA extracted from UM tumor specimens. For these experiments, de-identified residual samples were used. Given that the majority of specimens are obtained via FNAB, most tumor samples are exhausted by performing the 15-gene expression profile test and residual samples are limited.

As such, samples used in reproducibility experiments were not consecutive samples, but in each experiment, leftover samples from approximately the same time period were used. Samples were between 1 and 10 weeks old (from date of tissue receipt) and remained frozen after initial processing until reliability experiments.

Results

Inter-assay and intra-assay repeatability

To evaluate the repeatability of gene expression profiling and class assignment agreement on the same sample between separate PCR runs, DecisionDx-UM testing was performed on 16 samples on three consecutive days, resulting in 48 molecular classifications (Table 1). The class assignment concordance for each sample across all three days was 100% (eight Class 1A, three Class 1B, and five Class 2 tumors). Multiple regression analysis of the discriminant scores from the three runs showed an average R^2 value of 0.9944 (Fig. 2a). The majority of variation in discriminant scores between runs fell within the 95% confidence interval (−0.1809 to 0.1219), with an estimated bias of −0.0295 (Fig. 2b).

In a second reproducibility study, matched duplicate runs of samples used for proficiency testing or instrument verification at six time points during a one-year period were analyzed for inter-assay concordance (Table 1). Overall, reproducibility was evaluated on 46 samples run in duplicate during this one-year interval, and the discriminant scores and molecular classifications were compared for the matched samples. The molecular classifications

Table 1 Summary of results from repeatability and proficiency studies

Study	Design summary	Molecular class calls (n)	Concordance	Bias discriminant scores between replicates (95% CI)	Discriminant score R^2
Inter-assay (consecutive days)	16 samples, 1 instrument, 2 operators, 3 runs, 3 consecutive days, 1 manufacturing reagent lot	48	100%	−0.0295 (−0.1809-0.1219)	0.9944
Inter-assay (long term)	46 samples run on 2 separate days, 2 instruments, multiple runs, multiple operators, multiple manufacturing reagent lots	92	100%	0.0049 (−0.2816-0.2914)	0.9747
Intra-assay	12 tumors with 2 replicates on 2 plates each, 1 instrument, 1 operator, 3 runs, 3 consecutive days, 1 manufacturing reagent lot	48	100%	0.0145 (−0.1182-0.1472)	0.9934
Inter-site	29 samples, two instruments, two operators, 2 manufacturing reagent lots	58	100%	0.0233 (−0.1939-0.2405)	0.9818
Inter-operator/ instrument	28 samples, 2 instruments, 2 operators, 2 runs, 1 day, 1 manufacturing reagent lot	56	96% (C1 vs C2) 90% (C1A vs C1B)	−0.0540 (−0.3266 -0.2186)	0.9636

were 100% concordant for all samples (7 Class 1A, 15 Class 1B, and 24 Class 2 tumors). Regression analysis showed an R^2 of 0.9747 (Fig. 2c). The estimated bias in discriminant scores was 0.0049 and most variation in discriminant scores fell within the 95% confidence interval (−0.2816 to 0.2914) (Fig. 2d).

Intra-assay repeatability was tested by running two replicates of four samples on the same PCR card, and repeating this experiment on a second card. This was performed with three sets of four samples, resulting in 24 paired molecular classifications from 12 tumor specimens. Class assignment agreement was 100% for the four samples within each card and between the two cards (Table 1; five Class 1A, two Class 1B and five Class 2 tumors). The R^2 value from correlation analysis was 0.9934 (Fig. 2e). As shown on a Bland-Altman plot (Fig. 2f), all (24/24) of the paired intra-assay discriminant scores had differences that fell within the 95% confidence interval (−0.1182 to 0.1472) and the estimated bias was 0.0145.

Transfer of the test to a new laboratory location afforded the opportunity to test the inter-assay reliability of the test when performed in different laboratories. Twenty-nine samples were run at our CLIA-certified contract laboratory (St. Joseph's Hospital and Medical Center, Phoenix AZ) and a new Castle Biosciences, Inc. facility (Table 1). The DecisionDx-UM Class calls were 100% concordant between the two laboratories. The R^2 value of the correlation between discriminant scores was 0.9818 ($p < 0.001$) (Fig. 3a). The estimated bias was 0.0233 and 26/29 (90%) of the discriminant scores had an inter-lab difference that fell within the 95% confidence interval (−0.1939 to 0.2405; Fig. 3b).

Twenty-eight samples were run on two instruments by separate operators to analyze inter-instrument and −operator reliability (Table 1). Two Class 1 calls were discordant for their 1A versus 1B subclassification. One

discordant sample had a Class 1B result because the *RAB31/CDH1* expression fell just under the subclassification threshold, and its variability fell within the 95% confidence interval for *RAB31/CDH1* in reliability experiments. The remaining discordant case had a difference in *RAB31/CDH1* between runs that fell outside of this confidence interval and was thus an outlier. Class 1 vs. Class 2 calls were 96% concordant (27/28). The case that was discordant for Class 1 vs. Class 2 did not have any unique characteristic that could potentially explain the discrepancy and thus seems to represent an outlier. As shown in Fig. 3c, correlation analysis of the discriminant scores between the two instruments generated an R^2 value of 0.9636 ($p < 0.001$). The estimated bias was −0.0540 (95% CI = −0.3266 to 0.2186) and only 1 sample fell outside of this confidence interval (Fig. 3d).

Technical success of clinical testing

From January 2010 to May 2016, 5516 tumor specimens were tested. Of these, 4829 (88%) were FNABs and 687 (12%) were FFPE, the vast majority of which were 5-μm sections from enucleations and the remaining as FFPE cell blocks (Fig. 4a, Table 2). Gene expression profiling was successful for 96.35% (5315) of these tumors: 2305 (43.4%) were Class 1A, 1192 (22.4%) were Class 1B, and 1818 (34.2%) were Class 2 (Table 2, Fig. 4b-c).

Failure to generate a successful gene expression profile report can be due to i) the failure of multiple control and/or discriminating genes to amplify (multi-gene failure [MGF]), or ii) insufficient tumor cell density (<80%) within a manually dissectable area of FFPE tissue as determined by a pathologist, which results in rejection of the tumor sample prior to testing. Overall, 180 (3.3%) of the samples tested resulted in MGFs and 21 (0.4%) samples had insufficient tumor density (Table 2, Fig. 4c). Eighteen of the MGFs (10%) were related to out-of-specification FNAB specimens, meaning the FNABs

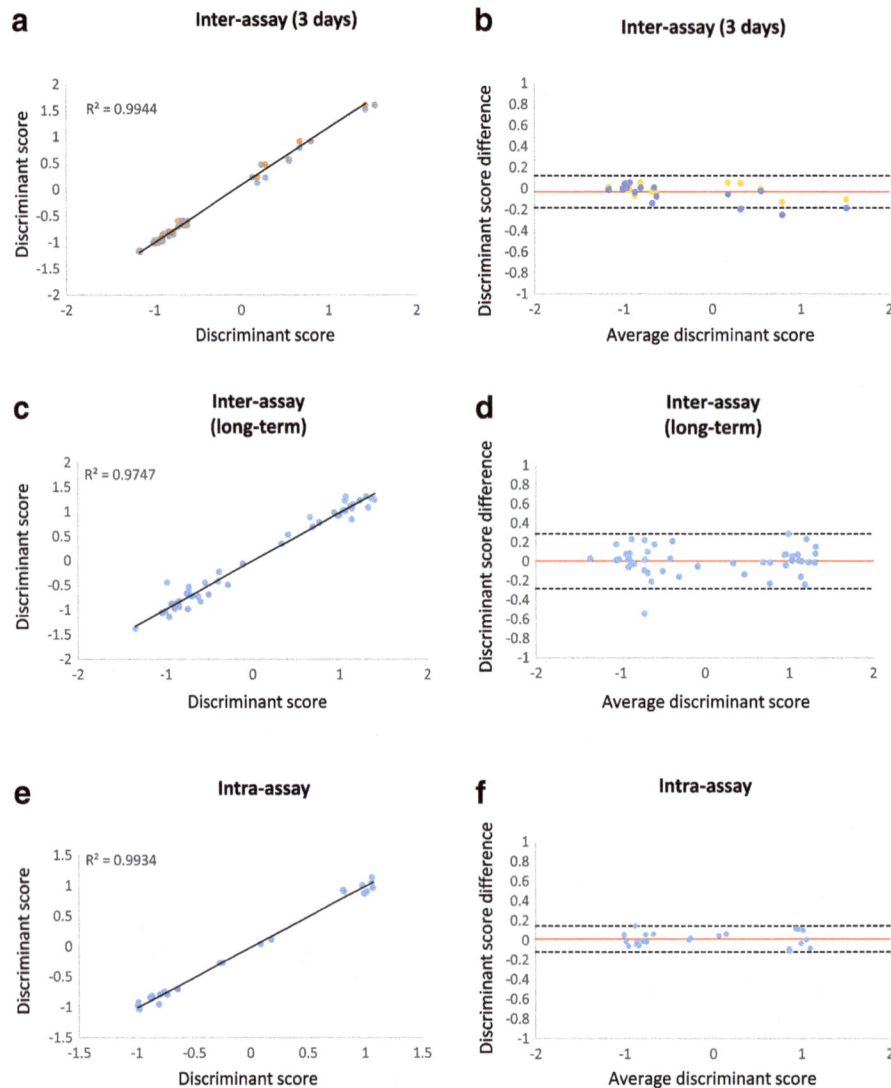

Fig. 2 Inter- and intra-assay reliability of DecisionDx-UM. **a** Inter-assay correlation of discriminant scores for 16 samples run on 3 consecutive days. **b** Bland-Altman plot showing the difference in discriminant scores between runs and the 95% confidence interval (*dashed lines*). The estimated bias (or mean difference in discriminant values) is represented as the *red line*. **c** Inter-assay correlation of discriminant scores of 46 samples run twice during a one-year period for proficiency testing or instrument verification. **d** Bland-Altman plot of proficiency testing and instrument verification samples. **e** Intra-assay correlation of discriminant scores of 12 samples tested in duplicate on two cards. **f** Bland-Altman plot showing differences in paired discriminant scores within each card

were received thawed and/or were not within the acceptable volume range (10-220 uL). Success rates for FNAB and FFPE tissues were similar. Testing was successful for 4678 (97%) out of 4829 FNABs, with only 151 (3%) experiencing MGFs (Table 2). Of the 666 FFPE tumors that passed the quality control assessment and went on to gene expression profile testing, 637 (96%) were successful and 29 (4%) had MGFs.

To determine if long distance shipment has an effect on the reliability of gene expression profiling we evaluated performance on international samples. Since 2010, 218 tumor samples from outside of the United States

have been tested; 202 (93%) were fresh-frozen FNABs from Canada and four other countries outside of North America and the remaining 16 (8%) samples were FFPE tissues that came from Canada and two countries outside of North America (data not shown). Only two MGFs occurred (both FNAB samples from Canada), resulting in 99% technical success for internationally shipped specimens.

Discriminant scores and confidence intervals
The discriminant score associated with the DecisionDx-UM Class reflects the inverse distance of the patient

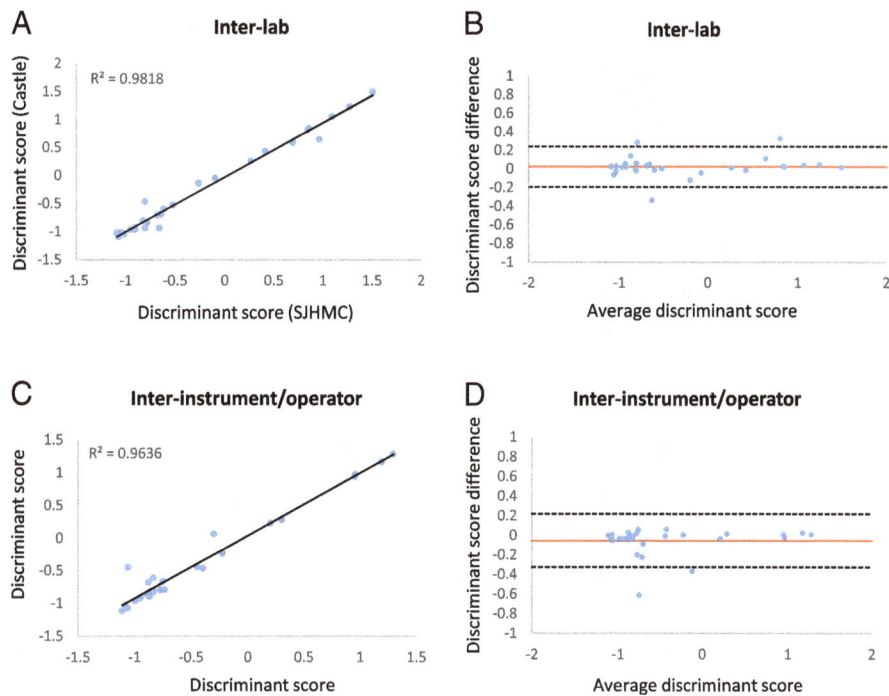

Fig. 3 Inter-lab and inter-instrument/operator reliability of DecisionDx-UM. **a** Correlation of 29 paired discriminant scores from samples run at two CLIA-certified laboratories. **b** Bland-Altman plot of the estimated bias (average difference between discriminant scores, *red line*) between labs and the 95% confidence interval (*dashed lines*). **c** Correlation analysis of 28 paired inter-instrument/operator discriminant values. **d** Bland-Altman plot paired inter-instrument/operator discriminant values

sample to the hyperplane. As of May 2016, the discriminant scores have ranged from −1.56808 to +1.70482 (Fig. 5). The average discriminant score for Class 1 was −0.81033 (95% CI = −0.256 to −1.365). The average discriminant score for Class 2 was 0.816144 (95% CI = 0.0528 to 1.567). A score between −0.1 to 0.1 is considered of reduced confidence and is reported clinically as such. However, a discriminant score with reduced confidence has not been associated with a different outcome than a normal confidence score [25], and the vast majority (~97%) of the discriminant scores reported clinically have been reported within the normal confidence range.

Pathologic characteristics of DecisionDx-UM-tested tumors

Associated de-identified pathological data was available for 527 FFPE tumors from enucleations tested between January 2010 and May 2016. The pathologic characteristics of these tumors are described in Table 3, with statistical analysis of correlation with molecular class presented in Table 4. Eighty-eight tumors (17%) were Class 1A, 201 (38%) were Class 1B, and 238 (45%) were Class 2. Class 2 tumors had significantly greater largest basal diameters (LBDs) than Class 1 tumors ($p < 0.0001$ by Mann-Whitney test). Compared to Class 1A tumors,

Class 1B tumors also had significantly greater LBDs (median of 14 mm vs 11.5 mm, $p = 0.008$ by Mann-Whitney test). Similarly, Class 2 tumors were significantly thicker than Class 1 tumors (median of 9.45 mm vs 7, $p < 0.0001$), and within Class 1, Class 1B tumors were significantly thicker than Class 1A tumors (median of 8 mm vs 6 mm, $p = 0.001$). A Class 1 signature was associated with predominantly spindle cell type, while a Class 2 signature was significantly associated with a mixed or predominantly epithelioid cell type ($p < 0.0001$ by Fisher's exact). Class 1A and 1B tumors had similar cell morphologies, while Class 2 tumors were significantly associated with a mixed/predominantly epithelioid cell type compared to Class 1B tumors ($p = 0.0002$ by Fisher's exact). There was no difference in ciliary body involvement between Class 1A and 1B tumors, but Class 2 tumors were more likely to have ciliary body involvement than Class 1A and 1B tumors ($p < 0.0001$ by Fisher's exact). There was no significant association with any molecular class and extra-ocular extension.

Discussion

Given the advances in molecular cancer diagnostics in the last decade, recommendations have been established to guide careful, thorough assessments of these tests [11, 27]. One of the major criteria for a clinically

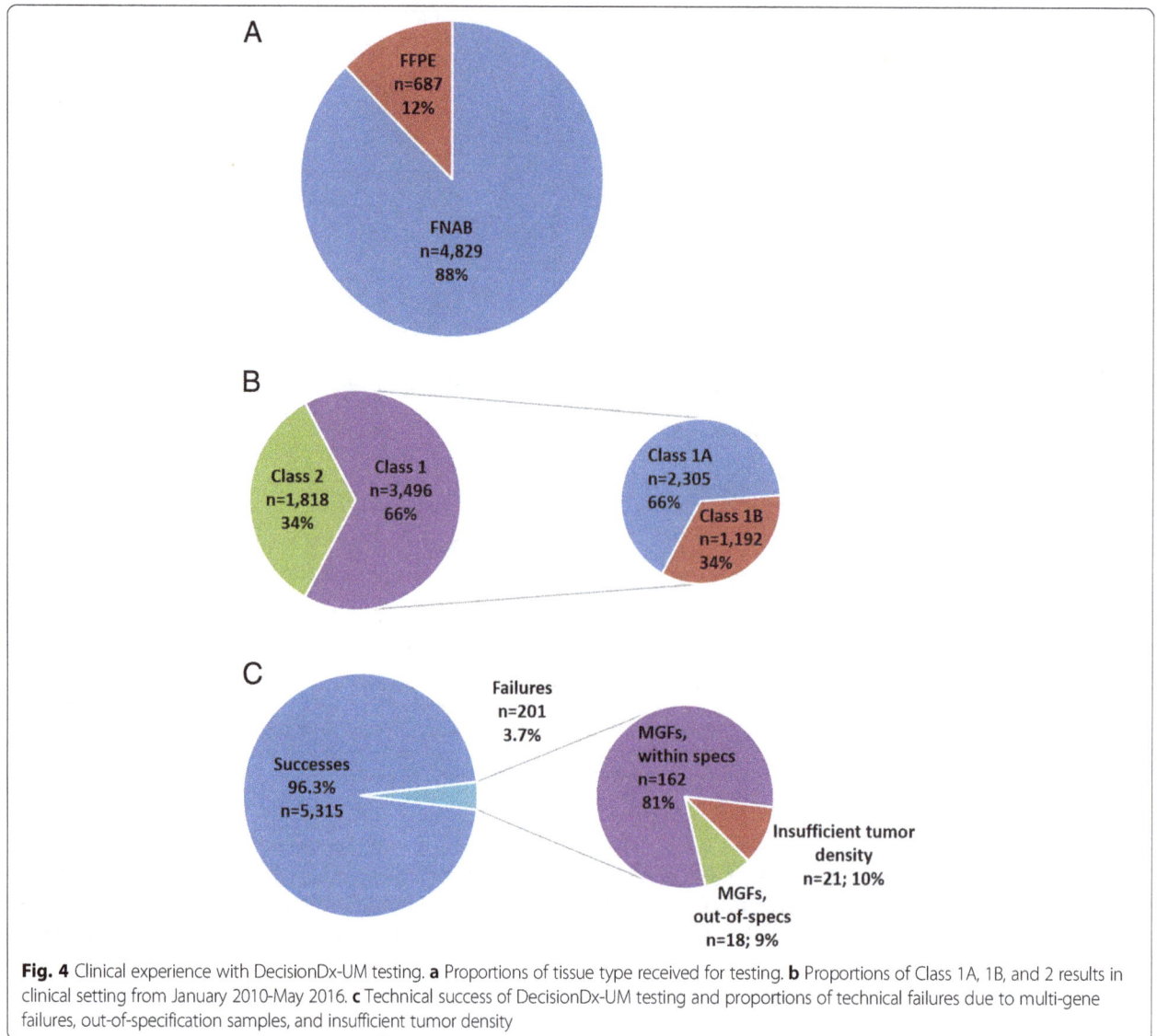

Fig. 4 Clinical experience with DecisionDx-UM testing. **a** Proportions of tissue type received for testing. **b** Proportions of Class 1A, 1B, and 2 results in clinical setting from January 2010-May 2016. **c** Technical success of DecisionDx-UM testing and proportions of technical failures due to multi-gene failures, out-of-specification samples, and insufficient tumor density

useful, well-validated assay is that the test must demonstrate analytic validity, which includes reliability and reproducibility of the test to measure the intended molecular analytes [11, 27]. In this study, we report on the analytic validity of the 15-gene expression profile test (DecisionDx-UM) as performed in a CLIA-certified clinical laboratory. Reproducibility and reliability were demonstrated through i) inter-assay concordance, ii) inter-assay concordance of samples used for proficiency testing and instrument verification throughout one year, iii) intra-assay concordance, iv) inter-lab concordance between two CLIA-certified laboratories, and v) inter-instrument/operator concordance. Molecular classifications by DecisionDx-UM were 100% concordant for four of these assessments, with only 3 discordant specimens out of the total 143 samples in the analytic experiments. The reported discriminant scores for the same tumor sample were highly correlated, as reflected by R^2 values

Table 2 Clinical experience of DecisionDx-UM testing

Sample Type	Received	Successfully reported	Multi-gene Failures (MGF)		Insufficient tissue
			within specs	Outside specs	
FNAB (n, % of row)	4829	4678 (97%)	133 (2.7%)	18 (0.3%)	N/A
FFPE (n,% of row)	687	637 (93%)	29 (4%)	N/A	21 (3%)
Total (n, % of row)	5516	5315 (96.3%)	180 (3.3%)		21 (0.4%)

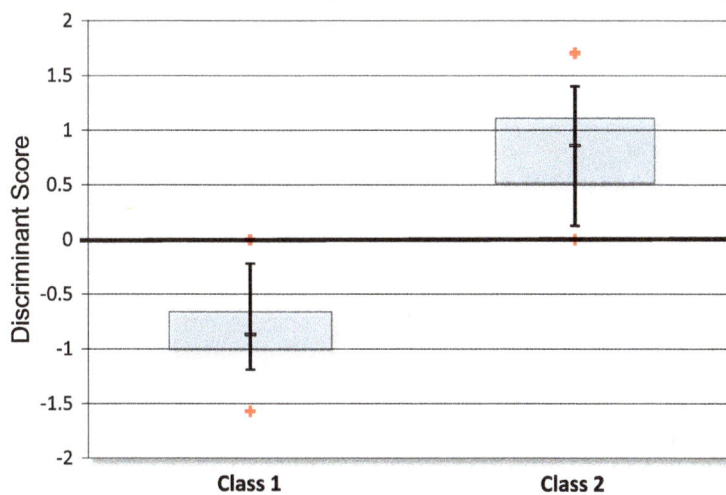

Fig. 5 Distribution of discriminant scores. The distribution of discriminant scores that have been reported clinically. The output of the SVM algorithm is negative for Class 1, but reported as a positive number. The 50th percentile is represented by the *blue box* and the *black bars* indicate the 90th percentile. The *blue line* is the median of each group and the red stars indicate the minimum and maximum observed scores of each Class

above 0.96 for the inter-assay, intra-assay, inter-instrument, and inter-lab experiments. Furthermore, the run-to-run, lab-to-lab, instrument-instrument, and intra-run variabilities between discriminant scores were all within acceptable limits that would not impact patient care. These results demonstrate that the DecisionDx-UM class assignment for the same tumor specimen is consistent within the same PCR card and when run on separate days in different PCR cards, even with several weeks in between runs. To our knowledge, this is the only report of

Table 3 Morphologic characteristics and correlation with molecular class result in enucleated cases

	Class 1A (*n* = 88, 17%)	Class 1B (*n* = 201; 38%)	Class 2 (*n* = 238, 45%)
Largest basal diameter (mm), median (range)	11.5 (1.5-28)	14 (1.1-35)	16 (1.4-39)
≤12 mm (n, %)	47 (53%)	75 (37%)	57 (24%)
> 12 mm (n, %)	29 (33%)	109 (54%)	165 (69%)
Not addressed (n, %)	12 (14%)	17 (9%)	16 (7%)
Tumor height (mm), median (range)	6 (0.4-20)	8 (0.5-29)	9.45 (1-36)
≤ 5.5 mm (n, %)	34 (39%)	47 (23.5%)	51 (21%)
> 5.5 mm (n, %)	42 (47%)	135 (67%)	166 (70%)
Not addressed	12 (14%)	19 (9.5%)	21 (9%)
Cell type (n, %)			
Spindle predominant	40 (45.5%)	92 (46%)	65 (27%)
Mixed/epithelioid predominant	40 (45.5%)	102 (51%)	158 (66%)
Not addressed	8 (9%)	7 (3%)	15 (6%)
Ciliary body involvement (n,%)			
No	35 (40%)	104 (52%)	84 (35%)
Yes	23 (26%)	45 (22%)	111 (47%)
Not addressed	30 (34%)	52 (26%)	43 (18%)
Extra-scleral/ocular extension (n,%)			
No	59 (67%)	145 (72%)	176 (74%)
Yes	14 (16%)	34 (17%)	42 (18%)
Not addressed	15 (17%)	22 (11%)	20 (8%)

Table 4 Statistical comparisons between molecular class and tumor pathology in enucleated cases

	Class 1 vs. Class 2	Class 1A vs. Class 1B	Class 1B vs. Class 2	Class 1A vs. Class 2
Largest basal diameter[a]	$p < 0.0001$	$p = 0.008$	$p = 0.0001$	$p < 0.0001$
Tumor height[a]	$p < 0.0001$	$p = 0.0015$	$p = 0.0085$	$p < 0.0001$
Cell type[b]	$p < 0.0001$	n.s.	$p = 0.0002$	$p = 0.001$
Ciliary body involvement[b]	$p < 0.0001$	n.s.	$p < 0.0001$	$p < 0.0001$
Extra-scleral/ocular extension	n.s.	n.s.	n.s.	n.s.

[a]Mann-Whitney test; [b]Fisher's exact test

analytic validity for any prognostic test for UM. Comparable analytic validation has not yet been reported for fluorescence in situ hybridization (FISH), microsatellite analysis (MSA), single nucleotide polymorphism (SNP) arrays, or multiplex-ligation probe amplification (MLPA), all of which can be used to detect monosomy 3 and other chromosomal copy number changes that have been associated with UM metastasis, or next-generation sequencing to detect mutations and chromosomal aberrations to estimate UM prognosis.

Gene expression profiling is one of the clinically significant variables for disease prognostication recommended by the 2017 AJCC staging guidelines [28], and as such, the DecisionDx-UM test is routinely used across the United States and has been clinically available since 2010. The prognostic test was developed after two distinct molecular subtypes of UM were identified and shown to have correlation with outcomes [7, 10, 29, 30]. A 15-gene RT-PCR test was developed to identify these UM molecular subtypes and prospectively validated in multiple studies [8, 9, 20, 21, 23]. As eye-sparing treatments are frequently utilized in the contemporary management of UM and enucleations are less common, the standard practice for physicians utilizing DecisionDx-UM is to collect a biopsy prior to or at the time of radioactive plaque or proton beam clip placement. Due to the lack of residual tissue aside from that obtained during biopsy, successful gene expression profiling on a single biopsy is critical. While the technical success of the 15-gene expression profile assay has been previously reported as ranging from 95 to 99% [8, 9, 19], many of the samples in those studies were tested in the research laboratory that developed the assay, which was then licensed by Castle Biosciences, Inc. in 2009. In this report, we demonstrate that 96.4% of 5516 samples that have been clinically tested at Castle Biosciences' laboratory generated successful molecular classification reports, establishing the consistency of technical success from the test. Of the unsuccessful tests, 39 out of 201 (19%) were due to samples outside of quality control specifications (for FNABs, incorrect volume and/or not frozen, $n = 18$; for FFPE tissues, insufficient tumor volume, $n = 21$). Thawed samples and those with insufficient/excessive

volume have been previously reported to be associated with technical failures of gene expression profiling [8]. The technical success rate of DecisionDx-UM testing is substantially higher than what has been previously reported for other molecular methods used in UM prognostication, including FISH, MSA, and array CGH, which range from 50 to 87% in much smaller sample sets [31–34].

Of the 5315 successful tests reported, 43.4% were Class 1A, 22.4% were Class 1B, and 34.2% were Class 2. Overall, these proportions are similar to class those reported in the Cooperative Ocular Oncology Group (COOG) study, which were 47% Class 1A, 13%, Class 1B and 40% Class 2 [9]. Likewise, other single- and multi-center studies that analyzed subsets of the clinically tested patients reported here have shown similar proportions of Class 1A, 1B, and 2 results [21, 23, 35].

Of the enucleation specimens tested for which there were associated pathology data, the proportion of Class 1 patients shifted to be predominately Class 1B vs. Class 1A, and the proportion of Class 2 tumors was also increased compared to the total clinical population. Given the significantly increased LBDs and thicknesses of enucleation specimens (i.e. those that necessitated removal of the globe), an increase in Class 2 and Class 1B tumor classification is not unexpected. Importantly, there were no significant differences between Class 1A and 1B tumors in terms of cell morphology, ciliary body involvement, or extraocular extension, underscoring the utility of molecular testing to delineate risk in these tumors that otherwise share similar pathologic features. Overall, the pathology and molecular class data in our clinically tested cohort reflect published reports that greater LBD and tumor thickness tend to be clinicopathologic features associated with more aggressive tumors [9, 20, 22, 23], and these riskier phenotypes are most frequently seen in Class 1B or Class 2 tumors. An advantage of gene expression profiling is that it reflects objective, intrinsic tumor biology, whereas measurements of LBD in particular can be subjective due to variation between observers and in techniques used for size measurement [36]. Additionally, cytopathologic analysis can be impaired by a high rate of insufficient cellularity from FNABs [19]. Several studies have shown that GEP is the most significant independent prognostic factor for metastatic risk when compared to clinicopathologic features, including LBD [9, 18–20, 22, 23, 37].

Conclusions

In summary, the results of these analytic performance data demonstrate the reproducibility and reliability of the DecisionDx-UM test. This is confirmed by the high correlation of discriminant scores and concordance of molecular classifications on samples subjected to repeat testing. The robust high technical success rate of the test on even small amounts of tissue obtained by FNAB has been maintained from the test's original development through clinical implementation and testing of more than 5000 patients, and represents an important aspect of testing, given that patients who receive eye-sparing radiotherapy, usually do not have the opportunity to be biopsied again after treatment.

Abbreviations

COOG: Collaborative Ocular Oncology Group; FFPE: Formalin-fixed, paraffin-embedded; FISH: Fluorescence in situ hybridization; FNAB: Fine needle aspirate biopsy; LBD: Largest basal diameter; MGF: Multi-gene failure; MLPA: Multiplex ligation probe amplification; MSA: Microsatellite analysis; UM: Uveal melanoma

Acknowledgements

Not applicable.

Funding

This study was sponsored by Castle Biosciences, Inc.

Authors' contributions

KMP, JW, KO, TP, JS, and FM generated the data. KMP, JW, JS, and FM analyzed the data. KMP, RC, and FM wrote the manuscript. All authors reviewed and approved the final manuscript.

Competing interests

All authors are employees and option holders at Castle Biosciences, Inc.

Author details

[1]Castle Biosciences, Inc., 820 S. Friendswood Drive, Suite 201, Friendswood, TX 77546, USA. [2]Castle Biosciences Laboratory, 3737 N. 7th St, Suite 160, Phoenix, AZ 85014, USA.

References

1. Singh AD, Topham A. Incidence of uveal melanoma in the United States: 1973-1997. Ophthalmology. 2003;110(5):956–61.
2. Collaborative Ocular Melanoma Study Group. The COMS randomized trial of iodine 125 brachytherapy for choroidal melanoma: V. Twelve-year mortality rates and prognostic factors: COMS report no. 28. Arch Ophthalmol. 2006; 124(12):1684–93.
3. Kivela T, Kujala E. Prognostication in eye cancer: the latest tumor, node, metastasis classification and beyond. Eye (Lond). 2013;27(2):243–52.
4. Kujala E, et al. Staging of ciliary body and choroidal melanomas based on anatomic extent. J Clin Oncol. 2013;31(22):2825–31.
5. Diener-West M, et al. Screening for metastasis from choroidal melanoma: the collaborative ocular melanoma study group report 23. J Clin Oncol. 2004;22(12):2438–44.
6. Eskelin S, et al. Tumor doubling times in metastatic malignant melanoma of the uvea: tumor progression before and after treatment. Ophthalmology. 2000;107(8):1443–9.
7. Onken MD, et al. Gene expression profiling in uveal melanoma reveals two molecular classes and predicts metastatic death. Cancer Res. 2004;64(20):7205–9.
8. Onken MD, et al. An accurate, clinically feasible multi-gene expression assay for predicting metastasis in uveal melanoma. J Mol Diagn. 2010;12(4):461–8.
9. Onken MD, et al. Collaborative ocular oncology group report number 1: prospective validation of a multi-gene prognostic assay in uveal melanoma. Ophthalmology. 2012;119(8):1596–603.
10. Onken MD, et al. Prognostic testing in uveal melanoma by transcriptomic profiling of fine needle biopsy specimens. J Mol Diagn. 2006;8(5):567–73.
11. Febbo PG, et al. NCCN task force report: evaluating the clinical utility of tumor markers in oncology. J Natl Compr Cancer Netw. 2011;9(Suppl 5):S1–32. quiz S33
12. Walsh PS, et al. Analytical performance verification of a molecular diagnostic for cytology-indeterminate thyroid nodules. J Clin Endocrinol Metab. 2012; 97(12):E2297–306.
13. Hu Z, et al. Analytical performance of a bronchial genomic classifier. BMC Cancer. 2016;16:161.
14. Vachani A, et al. Clinical utility of a bronchial genomic classifier in patients with suspected lung cancer. Chest. 2016;150(1):210–8.
15. Silvestri GA, et al. A bronchial genomic classifier for the diagnostic evaluation of lung cancer. N Engl J Med. 2015;373(3):243–51.
16. Duick DS, et al. The impact of benign gene expression classifier test results on the endocrinologist-patient decision to operate on patients with thyroid nodules with indeterminate fine-needle aspiration cytopathology. Thyroid. 2012;22(10):996–1001.
17. Alexander EK, et al. Preoperative diagnosis of benign thyroid nodules with indeterminate cytology. N Engl J Med. 2012;367(8):705–15.
18. Chappell MC, et al. Uveal melanoma: molecular pattern, clinical features, and radiation response. Am J Ophthalmol. 2012;154(2):227–32. e2
19. Correa ZM, Augsburger JJ. Sufficiency of FNAB aspirates of posterior uveal melanoma for cytologic versus GEP classification in 159 patients, and relative prognostic significance of these classifications. Graefes Arch Clin Exp Ophthalmol. 2014;252(1):131–5.
20. Correa ZM, Augsburger JJ. Independent prognostic significance of gene expression profile class and largest basal diameter of posterior Uveal melanomas. Am J Ophthalmol. 2016;162:20–7. e1
21. Demirci H, Ozkurt ZG, Slimani N, Cook R, Oelschlager K. Gene expression profiling test of uveal melanoma: prognostic validation. Las Vegas: American Society of Ophthalmic Plastic & Reconstructive Surgery Fall Scientific Symposium; 2015.

22. Walter SD, et al. Prognostic implications of tumor diameter in association with gene expression profile for Uveal melanoma. JAMA Ophthalmol. 2016; 134(7):734–40.

23. Plasseraud KM, et al. Clinical performance and management outcomes with the DecisionDx-UM gene expression profile test in a prospective multicenter study. Journal of Oncology. 2016;2016:1–9.

24. Aaberg TM Jr, et al. Current clinical practice: differential management of uveal melanoma in the era of molecular tumor analyses. Clin Ophthalmol. 2014;8:2449–60.

25. Harbour JW. A prognostic test to predict the risk of metastasis in uveal melanoma based on a 15-gene expression profile. Methods Mol Biol. 2014; 1102:427–40.

26. Office for Human Research Protections. 45 Code of Federal Regulations Part 46 (45 CFR 6). Department of Health and Human Services; 2009.

27. Simon RM, Paik S, Hayes DF. Use of archived specimens in evaluation of prognostic and predictive biomarkers. J Natl Cancer Inst. 2009;101(21):1446–52.

28. Kivela, T., et al., Uveal Melanoma, in American Joint Committee on Cancer (AJCC) Staging Manual, M.B. Amin, Edge, M.B., Greene, F.L., Byrd, D.R., Brookland, R.K., Washington, M.K., Gershenwald, J.E., Compton, C.C., Hess, K.R., Sullivan, D.C., Jessup, J.M., Brierley, J.D., Gaspar, L.E., Schilsky, R.L., Balch, C.M., Winchester, D.P., Asare, E.A., Madera, M., Gress, D.M., Meyer, L.R., Editor. 2017, Spring.

29. Onken MD, et al. Loss of heterozygosity of chromosome 3 detected with single nucleotide polymorphisms is superior to monosomy 3 for predicting metastasis in uveal melanoma. Clin Cancer Res. 2007;13(10):2923–7.

30. Worley LA, et al. Transcriptomic versus chromosomal prognostic markers and clinical outcome in uveal melanoma. Clin Cancer Res. 2007;13(5):1466–71.

31. Midena E, et al. In vivo detection of monosomy 3 in eyes with medium-sized uveal melanoma using transscleral fine needle aspiration biopsy. Eur J Ophthalmol. 2006;16(3):422–5.

32. Young TA, et al. Fluorescent in situ hybridization for monosomy 3 via 30-gauge fine-needle aspiration biopsy of choroidal melanoma in vivo. Ophthalmology. 2007;114(1):142–6.

33. Shields CL, et al. Chromosome 3 analysis of uveal melanoma using fine-needle aspiration biopsy at the time of plaque radiotherapy in 140 consecutive cases. Trans Am Ophthalmol Soc. 2007;105:43–52. discussion 52-3

34. Desjardins L, et al. FNA biopsies for genomic analysis and adjuvant therapy for uveal melanoma. Acta Ophthalmol. 2010;88:0.

35. Schefler A, et al. Ocular Oncology Study Consortium (OOSC) Report No. 2: Effect of Clinical and Pathologic Variables on Biopsy Complication Rates. San Francisco: American Association of Retina Specialists; 2016.

36. Augsburger JJ, et al. Accuracy of clinical estimates of tumor dimensions. A clinical-pathologic correlation study of posterior uveal melanomas. Retina. 1985;5(1):26–9.

37. Decatur CL, et al. Driver mutations in Uveal melanoma: associations with gene expression profile and patient outcomes. JAMA Ophthalmol. 2016; 134(7):728–33.

7

Frequency of rare and multi viral high-risk HPV types infection in cervical high grade squamous intraepithelial lesions in a non-native dominant middle eastern country: a polymerase chain reaction-based pilot study

Alia Albawardi[1], M. Ruhul Quddus[2], Shamsa Al Awar[3] and Saeeda Almarzooqi[1]* ⓘ

Abstract

Background: The incidence of abnormal cervical smears in the United Arab Emirates (UAE) is 3.6%. Data regarding specific high-risk HPV (hrHPV) genotypes are insufficient. Identification of hrHPV subtypes is essential to allow formulating effective vaccination strategies.

Methods: A total of 75 archival cervical cone biopsies with HSIL or higher lesions (2012–2016) were retrieved from a tertiary hospital, including HSIL ($n = 70$), adenocarcinoma in-situ ($n = 1$) and squamous cell carcinoma ($n = 4$). Five tissue sections (10-μ-thick each) were cut and DNA extracted using the QIAamp DNA FFPE Tissue Kit. GenomeMeTM's GeneNavTM HPV One qPCR Kit was used for specific detection of HPV 16 and 18; and non-16/18 samples were typed by GenomeMeTM's GeneNavTM HPV Genotyping qPCR Kit.

Results: Median age was 34 years (range 19–58) with 70% UAE Nationals. hrHPV detected were 16, 18, 31, 33, 35, 39, 45, 51, 52, 58, 59, 66 & 68. hrHPV testing was negative in 12% of cases. Most common types were HPV 16 (49%), HPV 31 (20%) and HPV 18 (6.6%). hrHPV 16 and/or 18 represented 56% and rare subtypes 32%. Co-infection was present in 16%. Eight cases had two-viral subtype infections and 4 cases had 3 subtype infections. Multi-viral HPV infection was limited to hrHPV 16, 18, 31 & 33 subtypes.

Conclusions: Infection by non HPV 16/18 is fairly common. A higher than expected incidence of rare subtype (20% hrHPV31) and multi-viral hrHPV (16%) were detected. This finding stresses the importance of this pilot study as currently only quadravalent vaccine is offered to control the HPV infection in the UAE population.

Keywords: Cervical cancer, HPV, Papillomaviridae, UAE

* Correspondence: saeeda.almarzooqi@uaeu.ac.ae
The results of this study were presented in part at the 106th Annual Meeting of the USCAP in March 2017, San Antonio, Texas, USA.
[1]Pathology Department, College of Medicine and Health Sciences, UAE University, Al Ain, United Arab Emirates
Full list of author information is available at the end of the article

Background

Cervical cancer is the third most common cancer in females in the United Arab Emirates as per 2014 cancer incidence report in the emirate of Abu Dhabi [1]. It is the fourth leading cause of cancer-related mortality in the UAE [2]. Human Papillomavirus (HPV) infection has been established as an etiologic agent in the pathogenesis of cervical neoplasia [3]. HPV infection is reported in 80% of the cases with low-grade squamous intraepithelial lesions (LSILs) and 90% of cases with high-grade squamous intraepithelial lesions (HSILs) [4].

The reported incidence of cervical abnormalities in cervical smears among women in the UAE is 3.6% in one study [5]. The author reported lesions including LSIL, HSIL, ASCUS (atypical squamous cells of undetermined significance) and glandular abnormalities. However, tissue biopsy confirmation of the findings was not reported by the investigators and characterization of HPV subtypes was not performed - [5]. A comparable overall incidence of 3.3% was also reported in a retrospective study performed on cervical Pap smears on 602 UAE and immigrant women in 2012. In this study ASCUS represented 1.8%, LSIL 1.2%, and HSIL 0.3%. The ASCUS:SIL ratio was 1.2 [6]. The ASCUS:SIL ratio at our lab was 1.9 in 2017 (non-published data).

Infrequent reports on studies identifying hrHPV types are available from the countries with somewhat similar geography and demography to the UAE. One such report included women presenting to an obstetrics and gynecology department at a hospital in Bahrain [7]. It reported the following epithelial abnormalities on Pap smears from 1082 women: LSIL 1.94%, HSIL 0.46%, ASCUS 0.18% and invasive lesions in 0.64%. The most common hrHPV type was HPV 16 and 52. In addition, HPV 18, 31, 33, 51, 44, 45, 56 and 59 were detected in their study population. The sample included both Bahraini women (32%) and other nationalities [7]. Hajja et al. has demonstrated the presence of hrHPV genotypes 16,18,45,62 and 53 in a smaller sample of 100 women attending a gynecology clinic in Bahrain [8]. In Saudi Arabia, the prevalence of HPV infection was 9.8% among Saudi women seen during routine screening [9]. The most common hrHPV were 68/73 (12%), HPV 18 (9.8%) and HPV 16 (7.3%) [9]. In a population based study performed on 799 Iranian women, cervical abnormalities were detected in about 5% of Pap smears. hrHPV genotypes were found to be HPV 16, 18, 31, 33, 51, 56 and 66 [10]. A molecular study conducted in Pakistan on a sample of normal cervical smears demonstrated the following hrHPV types in their sample: HPV 33 (8.33%), HPV 18 (6.25%) and HPV 16 (4.17%) [11].

In the ATHENA trial conducted in the USA on a large screening population, HPV 16 was reported as the most commonly associated hrHPV genotype with high-grade cervical lesions. In addition, the report also found an association of hrHPV 18 with half of the cases of in-situ and invasive adenocarcinoma of the uterine cervix [12].

Data regarding the exact prevalence of various hrHPV types in the UAE population are limited. In 2008, the Health Authority of Abu Dhabi (HAAD) introduced HPV vaccination to all female students between the ages of 15–17. In addition, regular screening is recommended every 3–5 years to women aged 25–65 [13]. Both FDA approved vaccines, e.g., quadrivalent (Gardasil, Merck) and bivalent (Cervarix, GlaxoSmithKline Biologicals) are approved and administered in the UAE. Gardasil vaccine targets HPV 6, 11, 16, and 18 with an aim to reduce the incidence of genital condylomas caused by HPV 6, 11 and cervical/vaginal/vulvar intraepithelial neoplasias (CINs, VAINs, VIN) and carcinomas caused by the most frequently implicated subtypes of hrHPV 16, 18. Cervarix is administered in the UAE for the prevention of cervical carcinoma that targets HPV 16 and 18 [14, 15].

Multiplex Real-Time Polymerase Chain Reaction-based (PCR) technique has recently been used to genotype hrHPV in the UAE population which allows simultaneous detection of multiple hrHPV genotypes [16].

Knowledge of the specific hrHPV subtypes in the UAE population would not only help guide the formulation of proper cancer screening recommendations, but also assist in directing vaccination program strategies should the infection patterns deviate from the known national/ regional/ and international epidemiologic data.

Methods
Subjects

Women diagnosed with cervical squamous intraepithelial neoplasias and cervical carcinomas were retrieved from the archives of the Department of Pathology at a tertiary care hospital (Tawam Hospital, Abu Dhabi) during the period from 2012 to 2016. Hematoxylin and eosin stained slides were reviewed by two of the investigators (MRQ and SAA) to confirm the diagnosis. Paraffin tissue blocks were retrieved on all cases except those with insufficient residual tissue. Cases were classified based on morphologic criteria for cervical neoplasia according to the World Health Organization (WHO) Classification of Tumors of Uterine Cervix [4]. Demographic and pathological data including age, nationality, pathological diagnosis and tumor-related histological features where applicable (histological subtype, tumor size, grade, stage) were all documented.

DNA extraction and HPV typing

Five representative tissue sections (each 10-μ-thick) were obtained from archival formalin fixed paraffin embedded (FFPE) tissue and placed in Eppendorf tubes. Sterile precautions were taken to avoid cross-contamination including changing cutting blades between cases and changing hand gloves. DNA was extracted using the QIAamp DNA FFPE Tissue Kit (QIAGEN Inc., Valencia, CA 91355, Cat No. 56404) at Women & Infants Hospital, Providence, RI, USA following the protocol recommended by the manufacturer. hrHPV genotyping was initially performed using multiplex PCR followed by Tag/Capsure probe hybridization at Memorial Hospital of Rhode Island, USA, a laboratory facility of Women & Infants Hospital. Subsequently the findings were ratified using a second detection method, GenomeMeTM's GeneNavTM HPV One qPCR Kit (GenomeMe, Richmond, BC, Canada) which specifically detected HPV 16 and18 and non-specially detected other rare subtypes. Subsequently all non-16/18 positive samples were typed on-site at GenomeMe, Canada, Richmond, BC, Canada using their GeneNavTM HPV Genotyping qPCR Kit.

Results

The study was based on a total of 75 cases including HSIL ($n = 70$), adenocarcinoma in-situ ($n = 1$) and invasive squamous cell carcinoma ($n = 4$). The median age for HSIL and higher lesions was 34 years (range 19–58 years). UAE nationals constituted 53 cases (70%) of the study sample. Overall, hrHPV types detected were 16, 18, 31, 33, 35, 39, 45, 51, 52, 58, 59, 66 and 68 (Table 1 and Fig. 1). Nine of 75 (12%) HSIL cases were negative for hrHPV. Most common types were HPV 16 (49%), HPV 31 (20%) and HPV 18 (6.6%). HPV 16 and 18 were identified in 56% and other types in 32%. Table 2 illustrates HPV distribution among

Table 1 Frequency of hrHPV types in 75 cases of HSIL/AIS/ Invasive carcinoma

Serotype detected	n^a (%)
HPV16	37 (49%)
HPV18	5 (6.6%)
HPV31	15 (20%)
HPV33	4 (5.3%)
HPV45	4 (5.3%)
HPV52	4 (5.3%)
HPV58	3 (4%)
HPV68	2 (2.6%)
HPV35	2 (2.6%)
HPV39	2 (2.6%)
HPV66	2 (2.6%)
HPV59	1 (1.3%)
HPV51	1 (1.3%)
Negative	9 (12%)
Two serotypes	8 (10.6%)
Three serotypes	4 (5.3%)

$^a n$ number of cases

different age groups. Patients between 25 and 45 years had a higher frequency of HPV 16 and 31. HPV 16 was present across all age groups. Co-infection was seen in 12 of the 75 cases (16%) (Table 3). Eight cases had two viral subtype infections and four cases had three subtype infections. Multi-viral HVP infection was limited to cases with HPV 16 ($n = 5$), 18 ($n = 2$), 33 ($n = 1$) & 31 ($n = 4$) only. Co-infection consisted of genotypes of the same species in four cases. The remaining cases were infected by a combination of HPV genotypes consisting of different species (67% of cases). The species detected in this study sample included α9 species (HPV 16, 31, 33, 52), α7 species (HPV 18, 39, 59, 68), α6 species (HPV 66) and α5 species (HPV 51).

The results of this study were presented in part at the 106th Annual Meeting of the USCAP in March 2017, San Antonio, Texas, USA [17].

Discussion

High-risk Human Papilloma Virus infection, the single most important etiologic agent for uterine cervical carcinomas, appears to show regional variation in the prevalence of its subtypes. Worldwide, the most common HPV genotypes are HPV 16/18 detected in up to 70% of cervical cancers [18]. The assumption that HPV 16 and 18 are also the most common genotypes in the UAE and other regions may not be accurate. Epidemiologic variability of infection pattern is more likely [19]. This is evident from various publications in the region and worldwide [9, 11].

The following reports published from Asia, South America, Europe, Africa, and North America also ratify this view. In Turkey, HPV 16 (20.7%) represented the most common HPV genotype in a screening sample of one million women. It was followed by HPV 51 (10.8%), 31 (8.7%), 52 (7.1%) and 18 (5.1%) [20]. Similarly, a Malaysian study found HPV 16, 52 and 58 to be the most common types in their study sample of 1293 women [21].

A study in Bahrain reported HPV 16 and 52 as the most common types [7]. In a similar study on 298 women in Kuwait, the authors screened ThinPrep smears during routine gynecological examinations and genotyped HPV using PCR-based technique [22]. The study found that HPV 16 was the most common HPV type (24.3%). Other frequent types included HPV 11 (13.8%), HPV 66 (11.2%), HPV 33 (9.9%), HPV 53 (9.2%), HPV 81 (9.2%), HPV 56 (7.9%) and HPV 18 (6.6%) [22]. In Saudi Arabia, a cross-sectional study of 417 women (mean age 41.9) attending routine gynecological evaluations were screened for hrHPV [9], revealing HPV DNA in 9.8% (41 cases) of the study sample. The majority of their cases (77%) were Saudi women. The most common hrHPV types were hrHPV68/73 (12.2%) followed by HPV 18 (9.8%) and HPV 16 (7.3%). There were only 41 positive cases for HPV from the 417 cases assessed. Other HPV types detected were HPV 31 (4.9%), HPV 51 (4.9%), HPV 52 (4.9%), HPV 39

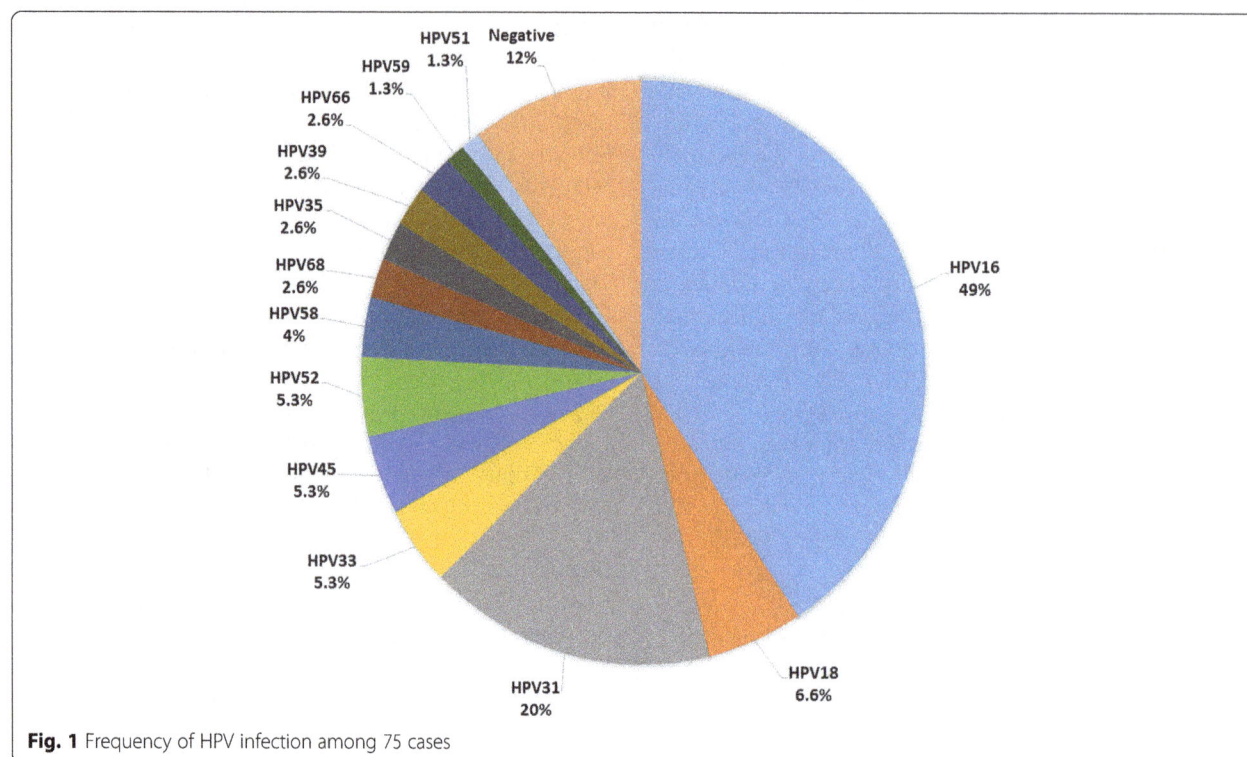

Fig. 1 Frequency of HPV infection among 75 cases

Table 2 HPV genotypes by age group

Age group	HPV genotypes
< 25	31
	16
25–34	58
	45
	33
	35 (n = 2)
	18 (n = 2)
	31 (n = 8)
	16 (n = 19)
35–44	18
	58 (n = 2)
	45(n = 2)
	31 (n = 4)
	16(n = 14)
45–54	45
	33
	18 (n = 2)
	16(n = 2)
+55	16

(2.4%), HPV 56 (2.4%) and HPV 58 (2.4%). The low-risk HPV types included HPV 6, 42, 53, 54, 11, 40, 70 and 74 in order of frequency [9]. The study, although offering a preview of the incidence of HPV in the Saudi population, may not hold true when a larger population based study is undertaken [9]. An Iranian study reported HPV 16 and 18 as the most common genotypes in their study population [10].

A study in Xinjiang (in north-western China) performed using routine Pap smear found that HPV 16, 58 and 39 are the most common genotypes [23]. In contrast, HPV 16 and 18 were the most common genotypes detected in a sample of 2309 cervical cancer patients in western China, followed by HPV 58, 53, and 33 [24]. Thus, even within the same country, there might be regional variations.

HPV 16 (38.9%) and HPV 58 (19.5%) were found to be the most common HPV genotype in cervical lesions and cervical cancer in the coastal region of Ecuador [25]. In the US, HPV 16 is the most common genotype in a screening population reported by the ATHENA trial [26]. In North America, HPV 16 constituted 5.8% and HPV 18 2.1% followed by HPV 52 2.0%. In contrast, in continental Europe HPV 16 constituted 4.8% and HPV 31 2.3% followed by HPV 18 0.9%. In African continent, HPV 16 (3.5%) and HPV 52 (2.4%) were the most prevalent types [27].

A recent study in the UAE on cases of ASCUS (atypical squamous cells of undetermined significance)

Table 3 HPV genotypes in cases of co-infection highlighing different HPV species in the 12 cases with co-infection

Case	HPV genotype	Co-infection1	Co-infection 2
1	33	68	
2	31	39	
3	31	52	
4	31	52	59
5	31	33	
6	18	51	52
7	18	33	66
8	16	66	
9	16	52	
10	16	68	
11	16	31	39
12	16	31	

α9 species

α7 species

α6 species

α5 species

demonstrated the presence of hrHPV in 17.9% of cases [28]. The authors also reported hrHPV 16 as the most common type isolated in ASCUS cases for patients aged 25–34 years. Interestingly the authors found that hrHPV 18 was more frequent in patients above 64 years. In addition, other hrHPV types were more frequent in their cases of ASCUS in patients between 25 and 45 years. The exact frequencies and genotypes, however, were not reported. The findings are in keeping with the current report showing hrHPV 18 as a less frequent hrHPV type in the UAE population [28]. Similarly, Krishnan and Thomas reported HPV 16 to be the most common HPV type in cases with abnormal Pap smear [29]. Likewise, hrHPV 18 was not the second most frequent type. The following hrHPV types (51, 31, 66, 56 and 59) were reported by all these authors [29].

Despite many publications on HPV genotypes in different regions, there are still some gaps in available data on different HPV genotypes in various geographic regions and even within different regions of the same country. This variability may reflect differences in geographic, ethnic, socio-cultural, and religious practices of the region. In a recent study in the USA found that HPV 16 was less prevalent in Hispanic and Black women compared to White women [26].

In the current study, HPV 16 was detected in the majority of cases (49%), whereas HPV 18 was detected only in 6.6% of the study sample, a significant deviation from what has been reported from the western world. Bruni et al. performed a meta-analysis on HPV infection prevalence dividing the studies into five geographic regions: worldwide, Americas, Africa, Asia and Europe. It included studies addressing both low and high risk HPV. They found that the most common HPV types worldwide were HPV 16 (3.2%) and HPV 18(1.4%) [27]. In northern America, HPV 16 constituted 5.8% and HPV 18 2.1% followed by HPV 52 2.0%. In contrast, in continental Europe HPV 16 constituted 4.8% and HPV 31 2.3% followed by HPV 18 0.9%. In African continent, HPV 16 3.5% and HPV52 2.4% were the most prevalent types [27].

The detection of HPV 31 in 20% of the samples examined in this study has potential implications in terms of vaccination strategies currently practiced here in the UAE. Currently, the two approved and available vaccines are the bivalent and the quadravalent vaccines which do not offer direct protection against HPV 31 [13–15]. Epidemiological studies are showing a trend of declining incidence of SIL and AIS in vaccinated subjects, and in addition, offering possible partial protection against some rare HPV types because of cross antigenicity [30]. Gardasil9, targets Types 6, 11, 16, 18, 31, 33, 45, 52, and 58 [31]. Thus, it appears reasonable to speculate that Gardasil9 might be a better alternative for the local population as HPV 31, detected in 20% of current study, is not one of the HPV subtypes to be directly protected by the two vaccines administered in the UAE currently.

Co-infection represented 16% of cases in the current study. It included cases infected with HPV 16, 18, 31, and 33. Infection with multiple species was present in 67% of the cases with co-infection. A study from India detected multiple genotypes in 23.41% of their HPV positive cases [32]. Interestingly, infection with multiple genotypes of α9 and α7species excluding HPV 16 and HPV 18 were associated with an increased risk of cervical cancer with an odds ratio of 5.3 and 2.5 respectively [32]. This finding is pertinent in formulating an effective vaccination strategy of any country or region. Quddus et al. detected co-infection in 32% of cases with adenosquamous carcinoma of the cervix in USA [33]. Hui et al. recently reported prevalence of multiviral HPV infection involving multiple anatomic sites of the lower female genital tract of the same individual and as high as 5 different subtypes of hrHPV were reported to be identified in an individual case in that series [34].

Ginindza et al. found that infection with multiple hrHPV increases in patients with decreased immunity.

In their study including HIV patients the prevalence of multiple hrHPV infection was 27.7% compared to 12.7% in non-HIV patients [35]. It has been postulated that co-infection may propel carcinogenesis based on the association of multiple HPV genotype infection with cervical carcinoma [35].

All these studies reveal considerable geographic variation within the region and also from the Western studies. Other studies in the region demonstrated different results. It also appears that the rare subtypes appear to be prevalent in this region with different cultural and religious backgrounds. As each country in this region, or for that matter any other region of the world, is governed by independent administration despite their proximity it is imperative that the exact prevalence of hrHPV in a particular country/region should be available for effective control of this disease.

The current pilot study is based on a limited number of samples. The finding ought to be ratified by larger, multicenter studies to get an actual overall incidence of the HPV subtypes in the country. The current study addressed cases that presented with HSIL or higher lesions. Thus, data on HPV type prevalence might be skewed toward the more aggressive lesions. One would argue that from a clinical perspective, the more aggressive lesions are those that need intervention to prevent progression and reduce the incidence of cervical cancer related mortality and morbidity. The sample of HSIL positivity might indicate that those cases with the less aggressive HPV types did not progress and may have resolved without progression. Thus, those cases would not need attention when vaccination and screening program recommendations are being implemented in the country.

The incidence of hrHPV among the UAE population emphasizes the need for qualified well-trained healthcare professionals and gynecologists, who can perform colposcopic examination, detect and manage the disease appropriately; unfortunately, that need that has not been met here as off yet as reported by Ghazal-Aswad et al. [36].

It is noteworthy to mention that even after using the most sensitive techniques available now, about 12% of UAE women studied did not show any detectable hrHPV in the tissues samples examined. This may imply that other carcinogenic factors may be responsible for these or there are more yet unrecognized hrHPV.

The current findings are significant for the UAE population where the quadrivalent vaccine is currently used. This entails the possibility of limited protection in at least 20% of cases infected with HPV 31. In addition, the presence of co-infection by different HPV species warrants recommendation of vaccines with a wider coverage. Results will impact future screening and prevention recommendation by the Cervical Cancer Prevention Taskforce. This study will serve as a foundation for a larger study which appears prudent to ratify our findings.

It is worth stating that risk of an HSIL lesion developing into invasive cancer depends to a large extent on the type of HPV. It has been shown that HPV 16 and 18 are detected in higher percentages in cases of invasive cervical squamous cell carcinoma in comparison to cases of LSIL. In addition, HPV 33 and 45 are similarly detected in invasive lesions. HPV 31 has an odds ratio of 3.4 of developing invasive cervical cancer. Thus, HPV type virulence is another consideration when vaccination and screening guidelines are addressed [3].

Conclusion

In conclusion, this pilot study illustrates that HPV 16 and 31 are the most frequent HPV genotypes in cervical neoplasia in the UAE population. Co-infection with multiple genotypes is present in 16% of cases and consists of different HPV subtypes. Should these findings hold true on a larger population-based study it would be imperative to introduce a vaccine which would offer direct protection against both common and some of the rare subtypes of HPV infection in the United Arab Emirates.

Abbreviations

ASCUS: Atypical squamous cells of undetermined significance; CIN: Cervical intraepithelial neoplasias; FFPE: Formalin fixed paraffin embedded; HAAD: Health Authority of Abu Dhabi; HPV: Human Papillomavirus; hrHPV: High-risk HPV; HSILs: High-grade squamous intraepithelial lesions; LSILs: Low- grade squamous intraepithelial lesions; PCR: Polymerase Chain Reaction-based; UAE: United Arab Emirates; VAIN: Vaginal intraepithelial neoplasias; VIN: Vulvar intraepithelial neoplasias; WHO: World Health Organization

Acknowledgements

We would like to acknowledge the technical assistance of Mr. Aktham Awad, Mr. Ahmed Shams and Ms. Dhanya Saraswathiamma. We are thankful to Ms. Hafsa Al Shebli for providing the ASCUS:SIL at Tawam Hospital. We also would like to acknowledge the assistance of Ms. Pamela Roberts for language editing and proofreading.

Funding

This work was supported by the College of Medicine and Health Sciences, United Arab Emirates University [grant# NP16-32, 2016].

Authors' contributions

ASA, SSA, MRQ and SAA designed the study. SSA and ASA collected data. SSA, ASA and MRQ reviewed slides and analyzed data. Laboratory tests for HPV were done under supervision of MRQ. SSA and MRQ drafted manuscript. All authors read and approved the final manuscript. Alia Saeed Albawardi (ASA), M. Ruhul Quddus (MRQ), Shamsa Abdulmanan Al Awar (SAA) and Saeeda Saleh Almarzooqi (SSA).

Competing interests

The authors declare that they have no competing interests.

Author details

[1]Pathology Department, College of Medicine and Health Sciences, UAE University, Al Ain, United Arab Emirates. [2]Department of Pathology, Women & Infants Hospital/Alpert Medical of Brown University, Providence, RI 02905, USA. [3]Obstetrics and Gynecology Department, College of Medicine and Health Sciences, UAE University, Al Ain, United Arab Emirates.

References

1. Health statistics 2015- Health Authority Abu Dhabi. Available from: https://www.haad.ae/HAAD/LinkClick.aspx?fileticket=gzx_WUkD27Y%3d&tabid=1516. Accessed 28 Aug 2017
2. International Agency of Research on Cancer, GLOBOCAN. Incidence and mortality data for the United Arab Emirates. 2008. Available from: http://globocan.iarc.fr/. Accessed 28 Aug 2017
3. IARC Monographs on the Evaluation of Carcinogenic Risks to Humans. IARC monographs 90-7: Studies of Cancer in Humans. Available from http://monographs.iarc.fr/ENG/Monographs/vol90/mono90-7.pdf. Accessed 25 Dec 2017
4. Stoler M, et al. Tumours of the uterine cervix. In: Kurman R, Carcangiu ML, Heerington CM, Young RH, editors. WHO Classification of Tumours of Female Reproductive Organs. 4th ed. Lyon: International Agency for Reseach on Cancer; 2014. p. 189–206.
5. Ghazal-Aswad S, Gargash H, Badrinath P, Al-Sharhan MA, Sidky I, Osman N, Chan NH. Cervical smear abnormalities in the United Arab Emirates: a pilot study in the Arabian Gulf. Acta Cytol. 2006;50(1):41–7.
6. Al Eyd GJ, Shaik RB. Rate of opportunistic pap smear screening and patterns of epithelial cell abnormalities in pap smears in ajman, United arab emirates. Sultan Qaboos Univ Med J. 2012;12(4):473–8.
7. Maqsood F, Arif W, Iqbal S, Bajwa ZI, Ali M. Prevalence of cervical abnormalities and co-existent human papilloma virus infection in a mixed Bahraini population. Annals of KEMU. 2011;17(3):256–61.
8. Hajjaj AA, Senok AC, Al-Mahmeed AE, Issa AA, Arzese AR, Botta GA. Human papillomavirus infection among women attending health facilities in the Kingdom of Bahrain. Saudi Med J. 2006;27(4):487–91.
9. AlObaid A, Al-Badawi IA, Al-Kadri H, Gopala K, Kandeil W, Quint W, Al-Aker M, DeAntonio R. Human papillomavirus prevalence and type distribution among women attending routine gynecological examinations in Saudi Arabia. BMC Infect Dis. 2014;14:643.
10. Eghbali SS, Amirinejad R, Obeidi N, Mosadeghzadeh S, Vahdat K, Azizi F, Pazoki R, Sanjdideh Z, Amiri Z, Nabipour I, Zandi K. Oncogenic human papillomavirus genital infection in southern Iranian women: population-based study versus clinic-based data. Virol J. 2012;9:194.
11. Aziz H, Iqbal H, Mahmood H, Fatima S, Faheem M, Sattar AA, Tabassum S, Napper S, Batool S, Rasheed N. Human papillomavirus infection in females with normal cervical cytology: Genotyping and phylogenetic analysis among women in Punjab,Pakistan. Int J Infect Dis. 2017;66:83–9. https://doi.org/10.1016/j.ijid.2017.11.009.
12. Monsonego J, Cox JT, Behrens C, Sandri M, Franco EL, Yap PS, Huh W. Prevalence of high-risk human papilloma virus genotypes and associated risk of cervical precancerous lesions in a large U.S. screening population: data from the ATHENA trial. Gynecol Oncol. 2015;137(1):47–54.
13. Health Authority of Abu Dhabi: Cervical Cancer Prevention Data. Available from: http://www.haad.ae/simplycheck/tabid/58/ctl/Details/Mid/387/ItemID/7/Default.aspx. Accessed 2 June 2015
14. Gardasil vaccine information. Available from: www.gardasil.com. Accessed 2 June 2015
15. Cervarix vaccine information. Available from: available from https://gskpro.com/en-gb/products/cervarix/. Accessed 4 June 2018
16. Tsakogiannis D, Diamantidou V, Toska E, Kyriakopoulou Z, Dimitriou TG, Ruether IG, Gortsilas P, Markoulatos P. Multiplex PCR assay for the rapid identification of human papillomavirus genotypes 16, 18, 45, 35, 66, 33, 51, 58, and 31 in clinical samples. Arch Virol. 2015;160(1):207–14.
17. Quddus MR, Albawardi A, Al-Awar S, Almarzooqi SSH. Frequency of Rare and Multi Viral High-Risk HPV Subtype Infection in Cervical Squamous and Glandular Lesions in an Immigrant Dominant Middle Eastern Country: A PCR-Based Study. Mod Pathol. 2017;30(Suppl 2):305A.
18. Castle PE, Maza M. Prophylactic HPV vaccination: past, present, and future. Epidemiol Infect. 2016;144(3):449–68. https://doi.org/10.1017/S0950268815002198.
19. Castellsagué X, Ault KA, Bosch FX, Brown D, Cuzick J, Ferris DG, Joura EA, Garland SM, Giuliano AR, Hernandez-Avila M, Huh W, Iversen OE, Kjaer SK, Luna J, Monsonego J, Muñoz N, Myers E, Paavonen J, Pitisuttihum P, Steben M, Wheeler CM, Perez G, Saah A, Luxembourg A, Sings HL, Velicer C. Human papillomavirus detection in cervical neoplasia attributed to 12 high-risk human papillomavirus genotypes by region. Papillomavirus Res. 2016;2:61–9. https://doi.org/10.1016/j.pvr.2016.03.002.
20. Gultekin M, Zayifoglu Karaca M, Kucukyildiz I, Dundar S, Boztas G, Turan HS, Hacikamiloglu E, Murtuza K, Keskinkilic B, Sencan I. Initial results of population based cervical cancer screening program using hpv testing in one million turkish women. Int J Cancer. 2017; https://doi.org/10.1002/ijc.31212.
21. Khoo SP, Bhoo-Pathy N, Yap SH, Anwar Shafii MK, Hairizan Nasir N, Belinson J, Subramaniam S, Goh PP, Zeng M, Tan HD, Gravitt P, Woo YL. Prevalence and sociodemographic correlates of cervicovaginal human papillomavirus (HPV) carriage in a cross-sectional, multiethnic, community-based female Asian population. Sex Transm Infect. 2017; https://doi.org/10.1136/sextrans-2017-053320.
22. Al-Awadhi R, Chehadeh W, Jaragh M, Al-Shaheen A, Sharma P, Kapila K. Distribution of human papillomavirus among women with abnormal cervical cytology in Kuwait. Diagn Cytopathol. 2013;41(2):107–14. https://doi.org/10.1002/dc.21778.
23. Mijit F, Ablimit T, Abduxkur G, Abliz G. Distribution of human papillomavirus (HPV) genotypes detected by routine pap smear in Uyghur-Muslim women from Karasay Township Hotan (Xinjiang, China). J Med Virol. 2015;87(11):1960–5. https://doi.org/10.1002/jmv.24240.
24. Li K, Yin R, Wang D, Li Q. Human papillomavirus subtypes distribution among 2309 cervical cancer patients in West China. Oncotarget. 2017;8(17):28502–9. https://doi.org/10.18632/oncotarget.16093.
25. Bedoya-Pilozo CH, Medina Magües LG, Espinosa-García M, Sánchez M, Parrales Valdiviezo JV, Molina D, Ibarra MA, Quimis-Ponce M, España K, Párraga Macias KE, Cajas Flores NV, Orlando SA, Robalino Penaherrera JA, Chedraui P, Escobar S, Loja Chango RD, Ramirez-Morán C, Espinoza-Caicedo J, Sánchez-Giler S, Limia CM, Alemán Y, Soto Y, Kouri V, Culasso ACA, Badano I. Molecular epidemiology and phylogenetic analysis of human papillomavirus infection in women with cervical lesions and cancer from the coastal region of Ecuador. Rev Argent Microbiol. 2017; https://doi.org/10.1016/j.ram.2017.06.004.
26. Montealegre JR, Peckham-Gregory EC, Marquez-Do D, Dillon L, Guillaud M, Adler-Storthz K, Follen M, Scheurer ME. Racial/ethnic differences in HPV 16/18 genotypes and integration status among women with a history of cytological abnormalities. Gynecol Oncol. 2017. doi: https://doi.org/10.1016/j.ygyno.2017.12.014.
27. Bruni L, Diaz M, Castellsagué X, Ferrer E, Bosch FX, de Sanjosé S. Cervical human papillomavirus prevalence in 5 continents: meta-analysis of 1 million women with normal cytological findings. J Infect Dis. 2010;202(12):1789–99. https://doi.org/10.1086/657321.
28. Fakhreldin M, Elmasry K. Improving the performance of reflex Human Papilloma Virus (HPV) testing in triaging women with atypical squamous cells of undetermined significance (ASCUS): A restrospective study in a tertiary hospital in United Arab Emirates (UAE). Vaccine. 2016;34(6):823–30. https://doi.org/10.1016/j.vaccine.2015.12.011.
29. Krishnan K, Thomas A. Correlation of cervical cytology with high-risk HPV molecular diagnosis, genotypes, and histopathology-A four year study from the UAE. Diagn Cytopathol. 2016;44(2):91–7. https://doi.org/10.1002/dc.23391.
30. Skinner SR, Apter D, De Carvalho N, Harper DM, Konno R, Paavonen J, Romanowski B, Roteli-Martins C, Burlet N, Mihalyi A, Struyf F. Human papillomavirus (HPV)-16/18 AS04-adjuvanted vaccine for the prevention of cervical cancer and HPV-related diseases. Expert Rev Vaccines. 2016;15(3):367–87. https://doi.org/10.1586/14760584.2016.1124763.
31. Wat is Gardasil9?. Available from: https://www.gardasil9.com/about-gardasil9/what-is-gardasil9/. Accessed 2 June 2015
32. Senapati R, Nayak B, Kar SK, Dwibedi B. HPV genotypes co-infections associated with cervical carcinoma: Special focus on phylogenetically related and non-vaccine targeted genotypes. PLoS One. 2017;12(11):e0187844. https://doi.org/10.1371/journal.pone.0187844.

33. Quddus MR, Manna P, Sung CJ, Kerley S, Steinhoff MM, Lawrence WD. Prevalence, distribution, and viral burden of all 15 high-risk human papillomavirus types in adenosquamous carcinoma of the uterine cervix: a multiplex real-time polymerase chain reaction-based study. Hum Pathol. 2014;45(2):303–9. https://doi.org/10.1016/j.humpath.2013.07.048.

34. Hui Y, Manna P, Ou J, Kerley S, Zhang C, Sung CJ, Lawrence WD, Quddus MR. High-risk human papilloma virus infection involving multiple anatomic sites of the female genital tract: a multiplex real-time polymerase chain reaction-based study. Hum Pathol. 2015;46:1376–81.

35. Ginindza TG, Dlamini X, Almonte M, Herrero R, Jolly PE, Tsoka-Gwegweni JM, Weiderpass E, Broutet N, Sartorius B. Prevalence of and Associated Risk Factors for High Risk Human Papillomavirus among Sexually Active Women, Swaziland. PLoS One. 2017;12(1):e0170189. https://doi.org/10.1371/journal.pone.0170189.

36. Ghazal-Aswad S, Badrinath P, Sidky I, Gargash H. Colposcopy services in the United Arab Emirates. J Low Genit Tract Dis. 2006;10(3):151–5.

8

Physical basis of the 'magnification rule' for standardized Immunohistochemical scoring of HER2 in breast and gastric cancer

Andreas H. Scheel[1][*], Frédérique Penault-Llorca[2], Wedad Hanna[3], Gustavo Baretton[4], Peter Middel[5,6], Judith Burchhardt[5], Manfred Hofmann[5], Bharat Jasani[7] and Josef Rüschoff[5,7]

Abstract

Background: Detection of HER2/neu receptor overexpression and/or amplification is a prerequisite for efficient anti-HER2 treatment of breast and gastric carcinomas. Immunohistochemistry (IHC) of the HER2 protein is the most common screening test, thus precise and reproducible IHC-scoring is of utmost importance. Interobserver variance still is a problem; in particular in gastric carcinomas the reliable differentiation of IHC scores 2+ and 1+ is challenging. Herein we describe the physical basis of what we called the 'magnification rule': Different microscope objectives are employed to reproducibly subdivide the continuous spectrum of IHC staining intensities into distinct categories (1+, 2+, 3+).

Methods: HER2-IHC was performed on 120 breast cancer biopsy specimens ($n = 40$ per category). Width and color-intensity of membranous DAB chromogen precipitates were measured by whole-slide scanning and digital morphometry. Image-analysis data were related to semi-quantitative manual scoring according to the magnification rule and to the optical properties of the employed microscope objectives.

Results: The semi-quantitative manual HER2-IHC scores are correlated to color-intensity measured by image-analysis and to the width of DAB-precipitates. The mean widths ±standard deviations of precipitates were: IHC-score 1+, 0.64 ± 0.1 μm; score 2+, 1.0 ± 0.23 μm; score 3+, 2.14 ± 0.4 μm. The width of precipitates per category matched the optical resolution of the employed microscope objective lenses: Approximately 0.4 μm (40×), 1.0 μm (10×) and 2.0 μm (5×).

Conclusions: Perceived intensity, width of the DAB chromogen precipitate, and absolute color-intensity determined by image-analysis are linked. These interrelations form the physical basis of the 'magnification rule': 2+ precipitates are too narrow to be observed with 5× microscope objectives, 1+ precipitates are too narrow for 10× objectives. Thus, the rule uses the optical resolution windows of standard diagnostic microscope objectives to derive the width of the DAB-precipitates. The width is in turn correlated with color-intensity. Hereby, the more or less subjective estimation of IHC scores based only on the staining-intensity is replaced by a quasi-morphometric measurement. The principle seems universally applicable to immunohistochemical stainings of membrane-bound biomarkers that require an intensity-dependent scoring.

Keywords: HER2/neu, Immunohistochemistry, Breast cancer, Gastric cancer, Magnification rule, Predictive biomarker

* Correspondence: andreas.scheel@uk-koeln.de
[1]Institute of Pathology, University Hospital Cologne, Kerpener Str. 62, 50937 Cologne, Germany
Full list of author information is available at the end of the article

Background

Targeting the HER2/neu pathway [1] has shown remarkable efficiency in the treatment of breast and gastric cancer [2, 3]. A prerequisite for specific treatment is the demonstration of HER2 receptor overexpression by immunohistochemistry (IHC) and/or *HER2/neu* gene amplification by in-situ hybridization (ISH) [4–6]. Although advanced DNA-sequencing techniques have been demonstrated to analyze panels of oncogenic genomic aberrations including amplification of HER2/neu [7], current testing guidelines are based on IHC and ISH only [4, 5]. Most algorithms use IHC as first screening test and ISH as second test for the confirmation of equivocal cases (IHC 2+). Thus, IHC plays a key-role for HER2 testing in the routine diagnostics of breast and gastroesophageal cancer.

Interpretation of HER2-IHC is, however, more or less subjective which causes overall disagreement rates of around 10% [8]. The main issue in breast cancer is false positive scoring while in gastric cancer false negative scoring is the major problem. In a retrospective central review of 187 HER2 stained breast cancer specimens from 10 pathological institutions 9.5% of the negative cases were reclassified as positive and 31.7% of the positive cases as negative [9]. In gastric cancer, a central review of 394 HER2 stained specimens from 19 French pathological institutions revealed a false positive rate of 5% but a false negative rate of 27.4% [10]. This problem has recently also been addressed by the panelists of the new HER2 testing guideline for gastric and gastroesophageal cancer [5]. It is stated that in particular reproducibility of 1+ and 2+ IHC scores can be low and the distinction between 1+ and 2+ is "challenging". However, it remains unclear to the reader how this particular scoring problem can be resolved in clinical practice.

From the perspective of our long-standing experience with HER2 testing, e.g., as the central lab for HERA [2] and ToGA [3] trials, we consider subjectivity in IHC-scoring as major source of discordant results between local and central testing. This is particularly true for false negative HER2 testing in gastric cancer. In contrast to breast cancer where ring-shaped membranous staining is crucial to score a case either positive (IHC 3+) or potentially positive (IHC2+), scoring in gastric cancer is solely based on intensity assessment by eye. Due to neurophysiological limitations it is practically impossible to objectively assess color-intensities alone unless other structural criteria, e.g. such as ring-shaped staining, are included [11–13].

In the context of the ToGA-study [3] we therefore developed a semiquantitative approach called 'magnification rule' (MR) that relates staining-intensity to the microscope magnification used to perceive it: Any

membranous staining that can be recognized at low magnification (2.5-5× objective lens) corresponds to IHC3+; if higher magnification (10×-20×) is needed to unequivocally identify stained membranes, IHC2+ is diagnosed. Any staining visible only at 40× objective lens represents an IHC1+ score [14, 15].

By using this rule the inter-observer consensus raised significantly from κ< 0.5 to κ=0.805 in a study on 547 gastric cancer specimens evaluated by six pathologists [15]. The finding was confirmed by a recent study which compared HER2 scoring by conventional light microscopy and by virtual microscopy and yielded inter-observer concordance values of up to κ=0.811 [16]. Thus, the MR has already been incorporated in national recommendations on HER2-testing in gastric cancer [6, 17]. This quasi-morphometric semiquantitative approach applies also to HER2-IHC scoring in breast cancer where it is used for the first step of scoring, i.e. the estimation of the color-intensity, before the second criterion, the ring-shape pattern of the staining, is assessed [15, 17].

The present study analyses the physical background of the MR using a series of 120 breast cancer samples immunostained for HER2. The data provide a physical basis of how the MR works to overcome subjectivity in the scoring of membrane-bound IHC-biomarkers.

Methods

Breast cancer biopsy specimens

One hundred and twenty specimens of invasive breast carcinoma (no special subtype; NST) were retrospectively investigated using routinely HER2 stained biopsies diagnosed within one year at the Institute of Pathology Nordhessen, Kassel, Germany (Example photomicrographs: Fig. 1, Additional file 1: Figure S1). HER2 status was determined according to the 2013 updated ASCO/CAP recommendations [4]. Accordingly, carcinomas classified as IHC 2+ were subsequently tested with dual-color chromogenic in situ hybridization (ISH) for amplification of the HER2/Neu Gene (INFORM HER2 Dual ISH DNA Probe Cocktail Assay, Ventana Medical Systems Inc., Tucson, USA). Anonymized cases were scored by three pathologists and the consensus score for each taken as the final IHC HER2 status.

IHC-staining and digital quantification

Immunohistochemistry (IHC) was performed using the 4B5 anti-HER2 primary antibody and a polymer-based detection system (UltraView DAB) on a BenchMark automated staining system (all by Ventana Medical Systems Inc., Tucson, USA). Peroxidase-conjugated secondary antibodies were used for chromogenic detecting by oxidizing 3,3′-Diaminobenzidin according to the manufactures protocol.

Magnification	40x	20x	10x	5x
Consensus Intensity-Score	'1+'	'2+'		'3+'
Num. Aperture	0.65 - 0.75	0.40 - 0.50	0.25 - 0.30	0.12 - 0.15
Resolution [µm]	0.40 - 0.46	0.60 - 0.75	1.0 - 1.20	2.0 - 2.50
DAB-Precipitate width ± SD [µm]	0.64 ± 0.1	1.0 ± 0.23		2.14 ± 0.4

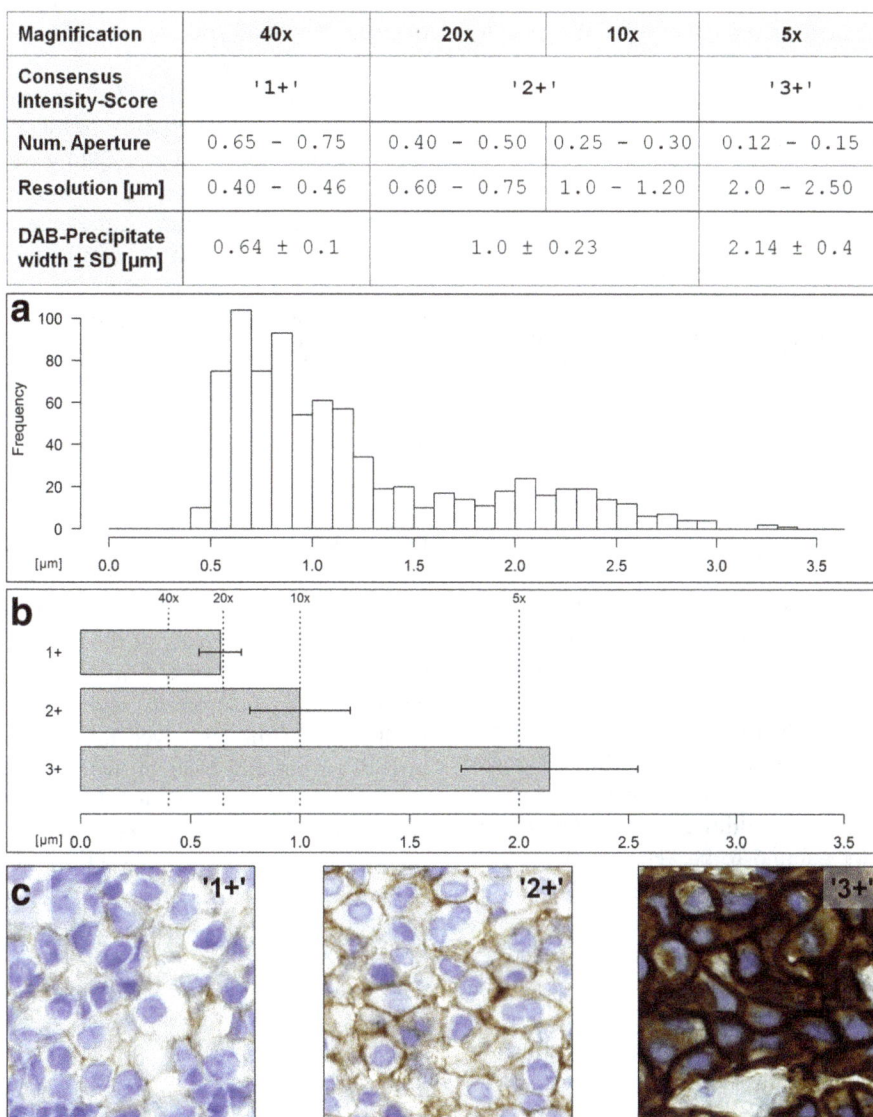

Fig. 1 Her2-IHC scoring categories reflect DAB-precipitate widths. Table: Microscope objectives have a fixed resolution that depends on the numerical aperture (Range: Values of common objectives). DAB-precipitates in HER2-IHC differ in width according to the intensity score. **a** histogram: Summary of 1200 DAB-precipitate-width measurements in µm. **b** bar chart: Mean DAB-width (bars) ±SD (antennae); resolution of standard microscope objectives (dashed lines). **c** images: Representative HER2-IHC stainings of invasive ductal breast carcinomas according to intensity score

IHC HER2 stained slides were digitized using a Pannoramic P250 whole slide scanner (3D Histech, Budapest, Hungary) at 5.11 pixel/µm. DAB-precipitate thickness was measured with 'ImageJ' image-analysis software [18]. The regions of interest (ROIs) were manually defined according to the following rules: 10 non-adjacent tumor cells were measured per specimen. For each cell, ROIs perpendicular to the precipitate were drawn at 4 positions, i.e. 40 measurements per specimen, 4800 measurements in total. DAB-precipitate intensities were calculated using a color deconvolution algorithm [19]. The mean ROI-length and color intensity was calculated for each cell. The 8bit grey-scale intensity-

values (0 = black, 256 = white) are as stated inverted, relative values to facilitate interpretation (0% = white, no staining; 100% black, full staining-intensity).

Microscope resolution

The resolution (d) of the objective of a light microscope is the minimum distance required to distinguish two adjacent points on a focal plane. In light microscopy d is determined by the numerical apertures (NA) of the microscope objectives and condenser and the wavelength of the employed light (λ) through Abbe's law $= \frac{\lambda}{2NA}$. NA is defined as $NA = n * \sin(\alpha)$ by the half-angle of the maximum cone of light that can pass through the objective (α) and the index of refraction (n) of the medium in which the objective is used, $d = \frac{\lambda}{2n \sin(\alpha)}$. For λ=600 nm, standard diagnostic microscope objectives yield the resolutions 5×: 2.0 µm (NA=0.14), 10×: 1.0 µm (NA=0.3), 20×: 0.6 µm (NA=0.5), 100×: 0.4 µm (NA=0.75).

Statistics

Statistics and statistical testing were performed using 'R' statistical programming language (http://www.r-project.org/). The data were found normally distributed and were tested using the Welch two-sample t-test. In all tests, the significance level was set to α = 1%.

Results

HER2-IHC scoring categories reflect the width of DAB-precipitates

In total, n = 120 cases of invasive breast carcinoma (no special subtype; NST) were analyzed which yielded 4800 individual measurements. The linear DAB-precipitates formed by the HER2-IHC were quantified. Plotting the width of the precipitates per cells as continuous histogram yielded a biphasic distribution (Fig. 1a). However, if the cells per case are aggregated by the arithmetic mean, three groups emerged that matched the manual scoring categories (Fig. 1b, Additional file 2: Figure S2). The mean widths were found to be: IHC-score 1+, 0.64 ± 0.1 µm; score 2+, 1.0 ± 0.23 µm; score 3+, 2.14 ± 0.4 µm. The differences between the three groups are statistically significant (p < 0.01). Thus, the scoring categories indicate groups of cases with perceivable differences in the widths of the DAB-precipitates.

The values were related to the optical resolutions of diagnostic microscope objectives. As predicted by the MR, precipitates of the scoring category 1+ are too narrow to be observable with a 10× microscopic lens and are delineated best by a 40× objective. Moreover, 2+ precipitates are broad enough to be visible at 10× but to narrow to be visible at 5×. Only 3+ precipitates were found broad enough to be readily recognizable if a 5× (or even a 2.5×) objective lens is used (Fig. 1). The forth scoring category, '0' was omitted, as the DAB-precipitates were found absent or insufficient for quantification.

Precipitate width and color intensity are correlated

Color intensity of the DAB-precipitates was determined using color deconvolution [19]. Similar to the precipitate width, the intensities of the three scoring categories were significantly different (p < 0.01) (Fig. 2). Moreover, a good linear correlation between width and intensity was noticed among scoring categories 1+ and 2+ (Pearson's r = 0.73). The intensity in scoring category 3+ was saturated (Additional file 3: Figure S3).

Precipitate width and color intensity do not differentiate between amplified and non-amplified cases in the IHC 2+ scoring category

All cases classified as IHC 2+ were subsequently tested for *HER2/neu* gene amplification by in situ hybridization (ISH). Among the study cases, 20 were ISH positive and 20 were ISH negative. The DAB-precipitate width showed a non-significant difference between the ISH positive cases (1.02 ± 0.23 µm) and the ISH negative cases (0.98 ± 0.22 µm, p = 0.02485). Indeed, histograms of the individual cells showed that the IHC 2+ ISH positive and IHC 2+ ISH negative cases feature almost completely overlapping precipitate widths (Additional file 2: Figure S2). No difference in the HER2-IHC color intensities was noticed between ISH negative and ISH positive cases either (p = 0.7493) (Fig. 2).

Discussion

HER2-IHC scores determined according to the 'magnification rule' (MR) were compared to image-analysis of width and color intensity of the DAB chromogen precipitates along the tumor cell membranes. The parameters were closely correlated and matched the optical resolutions of the employed microscope objectives. This provides a physical basis of the MR which was originally established as an empirical rule for standardized HER2-IHC scoring in gastric cancer.

HER2-IHC assays are based on peroxidase-coupled secondary antibodies that oxidize 3,3′-diaminobenzidine (DAB) into an insoluble, brownish precipitate at the spot of the bound epitope. As HER2 is confined to the cell-membrane, the reaction yields linear precipitates at the cell-boundaries. Technical aspects of HER2-IHC are robust and can be standardized by validated protocols, on-slide control tissue and external quality assessment [20–22] but interpretation of the resulting staining patterns may be challenging [4]: HER2-IHC scoring relies on subdividing the cases into categories based on staining-intensity (0, 1+, negative; 2+, equivocal, requires ISH-testing; 3+ positive) (Fig. 1, Additional file 1: Figure S1).

The human optical system is optimized to notice relative differences in color-intensity rather than absolute values. Visual stimuli are precortically processed in the retina through lateral inhibition which underlies varies optical illusions first described by Ernst Mach in 1865 as 'Mach bands' [12]. A given surface might appear brighter or darker depending on the luminosity of its surroundings [11, 13]. Accordingly, intensity-scores in histopathology are in general prone to subjectivity.

This is of particular importance in HER2-IHC scoring in gastric cancer, which is based solely on staining-intensity. In contrast, HER2-IHC scoring in breast cancer also includes the staining-pattern as the DAB-precipitates have to be ring-shaped to be considered as IHC 3+. In

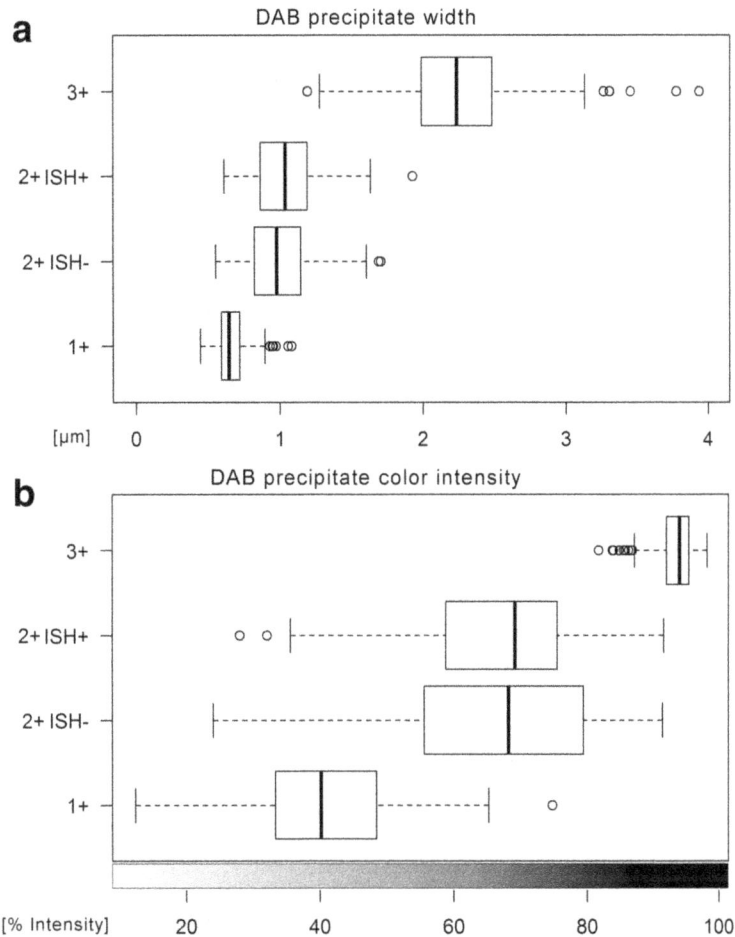

Fig. 2 Width and color intensity of HER2 are correlated. Immunohistochemistry of $n = 120$ cases of invasive ductal carcinoma of the mammary gland show that width of the linear DAB precipitates (**a**) and DAB color intensity (**b**) are correlated (8bit scale, inverted relative values). However, neither parameter discriminates IHC Score 2+ samples that are *Her2* amplified (ISH+) or not amplified (ISH-) by in situ hybridization

particular, inter-observer reproducibility of categories 1+ and 2+ scores can be low in gastric cancer. In two global clinical trials 6.4% (29/455) of cases with intestinal or mixed histology were found erroneously classified as HER2-IHC negative. In most of these cases ($n = 21$) initial scores were IHC 0 or IHC 1+ whereas central counter-testing revealed either IHC 2+ and ISH positivity ($n = 17$) or even IHC 3+ ($n = 4$). Four additional cases locally IHC 2+ FISH-negative were centrally ISH positive [23].

In a recent French study comprising 393 centrally re-evaluated gastric carcinomas false negative rate reached even 27.4% (20/73 HER2-IHC 2+). False positive rate was 5% (16/320) with an overall discordance rate of 9% [10].

In the present study it could be demonstrated that objectively measured widths and color intensities of the linear membranous precipitates correlate with the semi-quantitative intensity score manually assessed by MR. Utilizing this approach circumvents the need to interpret the staining just by color-intensity and constitutes a quasi-morphometric measurement.

Our data suggest that the MR might be applicable to other membrane-bound biomarkers as well. Indeed, inter-observer concordance of IHC-scoring of EGFR could be significantly improved within a round-robin test that included 11 international pathological laboratories [24]. The MR could also be included in the comprehensive 'Histo-Score' (H-Score) [25]. The H-Score incorporates all IHC-intensity categories and is frequently used to determine an optimal cut-point in IHC-scoring [26, 27]. The prerequisite to using the MR is that biological relevant scoring-categories have to be reflected by differences in the geometry of the histological stain that match the optical resolution windows of the microscope objectives. A given IHC-protocol could be optimized to match the appropriate intensity range.

The interrelation of DAB-width, -intensity and score might also form the basis for an image-analysis algorithm which mimics the magnification rule. Different approaches have been investigated for HER2-IHC image-analysis by using color intensities [28, 29] or geometric properties of the staining pattern [30]. Recent advances in digital image analysis have shown to increase of inter-observer agreement and decrease of the number of equivocally scored cases [31, 32].

Conclusions

IHC scoring by using the 'magnification rule' is a semi-quantitative procedure that circumvents neurophysiological restrictions of our visual system. It is based on physical interrelations and can be used to overcome subjectivity in HER2 IHC-testing, particularly in gastric cancer. It might also be applicable to other membrane-bound IHC-stainings. As a practical and easy-to-use method it has found wide application and was incorporated into national and international recommendation on HER2-IHC [6, 15, 17].

Additional files

Additional file 1: Figure S1. Example photomicrographs of HER2-IHC. Images depict scoring categories 1+, 2+ and 3+ at magnifications reflecting different microscope objectives (2.5× - 63×. Inserts: Magnified details, 4× additional magnification). Note that the linear DAB-precipitates in categories 1+ and 2+ are not perceivable at low power magnification (2.5×, 5×).

Additional file 2: Figure S2. Width of HER2 DAB-precipitates and result of in situ hybridization (ISH). Histograms of $n = 1200$ measurements in 40 cases per scoring category; estimated density (graphs).

Additional file 3: Figure S3. Scatter-plot of HER2 DAB-precipitates width and color intensity. For scoring intensities 1+ and 2+ (grey), width and intensity show a linear correlation ($r = 0.73$, dashed lined). Scoring category 3+ shows saturated intensity ($n = 1200$ measurements in 40 cases per scoring category).

Abbreviations

ASCO/CAP: American Society of Clinical Oncology / College of American Pathologists; DAB: Diaminobenzidine; HER2: The HER2 protein, i.e. human epidermal growth factor receptor 2; HER2/neu: The HER2/neu gene which encodes the HER2 protein; HERA: Acronym of the clinical phase 3 trial that tested adjuvant Trastuzumab in breast cancer, cf. Lancet. 2017; 389:1195-1205; IHC: Immunohistochemistry; ISH: In-situ hybridization; MR: Magnification rule; NA: Numerical aperture; ROI: Region of interest; SD: Standard deviation; ToGA: Acronym of the clinical phase 3 trial that tested adjuvant Trastuzumab in gastric cancer, cf. Lancet. 2010; 376:687-97; 0, 1+, 2+, 3 + : Categories of the scoring system for HER2-IHC interpretation; 4B5: Clone of the primary anti-HER2 antibodies used for HER2-IHC

Acknowledgements

We are much obliged to Sysmex (Norderstedt, Germany) for kindly providing us with the Pannoramic P250 whole slide scanner. We would like to thank Ulrike Hampacher and Heike Fliegel (Institute of Pathology Nordhessen, Kassel) for excellent technical assistance.

Funding

The study did not receive funding.

Authors' contributions

The magnification rule (MR) was conceived by JR. Usage of the MR in practical HER2-testing was tested and discussed by FPL, WH, GB, PM, MH, BJ and JR. The study was designed by AHS and JB under guidance of JR, PM and MH with support of FPL, WH and GB. Whole slide scanning was performed by JB and AHS. Manual HER2-scoring was done by JR, MH and PM. Image-analysis was done by AHS. Data-analysis was done by AHS under guidance of JR, PM, and BJ. The manuscript was drafted by AHS and JR. The manuscript was discussed with all coauthors and revised accordingly by AHS. The final version of the manuscript was agreed by all authors.

Competing interests

The authors declare that they have no competing interests.

Author details

[1]Institute of Pathology, University Hospital Cologne, Kerpener Str. 62, 50937 Cologne, Germany. [2]Département de Pathologie, Centre Jean-Perrin, 58, rue Montalembert, 392, 63011 Clermont-Ferrand cedex 1, BP, France. [3]Department of Laboratory Medicine and Pathobiology, University of Toronto, Toronto, Canada. [4]Institute of Pathology, University Hospital Dresden, Fetscherstr, 74, 01307 Dresden, Germany. [5]Institute of Pathology Nordhessen, Germaniastraße 7, 34119 Kassel, Germany. [6]Institute of Pathology, University Hospital Göttingen, Robert-Koch-Str. 40, 37075 Göttingen, Germany. [7]Targos Molecular Pathology GmbH, Germaniastraße 7, 34119 Kassel, Germany.

References

1. Yarden Y, Pines G. The ERBB network: at last, cancer therapy meets systems biology. Nat Rev Cancer. 2012;12:553–63.
2. Cameron D, Piccart-Gebhart MJ, Gelber RD, et al. 11 years' follow-up of trastuzumab after adjuvant chemotherapy in HER2-positive early breast cancer: final analysis of the HERceptin adjuvant (HERA) trial. Lancet. 2017; 389:1195–205.
3. Bang YJ, Van Cutsem E, Feyereislova A, et al. Trastuzumab in combination with chemotherapy versus chemotherapy alone for treatment of HER2-positive advanced gastric or gastro-oesophageal junction cancer (ToGA): a phase 3, open-label, randomised controlled trial. Lancet. 2010;376:687–97.
4. Wolff AC, Hammond ME, Hicks DG, et al. Recommendations for human epidermal growth factor receptor 2 testing in breast cancer: American Society of Clinical Oncology/College of American Pathologists clinical practice guideline update. J Clin Oncol. 2013;31:3997–4013.
5. Bartley AN, Washington MK, Ismaila N, Ajani JA. HER2 testing and clinical decision making in gastroesophageal adenocarcinoma: guideline summary from the College of American Pathologists, American Society for Clinical Pathology, and American Society of Clinical Oncology. J Oncol Pract. 2017;13:53–7.
6. Baretton G, Dietel M, Gaiser T, et al. HER2 testing in gastric cancer : results of a meeting of German experts. Pathologe. 2016;37:361–6.
7. Ross DS, Zehir A, Cheng DT, et al. Next-generation assessment of human epidermal growth factor receptor 2 (ERBB2) amplification status: clinical validation in the context of a hybrid capture-based, comprehensive solid tumor genomic profiling assay. J Mol Diagn. 2017;19:244–54.
8. Piccart-Gebhart MJ. St.Gallen International Breast Cancer Conference Primary Therapy of Early Breast Cancer Evidence, Controversies, Consensus; 11 - 14 Mar 2009; St. Gallen, Switzerland.
9. Orlando L, Viale G, Bria E, et al. Discordance in pathology report after central pathology review: implications for breast cancer adjuvant treatment. Breast. 2016;30:151–5.
10. Monges G, Terris B, Chenard M-P, et al. Assessment of HER2 status from an epidemiology study in tumor tissue samples of gastric and gastro-

esophageal junction cancer: Results from the french cohort of the HER-EAGLE study. JCO. 2013;31(4, Supplement S):26. http://ascopubs.org/doi/abs/10.1200/jco.2013.31.4_suppl.26.

11. Goldstein EB, editor. Blackwell handbook of perception. 4th ed. USA: Blackwell Publishers Inc; 2001. p. 53 ff.

12. Lotto RB, Williams SM, Purves D. Mach bands as empirically derived associations. Proc Natl Acad Sci U S A. 1999;96:5245–50.

13. Adelson EH. Perceptual organization and the judgment of brightness. Science. 1993;262:2042–4.

14. Rüschoff J, Dietel M, Baretton G, et al. HER2 diagnostics in gastric cancer-guideline validation and development of standardized immunohistochemical testing. Virchows Arch. 2010;457:299–307.

15. Rüschoff J, Hanna W, Bilous M, et al. HER2 testing in gastric cancer: a practical approach. Mod Pathol. 2012;25:637–50.

16. Behrens HM, Warneke VS, Böger C, et al. Reproducibility of Her2/neu scoring in gastric cancer and assessment of the 10% cut-off rule. Cancer Med. 2015;4:235–44.

17. Rakha EA, Starczynski J, Lee AH, Ellis IO. The updated ASCO/CAP guideline recommendations for HER2 testing in the management of invasive breast cancer: a critical review of their implications for routine practice. Histopathology. 2014;64:609–15.

18. Schneider CA, Rasband WS, Eliceiri KW. NIH image to ImageJ: 25 years of image analysis. Nat Methods. 2012;9:671–5.

19. Ruifrok AC, Johnston DA. Quantification of histochemical staining by colour deconvolution. Anal Quant Cytol Histol. 2001;23:291–9.

20. Choritz H, Büsche G, Kreipe H, et al. Quality assessment of HER2 testing by monitoring of positivity rates. Virchows Arch. 2011;459:283–9.

21. Vyberg M, Nielsen S, Røge R, et al. Immunohistochemical expression of HER2 in breast cancer: socioeconomic impact of inaccurate tests. BMC Health Serv Res. 2015;15:352.

22. Rüschoff J, Lebeau A, Kreipe H, et al. Assessing HER2 testing quality in breast cancer: variables that influence HER2 positivity rate from a large, multicenter, observational study in Germany. Mod Pathol. 2017;30:217–26.

23. Cunningham D, Shah MA, Smith D, et al. False-negative rate for HER2 testing in 738 gastric and gastroesophageal junction cancers from two global randomized clinical trials. J Clin Oncol. 2015;33(Supplement 3):16. http://ascopubs.org/doi/abs/10.1200/jco.2015.33.3_suppl.16.

24. Rüschoff J, Kerr KM, Grote HJ, et al. Reproducibility of immunohistochemical scoring for epidermal growth factor receptor expression in non-small cell lung cancer: round robin test. Arch Pathol Lab Med. 2013;137:1255–61.

25. Hirsch FR, Varella-Garcia M, Bunn PA Jr, et al. Epidermal growth factor receptor in non-small-cell lung carcinomas: correlation between gene copy number and protein expression and impact on prognosis. J Clin Oncol. 2003;21:3798–807.

26. Garon EB, Rizvi NA, Hui R, et al. Pembrolizumab for the treatment of non-small-cell lung cancer. N Engl J Med. 2015;372:2018–28.

27. Dolled-Filhart M, Roach C, Toland G, et al. Development of a companion diagnostic for Pembrolizumab in non-small cell lung cancer using immunohistochemistry for programmed death Ligand-1. Arch Pathol Lab Med. 2016;140:1243–9.

28. Ali HR, Irwin M, Morris L, et al. Astronomical algorithms for automated analysis of tissue protein expression in breast cancer. Br J Cancer. 2013;108:602–12.

29. Jeung J, Patel R, Vila L, Wakefield D, Liu C. Quantitation of HER2/neu expression in primary gastroesophageal adenocarcinomas using conventional light microscopy and quantitative image analysis. Arch Pathol Lab Med. 2012;136:610–7.

30. Laurinaviciene A, Dasevicius D, Ostapenko V, Jarmalaite S, Lazutka J, Laurinavicius A. Membrane connectivity estimated by digital image analysis of HER2 immunohistochemistry is concordant with visual scoring and fluorescence in situ hybridization results: algorithm evaluation on breast cancer tissue microarrays. Diagn Pathol. 2011;6:1746–596.

31. Helin HO, Tuominen VJ, Ylinen O, Helin HJ, Isola J. Free digital image analysis software helps to resolve equivocal scores in HER2 immunohistochemistry. Virchows Arch. 2016;468:191–8.

32. Nielsen SL, Nielsen S, Vyberg M. Digital image analysis of HER2 Immunostained gastric and gastroesophageal junction adenocarcinomas. Appl Immunohistochem Mol Morphol. 2017;25:320–8.

9

Evaluation of the correlation of MACC1, CD44, Twist1, and KiSS-1 in the metastasis and prognosis for colon carcinoma

Bo Zhu[1,2†], Yichao Wang[1,2†], Xiaolin Wang[1,2†], Shiwu Wu[1,2*], Lei Zhou[1,2], Xiaomeng Gong[1,2], Wenqing Song[1,2] and Danna Wang[1,2]

Abstract

Background: Metastasis-associated in colon cancer 1 (MACC1) has been reported to promote tumor cell invasion and metastasis. Cancer stem cells and epithelial-mesenchymal transition (EMT) have also been reported to promote tumor cell proliferation, invasion, and metastasis. KiSS-1, a known suppressor of metastasis, has been reported to be down-regulated in various tumors. However, the associations of MACC1, CD44, Twist1, and KiSS-1 in colonic adenocarcinoma (CAC) invasion and metastasis remain unclear. The purpose of this study is to investigate the roles of MACC1, CD44, Twist1, and KiSS-1 in CAC invasion and metastasis and their associations with each other and with the clinicopathological characteristics of CAC patients.

Methods: Immunohistochemistry and multivariate analysis were carried out to explore the expression of MACC1, CD44, Twist1, and KiSS-1 in 212 whole-CAC-tissue specimens and the corresponding normal colon mucosa tissues. Demographic, clinicopathological, and follow-up data were also collected.

Results: The results of this study showed MACC1, CD44, and Twist1 expression to be up-regulated, and KiSS-1 expression was down-regulated in CAC tissues. Positive expression of MACC1, CD44, and Twist1 was found to be positively correlated with invasion, tumor grades, and lymph- node-metastasis (LNM) stages and tumor-node-metastasis (TNM) stages for patients with CAC. Positive expression of KiSS-1 was inversely associated with invasion, tumor size, LNM stage, and TNM stage. The KiSS-1-positive expression group had significantly more favorable OS than did the KiSS-1-negative group. Univariate analysis indicated that overexpression of MACC1, CD44, and Twists1 was negatively associated with longer overall survival (OS) time, and there was a positive relationship between KiSS-1-positive expression and OS time for patients with CAC. Multivariate Cox analysis demonstrated that overexpression of MACC1, CD44, Twist1, and low expression of KiSS-1 and LNM and TNM stages were independent predictors of prognosis in patients with CAC.

Conclusions: The results in this study indicated that levels of expression of MACC1, CD44, Twist1, and KiSS-1 are related to the duration of OS in patients with CAC. MACC1, CD44, Twist1, and KiSS-1 may be suitable for use as biomarkers and therapeutic targets in CAC.

Keywords: CAC, MACC1, CD44, Twist1, KiSS-1

* Correspondence: wushiwu@bbmc.edu.cn
†Bo Zhu, Yichao Wang and Xiaolin Wang contributed equally to this work.
[1]Department of Pathology, The First Affiliated Hospital of Bengbu Medical College, Bengbu, China
[2]Department of Pathology, Bengbu Medical University, Bengbu, China

Background

Colorectal cancer (CRC) is the third most common cancer worldwide, with an estimated 1.4 million new cases in 2012 [1]. In China, CRC had an estimated 376,300 cases, which made it the fifth most common cancer in 2015 [2]. The most common causes of cancer treatment failure are relapse and metastasis. This may be related to an oncogene called metastasis-associated in colon cancer 1 (MACC1). In 2009, MACC1 was first found in colon cancer cell lines [3]. MACC1 is reported to combine with the mesenchymal-epithelial transition (MET) gene promoter and so participate in the hepatocyte growth factor/ mesenchymal-epithelial transition (HGF/MET) signaling pathway [3, 4]. MACC1 is also reported to not only promote tumor cell proliferation, invasion, and dissemination by inducing epithelial-mesenchymal transition (EMT) in vitro [5, 6] but also to induce tumor cell growth, invasion, and metastasis in vivo [3, 7]. It has been demonstrated that MACC1 should be defined as a prognostic and metastatic biomarker for various cancers [8].

Many more studies have ascribed tumor metastasis and recurrence to a subpopulation of tumor cells defined as cancer stem cells (CSCs, also called tumor-initiating cells). CSCs have the characteristics of self-renewal, proliferation, invasiveness, and metastasis. They are responsible for cancer initiation and natural resistance to therapy [8–12]. CD44 is not only a common biomarker of CSCs in cancers, such as colorectal cancer, lung cancer, and glioblastoma [13–15], but also a receptor of hyaluronan. CD44 levels are correlated with cell-to-extracellular matrix (ECM) adhesion, cell growth, and angiogenesis [16, 17].

It has been demonstrated that cancer cells can invade and metastasize after they lose epithelial features and gain a mesenchymal phenotype, which is called the epithelial-mesenchymal transition (EMT) [18, 19]. Twist1, which belongs to the highly conservative basic helix-loop-helix family, is a transcription factor. Twist1 is a pivotal regulator of EMT and reported to promote N-cadherin synthesis and inhibit E-cadherin expression [20, 21], thus causing profound morphological changes in tumor cells and expression of cell-matrix adhesion genes to induce tumor cell mobility and migration [22].

KiSS-1, which was originally identified in non-metastatic melanoma by analysis of subtractive hybridization, is widely considered a critical cancer metastasis suppressor gene [11, 23]. The KiSS-1 gene, which encodes a 145-amino-acid protein, can bind to the G protein-coupled receptor 54 (GPR54, also called KiSS-1R). KiSS-1 can control cell-cell adhesion by promoting E-cadherin expression and cell-matrix adhesion and cytoskeleton remodeling through inhibition of MMP expression [11, 24, 25]. KiSS-1 expression is also reported to suppress the metastatic potential of tumor cells but not tumorigenicity [25, 26]. Further studies have demonstrated that downregulation of KiSS-1 may be involved in the process of tumor invasiveness and metastasis [11, 25, 26].

The purpose of the current study is to assess the expression of MACC1, CD44, Twist1, and KiSS-1 in the colonic adenocarcinoma (CAC) tissues of patients and their associations between pathological characteristics and prognosis of patients with CAC. Immunohistochemistry was used to evaluate the expression of MACC1, CD44, Twist1, and KiSS-1 in CAC tissues and the corresponding adjacent normal colon mucosa tissues of patients with CAC.

Methods

Patients and tissue specimens

We collected the records of 212 patients (median age: 56.6 years; and range: 29–78 years) with CAC (rectal adenocarcinomas were excluded) diagnosed at the Department of Pathology at our hospital from January 2010 to December 2011. Because all outcomes had already taken place before the study began, it is retrospective. Patients who had any history of anti-cancer therapy were excluded. All patients with CAC provided written, extensively informed consent for their specimens to be used (including in hospital and out hospital). The study was carried out in accordance with the Declaration of Helsinki guidelines and approved by the Bengbu Medical College ethics committee (No. BBMCEC2016024). We collected patient data including complete clinicopathological, demographic, and follow-up data (follow-up at 3-month intervals through mobile phone or social applications). Overall survival (OS) time was computed from the date of radical surgery to date of death or to December 2016 (their mean OS: 53.3 months; and range: 22–72 months). TNM stages and LNM stages were calculated in accordance with the 8th edition of the guidelines issued by the American Joint Committee on Cancer (AJCC). Tumor grades were calculated in accordance with the standards issued by the World Health Organization (WHO). Specific clinicopathological characteristics are shown in Table 1.

Immunohistochemistry

All tissues were fixed in 10% buffered formalin solution and then embedded in paraffin. All tissues were then cut into 4-μm-thick sections. Immunostaining was conducted using the Elivision™ Plus method, and the procedure was performed in accordance with the kit instructions. Samples were deparaffinized using routine methods and dehydrated using xylene and alcohol. Methanol containing 3% H_2O_2 solution was used for blocking endogenous peroxidase activity, and citrate buffer was used to repair antigen. Goat serum was used for blocking. MACC1 (rabbit polyclonal antibody, Santa Cruz Biotechnology, US), CD44 (mouse monoclonal antibody, Abcam, US), Twist1 (mouse monoclonal antibody, Abcam, US), and KiSS-1

Table 1 Patients characteristics

Patients characteristics	Frequency (n)	Percentage (%)
Gender		
Male	142	67.0
Female	70	33.0
Ages		
≤ 60	134	63.2
> 60	78	36.8
Size		
≤ 2.0 cm	33	15.6
> 2.0 cm, ≤5.0 cm	110	51.9
> 5.0 cm	69	32.5
Location		
Ascending	42	19.8
Transverse	64	30.2
Descending	33	15.6
Sigmoid	73	34.4
Gross type		
Ulcerative	65	30.7
Infiltrating	46	21.7
Polypoid	68	32.1
Colloid	33	15.6
Invasion		
Submucosa	36	17.0
Muscularis	64	30.2
Subserosa[a]	101	47.6
Visceral peritoneum[b]	11	5.2
Grade		
Well	32	15.1
Moderate	135	63.7
Poor	45	21.2
Lymph node metastasis stages		
N0	136	64.2
N1	70	33.0
N2	6	2.8
TNM stage		
I	69	32.5
II	67	31.6
III	76	35.8

[a]The tumor has grown through the muscularis propria and into the subserosa, which is thin layer of connective tissue beneath the outer layer of some parts of the large intestine, or it has grown into tissues surrounding the colon. [b] The tumor has grown into the surface of the visceral peritoneum, which means it has grown through all layers of the colon, or the tumor has grown into or has attached to other organs or structures

(mouse monoclonal antibody, Santa Cruz Biotechnology, US) primary antibodies were added, and then all sections were incubated overnight at 4 °C. Then enhancer (reagent

A) and reagent B were added. The images were allowed to develop in diaminobenzidine (DAB) substrate. Finally, all sections were re-dyed with hematoxylin and mounted with gum.

Assessment of immunostaining

Ten randomly selected high-power-field (HPF) fields of every CAC section were selected to forestall any intratumoral heterogeneity of marker expression. In accordance with percentage of positive cells and positive intensity, immunostaining results were multiplied using intensity scores (0 points means none; 1 point means weak staining; 2 points means moderate staining; 3 point means strong staining) and percentage scores (1 point is positive cells ≤10%; 2 points is 10% < positive cells ≤50%; 3 points is 50% < positive cells ≤75%; 4 points is positive cells > 75%) which ranged from 0 to 12 [8, 11]. Here > 2 points was considered indicative of positive expression. For slices positive for all of biomarkers, the average score of all sections was taken.

Statistical analysis

All data were analyzed using SPSS 19.0 software (Chicago, IL, US). Countable data were subjected to the Chi-square test for comparisons between two groups. Multivariate logistic regression analysis was performed to establish the relative factors for metastasis. Univariate OS analysis was carried out using the Kaplan-Meier method with log-rank test. Multivariate OS analysis was carried out using Cox regression model test. $P < 0.05$ was considered indicative of statistically significant differences.

Results

Associations between MACC1, CD44, Twist1, and KiSS-1 in cancer tissues of patients and clinicopathological characteristics

As shown in Fig. 1a, b, MACC1-positive expression was mainly confined to the cytoplasm. The positive expression of MACC1 in the CAC specimens (61.3%, 130/212) was significantly higher than in the normal colon mucosa specimens (7.1%, 15/212; $P < 0.001$). The immunostaining results indicated that positive expression of MACC1 in CAC was positively correlated with invasion, tumor differentiation, LNM stages, and TNM stages (Table 2).

As shown in Fig. 1c, d, CD44 positive expression was mainly confined to the cell membrane and cytoplasm. Similar to MACC1, the positive expression of CD44-positive expression in CAC tissues (54.7%, 116/212) was significantly greater than in the normal colon mucosa tissues (16.5%, 35/212; $P < 0.001$). The results also demonstrated that positive expression of CD44 in CAC was positively correlated with invasion, tumor differentiation, LNM stages, and TNM stages (Table 2).

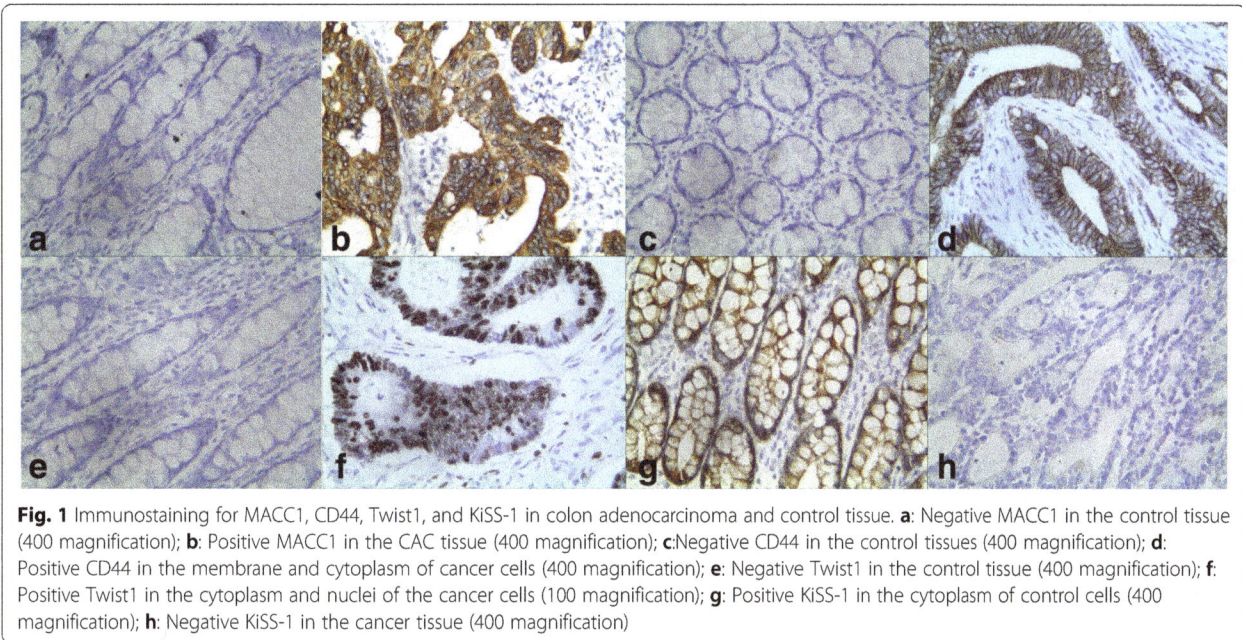

Fig. 1 Immunostaining for MACC1, CD44, Twist1, and KiSS-1 in colon adenocarcinoma and control tissue. **a**: Negative MACC1 in the control tissue (400 magnification); **b**: Positive MACC1 in the CAC tissue (400 magnification); **c**:Negative CD44 in the control tissues (400 magnification); **d**: Positive CD44 in the membrane and cytoplasm of cancer cells (400 magnification); **e**: Negative Twist1 in the control tissue (400 magnification); **f**: Positive Twist1 in the cytoplasm and nuclei of the cancer cells (100 magnification); **g**: Positive KiSS-1 in the cytoplasm of control cells (400 magnification); **h**: Negative KiSS-1 in the cancer tissue (400 magnification)

As shown in Fig. 1e, f, Twist1 expression was mainly confined to the cytoplasm and nuclei. The expression of Twist1 in CAC tissues (64.2%, 136/212) was significantly greater than in the normal colon mucosa tissues (9.4%, 20/212; $P < 0.001$). The results also showed that Twist1 expression in CAC was significantly closely associated with tumor differentiation, gross type, invasion, LNM stages, and TNM stages (Table 2).

As shown in Fig. 1g, h, KiSS-1-positive expression was mainly confined to the cytoplasm. The positive expression of KiSS-1 in CAC tissues (40.1%, 82/212) was significantly lower than in the normal colon mucosa tissues (94.3%, 200/212; $P < 0.001$). The results indicated that positive expression of KiSS-1 was inversely correlated with tumor size, invasion, LNM stages, and TNM stages (Table 2).

Associations among MACC1, CD44, Twist1, and KiSS-1 in CAC

The association between KiSS-1 expression and MACC1, CD44, and Twist1 expression was found to be negative ($r = -0.437$; $r = -0.397$; $r = -0.251$; respectively; $P < 0.001$) (Table 3). The association between MACC1 expression and CD44 expression and Twist1 expression was found to be positive ($r = 0.270$, $P < 0.001$; $r = 0.315$, $P < 0.001$). The association between CD44 expression and Twist1 expression was found to be positive ($r = 0.150$, $P = 0.029$) (Table 3).

Metastasis

Univariate metastasis analysis indicated that invasion was positively correlated with LNM stages ($P < 0.05$). Multivariate metastasis logistic analysis suggested that overexpression of MACC1, CD44, Twist1, and down-regulation of KiSS-1 and invasion were both significantly closely associated with LNM (Table 4).

Survival analysis

As shown in Fig. 2a, univariate OS analysis indicated that the OS time of MACC1+ (47.8 ± 12.5 months) for patients with CAC was significantly shorter than that of MACC1- for patients (62.0 ± 9.6 months; log-rank = 61.757, $P < 0.001$). As shown in Fig. 2b, the univariate OS time of CD44+ (46.8 ± 12.9 months) was significantly lower than in CD44- patients (61.2 ± 8.9 months; log-rank = 54.938, $P < 0.001$). As shown in Fig. 2c, the univariate OS time of Twist1+ patients (49.7 ± 13.0 months) was significantly lower than in Twist1- patients (59.7 ± 11.5 months; log-rank = 24.306, $P < 0.001$). As shown in Fig. 2d, the univariate OS time of KiSS-1+ patients (64.7 ± 4.9 months) was significantly greater than that of KiSS-1- patients (45.7 ± 11.6 months; log-rank = 115.258, $P < 0.001$). As shown in Fig. 2e, the univariate OS time of the combination of KiSS-1 negative expression and MACC1+, CD44+, and Twist1+ positive expression patients was significantly lower than that in KiSS-1 positive expression and MACC1-, CD44-, and Twist1- (log-rank = 84.625, $P < 0.001$). The univariate OS time was also significantly closely associated with the following other clinicopathological characteristics, invasion ($P = 0.002$, log-rank = 14.868; Fig. 2f), LNM stages ($P < 0.001$, log-rank = 325.068; Fig. 2g), and TNM stages ($P < 0.001$, log-rank = 152.179; Fig. 2h) (Table 5).

Table 2 The correlation between MACC1, or CD44, or Twist1, or KiSS-1 and clinicopathological characteristics in colon adenocarcinoma

Variable	MACC1 Negative	Positive	P	CD44 Negative	Positive	P	Twist1 Negative	Positive	P	KiSS-1 Negative	Positive	P
Gender			0.239			0.929			0.783			0.564
Male	51	91		64	78		50	92		87	55	
Female	31	39		32	38		26	44		40	30	
Age (years)			0.263			0.927			0.775			0.833
≤60	48	86		61	73		49	85		81	53	
>60	34	44		35	43		27	51		46	32	
Size (cm)			0.081			0.375			0.085			<0.001
≤2.0	10	23		14	19		10	23		16	17	
>2.0, ≤5.0	38	72		46	64		34	76		80	30	
>5.0	34	35		36	33		32	37		31	38	
Location			0.863			0.156			0.507			0.526
Ascending	17	25		21	21		13	29		21	21	
Transverse	22	42		25	39		22	42		39	25	
Descending	13	20		11	22		10	23		21	12	
Sigmoid	30	43		39	34		31	42		46	27	
Gross type			0.056			0.406			0.002			0.929
Ulcerative	27	38		35	30		31	34		37	28	
Infiltrating	10	36		20	26		6	40		28	17	
Polypoid	29	39		28	40		25	43		41	27	
Colloid	16	17		13	20		14	19		21	12	
Invasion			0.035			0.040			0.002			0.003
Submucosa	20	16		21	15		19	17		13	23	
Muscularis	19	45		29	35		30	34		38	26	
Subserosa	41	60		45	56		25	76		66	35	
Visceral peritoneum	2	9		1	10		2	9		10	1	
Grade			0.032			0.024			<0.001			0.745
Well	18	14		20	12		19	13		18	14	
Moderate	52	83		62	73		53	82		80	55	
Poor	12	33		14	31		4	41		29	16	
LNM stages			<0.001			<0.001			<0.001			<0.001
N0	71	65		85	51		64	72		60	76	
N1	11	59		11	59		12	58		61	9	
N2	0	6		0	6		0	6		6	0	
TNM stage			<0.001			<0.001			<0.001			<0.001
I	37	32		47	22		40	29		23	46	
II	34	33		38	29		24	43		37	30	
III	11	65		11	65		12	64		67	9	

Multivariate analysis suggested that MACC1, CD44, Twist1, and KiSS-1 expression, LNM stages, and TNM stages should be considered independent predictors affecting patient survival (Table 6).

Discussion

Colon cancer is a common malignant tumor of the digestive system. Its high heterogeneity makes it difficult to fully evaluate the comprehensiveness and effectiveness of any

Table 3 Correlation among MACC1, CD44, Twist1 and KiSS-1 in CAC

Variable	MACC1 Negative	MACC1 Positive	r	P	CD44 Negative	CD44 Positive	r	P	KiSS-1 Negative	KiSS-1 Positive	r	P
MACC1							0.270	< 0.001[a]			−0.437	< 0.001[b]
Negative					51	31			27	55		
Positive					45	85			100	30		
CD44			0.270	< 0.001[a]							−0.397	< 0.001[b]
Negative	51	45							37	59		
Positive	31	85							90	26		
Twist1			0.315	< 0.001[a]			0.150	0.029[a]			−0.251	< 0.001[b]
Negative	45	31			42	34			33	43		
Positive	37	99			54	82			94	42		

[a]positive correlation, [b]negative correlation

biomarker. Previous studies have demonstrated that MACC1 can promote tumor cell proliferation and migration [3, 4]. In this study, our findings indicated that positive expression of MACC1 in CAC was positively correlated with invasion and tumor differentiation and LNM and TNM stages. Positive expression of MACC1 was found to be significantly closely associated with lower OS time when compared with MACC1 negative. These findings demonstrated that MACC1 was considered an effective biomarker for invasion and metastasis, as well as a predictor for prognosis [3–8, 27, 28].

CD44 was initially considered an adhesion molecule capable of regulating cell-ECM adhesion, invasion, and metastasis [16, 17]. CD44 overexpression has been found to be correlated with tumorigenesis and to predict a poor response to anti-cancer therapy [8, 15]. The results recorded in this study also demonstrated that positive expression of CD44 in CAC was positively correlated with tumor differentiation, invasion, LNM stages, and TNM stages. CD44+ patients showed shorter OS times than CD44- patients. Several other studies have explored the metastatic and prognostic significance of CD44, and they produced similar results [16, 17]. These findings confirmed that CD44 may be an effective biomarker for predicting the invasion and metastasis of CAC and may predict prognosis.

EMT is believed to be involved in a series of fundamental biological behaviors, such as growth, motility, invasion, adhesion, metastasis, and recurrence. Twist1, which consists of two exons and one intron, is a pivotal transcriptional factor in EMT. The results of this study showed the expression of Twist1 in CAC to be positively associated with tumor differentiation, gross type, invasion, and LNM stages and TNM stages. Twist1+ patients showed significantly shorter OS than Twist1- patients. Because the infiltrating type of CAC tends to develop more rapidly than other types of CAC, which could suggest that Twist1 is a valuable biomarker for more aggressive CAC. In this way, our findings support the conclusion that Twist1 may be a reliable biomarker of CAC, particularly in predicting progression, metastasis, and prognosis.

KiSS-1 is considered a metastatic suppressor in many cancers [11, 25, 26]. Results have demonstrated that the normal expression of KiSS-1 can suppress tumor cell growth, motility, and migration. The results of this study indicated a negative correlation between positive expression of KiSS-1 and tumor size, invasion, LNM stage, or TNM stage. KiSS-1+ patients were significantly associated with longer OS time when compared with KiSS-1- patients. These findings suggested that KiSS-1 should be considered as a potential predictor for progression and metastasis of CAC, as well as prognosis [11, 25, 26, 29].

Table 4 Univariate analysis and multivariate analysis of factors affecting lymph node metastasis

Variables	Categories	Univariate analysis P	Multivariate analysis HR	95% CI	P
Invasion	Subserosa/ Visceral peritoneum[a]	< 0.001	12.336	1.264-120.427	0.031
MACC1	Negative/Positive	< 0.001	2.956	1.222-7.149	0.016
CD44	Negative/Positive	< 0.001	6.496	2.858-14.767	< 0.001
Twist1	Negative/Positive	< 0.001	3.951	1.673-9.331	0.002
KiSS-1	Negative/Positive	< 0.001	0.271	0.110-0.666	0.004

[a]Subserosa: The tumor has grown through the mucosa and into the subserosa; Visceral peritoneum: The tumor has grown into the surface of the visceral peritoneum, which means it has grown through all layers of the colon, or the tumor has grown into or has attached to other organs or structures

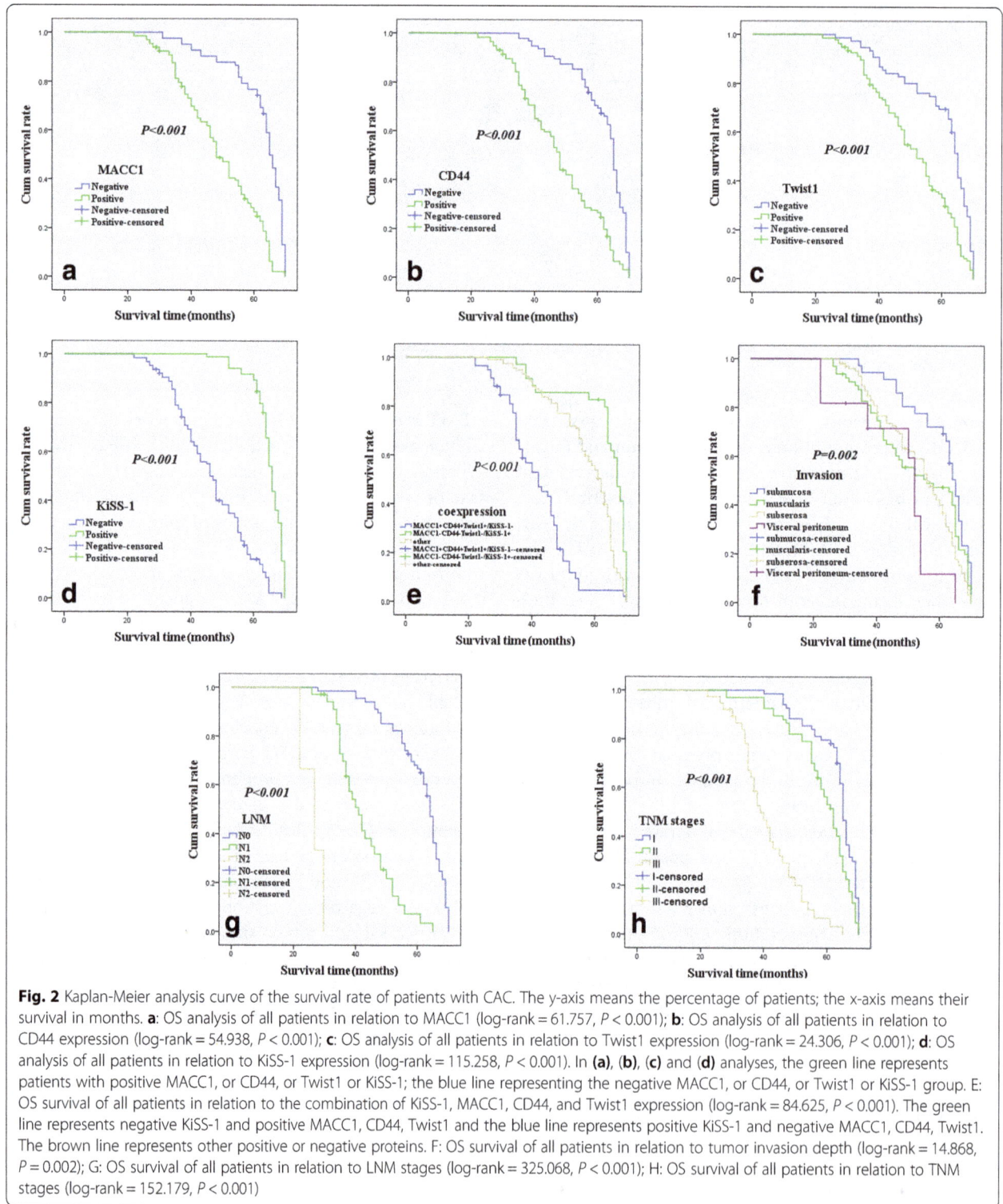

Fig. 2 Kaplan-Meier analysis curve of the survival rate of patients with CAC. The y-axis means the percentage of patients; the x-axis means their survival in months. **a**: OS analysis of all patients in relation to MACC1 (log-rank = 61.757, $P < 0.001$); **b**: OS analysis of all patients in relation to CD44 expression (log-rank = 54.938, $P < 0.001$); **c**: OS analysis of all patients in relation to Twist1 expression (log-rank = 24.306, $P < 0.001$); **d**: OS analysis of all patients in relation to KiSS-1 expression (log-rank = 115.258, $P < 0.001$). In **(a)**, **(b)**, **(c)** and **(d)** analyses, the green line represents patients with positive MACC1, or CD44, or Twist1 or KiSS-1; the blue line representing the negative MACC1, or CD44, or Twist1 or KiSS-1 group. E: OS survival of all patients in relation to the combination of KiSS-1, MACC1, CD44, and Twist1 expression (log-rank = 84.625, $P < 0.001$). The green line represents negative KiSS-1 and positive MACC1, CD44, Twist1 and the blue line represents positive KiSS-1 and negative MACC1, CD44, Twist1. The brown line represents other positive or negative proteins. F: OS survival of all patients in relation to tumor invasion depth (log-rank = 14.868, $P = 0.002$); G: OS survival of all patients in relation to LNM stages (log-rank = 325.068, $P < 0.001$); H: OS survival of all patients in relation to TNM stages (log-rank = 152.179, $P < 0.001$)

In the current study, univariate analysis indicated that invasion, LNM, TNM stages, and expression of MACC1, CD44, Twist1, and KiSS-1 were significantly closely associated with duration of OS in patients with CAC. Multivariate OS analysis showed that LNM stages, TNM stages, positive expression of MACC1, CD44, Twist1, and KiSS-1 were independent predictors affecting patient survival. Multivariate metastasis logistic analysis showed expression of MACC1, CD44, Twist1, and KiSS-1, and invasion to be significantly closely associated with metastasis of CAC.

Table 5 Results of univariate analyses of overall survival (OS) time

Variable	n	Mean OS (months)	Log-rank	P value
MACC1			61.757	< 0.001
Negative	82	62.0 ± 9.6		
Positive	130	47.8 ± 12.5		
CD44			54.938	< 0.001
Negative	96	61.2 ± 8.9		
Positive	116	46.8 ± 12.9		
Twist1			24.306	< 0.001
Negative	76	59.7 ± 11.5		
Positive	136	49.7 ± 13.0		
KiSS-1			115.258	< 0.001
Negative	127	45.7 ± 11.6		
Positive	85	64.7 ± 4.9		
Gender			0.070	0.792
Male	142	54.0 ± 12.4		
Female	70	52.0 ± 15.2		
Ages (year)			0.206	0.650
≤ 60	134	54.3 ± 12.7		
> 60	78	51.7 ± 14.4		
Size (cm)			5.887	0.053
≤ 2.0	33	55.0 ± 13.4		
> 2.0, ≤5.0	110	51.0 ± 12.7		
> 5.0	69	56.2 ± 13.9		
Location			7.503	0.057
Ascending	42	54.3 ± 14.0		
Transverse	64	51.4 ± 13.4		
Descending	33	52.3 ± 13.3		
Sigmoid	73	54.9 ± 13.0		
Type			3.781	0.286
Ulcerative	65	55.3 ± 13.0		
Infiltrating	46	51.8 ± 13.4		
Polypoid	68	52.6 ± 14.0		
Colloid	33	53.2 ± 12.7		
Invasion			14.868	0.002
Submucosa	36	60.2 ± 9.9		
Muscularis	64	52.1 ± 14.7		
Subserosa	101	52.7 ± 12.5		
Visceral peritoneum	11	43.2 ± 14.4		
Grade			3.544	0.170
Well	32	56.1 ± 14.1		
Moderate	135	53.7 ± 13.0		
Poor	45	50.1 ± 13.5		
LNM stages			325.068	< 0.001

Table 5 Results of univariate analyses of overall survival (OS) time *(Continued)*

Variable	n	Mean OS (months)	Log-rank	P value
N0	136	60.6 ± 8.8		
N1	70	41.5 ± 9.1		
N2	6	26.3 ± 3.6		
TNM stage			152.179	< 0.001
I	69	62.7 ± 7.4		
II	67	58.4 ± 9.7		
III	79	40.3 ± 9.7		

These findings also demonstrated that MACC1, CD44, Twist1, and KiSS-1 should be considered to be useful biomarkers for predicting the invasion and metastasis of CAC, as well as a predictor for prognosis.

There were some differences between our results and previous findings. This may be related to the use of different biomarkers, different immunohistochemical methods, or even different patients (such as Wang W. et al., who reported that KiSS-1 expression was statistically significantly higher in colorectal cancer tissue than in corresponding adjacent normal mucosa [30], Wu Q. et al. reported that CD44 expression was not associated with LNM in multivariate logistic regression analysis [17], and Yusup A. et al. reported that Twist1 expression was not correlated with survival [31]). However, we demonstrated that MACC1, CD44, Twist1, and KiSS-1 expression were associated with metastasis and prognosis of CAC. CSCs may indicate the initiation, progression, and metastasis of CAC. Their capacity for self-renewal, proliferation, and multiple forms of differentiation allow CSCs to induce EMT and so promote invasion and metastasis. CD44 is an adhesion molecule that can regulate cell-matrix adhesion. CD44 overexpression is beneficial to CAC progression and metastasis. During cancer progression, MACC1 overexpression should inhibit cancer cell apoptosis and promote cancer cell EMT via HGF/MET pathways [32, 33]. Twist1 overexpression could further promote the cancer cell EMT process through regulating E-cadherin, N-cadherin, and MMP expression [21, 34]. Thus, EMT could induce cancer cell motility, migration, and even metastasis. Aberrant

Table 6 Results of multivariate analyses of overall survival (OS) time

Variable	B	SE	P	RR	95% CI
MACC1	1.070	0.198	< 0.001	2.917	1.978–4.301
CD44	0.512	0.176	0.004	1.669	1.183–2.357
Twist1	0.348	0.176	0.048	1.417	1.003–2.000
KiSS-1	−1.368	0.201	< 0.001	0.255	0.172–0.377
LNM stages	0.801	0.368	0.029	2.229	1.084–4.581
TNM stages	0.630	0.260	0.015	1.877	1.127–3.124

expression of KiSS-1 could decrease or lower its ability to inhibit cancer cell invasion and metastasis [11, 25, 26].

Conclusions

This study demonstrated that expression levels of MACC1, CD44, Twist1, and KiSS-1 are related to duration of OS among patients with CAC. In this way, MACC1, CD44, Twist1, and KiSS-1 could serve as valuable biomarkers in CAC and may be helpful for the metastasis and prognosis for CAC.

Acknowledgements
We thank all staffs at the Department of Pathology of our hospital for assistance with data and project management.

Funding
This work was supported by the Nature Science Foundation of Anhui Province (No.1708085MH230) and the Nature Science Key Program of Bengbu Medical College (No.BYKY1711ZD) and Key projects of support program for outstanding young talents in Colleges and Universities of Anhui Province (No. gxyqZD2016160) and the Nature Science Key Program of College and University of Anhui Province (No.KJ2018A1029).

Authors' contributions
WSW, ZB, WYC and WXL carried out the design, analysis of pathology and drafted the manuscript. ZL, GXM, and SWQ carried out sample collection an coordination. WDN performed the immunohistochemistry. All authors read and approved the manuscript.

Competing interests
The authors declare that they have no competing interests.

References
1. Torre LA, Bray F, Siegel RL, Ferlay J, Lortet-Tieulent J, Jemal A. Global cancer statistics, 2012. CA Cancer J Clin. 2015;65:87–108.
2. Chen W, Zheng R, Baade PD, Zhang S, Zeng H, Bray F, Jemal A, Yu XQ, He J. Cancer statistics in China, 2015. CA Cancer J Clin. 2016;66:115–32.
3. Stein U, Walther W, Arlt F, Schwabe H, Smith J, Fichtner I, Birchmeier W, Schlag PM. MACC1, a newly identified key regulator of HGF-MET signaling, predicts colon cancer metastasis. Nat Med. 2009;15:59–67.
4. Stein U, Smith J, Walther W, Arlt F. MACC1 controls mMet: what a difference an Sp1 site makes. Cell Cycle. 2009;8:2467–9.
5. Koelzer VH, Herrmann P, Zlobec I, Karamitopoulou E, Luqli A, Stein U. Heterogeneity analysis of metastasis associated in colon cancer 1 (MACC1) for survival prognosis of colorectal cancer patients: a retrospective cohort study. BMC Cancer. 2015;15:160.
6. Wang L, Wu Y, Lin L, Liu P, Huang H, Liao W, Zheng D, Zuo Q, Sun L, Huang N, Shi M, Liao Y, Liao W. Metastasis-associated in colon cancer-1 upregulation predicts a poor prognosis of gastric cancer, and promotes tumor cell proliferation and invasion. Int J Cancer. 2013;133:1419–30.
7. Chundong G, Uramoto H, Onitsuka T, Shimokawa H, Iwanami T, Nakagawa M, Oyama T, Tanaka F. Molecular diagnosis of MACC1 status in lung adenocarcinoma by immunohistochemical analysis. Anticancer Res. 2011;31:1141–5.
8. Zhou L, Yu L, Zhu B, Wu S, Song W, Gong X, Wang D. Metastasis-associated in colon cancer-1 and aldehyde dehydrogenase 1 are metastatic and prognostic biomarker for non-small cell lung cancer. BMC Cancer. 2016;16(1):876.
9. Park IH, Zhao R, West JA, Yabuuchi A, Huo H, Ince TA, Lerou PH, Lensch MW, Daley GQ. Reprogramming of human somatic cells to pluripotency with defined factors. Nature. 2008;451:141–6.
10. Yu J, Vodyanik MA, Smuga-Otto K, Antosiewicz-Bourget J, Frane JL, Tian S, Nie J, Jonsdottir GA, Ruotti V, Stewart R, Slukvin II, Thomson JA. Induced pluripotent stem cell lines derived from human somatic cells. Science. 2007;318:1917–20.
11. Yu L, Zhu B, Wu S, Zhou L, Song W, Gong X, Wang D. Evaluation of the correlation of vasculogenic mimicry, ALDH1, KiSS-1, and MACC1 in the prediction of metastasis and prognosis in ovarian carcinoma. Diagn Pathol. 2017;12:23.
12. Lu G, Zhou L, Song W, Wu S, Zhu B, Wang D. Expression of ORAOV1, CD133 and WWOX correlate with metastasis and prognosis in gastric adenocarcinoma. Int J Clin Exp Pathol. 2017;10:8916–24.
13. Fang C, Fan C, Wang C, Huang Q, Meng W, Yu Y, Yang L, Peng Z, Hu J, Li Y, Mo X, Zhou Z. CD133+CD54+CD44+ circulating tumor cells as a biomarker of treatment selection and liver metastasis in patients with colorectal cancer. Oncotarget. 2016;7:77389–403.
14. Choi SI, Kim SY, Lee JH, Kim JY, Cho EW, Kim IG. Osteopontin production by TM4SF4 signaling drives a positive feedback autocrine loop with the STAT3 pathway to maintain cancer stem cell-like properties in lung cancer cells. Oncotarget. 2017;8:101284–97.
15. Wang HH, Liao CC, Chow NH, Huang LL, Chuang JI, Wei KC, Shin JW. Whether CD44 is an applicable marker for glioma stem cells. Am J Transl Res. 2017;9:4785–806.
16. Iseki Y, Shibutani M, Maeda K, Nagahara H, Ikeya T, Hirakawa K. Significance of E-cadherin and CD44 expression in patients with unresectable metastatic colorectal cancer. Oncol Lett. 2017;14:1025–34.
17. Wu Q, Yang Y, Wu S, Li W, Zhang N, Dong X, Ou Y. Evaluation of the correlation of KAI1/CD82, CD44, MMP7 and β-catenin in the prediction of prognosis and metastasis in colorectal carcinoma. Diagn Pathol. 2015;10:176.
18. Yang D, Sun Y, Hu L, Zheng H, Ji P, Pecot CV, Zhao Y, Reynolds S, Cheng H, Rupaimoole R, Cogdell D, Nykter M, Broaddus R, Rodriguez-Aguayo C, Lopez-Berestein G, Liu J, Shmulevich I, Sood AK, Chen K, Zhang W. Integrated analyses identify a master microRNA regulatory network for the mesenchymal subtype in serous ovarian cancer. Cancer Cell. 2013;23:186–99.
19. Mitra R, Chen X, Greenawalt EJ, Maulik U, Jiang W, Zhao Z, Eischen CM. Decoding critical long non-coding RNA in ovarian cancer epithelial-to-mesenchymal transition. Nat Commun. 2017;8:1604.
20. Duan Y, He Q, Yue K, Si H, Wang J, Zhou X, Wang X. Hypoxia induced Bcl-2/Twist1 complex promotes tumor cell invasion in oral squamous cell carcinoma. Oncotarget. 2016;8:21–39.
21. Zhou L, Yu L, Zhu B, Wu S, Song W, Gong X, Wang D. Vasculogenic mimicry and expression of Twist1 and KAI1 correlate with metastasis and prognosis in lung squamous cell carcinoma. Int J Clin Exp Pathol. 2017;10:7542–50.
22. Shamir ER, Pappalardo E, Jorgens DM, Coutinho K, Tsai WT, Aziz K, Auer M, Tran PT, Bader JS, Ewald AJ. Twist1-induced dissemination preserves epithelial identity and requires Ecadherin. J Cell Biol. 2014;204:839–56.
23. Welch DR, Chen P, Miele ME, McGary CT, Bower JM, Stanbridge EJ, Weissman BE. Microcell-mediated transfer of chromosome 6 into metastatic human C8161 melanoma cells suppresses metastasis but does not inhibit tumorigenicity. Oncogene. 1994;9:255–62.
24. Navenot JM, Fujii N, Peiper SC. Activation of rRho and rRho-associated kinase by GPR54 and KiSS1 metastasis suppressor gene product induces changes of cell morphology and contributes to apoptosis. Mol Pharmacol. 2009;75:1300–6.
25. Quevedo EG, Aguilar GM, Aguilar LA, Rubio SA, Martínez SE, Rodríguez IP, Corona JS, Morán MI, Gómez RC, Moguel MC. Polymorphisms rs12998 and rs5780218 in KiSS1 suppressor metastasis gene in Mexican patients with breast cancer. Dis Markers. 2015;2015:365845.

26. Song W, Zhou L, Gong X, Wu S, Yu L, Zhu B, Wang D. Expression of ORAOV1, ABCG2, and KiSS-1 associate with prognosis in laryngeal squamous cell carcinoma. Int J Clin Exp MedInt J. Clin Exp Med. 2017; 10:14623–31.

27. Yang YP, Ou JH, Chang XJ, Lu YY, Bai WL, Dong Z, Wang H, An LJ, Xu ZX, Wang CP, Zeng Z, Hu KQ. High intratumoral metastasis-associated in colon cancer-1 expression predicts poor outcomes of cryoablation therapy for advanced hepatocellular carcinoma. J Transl Med. 2013;11:41.

28. Hu H, Tian D, Chen T, Han R, Sun Y, Wu C. Metastasis-associated in colon cancer 1 is a novel survival-related biomarker for human patients with renal pelvis carcinoma. PLoS One. 2014;9:e100161.

29. Cao F, Chen L, Liu M, Lin W, Ji J, You J, Qiao F, Liu H. Expression of preoperative KISS1 gene in tumor tissue with epithelial ovarian cancer and its prognostic value. Medicine (Baltimore). 2016;95:e5296.

30. Wang W, ZI Y, Okugawa Y, Inoue Y, Tanaka K, Toiyama Y, Shimura T, Okigami M, Kawamoto aA, Hiro J, Saiqusa S, Mohri Y, Uchida K, Kusunoki M. Loss of the metastasis suppressor gene KiSS1 is associated with lymph node metastasis and poor prognosis in human colorectal cancer. Oncol Rep. 2016;30:1449–54.

31. Yusup A, Huji B, Fang C, Wang F, Dadihan T, Wang HJ, Upur H. Expression of trefoil factors and Twist1 in colorectal cancer and their correlation with metastatic potential and prognosis. World J Gastroenterol. 2017;23:110–20.

32. Lu G, Zhou L, Zhang X, Zhu B, Wu S, Song W, Gong X, Wang D, Tao Y. The expression of metastasis-associated in colon cancer-1 and KAI1 in gastric adenocarcinoma and their clinical significance. World J Surg Oncol. 2016;14:276.

33. Burock S, Herrmann P, Wendler I, Niederstrasser M, Wernecke KD, Stein U. Circulating metastasis associated in colon cancer 1 transcripts in gastric cancer patient plasma as diagnostic and prognostic biomarker. World J Gastroenterol. 2015;21:333–41.

34. Yang J, Mani SA, Donaher JL, Ramaswamy S, Itzykson RA, Come C, Savagner P, Gitelman I, Richardson A, Weinberg RA. Twist, a master regulator of morphogenesis, plays an essential role in tumor metastasis. Cell. 2004;117:927–39.

10

PD-L1 in pancreatic ductal adenocarcinoma: a retrospective analysis of 373 Chinese patients using an in vitro diagnostic assay

Xiaolong Liang[1], Jian Sun[1], Huanwen Wu[1], Yufeng Luo[1], Lili Wang[1], Junliang Lu[1], Zhiwen Zhang[1], Junchao Guo[2*], Zhiyong Liang[1*] and Tonghua Liu[1*]

Abstract

Background: Programmed death ligand 1 (PD-L1) has shown potential as a therapeutic target in numerous solid tumors. Its prognostic significance has also been established in pancreatic ductal adenocarcinoma (PDAC). The present study aimed to explore PD-L1 expression in PDAC cases in a large Chinese cohort using an in vitro diagnostic (IVD) assay to provide further insight into the potential value of programmed cell death protein 1 (PD-1) as a therapeutic target.

Methods: Three hundred seventy-three PDAC patients were retrospectively recruited in this study. Tissue microarray (TMA) blocks were made from available formalin-fixed and paraffin-embedded (FFPE) tumor and matched adjacent tissue specimens. We evaluated PD-L1 protein expression via immunohistochemistry (IHC) using a U.S. Food and Drug Administration (FDA)-approved IVD assay. The relationships between PD-L1 positivity and both clinicopathological characteristics and patient prognosis were analyzed. PD-1 expression and clinicopathological significance were also evaluated.

Results: PD-L1 and PD-1 positivity were observed in 3.2% and 7.5% of cases, respectively. PD-L1 showed a predominantly membranous pattern in tumor cells, while no positive PD-L1 staining was observed in normal regions. Statistical analyses revealed that PD-L1 expression was associated with lymph node metastasis. PD-L1 positivity was a prognostic indicator of progression-free survival (PFS) and overall survival (OS) in univariate analyses, but only PFS remained statistically significant in multivariate analysis. PD-1 expression was detected in lymphocytes and was not associated with any clinicopathological feature except a history of pancreatitis.

Conclusions: The PD-L1 positivity rate is low in PDAC when evaluated using a companion diagnostic assay. It remains an independent prognostic factor for poor PFS.

Keywords: Pancreatic, PD-L1, Immunohistochemistry, Prognosis

* Correspondence: gjcpumch@163.com; liangzhiyong1220@yahoo.com;
Tonghua_liu@163.com
[2]Department of General Surgery, Peking Union Medical College Hospital,
Peking Union Medical College and Chinese Academy of Medical Sciences,
No. 1 Shuai Fu Yuan, Wangfujing, Beijing 100730, People's Republic of China
[1]Department of Pathology, Peking Union Medical College Hospital, Peking
Union Medical College and Chinese Academy of Medical Sciences, No. 1
Shuai Fu Yuan, Wangfujing, Beijing 100730, People's Republic of China

Background

Pancreatic ductal adenocarcinoma (PDAC) is one of the deadliest malignancies of the digestive system. Presently, the median survival for PDAC patients is measured in months; and the five-year survival for the unstratified patient group is less than 5% [1] despite radical surgery and chemotherapeutic regimens. Therefore, novel therapeutic strategies to tackle this drastic situation are urgently needed.

Programmed cell death protein 1 (PD-1), also known as B7–1, and its ligand, programmed death ligand 1 (PD-L1), also known as B7-H1, constitute a pair of corresponding regulatory receptors on the membrane of T cells and tumor cells, respectively. The role of the PD-1/PD-L1 pathway in the immune system, where it suppresses T cell activation and results in the loss of inhibitory function against tumors has been well elucidated and was recently summarized in a review by Vassiliki [2]. Meanwhile, the PD1/PD-L1 pathway and its relationship with cancer development and clinical outcomes have also been studied extensively [3, 4]. Moreover, blocking PD1/PD-L1 signaling has shown promising results in a broad spectrum of solid tumors, including pancreatic cancer [5, 6].

Analyses of PD-L1 expression in pancreatic cancer have yielded drastically variable results [7–12]. The expression rates range from 12.5% using a 5% cut-off point to 100%, where 60% to 90% of the tumor cells in each specimen were positive [13]. While the existing data suggest that PD-L1 is an indicator of an unfavorable prognosis, the association between PD-L1 positivity and clinicopathological parameters is less consistent [7, 10–12]. Further, most previous studies have adopted various but low cut-off values (ranging from 5%–10%) for determination of PD-L1 positivity, which has raised concerns about the validity of PD-L1 as a potential therapeutic target in PDAC.

In the present study, we aimed to assess the expression of PD-L1 in PDAC and its relationship with patient outcomes in a large Chinese cohort. We adopted a U.S. Food and Drug Administration (FDA)-approved in vitro diagnostics (IVD) assay (Roche SP263) and a manufacturer-validated cut-off value (25%) to provide additional information for the potential value of PD-L1 as a therapeutic target in PDAC patients. Meanwhile, PD-1 expression levels in PDAC tissue were also investigated.

Methods

Patient enrollment

A consecutive series of patients who underwent surgical resection of a pancreatic mass at Peking Union Medical College Hospital (PUMCH) from September 2008 to July 2014 with a histologically established diagnosis of PDAC based on the WHO 2010 classification [14] were retrospectively recruited in our study. Patient information, including gender, age, smoking history, alcohol consumption, previous medical history (diabetes mellitus and chronic pancreatitis), family history of PDAC, clinical symptoms, clinical staging, treatment received, progression-free survival (PFS), and overall survival (OS), were obtained from medical records. Pathological diagnoses were acquired from the pathology database. Clinical staging was based on the tumor-node-metastasis staging system outlined in the seventh edition of the American Joint Commission on Cancer [15]. PFS was defined as the period from the time of surgery to the establishment of tumor recurrence by medical imaging. OS was defined as the period from the time of surgery to patient death.

All subjects gave consent at the time of clinical intervention for future use of data/material for research purposes. Obtaining additional informed consent was not required for this retrospective study. The present study was approved by the Institutional Review Board of Peking Union Medical College Hospital (No. S-K118).

Tissue microarray (TMA)

Representative, formalin-fixed, paraffin-embedded (FFPE) tissue blocks from the enrolled cases were retrieved from the tissue sample library of the pathology department of PUMCH along with the corresponding archived H&E slides. Representative tumor and non-tumor regions were identified by an experienced pathologist, and the regions of interest were annotated in the tissue block as the donor sites. A one-millimeter core needle was used for puncture. The puncture, transfer, and planting of tissue cores to the receiver block were performed using a semi-automated TMA construction system (Quick-Ray UT-06, UNITMA, Korea) according to the manufacturer's instructions.

Immunohistochemistry (IHC)

Four-micrometer-thick TMA sections were made from the TMA blocks and mounted on microscope slides. For PD-L1, the IHC staining was carried out on a Ventana Benchmark XT autostainer (Ventana, Tucson, AZ, USA) using an FDA-approved assay (Roche, SP263) following the manufacturer's manual, which was acquired from Roche Diagnostics Co. (Shanghai, China). For PD-1, the TMA slides were air dried, incubated at 60 degrees Celsius for 20 min, deparaffinized in xylene, and hydrolyzed in gradient alcohol. Antigen retrieval was accomplished through hyperbaric/microwave treatment in citric acid-EDTA at 95 degrees Celsius for 15 min. Nonspecific epitopes were then blocked with 10% goat serum. PD-1 antibody (rabbit monoclonal) was purchased from Zhongshan Gold Bridge (Beijing, China).

Interpretation of IHC results

For PD-L1, the percentage of tumor cells with membranous staining was documented; positivity was defined as ≥25% of tumor cells showing membranous staining [16], and the statistics at different cut-offs (5% and 10%) were also documented. PD-1 positivity was defined as membranous or cytoplasmic staining in ≥1% of the tumor-infiltrating lymphocytes (TILs) [17]. All slides were evaluated by two experienced pathologists who had no prior knowledge of the selected cases. When discordance in interpretation occurred, the examiners discussed the results until they reached an agreement.

Validation of the TMA IHC assay for PD-L1 and PD-1 expression

Given the concerns about the representativeness of the TMA, we set up a validation assay for PD-L1 and PD-1. For PD-L1, all cases that were classified as PD-L1-positive and 10 PD-L1-negative cases were selected. For PD-1, donor blocks from seventeen PD-1-positive cases and twelve PD-1-negative cases were recruited, and whole sections were made. PD-L1 or PD-1 expression was probed under the conditions described above. For PD-L1, the percentage of tumor cells with membranous staining was documented for each whole section. Consistency between the TMA and whole section staining was measured using the kappa value at different cut-off points (5%, 10%, and 25%). For PD-1, the whole-section slides were interpreted using the 1% cut-off value; the kappa values for the TMA and the whole section are provided.

Statistical analysis

All data were processed using SPSS software (version 20.0, IBM SPSS software). Numerical data were examined with a K-S test for Gaussian distribution. Student's t-test was used to detect differences in normally distributed numeric parameters. Meanwhile, the means and standard deviations were calculated. For categorical data or numerical data that were not normally distributed, a chi-square test or Spearman rank correlation test was used to analyze the relationship. The prognostic data were analyzed using a Kaplan-Meier analysis and Cox Regression. Survival curves were plotted. Factors yielding a $p < 0.1$ in the univariate analysis or considered clinically important were included in the multivariate analysis for PFS and OS. Missing data were not included in the statistical calculation. A $p < 0.05$ was considered statistically significant.

Results

Demographic characteristics of the patients

Three hundred seventy-three patients were evaluated in our study. Of these patients, 215 males and 158 females were included. The median age was 61 years, ranging from 29 to 82 years. In total, 132 and 65 patients had

histories of smoking and alcohol consumption, respectively. Only one patient had a history of pancreatitis, and five patients reported a family history of PDAC. White blood cell count, differentiation, and lymph node metastasis were also evaluated. The demographic characteristics of the enrolled patients are summarized in Table 1.

Expression of PD-L1/PD-1 in PDAC tissues

Of the 373 cases, 12 (3.2%) were positive for PD-L1 expression in cancer tissue using the 25% cut-off point. The number of PD-L1-positive cases increased to 22 (5.9%) and 33 (8.8%) when the cut-off points of 10% and 5%, respectively, were applied. However, no PD-L1 staining was observed in the normal tissue. Twenty-seven (7.5%) cases showed PD-1 expression in lymphocytes (Fig. 1). Moreover, no samples were positive for both PD-1 and PD-L1 at the same time.

Association between PD-L1/PD-1 expression and clinico-pathological parameters

No relationship was observed between the expression of PD-L1 and clinical features, such as gender, age, smoking, drinking, history of pancreatitis, or family history of PDAC. However, the association between PD-L1 expression and lymph node metastasis was marginally significant ($p = 0.058$). On the other hand, PD-1 expression was only related to a history of pancreatitis but not to any other parameters that we evaluated.

PD-L1 expression was associated with PDAC patient prognosis

Univariate analyses suggested that common bile duct invasion ($p = 0.026$), lymph node metastasis ($p = 0.005$), and PD-L1 expression ($p = 0.003$) were prognostic indicators of unfavorable PFS. The latter two factors remained statistically significant in multivariate analyses (lymph node metastasis, $p = 0.012$; PD-L1 positivity, $p = 0.003$). Meanwhile, lymph node metastasis ($p = 0.001$) and PD-L1 positivity ($p = 0.002$) were also prognostic indicators of poor OS in univariate analyses. However, only lymph node invasion retained statistical significance in multivariate analysis ($p = 0.010$) for OS, and PD-L1 positivity ($p = 0.079$) only showed a trend toward significance without reaching statistical significance (Table 2). In Kaplan-Meier tests, the PD-L1-positive arm showed significantly inferior OS and PFS than did the negative arm (Fig. 2). Using lower cut-off points narrowed the survival gap between the two arms, although the differences remained statistically significant (Additional file 1: Table S2).

Consistency of PD-L1/PD-1 staining between TMA and whole sections

Twenty-two and twenty-seven cases were included in the validation sets for PD-L1 and PD-1, respectively.

Table 1 Association between clinicopathological parameters and PD-L1 expression in 373 PDAC patients

Clinicopathological characteristics	Total	PD-1		p value	PD-L1		p value
		Positive	Negative		Positive	Negative	
total	373	27	346		12	361	
Age (years)	373			0.924			0.550
Mean ± SD		60.12 ± 9.96	59.93 ± 9.39		58.42 ± 8.38	60.16 ± 9.96	
Gender				0.561			0.067
male	215	17	198		10	205	
female	158	10	148		2	156	
Smoking				0.568			0.772
yes	132	11	121		4	128	
no	238	16	222		6	232	
Drinking				0.236			0.139
yes	65	7	58		0	65	
no	305	20	285		10	295	
History of pancreatitis				**0.001**			0.868
yes	1	1	0		0	1	
no	370	26	344		10	360	
Family history				0.528			0.371
yes	5	0	5		0	5	
no	366	27	339		10	356	
WBC (×10^9)				0.891			0.750
>10	30	2	28		1	29	
4–10	245	21	224		6	239	
<4	19	2	17		1	18	
Tumor differentiation				0.150			0.820
moderate /poor	307	20	287		10	297	
well	59	7	52		1	58	
pT				0.494			0.586
1	2	0	2		0	2	
2	18	0	18		1	17	
3	340	26	314		10	330	
4	8	1	7		0	8	
Clinical staging				1.000			1.000
1	10	0	10		0	10	
2	329	25	304		11	318	
3	13	1	12		0	13	
4	15	1	14		0	15	
Lymph node metastasis				0.759			0.058
yes	192	13	179		8	184	
no	90	7	83		0	90	
Lymphovascular invasion				1.000			1.000
yes	28	2	26		0	28	
no	135	11	124		4	131	

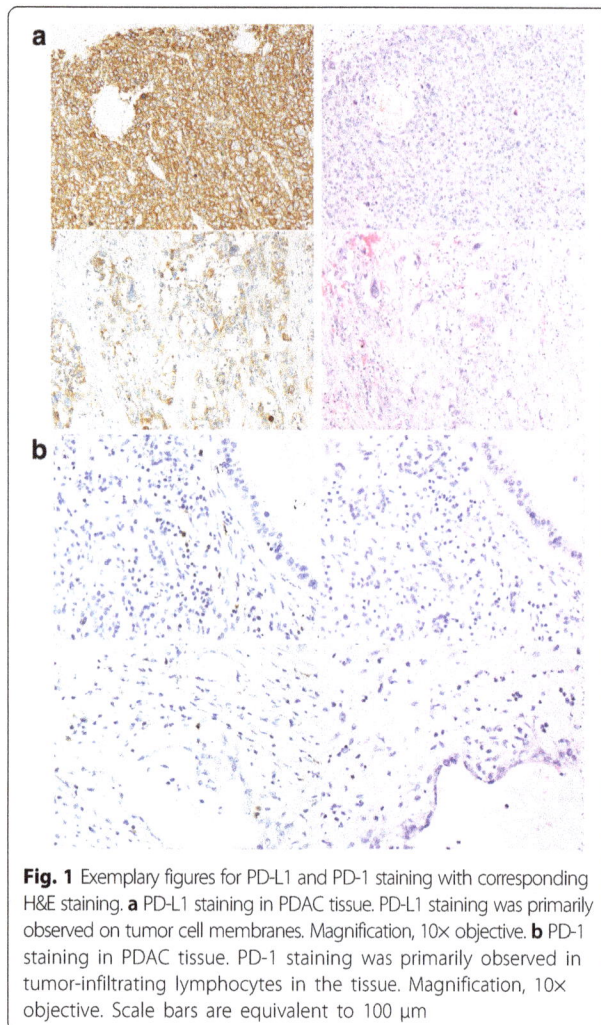

Fig. 1 Exemplary figures for PD-L1 and PD-1 staining with corresponding H&E staining. **a** PD-L1 staining in PDAC tissue. PD-L1 staining was primarily observed on tumor cell membranes. Magnification, 10× objective. **b** PD-1 staining in PDAC tissue. PD-1 staining was primarily observed in tumor-infiltrating lymphocytes in the tissue. Magnification, 10× objective. Scale bars are equivalent to 100 μm

The percentages of PD-L1-positive tumor cells in the TMA and in the corresponding whole sections are listed in Additional file 1: Table S3. At 25% and 10% cut-off points, one case (4.5%) that was negative in the TMA was found to be positive in the whole section. The number of inconsistent cases increased to 4 (18%) at the 5% cut-off point. The inconsistent cases were all positive in the whole sections but negative in the TMA. The kappa values of TMA and whole section samples at 5%, 10%, and 25% cut-off points were 0.621, 0.908, and 0.908, respectively. A related-samples Wilcoxon signed rank test yielded $p = 0.281$. PD-1 interpretations were 100% consistent in the TMA and whole sections (kappa = 1).

Discussion

In the present study, we recruited 373 cases to evaluate the clinicopathological significance of PD-1/PD-L1 expression in PDAC. To the best of our knowledge, this is the largest PDAC cohort enrolled for evaluation of PD-1/PD-L1 expression.

Among the 373 patients recruited, only 12 (3.2%) were interpreted as PD-L1-positive according to the prespecified criteria. In the literature, the positive rates mainly ranged from 39.2% to 49.4% [8–10], although Lu et al. reported that 60% to 90% of tumor cells were positive in all 13 (100%) pancreatic cancer cases analyzed [13]. In contrast, in a study by Soares et al., the authors found that only 3 of 25 (12.5%) pancreatic cancer cases were positive for PD-L1 expression. In the present study, when the cut-off value was lowered to 5%, the corresponding positivity increased to 8.8%, which was quite comparable to that reported by Soares et al.

The difference in PD-L1 positivity rates in the literature and our study is only partly attributable to the different cut-off points used. Lu et al., who used an FDA-approved anti-PD-L1 monoclonal antibody (clone 28–8) in their study, suggested that the difference in positivity rates could be a result of variable antibody sensitivity and specificity [13]. In the present study, we adopted another FDA-approved in vitro diagnostic (IVD) assay for evaluation of PD-L1 expression in the PDAC cases. By using a standardized and fully automatic staining protocol following the pre-validated operating procedure provided by the manufacturer, our data tended to be quite reliable, and according to our validation set, replicable. Therefore, antibody quality could not seemingly be blamed for any differences. In fact, pancreatic cancer is considered rather nonimmunogenic [18], which was also supported by the sparse presentation of PD-1-positive (7.5%) TILs in our cases. The non-immunogenicity of pancreatic cancer explains the low positivity rate of T-cell regulators, such as PD-L1, in our study. In a recent study, exposure to an irradiated, granulocyte-macrophage-colony-stimulating factor (GM-CSF)–secreting, allogeneic PDAC vaccine significantly stimulated the expression of PD-L1 in tumor cells from PDAC patients [19]. Based on these findings, we postulate that immunogenic exposure in the individuals might have contributed to the differential expression of immunomodulators by tumor cells. Information about vaccination and patient allergy history could provide some insight into this issue, and further investigation is warranted.

On the other hand, applying a cut-off value of 5–10% means that even when more than 90% of the tumor cells do not express PD-L1, the case is still classified as PD-L1-positive. This raises concern about the efficacy of the marker to predict the PD-1/PD-L1 inhibitor response, although the lower cut-off points have well justified their usefulness in prognostic applications. As the assay adopted in the present study was developed in conjunction with therapeutic regimens for uroepithelial carcinomas only, our results might better reflect actual therapeutic indications for PD-L1 status than those of

Table 2 Univariate and multivariate analyses of prognostic factors for PFS and OS

Characteristics	p (Univariate analysis)		p (Multivariate analysis)	
	PFS	OS	PFS	OS
Gender	0.572	0.579		
Smoking	0.480	0.858		
Smoking index	0.347	0.183		
Drinking	0.780	0.208		
Diabetes mellitus	0.888	0.829		
Digestive presentation	0.895	0.060		0.125
WBC count	0.072	0.484	0.068	
Neoadjuvant chemotherapy	0.695	0.731		
Histological grading	0.074	0.082	0.125	0.089
Position	0.087	0.572	0.660	
Pancreatic capsule invasion	0.382	0.797		
Vascular invasion	0.350	0.270		
Common bile duct invasion	**0.026**	0.268	0.251	
Lymph node invasion	**0.005**	**0.001**	**0.012**	**0.010**
Neuroinvasion	0.809	0.218		
Post-operative chemotherapy	0.478	0.338		
PD-1	0.939	0.160		
PD-L1	**0.003**	**0.002**	**0.003**	0.079

PFS: progression free survival; OS: Overall survival; HR: Hazard ratio;

previous studies because a higher cut-off value was applied. In this regard, the most important value of the present study lies in the fact that we are alerting clinicians to the possible low percentage of PDAC patients who might be responsive to PD-1/PD-L1 inhibitor therapy. Regardless, such speculation requires further analyses in association with PDAC patient treatment schemes in future clinical trials.

PD-L1 has been found to be associated with poor prognosis in non-small cell lung cancer (NSCLC) [20], breast cancer [21], esophageal squamous cell carcinoma [22], and urothelial carcinoma [23]. PD-L1 positivity also

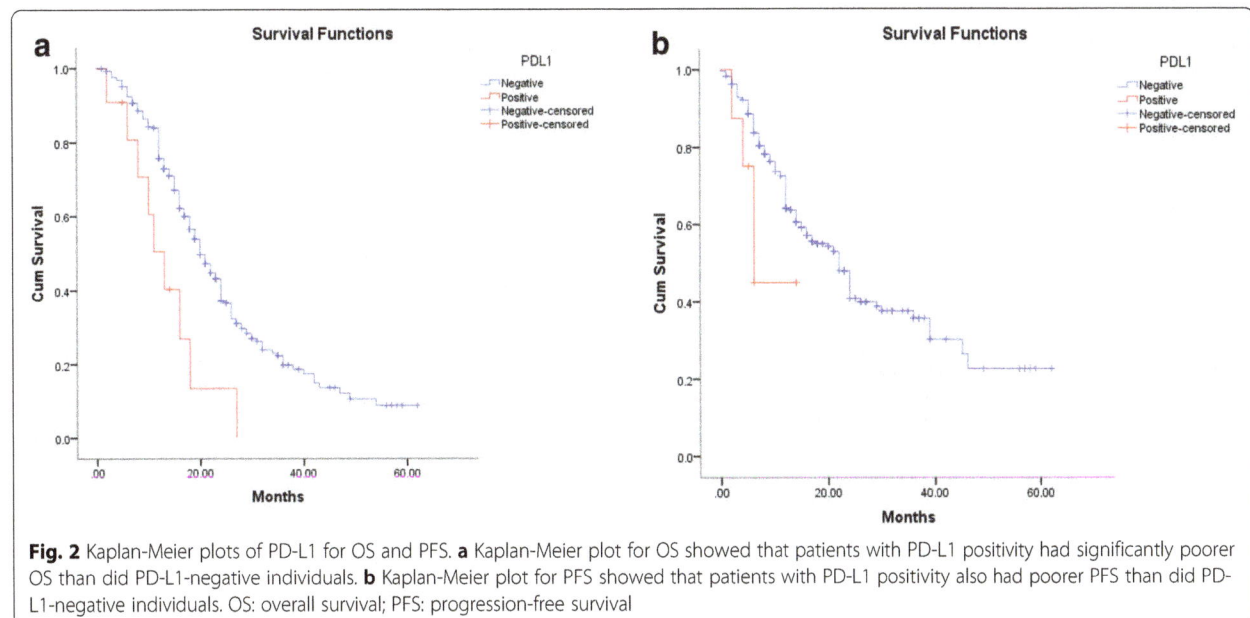

Fig. 2 Kaplan-Meier plots of PD-L1 for OS and PFS. **a** Kaplan-Meier plot for OS showed that patients with PD-L1 positivity had significantly poorer OS than did PD-L1-negative individuals. **b** Kaplan-Meier plot for PFS showed that patients with PD-L1 positivity also had poorer PFS than did PD-L1-negative individuals. OS: overall survival; PFS: progression-free survival

predicted aggressiveness in melanoma [24] and recurrence in clear cell renal cell carcinoma [25].

In our cohort, survival analyses demonstrated that the prognosis of PD-L1-positive cases was significantly poorer than that of the PD-L1-negative cases regarding both PFS and OS ($p < 0.05$). Regretfully, PD-L1 was only an independent prognostic factor for PFS. When testing for the prognostic significance of PD-L1 for OS in multivariate analysis, the p-value did not reach statistical significance, likely due to the small number of PD-L1-positive cases.

The main limitation of the present study lies in the small area studied for each specimen, which was imposed by the TMA-based assay. Although PD-L1 heterogeneity has not been revealed in PDAC, it has been reported in several types of solid tumors [26, 27]. The representativeness of the TMA cores may thus raise certain concerns. To tackle this issue, we set up a validation set using representative whole sections. Our data suggested that when the 25% cut-off point was applied, only one of 22 (4.5%) cases had inconsistent results between the TMA and corresponding whole section. This finding suggests that the PD-L1 positivity rate could be underestimated in this study due to the small area that could be examined using TMA. However, such an underestimation may be limited to a relatively low extent. However, studies using more representative whole tissue blocks are desired.

Conclusion
The PD-L1 positivity rate is low in PDAC when evaluated using a companion diagnostic assay. However, PD-L1 positivity remains an independent prognostic factor for poor PFS.

Abbreviations
FDA: Food and Drug Administration; FFPE: Formalin-fixed, paraffin-embedded; IHC: Immunohistochemistry; IVD: In vitro diagnostics; OS: Overall survival; PD-1: Programmed cell death protein 1; PDAC: Pancreatic ductal adenocarcinoma; PD-L1: Programmed death-ligand 1; PFS: Progression-free survival; PUMCH: Peking Union Medical College Hospital; TIL: Tumor-infiltrating lymphocyte; TMA: Tissue microarray; WHO: World Health Organization

Acknowledgments
Not applicable.

Funding
This study was supported by the Chinese Academy of Medical Science Innovation Fund for Medical Science (CIFMS, grant No. 2016-I2M-1-002).

Authors' contributions
LXL conducted the study and drafted the manuscript, and SJ and WHW evaluated the H&E slides for case enrollment and TMA preparation. LYF was responsible for the IHC procedures. WLL and ZZW interpreted the IHC results. GJC provided the clinical information of the patients and the follow data. ZZW also analyzed the data. LJL and GJC revised the manuscript. LZY and LTH supervised the study, provided necessary resources, and contributed intellectually by providing valuable advice on data interpretation and presentation. All authors read and approved the final manuscript.

Competing interests
The authors declare that they have no competing interests.

References
1. Deer EL, Gonzalez-Hernandez J, Coursen JD, Shea JE, Ngatia J, Scaife CL, Firpo MA, Mulvihill SJ. Phenotype and genotype of pancreatic cancer cell lines. Pancreas. 2010;39(4):425–35. https://doi.org/10.1097/MPA.0b013e3181c15963.
2. Boussiotis VA. Molecular and biochemical aspects of the PD-1 checkpoint pathway. N Engl J Med. 2016;375(18):1767–78. https://doi.org/10.1056/NEJMra1514296.
3. Soares KC, Rucki AA, Wu AA, Olino K, Xiao Q, Chai Y, Wamwea A, Bigelow E, Lutz E, Liu L, Yao S, Anders RA, Laheru D, Wolfgang CL, Edil BH, Schulick RD, Jaffee EM, Zheng L. PD-1/PD-L1 blockade together with vaccine therapy facilitates effector T cell infiltration into pancreatic tumors. Journal of immunotherapy (Hagerstown, Md : 1997). 2015;38(1):1–11. https://doi.org/10.1097/cji.0000000000000062.
4. Wang X, Bao Z, Zhang X, Li F, Lai T, Cao C, Chen Z, Li W, Shen H, Ying S. Effectiveness and safety of PD-1/PD-L1 inhibitors in the treatment of solid tumors: a systematic review and meta-analysis. Oncotarget. 2017; https://doi.org/10.18632/oncotarget.18316.
5. Soares KC, Rucki AA, Wu AA, Olino K, Xiao Q, Chai Y, Wamwea A, Bigelow E, Lutz E, Liu L, Yao S, Anders RA, Laheru D, Wolfgang CL, Edil BH, Schulick RD, Jaffee EM, Zheng L. PD-1/PD-L1 blockade together with vaccine therapy facilitates effector T-cell infiltration into pancreatic tumors. Journal of immunotherapy (Hagerstown, Md : 1997). 2015;38(1):1–11. https://doi.org/10.1097/cji.0000000000000062.
6. Winograd R, Byrne KT, Evans RA, Odorizzi PM, Meyer AR, Bajor DL, Clendenin C, Stanger BZ, Furth EE, Wherry EJ, Vonderheide RH. Induction of T-cell immunity overcomes complete resistance to PD-1 and CTLA-4 blockade and improves survival in pancreatic carcinoma. Cancer immunology research. 2015;3(4):399–411. https://doi.org/10.1158/2326-6066.cir-14-0215.
7. Nomi T, Sho M, Akahori T, Hamada K, Kubo A, Kanehiro H, Nakamura S, Enomoto K, Yagita H, Azuma M, Nakajima Y. Clinical significance and therapeutic potential of the programmed death-1 ligand/programmed death-1 pathway in human pancreatic cancer. Clinical cancer research : an official journal of the American Association for Cancer Research. 2007;13(7):2151–7. https://doi.org/10.1158/1078-0432.CCR-06-2746.
8. Geng L, Huang D, Liu J, Qian Y, Deng J, Li D, Hu Z, Zhang J, Jiang G, Zheng S. B7-H1 up-regulated expression in human pancreatic carcinoma tissue

associates with tumor progression. J Cancer Res Clin Oncol. 2008;134(9):1021–7. https://doi.org/10.1007/s00432-008-0364-8.

9. Chen XL, Yuan SX, Chen C, Mao YX, Xu G, Wang XY. Expression of B7-H1 protein in human pancreatic carcinoma tissues and its clinical significance. Ai zheng = Aizheng = Chinese journal of cancer. 2009;28(12):1328–32.

10. Wang L, Ma Q, Chen X, Guo K, Li J, Zhang M. Clinical significance of B7-H1 and B7-1 expressions in pancreatic carcinoma. World J Surg. 2010;34(5):1059–65. https://doi.org/10.1007/s00268-010-0448-x.

11. Diana A, Wang LM, D'Costa Z, Allen P, Azad A, Silva MA, Soonawalla Z, Liu S, McKenna WG, Muschel RJ, Fokas E. Prognostic value, localization and correlation of PD-1/PD-L1, CD8 and FOXP3 with the desmoplastic stroma in pancreatic ductal adenocarcinoma. Oncotarget. 2016;7(27):40992–1004. https://doi.org/10.18632/oncotarget.10038.

12. Wang Y, Lin J, Cui J, Han T, Jiao F, Meng Z, Wang L. Prognostic value and clinicopathological features of PD-1/PD-L1 expression with mismatch repair status and desmoplastic stroma in Chinese patients with pancreatic cancer. Oncotarget. 2017;8(6):9354–65. https://doi.org/10.18632/oncotarget.14069.

13. Lu C, Paschall AV, Shi H, Savage N, Waller JL, Sabbatini ME, Oberlies NH, Pearce C, Liu K. The MLL1-H3K4me3 Axis-mediated PD-L1 expression and pancreatic cancer immune evasion. JNCI: journal of the National Cancer Institute 109 (6):djw283-djw283. 2017; https://doi.org/10.1093/jnci/djw283.

14. Bosman FCF, Hruban RH. WHO classification of tumours of the digestive system. Lyon, France: IARC Press; 2010.

15. Edge SB, Compton CC. The American joint committee on cancer: the 7th edition of the AJCC cancer staging manual and the future of TNM. Ann Surg Oncol. 2010;17(6):1471–4. https://doi.org/10.1245/s10434-010-0985-4.

16. Powles T, O'Donnell PH, Massard C, et al. Efficacy and safety of durvalumab in locally advanced or metastatic urothelial carcinoma: updated results from a phase 1/2 open-label study. JAMA Oncology. 2017;3(9):e172411. https://doi.org/10.1001/jamaoncol.2017.2411.

17. Zhang J, Fang W, Qin T, Yang Y, Hong S, Liang W, Ma Y, Zhao H, Huang Y, Xue C, Huang P, Hu Z, Zhao Y, Zhang L. Co-expression of PD-1 and PD-L1 predicts poor outcome in nasopharyngeal carcinoma. Medical oncology (Northwood, London, England). 2015;32(3):86. https://doi.org/10.1007/s12032-015-0501-6.

18. Clark CE, Beatty GL, Vonderheide RH. Immunosurveillance of pancreatic adenocarcinoma: insights from genetically engineered mouse models of cancer. Cancer Lett. 2009;279(1):1–7. https://doi.org/10.1016/j.canlet.2008.09.037.

19. Lutz ER, AA W, Bigelow E, Sharma R, Mo G, Soares K, Solt S, Dorman A, Wamwea A, Yager A, Laheru D, Wolfgang CL, Wang J, Hruban RH, Anders RA, Jaffee EM, Zheng L. Immunotherapy converts nonimmunogenic pancreatic tumors into immunogenic foci of immune regulation. Cancer immunology research. 2014;2(7):616–31. https://doi.org/10.1158/2326-6066.cir-14-0027.

20. Igawa S, Sato Y, Ryuge S, Ichinoe M, Katono K, Hiyoshi Y, Otani S, Nagashio R, Nakashima H, Katagiri M, Sasaki J, Murakumo Y, Satoh Y, Masuda N. Impact of PD-L1 expression in patients with surgically resected non-small-cell lung cancer. Oncology. 2017; https://doi.org/10.1159/000458412.

21. Botti G, Collina F, Scognamiglio G, Rao F, Peluso V, De Cecio R, Piezzo M, Landi G, De Laurentiis M, Cantile M, Di Bonito M. Programmed death ligand 1 (PD-L1) tumor expression is associated with a better prognosis and diabetic disease in triple negative breast cancer patients. Int J Mol Sci. 2017;18(2) https://doi.org/10.3390/ijms18020459.

22. Ohigashi Y, Sho M, Yamada Y, Tsurui Y, Hamada K, Ikeda N, Mizuno T, Yoriki R, Kashizuka H, Yane K, Tsushima F, Otsuki N, Yagita H, Azuma M, Nakajima Y. Clinical significance of programmed death-1 ligand-1 and programmed death-1 ligand-2 expression in human esophageal cancer. Clinical cancer research : an official journal of the American Association for Cancer Research. 2005;11(8):2947–53. https://doi.org/10.1158/1078-0432.CCR-04-1469.

23. Bellmunt J, de Wit R, Vaughn DJ, Fradet Y, Lee JL, Fong L, Vogelzang NJ, Climent MA, Petrylak DP, Choueiri TK, Necchi A, Gerritsen W, Gurney H, Quinn DI, Culine S, Sternberg CN, Mai Y, Poehlein CH, Perini RF, Bajorin DF. Investigators K- (2017) Pembrolizumab as second-line therapy for advanced urothelial carcinoma. N Engl J Med. 376(11):1015–26. https://doi.org/10.1056/NEJMoa1613683.

24. Abdul Karim L, Wang P, Chahine J, Kallakury B. PD-L1 IHC assays in melanoma. Histopathology. 2017; https://doi.org/10.1111/his.13174.

25. Giraldo NA, Becht E, Vano Y, Petitprez F, Lacroix L, Validire P, Sanchez-Salas R, Ingels A, Oudard SM, Moatti A, Buttard B, Bourras S, Germain C, Cathelineau X, Fridman WH, Sautes-Fridman C. Tumor-infiltrating and peripheral blood T cell Immunophenotypes predict early relapse in localized clear cell renal cell carcinoma. Clinical cancer research : an official journal of the American Association for Cancer Research. 2017; https://doi.org/10.1158/1078-0432.CCR-16-2848.

26. Dill EA, Gru AA, Atkins KA, Friedman LA, Moore ME, Bullock TN, Cross JV, Dillon PM, Mills AM. PD-L1 expression and Intratumoral heterogeneity across breast cancer subtypes and stages: an assessment of 245 primary and 40 metastatic tumors. Am J Surg Pathol. 2017;41(3):334–42. https://doi.org/10.1097/pas.0000000000000780.

27. Casadevall D, Clave S, Taus A, Hardy-Werbin M, Rocha P, Lorenzo M, Menendez S, Salido M, Albanell J, Pijuan L, Arriola E. Heterogeneity of tumor and immune cell PD-L1 expression and lymphocyte counts in surgical NSCLC samples. Clinical lung cancer. 2017; https://doi.org/10.1016/j.cllc.2017.04.014.

11

Level of mitoses in non-muscle invasive papillary urothelial carcinomas (pTa and pT1) at initial bladder biopsy is a simple and powerful predictor of clinical outcome: a multi-center study in South Korea

Ji Eun Kwon[2], Nam Hoon Cho[3], Yeong-Jin Choi[4], So Dug Lim[5], Yong Mee Cho[6], Sun Young Jun[7], Sanghui Park[8], Young A. Kim[9], Sung-Sun Kim[10], Mi Sun Choe[11], Jung-dong Lee[12], Dae Yong Kang[12], Jae Y. Ro[13] and Hyun-Jung Kim[1*]

Abstract

Background: Histologic grade is the most important predictor of the clinical outcome of non-muscle invasive (Ta, T1) papillary urothelial carcinoma (NMIPUCa), but its ambiguous criteria diminish its power to predict recurrence/progression for individual patients. We attempted to find an objective and reproducible histologic predictor of NMIPUCa that correlates well with the clinical outcome.

Methods: A total of 296 PUCas were collected from the Departments of Surgical Pathology of 11 institutions in South Korea. The clinical outcome was grouped into no event (NE), recurrence (R), and progression (P) categories. All 25 histological parameters were numerically redefined. The clinical pathology of each case was reviewed individually by 11 pathologists from 11 institutions based on the 2004 WHO criteria and afterwards blindly evaluated by two participants, based on our proposed parameters. Univariate and multivariate logistic regression analyses were performed using the R software package.

Results: The level of mitoses was the most reliable parameter for predicting the clinical outcome. We propose a four-tiered grading system based on mitotic count (> 10/10 high-power fields), nuclear pleomorphism (smallest-to-largest ratio of tumor nuclei >20), presence of divergent histology, and capillary proliferation (> 20 capillary lumina per papillary core).

Conclusions: The level of mitoses at the initial bladder biopsy and transurethral resection (TUR) specimen appeared to be an independent predictor of the Ta PUCa outcome. Other parameters include the number of mitoses, nuclear pleomorphism, divergent histology, and capillary proliferation within the fibrovascular core. These findings may improve selection of patients for a therapeutic strategy as compared to previous grading systems.

Keywords: Predictor, Clinical outcome, Mitotic level, Papillary urothelial carcinoma, Predictor

* Correspondence: hjkim@paik.ac.kr
[1]Department of Pathology, Inje University Sanggye Paik Hospital, 1342, Dongilro, Nowon-gu, Seoul, South Korea
Full list of author information is available at the end of the article

Background

Non-muscle invasive papillary urothelial carcinomas (NMIPUC) of the urinary bladder, with tumors staged as non-invasive intraepithelial (Ta) or tumors with invasion of the lamina propria/submucosa (T1), are known to recur frequently (in up to 70% of cases), and occasionally (in up to 40% of cases) progress [1]. The European Association of Urology (EAU) guidelines for NMIPUC-(pTa/T1) of the bladder proposed risk stratification for progression into low-, intermediate-, and high-risk groups [2]. The same guideline stated that the patients in different groups should be managed using different strategies. Besides stage (Ta vs. T1), size (< 3 cm vs. $\geq$ 3 cm), number of papillary tumors (single vs. multiple), concurrent carcinoma in situ (CIS), and a history of recurrence, the best estimator of risk is the histological grade. The four existing grading systems (1973 World Health Organization [WHO], 1998 International Society of Urologic Pathology [ISUP]/2004 WHO, Cheng et al. [3, 4], and 2016 WHO classifications) have divided PUCs based on subjective morphological parameters, which has led to a high interobserver/intraobserver variability in diagnoses made by pathologists, as well as lower predictive power in management by urologists [5]. In view of this, alternative grading systems have been sought to improve the grading discrepancy [6]. Many studies on immunohistochemical and molecular markers have been conducted to reduce the subjectivity of the histological grading systems, but the markers studied have been declared as having no potential for playing a role in grading schemes [7–12].

The present study was conducted to identify more objective and reproducible histological predictors that may correlate well with the clinical outcome, and compare these to the previous histological grading systems. Eleven uropathologists evaluated light microscopic histological parameters together in three rounds, using a multihead microscope. Through this study, vigorous attempts were made to select all possible histological parameters as countable variables. Each parameter was evaluated using univariate and multivariate analyses, to determine whether these variables had statistically significant effect in predicting the clinical outcome.

Methods

Patient selection

Surgically removed NMIPUCs of the urinary bladder were collected from the surgical pathology archives of 11 institutions in South Korea. The inclusion criteria were as follows: (1) pTa or pT1 stage at the initial bladder biopsy; and (2) a 5-year minimum follow-up period for non-event (NE) cases. The exclusion criteria, on the other hand, were as follows: (1) a prior history or the concurrent presence of urothelial carcinoma either in

the ureter or in the renal pelvis; and (2) evidence of associated urothelial carcinoma in situ. A total of 296 cases were retrieved (Ta, 178; T1, 118). The number of cases contributed by each institute was 95, 47, 38, 22, 21, 21, 17, 15, 14, 4, and 2.

Clinical parameters

The retrieved cases were classified into three clinical subgroups: no event (NE), recurrence (R), and progression (P). NE was defined as cases with no evidence of tumor on the follow-up imaging study, urine cytology, or cystoscopy for at least 5-year follow-up duration; R was defined as cases showing a new tumor occurrence with the same or lower stage at least 3 months after the initial resection; and P was defined as a cases showing new tumor development with a higher stage than the initial stage, or metastasis to the lymph nodes or other organs. We collected clinical information on the patients from the medical records, including 1) age, 2) sex, 3) site, number, and size/volume of tumor in first biopsy, 4) interval to the 2nd event, 5) number of recurrences, 6) the type of final operation, 7) survival, 8) cause of death, and 9) site of metastasis. All types of specimens (cystoscopic biopsy, cold-cup biopsy, transurethral resection of bladder tumor) were included, but were not defined separately. However, there was no partial or radical cystectomy specimen (as an initial biopsy) among the 296 cases. The number of tumors was divided into two groups: single vs. multiple. The tumor size was also divided into two groups: $\leq$ 3 cm vs. > 3 cm. The distribution of each group is shown in Table 1.

Histological evaluation

For microscopic examination, hematoxylin and eosin (H&E)-stained glass slides of formalin-fixed, paraffin-embedded tissue of the tumors were retrieved. Interobserver discrepancy had been solved through several round-table multihead microscopic examinations involving 11 pathologists from 11 institutions, during which consensus opinion was reached. Although the proper muscle inclusion was not verified by the reviewers in all samples, 11 contributors had reviewed the original

Table 1 Clinical characteristics of the patients

	Stage	
	Ta (n = 178)	T1 (n = 118)
Clinical subgroup (NE/R/P)	73/69/37	32/50/30
Age (mean)	65	68
Sex (M/F)	138/40	93/25
Number of tumor (single vs. multiple)	99/79	46/70[a]
Size ($\leq$3 cm vs. > 3 cm)	130/48	68/50

NE No event, R Recurrence, P Progression
[a]not available in 2 cases

diagnosis and pathological stage, not only by a slide review, but also from the surgical records. The 2nd biopsy was routinely performed 3 months later for check-up of incomplete resection (i.e., residual tumor). Even if the initial diagnosis was NMIPUCa (Ta, T1), the cases with a short-interval change in the T stage were excluded and were regarded as an inaccurate diagnosis. The clinical pathology of each case was reviewed individually by 11 pathologists from 11 institutions based on the 2004 WHO criteria and was afterward blindly evaluated by two participants, based on our proposed parameters. The histological parameters that were examined are shown in Table 2 and Figs. 1 and 2. For prediction comparison, the previous grading systems, i.e., the 2004 WHO grading, Papillary urothelial neoplasm low malignant potential (PUNLMP) /Low grade (LG) /High grade (HG), 1973 WHO, Transitional cell carcinoma (TCC) grade 1/2/3, and Cheng et al., grade 1/2/3/4, were utilized [3, 4].

Statistical analysis

All of the aforementioned parameters were evaluated in two paired comparison groups (i.e., R vs. NE and P vs. NE) at each stage. To identify the factors influencing R and/or P, univariate and multivariate logistic regression analyses were performed. To investigate the diagnostic utility of the new grading system, it was compared with the previous grading systems by area under the curve (AUC) of receiver operating characteristics (ROC) curves. All the statistical analyses were performed in the R software package (R version 3.1.2, R Foundation for Statistical Computing, Vienna, Austria; <http://www.R-project.org/>).

Results

Univariate analysis

For PUC-Ta, among morphologic variables, the number (odds ratio [OR] 0.34 [95% confidence interval, CI: 0.17-0.67]; p-value = 0.002), size (OR 2.27 [95% CI: 1.05-5.07]; p-value = 0.0399), mitotic count (OR 1.03 [95% CI: 1.00-1.07]; p-value = 0.0468), mitotic level (OR 1.09 [95% CI: 0.24-4.83]; p-value = 0.010), and capillary proliferation in fibrovascular cores (OR 1.05 [95% CI: 1.01-1.10]; p-value = 0.0136) were associated with tumor recurrence. Nuclear pleomorphism showed borderline significance for association with recurrence of PUC-Ta (Table 3). The factors associated with PUC-Ta progression included patient age, cell density, nuclear pleomorphism, hyperchromasia, nuclear groove, prominent nucleoli, necrosis, mitotic count, mitotic level. Capillary proliferation and apoptosis had borderline statistical significance (Table 4). For PUC-T1, the whorling pattern was associated with recurrence and the mitotic level showed borderline significant association

with recurrence. Divergent histology was associated with progression only (Additional file 1: Tables S1 and S2).

Proposal of new grading system using more objective and fewer histological variables for predicting clinical outcome

Based on the univariate analysis results, three grades were designed for prediction of the biological behavior of PUC-Ta. The univariate analysis results for PUC-T1 revealed that only tumor stage influenced the biological behavior. Thus, once the tumor had invaded the lamina propria/submucosa, the histological parameters had an insignificant impact on the clinical outcome. Therefore, our new grading system was designed focusing on the prediction of PUC-Ta tumors. To design a new grading system with more objective and reproducible, yet simpler parameters, we chose mitotic level, mitotic count, capillary proliferation, and nuclear pleomorphism as important histological parameters, based on the univariate analysis. All four of these parameters not only had a statistically significant influence on both recurrence and progression of PUC-Ta, but were also quantifiable. Additionally, divergent histology was also selected as one of the parameters in our grading system; even though it showed an insignificant p-value in both recurrence and progression of PUC-Ta, it was statistically significant in terms of progression in PUC-T1 tumors.

Because the mitotic level appeared to be the most important morphological parameter based on the univariate analysis, the mitotic level was set as the first step in our proposed new grading system. Grades 1, 2, and 3 were assigned based on mitotic level, i.e., level 1, level 2, and level 3, respectively. In cases with any additional unfavorable histological features, including increased mitotic count (> 10/10 high-power fields), significant nuclear pleomorphism (smallest-to largest-ratio of tumor nuclei of >20), presence of divergent histology, and significant capillary proliferation (> 20 capillary lumina per papillary core), the tumors were upgraded: for example, grade 1 became grade 2, grade 2 became grade 3, and grade 3 became grade 4. We designed three similar but slightly different grading schemes.

Comparison of our proposed grading system with previous grading systems

To investigate the diagnostic and prognostic utility of our proposed grading system, we compared the previous grading systems by comparison of AUC values in each system. All the statistical analyses were performed with adjustments for age, gender, tumor size, and number of tumors, to exclude the impact of factors other than histological parameters. For the prediction of recurrence of PUC-Ta, the AUCs of three previous grading systems

Table 2 Histologic parameters evaluated in this study

Variables	Definition	Category	Explanation of category
Papillary fusion	Fusion of papillae with forming confluent and complex papillary cores	1	<1/3 area
		2	1/3 ~ 2/3 area
		3	>2/3 area
Umbrella cells	Area with preserved umbrella cells	1	>50% area
		2	5-50% area
		3	<5% area
Discohesiveness	Detached cells from papillae	1	<1/3 area
	Refer to Additional file 1: Figure S1.	2	1/3 ~ 2/3 area
		3	>2/3 area
Cell density		1	<1/3 areas show more than 2 times normal density
		2	1/3 ~ ≤2/3 area shows more than 2 times of normal density
		3	>2/3 area show more than 2 times normal density or >5% area shows more than 3 times normal density
Nuclear pleomorphism	Size of smallest nuclei vs. largest nuclei(regardless of tangential sectioning)	1	<3
		2	3 ≤ and <8
		3	8 ≤ and <20
		4	≥20
Multinucleated giant cells	Presence of bi-or multinucleated nuclei	0	Absence
		1	Presence
Loss of polarity	Proportion of cells deviating from the vertical alignment shown in normal urothelium	1	<5%
		2	5-50%
		3	>50%
Hyperchromasia	Semiquantitative degree of nuclear hyperchromasia	1	diffusely mild
		2	diffusely moderate or focally strong
		3	diffusely strong
Nuclear groove	Proportion of tumor cells without identifiable nuclear grooves	1	<5%
		2	5-50%
		3	> 50%
Prominent nucleoli	Proportion of cells having prominent nuclei (recognizable under 10× medium power)	1	<5%
		2	5-50%
		3	>50%
Whorling pattern	Refer to Additional file 1: Figure S1.	0	absent
		1	present
Necrosis	Degree of necrosis	1	singly spotted
		2	focally grouped or multifocally spotted
		3	surface necrosis of nests
		4	confluent necrosis
Divergent histology	Presence and number of glandular, squamous or micropapillary differentiation	0	absence
		1	1
		2	2
		3	3
Mitotic count	Number of mitosis/ 10 consecutive HPFs in most mitotically active area	CON	

Table 2 Histologic parameters evaluated in this study *(Continued)*

Mitotic count-CAT	Group of mitotic count	1	0-2
		2	3-7
		3	8-15
		4	≥16
Mitotic level	Most highest level of mitotic figures, from base to the top of the papilla(low 1/3, mid1/3, and high 1/3)	1	<1/3 or no mitosis
		2	1/3-2/3
		3	>2/3
Apoptosis	Number of apoptotic bodies in most active area/one HPF	1	<10
		2	10-100
		3	>100
Capillary proliferation	Number of capillary in one papillary core	CON	

CAT Categorical variable, *CON* Continuous variable, *HPF(s)* High power field(s)

were less than 0.7, whereas the AUCs of our proposed grading systems were over 0.7, and it was statistically significant (*p*-value <0.05). However, the differences between them were not statistically significant (Table 5). As for the prediction of progression of PUC-Ta, the AUCs of all of the previous and new grading systems were all larger than 0.7 (*p*-value <0.05) (Additional file 1: Figure S1).

Discussion

In this study, we attempted to find an objective and reproducible histologic predictor of NMIPUCa that correlates well with the clinical outcome and to compare these to the previous histological grading systems. We found that the level of mitoses at the initial bladder biopsy was an independent predictor of the Ta PUCa outcome; the number of mitoses, nuclear pleomorphism, divergent histology, and capillary proliferation within the fibrovascular core were also significant factors.

The EAU guideline proposed a three-risk group stratification. In addition to the tumor stage, tumor size, number of tumors, and association with CIS, histological grade was an important parameter for predicting progression [2, 5]. The 2004 and 2016 WHO grading systems had been modified from 1973 WHO classification; recently, in 2012, Cheng et al. developed a modified system. These systems are similar, but show slight variation. Each parameter was measured without well-defined criteria and has led to suboptimal reproducibility [13–15]. Each parameter was rated in terms of severity (mild/moderate/severe) or frequency (rare/occasionally/frequently). In routine pathology practice, pathologists often encounter a PUC of the bladder showing high mitotic activity, but only mild nuclear atypia and minimal loss of polarity, or in contrast, a case showing moderate nuclear pleomorphism and mild to moderate loss of

polarity, but without discernible mitotic activity. In those cases, grading was not straightforward, because there was no priority finding depending on the weighted value among the many criteria, which complicated the grading assignment, and resulted in low reproducibility.

We attempted to develop a simple and reproducible grading system that could predict the clinical outcome in NMIPUC of the bladder. In this study, we included only cases with available initial-biopsy specimens and cases with no concurrent CIS. Initially all 11 uropathologists evaluated all histologic parameters using individual light microscopes, for three rounds. Twenty-five histological features with their numerical parameters (e.g., categorized grade or absolute number), including mitotic level and number of mitoses, level of apoptosis, necrosis, whirling appearance, and capillary proliferation, which had not been evaluated prior to this study, were selected, as well as other histological factors mentioned in the literature. Thereafter, two pathologists blindly evaluated all 296 cases to determine interobserver reproducibility. Some parameters appeared to be influenced by fixation and stain conditions. Therefore, intranuclear groove and nucleolar prominence, which may be produced by procedural artifacts, were considered as low-priority parameters.

In the univariate analysis of T1-stage tumors, only a divergent histology correlated with progression. We considered that the pathological stage-factor, with the presence of stromal (lamina propria/submucosal) invasion, was the most important factor dictating biological behavior from among the histological factors. This finding was in accordance with the WHO recommendation that grading is performed only for noninvasive PUC (PUC-Ta), and with other reports in the literature [16]. Therefore, in this study, the construction of the histological predictive model was limited to noninvasive (Ta) tumors, with exclusion of T1 tumors.

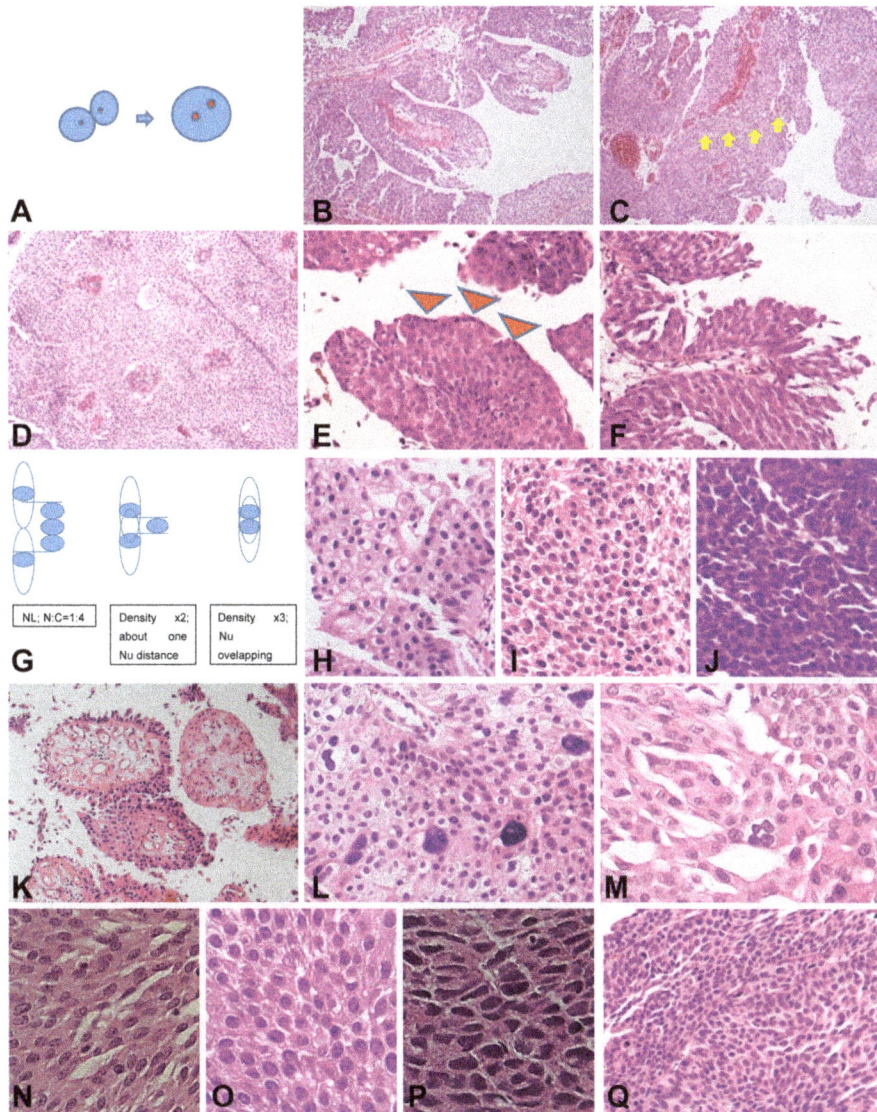

Fig. 1 (1) Representative images of histological parameters evaluated in this study. **a** Schematic figure of papillary fusion. **b** Delicate papillae with no fusion. **c** Papillary fusion (the arrow marks an imaginary fusion line). **d** Confluent fusion of papillae. **e** Presence of umbrella cells (arrowhead). **f** Absence of umbrella cells. **g** Schematic figure for the estimation of cell density based on the distance between cells. **h** Cell density score 1. **i** Cell density score 2. **j** Cell density score 3. **k** Discohesiveness (**l**). Nuclear pleomorphism category 4 based on a difference between the smallest and the biggest nucleus of the tumor cells of about 20-fold. **m** Multinucleated giant cells. **n** Mild nuclear hyperchromasia. **o** Moderate nuclear hyperchromasia. **p** Severe nuclear hyperchromasia. **q** Polarity loss score 2

Unlike T1 tumors, Ta tumors had many clinical and histologic parameters that influenced the clinical outcome. Among the clinical factors, the number and size of tumors correlated with recurrence, while patient's age was associated with progression. In terms of histological factors, mitotic count, mitotic level, and capillary proliferation correlated with recurrence. Cell density, nuclear pleomorphism, hyperchromasia, nuclear groove, prominent nucleoli, necrosis as well as mitotic count and level correlated with progression. Apoptosis and capillary proliferation disclosed borderline significance for progression.

It is worth noting that mitotic count showed the highest OR in the prediction of both recurrence and progression of PUC-Ta. In the early twenty-first century, many studies had focused on mitotic index (Ki-67, AgNO3) of Ta/T1 urothelial carcinomas, and have reported those as associated with tumor recurrence [17–19]. However, the impact of mitosis has not been fully evaluated for use, or has not been applied with a detailed cutoff-value in the grading system, in contrast to other epithelial cancers in other organs (low vs. high serous carcinoma of the ovary, histological grade of breast cancer and etc.) [20, 21]. Our

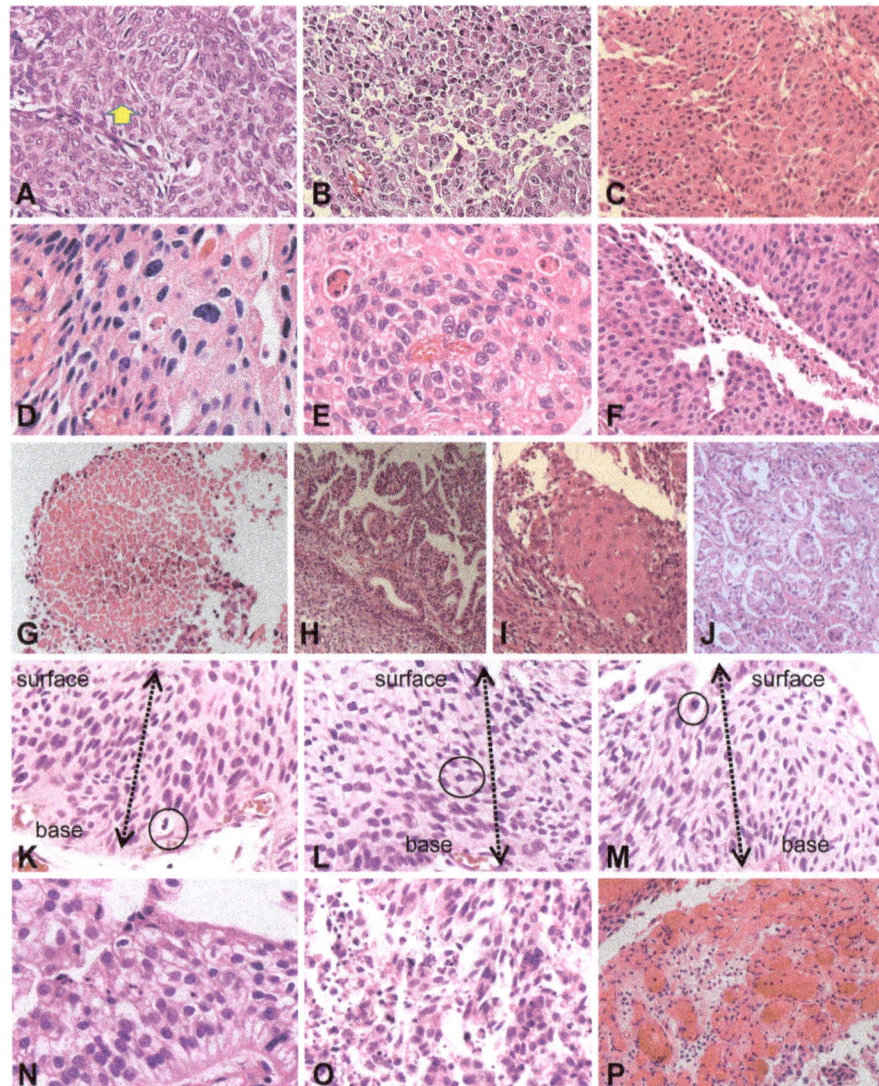

Fig. 2 (2) Further representative images of histological parameters evaluated in this study. **a** Example of a nuclear groove (arrow). **b** Prominent nucleoli. **c** Whorling pattern. **d** Single spotty necrosis (arrow). **e** Multifocal group necrosis (arrows). **f** Surface necrosis. **g** Confluent necrosis. **h** Glandular differentiation. **i** Squamous differentiation. **j** Micropapillary differentiation. **k** Mitosis level 1. **l** Mitosis level 2. **m** Mitosis level 3. **n** Apoptosis score 1. **o** Apoptosis score 3. **p** Capillary proliferation in fibrovascular core of papilla

results indicated that mitotic count should be integrated in the histological grading of PUC.

The importance of mitotic count has previously been emphasized for histological grading of NMIPUCa [22, 23]. Pich et al. showed that a high proliferative index is the most important recurrence-predictor among LMP and low-grade tumors [24]. Akkalp et al. also emphasized that higher mitotic activity (> 5/single high-power field) is a strong predictor for recurrence in Ta PUCa [25]. The studies indicate that proliferative activity can play an adjunctive role in histologic grading (even in low grade tumors) and prediction of recurrence or invasiveness, as also shown in this study. However, the criteria for proliferative activity were variable, including a mitotic count per one or 10 high power fields in any level of the neoplastic epithelium, and cut-off values for AgNOR and Ki-67. Considering that urothelial neoplasms are bulky, mitotic counting in high-power fields might be inconsistent and discordant.

Mitotic level has not received much attention either. The upper level of mitosis (level 3 mitosis) correlated with increased mitotic count and worse clinical outcome in our cohort. If a bulky mass is evaluated for the level of mitosis, the mitotic-specific marker, phospohistamine H3 (PHH3), can be useful for rapid detection of the mitotic level. PHH3 has been used for grading of upper-tract urothelial carcinoma [26]. Since the mitotic level and count were measurable, reproducible, and the most

Table 3 Univariate analysis of factors associated with recurrence of PUC-Ta

Variable	Category	Odds ratio	95% Confidence Interval	P-value
Age		1.00	0.97-1.03	0.9401
Sex	man vs. woman	1.11	0.50-2.47	0.7908
No of tumor		0.34	0.17-0.67	0.0021*
Size of tumor		2.27	1.05-5.07	0.0399*
Papillary fusion	2 vs 1	1.50	0.65-3.50	0.3430
	3 vs 1	1.60	0.74-3.50	0.2348
Umbrella cell	2 vs. 1	0.95	0.44-2.07	0.9020
	3 vs. 1	1.19	0.52-2.75	0.6723
Discohesiveness	2 vs. 1	1.93	0.80-4.78	0.1480
	3 vs. 1	1.57	0.71-3.53	0.2682
Cell density	2 vs. 1	1.62	0.69-3.88	0.2737
	3 vs. 1	0.88	0.37-2.08	0.7719
Nuclear pleomorphism	2 vs. 1	0.47	0.21-1.03	0.0621
	3 vs. 1	0.39	0.14-1.03	0.0599
	4 vs. 1	3.84	0.58-76.11	0.2324
Multinucleated giant cell	1 vs. 0	1.14	0.58-2.24	0.7041
Loss of polarity	2 vs. 1	1.03	0.41-2.59	0.9557
	3 vs. 1	0.82	0.29-2.26	0.6981
Hyperchromasia	2 vs. 1	1.36	0.67-2.79	0.3904
	3 vs. 1	0.97	0.26-3.47	0.9604
Nuclear groove	2 vs. 1	1.83	0.86-3.96	0.1184
	3 vs. 1	1.60	0.65-3.99	0.3079
Prominent nucleoli	2 vs. 1	1.12	0.56-2.23	0.7491
	3 vs. 1	0.81	0.15-3.90	0.7903
Whorling pattern	1 vs. 0	1.07	0.55-2.11	0.8327
Necrosis	2 vs 1	0.98	0.39-2.48	0.9694
	3 vs 1	0.77	0.21-2.58	0.6680
	4 vs 1	1.47	0.54-4.14	0.4490
Divergent histology		2.04	0.73-8.10	0.2172
Mitotic count		1.03	1.00-1.07	0.0468*
Mitotic count (CAT)	2 vs. 1	4.62	1.89-11.98	0.0011
	3 vs. 1	2.52	0.94-6.95	0.0684
	4 vs. 1	3.15	1.22-8.46	0.0193*
Mitotic level	2 vs. 1	2.13	0.83-5.70	0.1229
	3 vs. 1	4.44	1.88-11.18	0.0010*
Apoptosis	2 vs 1	1.15	0.53-2.50	0.7246
	3 vs 1	1.09	0.24-4.82	0.9116
Capillary proliferation		1.05	1.01-1.10	0.0136*

No Number, *CAT* Categorical variable; *P < 0.05

statistically significant parameters in our univariate analysis, we strongly recommended that these factors should be included as essential parameters in histological grading of PUC, even though identifying mitoses in an entire specimen requires marked effort.

HG tumors in the WHO 2004 and 2016 classification cover wide ranges of tumors from immediately above low-grade to highly anaplastic tumors. Recently, Cheng and his colleges suggested a four-tiered grading system that included grade 4, which consisted of an anaplastic group,

Table 4 Univariate analysis of factors associated with progression of PUC- Ta

Variable	Category	Odds ratio	95% Confidence Interval	P-value
Age		1.05	1.01-1.09	0.0095*
Sex	man vs. woman	1.06	0.46-2.7	0.8893
No of tumor		0.61	0.29-1.27	0.1856
Size of tumor		1.40	0.62-3.03	0.4012
Papillary fusion	2 vs 1	1.27	0.52-3.04	0.5871
	3 vs 1	0.89	0.36-2.13	0.8044
Umbrella cell	2 vs. 1	1.82	0.64-5.13	0.2590
	3 vs. 1	2.71	0.96-7.62	0.0591
Discohesiveness	2 vs. 1	1.30	0.49-3.26	0.5841
	3 vs. 1	1.38	0.58-3.2	0.4579
Cell density	2 vs. 1	2.02	0.56-9.58	0.3165
	3 vs. 1	5.40	1.73-23.89	0.0093*
Nuclear pleomorphism	2 vs. 1	0.72	0.26-2.06	0.5331
	3 vs. 1	3.18	1.25-8.68	0.0180*
	4 vs. 1	1.46	0.19-7.53	0.6683
Multinucleated giant cell	1 vs. 0	1.56	0.75-3.24	0.2337
Loss of polarity	2 vs. 1	1.17	0.35-3.86	0.798
	3 vs. 1	2.70	0.82-8.93	0.104;
Hyperchromasia	2 vs. 1	2.42	1.16-5.2	0.0200*
	3 vs. 1	1.75	0.71-4.32	0.2206
Nuclear groove	2 vs. 1	9.26	3.44-26.31	0.0000*
	3 vs. 1	5.28	1.68-23.39	0.0105*
Prominent nucleoli	2 vs. 1	0.00	NA	0.9889
	3 vs. 1	0.37	0.14-0.87	0.0314*
Whorling pattern	1 vs. 0	1.25	0.26-4.87	0.7550
Necrosis	2 vs 1	2.04	0.70-5.59	0.1747
	3 vs 1	5.58	2.00-15.73	0.0010*
	4 vs 1	2.47	0.83-6.90	0.0903
Divergent histology		1.70	0.68-3.98	0.2222
Mitotic count		1.06	1.03-1.09	0.0000*
Mitotic count(CAT)	2 vs. 1	8.72	2.1-59.47	0.0076*
	3 vs. 1	8.45	1.8-60.71	0.0124*
	4 vs. 1	24.80	6.59-162.78	0.0000*
Mitotic level	2 vs. 1	7.20	1.23-136.92	0.0689
	3 vs. 1	15.51	3.1-282.16	0.0083*
Apoptosis	2 vs 1	2.18	0.97-4.84	0.0559
	3 vs 1	3.40	0.94-11.44	0.0501*
Capillary proliferation		1.03	1-1.07	0.0673

NA Not available, *CAT* Categorical variable; *P < 0.05

and separating this group from the usual HG [3, 4, 27]. Because we agreed with the assignment of such an upper grade, the second step of our newly proposed grading scheme was focused on the selection of a more aggressive group. Four additional histological parameters (mitotic count, nuclear pleomorphism capillary proliferation, and divergent histology) were used. We assigned tumors as grade 4 when high-level mitosis, with more than 10 mitoses per 10 high-power fields, and any of the following were present: divergent histology, nuclear pleomorphism of more than 20-fold, and more than 20 capillary lumens per papillary core. The other two upgrading schemes

Table 5 Comparison of AUC for predicting PUC-Ta tumor recurrence between previous grading systems and our proposed grading system

Old_grades	AUC-Old_grades (se)	Proposed_grade	AUC-Proposed_grade	Old vs. new grade p-value
#1	0.686 (0.044)	1	0.709 (0.043)	0.3188
		2	0.715 (0.043)	0.2784
		3	0.703 (0.044)	0.4289
#2	0.688 (0.045)	1	0.709 (0.043)	0.3800
		2	0.715 (0.043)	0.3215
		3	0.703 (0.044)	0.5003
#3	0.685 (0.045)	1	0.709 (0.043)	0.2809
		2	0.715 (0.043)	0.2516
		3	0.703 (0.044)	0.3599

#1:2004 WHO grading system (low grade/high grade); #2: 1973 WHO grading system (TCC grade 1,2, and 3); #3:Cheng et al. 's grading system [G1/G2/G3/G4-Anaplastic]

(grade 1 to grade 2, and grade 2 to grade 3) were similar, but slightly different from this scheme.

Capillary proliferation has been evaluated in terms of the number of capillary lumina per papillary core that was cross-sectioned, and microvessel density (MVD) has been studied as a prognostic factor in many solid tumors [28, 29]. MVD could not be determined in this study, because endothelial marker immunostaining was performed in a limited number of cases of Ta tumors. However, we evaluated the light microscopic neovascularization by counting the number of capillary lumina in the most vaso-proliferative papillary core. The presence of more than 20 capillary lumina was correlated with a worse clinical outcome.

A divergent histology was defined as identifiable histological features differing from the usual urothelial carcinoma. A significant number of high-grade urothelial carcinomas demonstrated glandular or squamous differentiation. In this study, tumors with divergent histology showed a worse clinical outcome than those that were pure urothelial carcinomas. The divergent histology could represent a dedifferentiation with molecular events resulting in a gain of function. Cheng et al. classified tumors with divergent differentiation, such as the nested variant, micropapillary variant, plasmacytoid variant, sarcomatoid carcinoma, small-cell carcinoma, large-cell undifferentiated carcinoma, and pleomorphic giant cell carcinoma, as grade 4 tumors [3]. In our univariate analyses, divergent histology was associated with progression of PUC-T1, but it showed less statistical significance in PUC-Ta, with a *P*-value of 0.2. Most histological parameters played no significant roles in the clinical outcome of PUC-T1, except for divergent histology. This indicated that the presence of divergent differentiation should be considered, particularly in invasive carcinoma. The reason for the reduced significance of divergent histology in the prediction of clinical outcome in PUC-Ta may be related to the low frequency of Ta stage tumors. Aggressive tumors with a divergent

histology were more apparent in the invasive stage (T1) and were not usually detected at the Ta stage. Thus, we included divergent histology as one of adverse histological parameters for upgrading. Large cohort studies of PUC-Ta with a significant number of tumors with divergent histologic differentiation may be needed to verify whether this parameter has a clear biological impact.

Necrosis or apoptosis may be detected easily in a low-power view, but differentiation between these two features was not easy. In addition, degeneration of the papillary cores with dystrophic calcification could be confused with necrosis.

The newly proposed grading system designed here was compared with previous grading systems. Even though the difference in the AUCs between them was not statistically significant, the AUCs of the new grading system were larger than those of the previous grading systems for the prediction of PUC-Ta recurrence. The former AUC was more than 0.7 ($p < 0.05$), but that of the latter was less than 0.7. In addition, our proposed grading system was focused on only few, but the most powerful histological parameters, which are not descriptive or subjective, are rather quantifiable and are more reproducible, for practical use. Therefore, our system may be a better option to use as a grading system if it has a similar power for the prediction of the clinical outcome of PUC-Ta.

Because this study was not prospectively designed, with a controlled biopsy protocol and treatment, the treatment factors cannot be considered in the clinical outcome. Resection only vs. intravesical chemo/Bacille de Calmette-Guérin (BCG) treatment cannot be separately reviewed among the same grade and stage tumors. However, this study is valuable because it provided a comprehensive analysis of all histological parameters, including mitotic level and count, through a nationwide multicenter study, involving experienced uropathologists.

Although diagnostic improvement should be verified by means of a kappa value, we were unable to do so in this study. In the near future, we will collect "gray zone" tumors, with divergent designations by pathologists, and apply the new grading system to determine whether it allows improved diagnosis.

Conclusion

The mitotic level based on the initial biopsy appears to be an independent predictor of the PUCa-Ta outcome. This finding could potentially help distinguish between low and high grade tumors in borderline lesions. Therefore, this result may help in selecting patients for a therapeutic strategy, based on the initial biopsy of NMI-PUC of the bladder.

Abbreviations
AUC: Area under the curve; CIS: Carcinoma in situ; EAU: European Association of Urology; H&E: Hematoxylin and eosin; HPF: High power field; ISUP: International Society of Urologic Pathology; LMP/LG/HG: Papillary urothelial neoplasm low malignant potential/low grade/high grade; MVD: Microvessel density; NE: No event R; recurrence, P; progression; NMIPUC: Non-muscle invasive papillary urothelial carcinoma; PHH3: Phospohistamine H3; PUC: Papillary urothelial carcinoma; ROC: Receiver operating characteristics; T1: Invasion of the lamina propria/submucosa; Ta: Non-invasive intraepithelial; WHO: World Health Organization

Acknowledgments
Not applicable.

Funding
The Korean Society of Urology Oncology supported the cost for data collection, labor costs, statistical analysis, and publication costs (KUOS 2014-05). Inje University Research Foundation supported labor costs and publication costs (20100557).

Authors' contributions
H-J.K carried out project development, study design, data collection, and manuscript writing. J-E.K designed the study, performed the scaling criteria for each histological parameter, slide review, data collection, and statistics, and summarized the results. N.H.C and J.Y.R supervised the study design. Y-J.C, S.D.L, Y.M.C, S.Y.J, S.P, Y.A.K, S-S.K, and M.S.C contributed to data collection. J-D.L and D.Y.K conducted statistical analysis with R software. All authors read and approved the final manuscript.

Competing interests
The authors declare that they have no competing interests.

Author details
[1]Department of Pathology, Inje University Sanggye Paik Hospital, 1342, Dongilro, Nowon-gu, Seoul, South Korea. [2]Department of Pathology, Ajou University school of Medicine, Suwon, South Korea. [3]Department of Pathology, Yonsei Medical College of Medicine, Seoul, South Korea. [4]Department of Pathology, Seoul St Mary's Hospital, The Catholic University, Seoul, South Korea. [5]Department of Pathology, Konkuk University Medical center, Konkuk University School of Medicine, Seoul, South Korea. [6]Department of Pathology, Asan Medical Center, Ulsan College of Medicine, Seoul, South Korea. [7]Department of Pathology, Inchun St. Mary's Hospital, The Catholic University, Incheon, South Korea. [8]Department of Pathology, College of Medicine, Ewha Womens University, Seoul, South Korea. [9]Department of Pathology, SMG-SNU Boramae Medical Center, Seoul, South Korea. [10]Departments of Pathology, Chonnam National University Medical school, Gwangju, South Korea. [11]Department of Pathology, Keimyung University School of Medicine, Daegu, South Korea. [12]Office of Biostatistics, Ajou University, School of Medicine, Suwon, South Korea. [13]Department of Pathology, Houston Methodist Hospital, Weill Medical College of Cornell University, New York, USA.

References
1. Sylvester RJ, van der Meijden AP, Oosterlinck W, Witjes JA, Bouffioux C, Denis L, et al. Predicting recurrence and progression in individual patients with stage Ta T1 bladder cancer using EORTC risk tables: a combined analysis of 2596 patients from seven EORTC trials. Eur Urol. 2006;49:466–77. discussion 475-7
2. Babjuk M, Böhle A, Burger M, Capoun O, Cohen D, Compérat EM, et al. EAU guidelines on non-muscle-invasive urothelial carcinoma of the bladder: update 2016. Eur Urol. 2017;71:447–61.
3. Cheng L, MacLennan GT, Lopez-Beltran A. Histologic grading of urothelial carcinoma: a reappraisal. Hum Pathol. 2012;43:2097–108.
4. Cheng L, Lopez-Beltran A, Bostwick DG. Grading of bladder cancer. Bladder pathology. Hoboken: Willey-Blackwell; 2012. p. 161–87.
5. MacLennan GT, Kirkali Z, Cheng L. Histologic grading of noninvasive papillary urothelial Neoplasms. Eur Urol. 2007;51:889–98.
6. Shim JW, Cho KS, Choi YD, Park YW, Lee DW, Han WS, et al. Diagnostic algorithm for papillary urothelial tumors in the urinary bladder. Virchows Arch. 2008;452:353–62.
7. Van Rhijn BWG, Vis AN, Van der Kwast TH, Kirkel WJ, Radvanyi F, Ooms EC, et al. Molecular grading of Urothelial cell carcinoma with fibroblast growth factor receptor 3 and MIB-1 is superior to pathologic grade for the prediction of clinical outcome. J Clin Oncol. 2003;21:1912–21.
8. Birkhahn M, Mitra AP, Williams AJ, Lam G, Ye W, Datar RH, et al. Predicting recurrence and progression of noninvasive papillary bladder cancer at initial presentation based on quantitative gene expression profiles. Eur Urol. 2010;57:12–20.
9. Aron M, Luthringer DJ, McKenney JK, Hansel DE, Westfall DE, Parakh R, et al. Utility of a triple antibody cocktail intraurothelial neoplasm-3 (IUN-3-CK20/CD44s/p53) and α-methylacyl-CoA racemase (AMACR) in the distinction of urothelial carcinoma in situ (CIS) and reactive urothelial atypia. Am J Surg Pathol. 2013;37:1815–23.
10. Raspollini MR, Minervini A, Lapini A, Lanzi F, Rotellini M, Baroni G, et al. A proposed score for assessing progression in pT1 high-grade Urothelial carcinoma of the bladder. Appl Immunohistochem Mol Morphol. 2013;21:218–27.
11. Rajcani J, Kajo K, Adamkov M, Moravekova E, Lauko L, Felcanova D, et al. Immunohistochemical characterization of urothelial carcinoma. Brastisl Lek Listy. 2013;114:431–8.
12. Amin MB, Trpkov K, Lopez-Beltran A, Grignon D. Members of the ISUP Immunohistochemistry in diagnostic Urologic pathology group. Best practices recommendations in the application of immunohistochemistry in the bladder lesions. Report from the International Society of Urologic Pathology consensus conference. Am J Surg Pathol. 2014;38:e20–34.
13. Tuna B, Yörükoglu K, Duzcan E, Sen S, Nese N, Sarsık B, et al. Histologic grading of urothelial; papillary neoplasms: impact of combined grading (two-numbered grading system) on reproducibility. Virchows Arch. 2011; 458:659–64.

Level of mitoses in non-muscle invasive papillary urothelial carcinomas (pTa and pT1) at initial bladder biopsy...

101

14. Gonul II, Poyraz A, Unsal C, Acar C, Alkibay T. Comparison of 1998 WHO/ISUP and 1973 WHO classifications for interobserver reliability in grading of papillary urothelial neoplasm of the bladder. Pathological evaluation of 258 cases. Urol Int. 2007;78:338–44.

15. Bol MG, Baak JP, Buhr-Wildhagen S, Kruse AJ, Kjellevold KH, Janssen EA, et al. Reproducibility and prognostic variability of grade and lamina propria invasion in stages Ta, T1 urothelial carcinoma of the bladder. J Urol. 2003; 169:1291–4.

16. Reuter VE, Comperat E, Algava F, et al. Non-invasive urothelial lesions. In: Moch H, Humphrey PA, Ulbright TM, Reuter VE, editors. WHO classification of tumors of the urinary system and male genital organs. 4th ed. Lyon: IARC; 2016. p. 99–107.

17. Bol MG, Baek JP, de Bruin PC, Rep S, Marx W, Bos S, et al. Improved objectivity of grading of T_{A1} transitional cell carcinomas of the urinary bladder by quantitative nuclear and proliferation related factors. J Clin Pathol. 2001;54:854–9.

18. Oosterhuis JW, Schapers RF, Janssen-Heijien ML, Smeets AW, Pauwels RP. MIB-1 as a proliferative marker in transitional cell carcinoma of the bladder. Clinical significance and comparison with other prognostic factors. Cancer. 2000;88:2598–605.

19. Malpica A, Deavers MT, Lu K, Bodurka DC, Atkinson EN, Gershenson DM, et al. Grading ovarian serous carcinoma using a two-tier system. Am J Surg Pathol. 2004;28:496–504.

20. Robbins P, Pinder S, de Klerk N, Dawkins H, Harvey J, Sterrett G, et al. Histological grading of breast carcinomas: a study of interobserver agreement. Hum Pathol. 1995;26:873–9.

21. Mangurud OM, Gudlaugsson E, Skaland I, Tasdemir I, Dalen I, van Diermen B, et al. Prognostic comparison of proliferation makers and World Health Organization 1973/2004 grade in urothelial carcinoma of the urinary bladder. Hum Pathol. 2014;45:1496–503.

22. Watts KE, Montironi R, Mazzucchelli R, van der Kwast T, Osunkoya AO, Stephenson AJ, et al. Clinicopathologic characteristics of 23 cases of invasive low grade papillary urothelial carcinoma. Urologia. 2012;80:361–6.

23. Goyal S, Singl UR, Sharma S, Kaur N. Correlation of mitotic indices, AgNor count, Ki-67 and Bcl-2 with grade and stage in papillary urothelial bladder cancer. Urol J. 2014;11:1238–47.

24. Pich A, Chiusa L, Formiconi A, Galliano D, Bortolin P, Comino A, et al. Proliferative activity is the most significant predictor of recurrence in noninvasive papillary urothelial neoplasms of low malignant potential and grade 1 papillary carcinomas of the bladder. Cancer. 2002;95:784–90.

25. Akkalp AK, OPnur O, Tetikkurt US, Tolga D, Özsoy S, Müslümanoğlu AY. Prognostic significance of mitotic activity in noninvasive, low grade, papillary urothelial carcinoma. Anal Quant Cytopathol Histopathol. 2016;38:23–30.

26. Solomides CC, Birbe R, Nicolau N, Bagley D, Bibbo M. Does mitosis- specific marker phophohistone H3 help the grading of upper tract urothelial carcinomas in cell blocks? Acta Cytol. 2012;56:285–8.

27. Van Rhijn WG, Musquera M, Liu L, Vis AN, Zuiverloon TC, van Leenders GJ, et al. Molecular and clinical support for a four-tiered grading system for bladder cancer based on the WHO 1973 and 2004 classifications. Mod Pathol. 2014;154:1–11.

28. Santos L, Costa C, Pereira S, Koch M, Amaro T, Cardoso F, et al. Neovascularization is a prognostic factor of early recurrence in T1/G2 urothelial bladder tumors. Ann Oncol. 2003;14:1419–24.

29. Jang TJ, Kim SW, Lee KS. The expression of pigment epithelium-derived factor in bladder transitional cell carcinoma. Korean J Pathol. 2012;46:261–5.

12

Consistency of tumor and immune cell programmed cell death ligand-1 expression within and between tumor blocks using the VENTANA SP263 assay

Paul Scorer[1*], Marietta Scott[1], Nicola Lawson[1], Marianne J. Ratcliffe[2], Craig Barker[1], Marlon C. Rebelatto[3] and Jill Walker[2]

Abstract

Background: Several anti-programmed cell death-1 (PD-1) and anti-programmed cell death ligand-1 (PD-L1) therapies have shown encouraging safety and clinical activity in a variety of tumor types. A potential role for PD-L1 testing in identifying patients that are more likely to respond to treatment is emerging. PD-L1 expression in clinical practice is determined by testing one tumor section per patient. Therefore, it is critical to understand the impact of tissue sampling variability on patients' PD-L1 classification.

Methods: Resected non-small cell lung cancer (NSCLC), head and neck squamous cell carcinoma (HNSCC) and urothelial carcinoma (UC) tissue samples (five samples per tumor type) were obtained from commercial sources and two tumor blocks were taken from each. Three sections from each block (~ 100 μm apart) were stained using the VENTANA PD-L1 (SP263) assay, and scored based on the percentage of PD-L1-staining tumor cells (TCs) or tumor-infiltrating immune cells (ICs) present. Each section was categorized as PD-L1 high or low/negative using a variety of cut-off values, and intra-block and intra-case (between blocks of the same tumor) concordance (overall percentage agreement [OPA]) were evaluated. An additional 200 commercial NSCLC samples were also analyzed, and intra-block concordance determined by scoring two sections per sample (≥70 μm apart).

Results: Concordance in TC PD-L1 classification was high at all applied cut-offs. Intra-block and intra-case OPA for the 15 NSCLC, HNSCC or UC samples were 100% and 80–100%, respectively, across all cut-offs; intra-block OPA for the 200 NSCLC samples was 91.0–98.5% across all cut-offs. IC PD-L1 classification was less consistent; intra-block and intra-case OPA for the 15 NSCLC, HNSCC or UC samples ranged between 70 and 100% and between 60 and 100%, respectively, with similar observations in the intra-block analysis of the 200 NSCLC samples.

Conclusions: These results show the reproducibility of TC PD-L1 classification across the depth of the tumor using the VENTANA PD-L1 (SP263) assay. Practically, this means that treatment decisions based on TC PD-L1 classification can be made confidently, following analysis of one tumor section. Although more variable than TC staining, consistent IC PD-L1 classification was also observed within and between blocks and across cut-offs.

Keywords: PD-L1, Heterogeneity, Assay, Concordance, Consistency, Reproducibility, Immunohistochemistry, SP263, Intra-block, Intra-case

* Correspondence: Paul.Scorer@astrazeneca.com
[1]Precision Medicine Laboratories, Precision Medicine and Genomics, IMED Biotech Unit, AstraZeneca, HODGKIN, C/O B310 Cambridge Science Park, Milton Road, Cambridge CB4 0WG, UK
Full list of author information is available at the end of the article

Background

Many tumors evade detection by the immune system by exploiting inhibitory pathways (checkpoints) that suppress antitumor responses [1]. Antibodies have been developed that target these checkpoints with the aim of restoring antitumor immune activity. One of the most promising targets is the programmed cell death-1 (PD-1) / programmed cell death ligand-1 (PD-L1) checkpoint pathway, which negatively regulates effector T-cell activity, inhibiting antitumor immune responses and thereby promoting tumor immune evasion [2, 3].

The anti-PD-1 therapies pembrolizumab and nivolumab and the anti-PD-L1 agents durvalumab, atezolizumab and avelumab have demonstrated antitumor activity and manageable safety profiles across different tumor types [4–15]. Evidence suggests that these types of therapies are associated with higher response rates in patients whose tumors have high PD-L1 expression compared to those with low/no PD-L1 expression [4, 5, 10, 16–18]. Some of these agents are now available with companion or complementary PD-L1 diagnostic assays in various indications [19–22]; use of these assays aims to inform treatment decisions by identifying patients who are most likely to respond to treatment.

The clinical assessment of PD-L1 status relies on testing one formalin-fixed paraffin-embedded (FFPE) section per patient. Selection of a tumor section for biomarker analysis, including testing for PD-L1, may be random or dependent on factors such as sample quality or tumor tissue availability. Variations in the populations of PD-L1-staining tumor cells (TCs) and/or tumor-infiltrating immune cells (ICs) within a tumor could potentially impact the classification of the tumor as PD-L1-high or PD-L1-low/negative.

Cellular architecture and IC infiltration can vary throughout the tumor; however, the impact of this on PD-L1 expression levels and, more importantly, the PD-L1 status used in assessing patient suitability for certain treatments, is not fully understood. A study by Rehman et al. investigating the heterogeneity of PD-L1 expression in non-small cell lung cancer (NSCLC) tumor samples showed variability in PD-L1 expression between fields of view on the same slide (91% variance for TCs), but minimal heterogeneity between different blocks of the same tumor (94% concordance for TCs) [23]. However, while the Rehman et al. study provides information about intra-section and intra-case heterogeneity, the variability within a single tissue block (intra-block) was not investigated.

Data on intra-block and intra-case concordance in PD-L1 classification are available for the VENTANA PD-L1 (SP142) assay, and the Dako PD-L1 IHC 28–8 PharmDx and PD-L1 IHC 22C3 PharmDx assays, in NSCLC and urothelial carcinoma (UC) tissue samples

[24–27]. The objective of our study was to assess the intra-block and intra-case concordance in PD-L1 staining of TC and IC populations using the VENTANA PD-L1 (SP263) assay. Tissue samples from NSCLC, head and neck squamous cell carcinoma (HNSCC) and UC were assessed.

Methods

Tumor samples, preparation and staining, and assessment of 15 NSCLC, HNSCC or UC samples

For this study, FFPE samples of resected tissue from primary NSCLC, HNSCC and UC tumors were obtained from commercial sources (Avaden Biosciences, Seattle WA, USA). Appropriate patient consents for sample use were in place. To ensure the sample cohort covered a wide range of PD-L1 TC expression, FFPE sections were acquired for 20 cases from each indication (60 cases in total) and stained with the VENTANA PD-L1 (SP263) assay. Five representative cases were then selected from each indication (15 cases in total). The 15 selected cases included six cases with PD-L1 expression in > 70% of TCs, six cases with PD-L1 expression in 20–50% of TCs, and three cases with little or no PD-L1 expression in TCs. This selection was performed independently, prior to circulation of the slides to the study pathologist. The 15 cases were selected primarily on TC content and PD-L1 expression in TCs; the IC content and PD-L1 expression in ICs were assessed for confirmation that ICs would be present for analysis. From the 15 cases entered into the study, 14 had PD-L1 expression in < 10% of ICs and one had PD-L1 expression in > 20% of ICs.

Following the initial screening, two large tumor resection blocks were taken from each case (30 blocks in total). The samples were sectioned serially at 4 μm on to Superfrost Plus slides, dried at room temperature or 37 °C overnight and then baked at 56 °C for 1 h. Fifty-one serial sections were cut fresh from each block (Fig. 1) and cut sections were stored in slide storage boxes with close-fitting lids at − 20 °C until stained (within 1 month). Sections "Background" and 51 from each block were stained with hematoxylin and eosin to confirm that tumor was present in all serial sections, and to ensure there were enough TCs in the sections to provide an accurate estimate of PD-L1 expression. Sections "Methods", 25 and 50 from each block were stained using the VENTANA PD-L1 (SP263) assay with the VENTANA OptiView DAB IHC Detection Kit on the automated VENTANA BenchMark ULTRA platform. The sections were ~ 100 μm apart.

Stained sections were assessed by a single, certified pathologist, trained in PD-L1 immunohistochemistry interpretation (TCs and ICs) by VENTANA. To minimize bias, the pathologist was blind with respect to the case, block and section number being scored. The total percentage of TCs

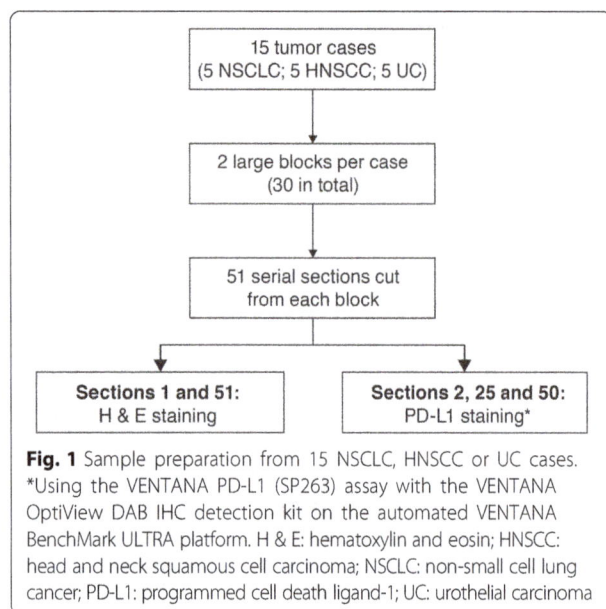

Fig. 1 Sample preparation from 15 NSCLC, HNSCC or UC cases. *Using the VENTANA PD-L1 (SP263) assay with the VENTANA OptiView DAB IHC detection kit on the automated VENTANA BenchMark ULTRA platform. H & E: hematoxylin and eosin; HNSCC: head and neck squamous cell carcinoma; NSCLC: non-small cell lung cancer; PD-L1: programmed cell death ligand-1; UC: urothelial carcinoma

from Stage I–IV primary tumors (Asterand, MI, USA; ProteoGenex, CA, USA; Tissue Solutions, CA, USA) were available as part of a larger comparative study [29]. The methodology for preparation and assessment of these samples was published previously [29]. Fresh sections were cut from each block, 7 months apart, to simulate repeat testing in a clinical setting. The sections were cut at a minimum of 70 μm separation, and were stained using the VENTANA PD-L1 (SP263) assay. These samples were read by a single blinded pathologist trained by VENTANA in a Clinical Laboratory Improvement Amendments (CLIA) program certified laboratory (Hematogenix, IL, USA). The mean washout period between assessments of the two sections from the same sample was 258 days (range 242–287). PD-L1 positivity was scored as follows: for TCs, scores of > 25% were recorded in 10% increments and scores of ≤25% were recorded as < 1%; 1–4%, 5–9, 10, 20% or 25%; for ICs, scores of > 10% were recorded in 10% increments and scores of ≤10% were recorded as 0, 1, 5% or 10%.

or ICs that stained positive for PD-L1 was recorded. Scoring of TC membrane positivity or IC positivity was performed as per the SP263 scoring algorithm and interpretation guide [28]. Scores of > 10% were recorded in 5% increments; scores of ≤10% were recorded as < 1%; 1–4%, 5–9 and 10% (Fig. 2).

Staining and assessment of additional 200 NSCLC samples

In addition to the 15 NSCLC, HNSCC or UC cases described above, 200 commercial NSCLC patient samples

Statistical analysis: Intra-block and intra-case assessment of 15 NSCLC, HNSCC or UC samples

For the 15 NSCLC, HNSCC or UC cases, TC and IC PD-L1 expression scores from the three sections of each block were recorded (90 TC and 90 IC scores in total; Additional file 1). Multiple clinically relevant diagnostic cut-offs (Table 1) [4, 8, 10–13, 17, 19–22, 30–33] were then applied to the TC and IC scores, and each section was classified as being above or below each cut-off value

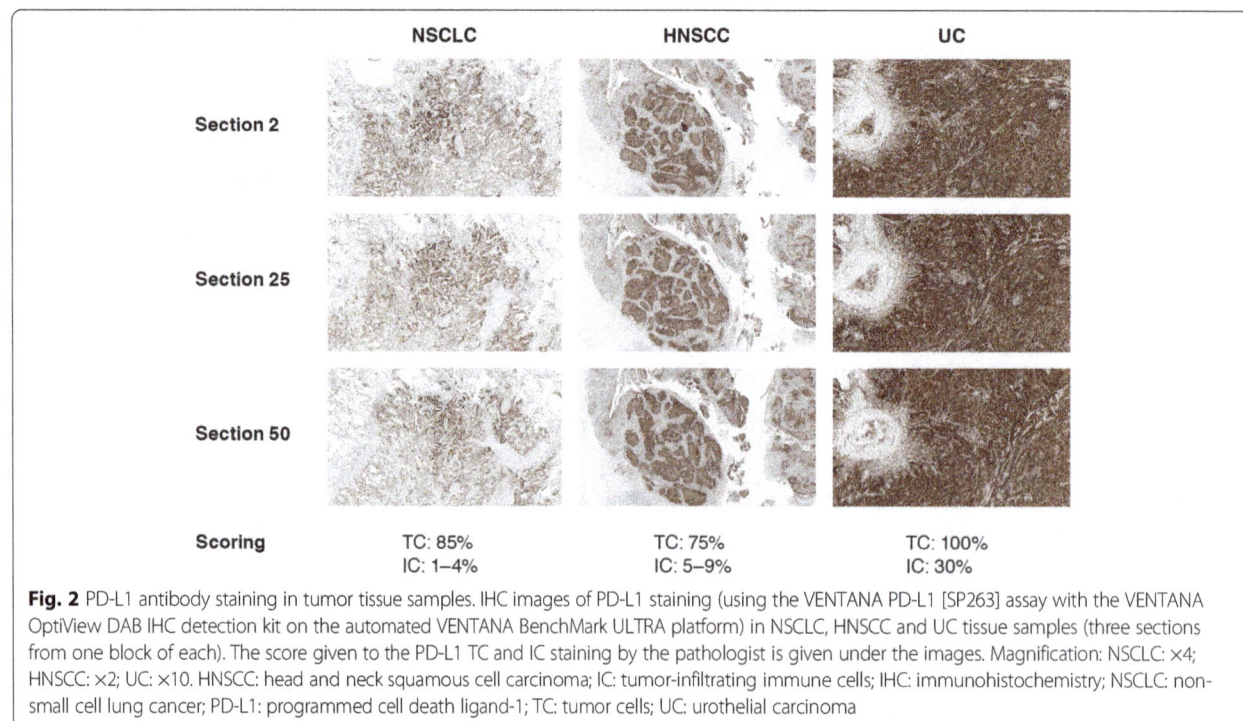

Fig. 2 PD-L1 antibody staining in tumor tissue samples. IHC images of PD-L1 staining (using the VENTANA PD-L1 [SP263] assay with the VENTANA OptiView DAB IHC detection kit on the automated VENTANA BenchMark ULTRA platform) in NSCLC, HNSCC and UC tissue samples (three sections from one block of each). The score given to the PD-L1 TC and IC staining by the pathologist is given under the images. Magnification: NSCLC: ×4; HNSCC: ×2; UC: ×10. HNSCC: head and neck squamous cell carcinoma; IC: tumor-infiltrating immune cells; IHC: immunohistochemistry; NSCLC: non-small cell lung cancer; PD-L1: programmed cell death ligand-1; TC: tumor cells; UC: urothelial carcinoma

Table 1 Comparison of approved PD-L1 diagnostic assays and PD-L1 cut-offs in NSCLC, HNSCC and UC

	VENTANA SP263 [19, 30]	Dako 22C3 [21]	Dako 28–8 [20]	VENTANA SP142 [22]
Developed as companion diagnostic assay for:	Durvalumab (AstraZeneca/ MedImmune)[a]	Pembrolizumab (Merck Sharp & Dohme)	Nivolumab (Bristol-Myers Squibb)	Atezolizumab (Genentech/Roche)
Compartment	TC; TC or IC	TC; TC & IC	TC	TC or IC; IC
PD-L1 cut-off NSCLC	≥25% TC [30]	≥50% TC - 1 L [21, 31] ≥1% TC - 2 L [31]	≥1%, ≥5%, ≥10% TC [8]	≥50% TC or ≥ 10% IC [13, 22]
PD-L1 cut-off HNSCC	≥25% TC [30]	≥1, ≥50 CPS[b] [17]	≥1%, ≥5%, ≥10% TC [10]	–
PD-L1 cut-off UC	≥25% TC or IC [4]	≥10 CPS[b] [32]	≥1%, ≥5% TC [11]	≥5% IC [12, 22]
FDA regulatory status	Approved complementary diagnostic in UC	Approved companion diagnostic in NSCLC	Approved complementary diagnostic in NSCLC	Approved complementary diagnostic in NSCLC and UC

[a]VENTANA SP263 is also approved for use with nivolumab and pembrolizumab in NSCLC patients (CE mark only; not FDA approved) [19]
[b]Previously reported as, and equivalent to ≥1%, ≥10% or ≥ 50% CPS [33]
CPS combined positive score evaluating both TC and IC, HNSCC head and neck squamous cell carcinoma, IC tumor-infiltrating immune cell, NSCLC non-small cell lung cancer, PD-L1 programmed cell death ligand-1, TC tumor cell, UC urothelial carcinoma

(PD-L1 high or low/negative status, respectively). The applied cut-offs were: ≥50%, ≥25%, ≥10% and ≥ 1% for TCs; ≥25%, ≥10%, ≥5% and ≥ 1% for ICs.

A block was classified as discordant if there was any variation in the diagnostic results (PD-L1 status) for any of its three sections. Intra-case comparisons were the same as intra-block comparisons, with the exception that six sections in total were compared per case (three sections per block; two blocks per case). Overall percentage agreement (OPA) within blocks (intra-block) and between blocks (intra-case) was calculated at each cut-off.

Statistical analysis: Intra-block analysis of 200 NSCLC cases
The analysis plan for the 200 NSCLC cases was published previously [29]. OPA, negative percentage agreement (NPA) and positive percentage agreement (PPA) [34] were calculated at multiple clinically relevant cut-offs (≥50%, ≥25%, ≥10% and ≥ 1%) for the two sections from each block. For each metric, the lower boundary of the 95% confidence interval (CI) was calculated with no upper bound, using the Clopper-Pearson method [35].

Results
Sample demographics
The patient demographics for the 15 NSCLC, HNSCC or UC cases are presented in Table 2. Patient age at the time of surgery ranged between 49 and 82 years. The tumor samples analyzed were at different stages of disease; NSCLC: Stage IB–IIIA; HNSCC: Stage I–III; UC: Stage II–IV. Sample age at the time of analysis ranged from 1 to 13 years. The patient demographics for the 200 NSCLC samples have been presented previously [36]. Thirty-eight percent were Stage I, 36% were Stage II and 21% were Stage III.

Intra-block concordance in PD-L1 classification
In the analysis of TCs, PD-L1 classification (above or below the cut-off) was consistent within tissue blocks for all the applied cut-offs (TC intra-block OPA was 100%) (Table 3).

PD-L1 classification was less consistent in the analysis of ICs. IC intra-block OPA ranged between 70 and 100% across all tumor types at the ≥1%, ≥5% and ≥ 10% cut-offs. However, OPA was 100% across all tumor types at the ≥25% cut-off (Table 3), reflective of the fact that the majority (14/15) of cases had IC staining scored below 25% (Additional file 1). The percentage of PD-L1-staining ICs between sections of the discordant blocks varied by no more than one scoring category (~ 5%), and the differences in PD-L1 scoring were either: < 1% vs 1–4%; 1–4% vs 5–9% or 5–9% vs 10% (Additional file 1).

These results were supported by the analysis of 200 additional NSCLC cases. In this much larger cohort, the minimum intra-block TC OPA was 91.0% (at the ≥1% cut-off); TC PPA and NPA were > 90 and > 80%, respectively, at all cut-offs (range: 81.4–100.0% across both PPA and NPA) (Table 4 and Fig. 3). The highest agreement was observed at the ≥25% cut-off (OPA: 98.5%; PPA: 96.7%; NPA: 100.0%).

PD-L1 classification in ICs was less consistent across this larger sample set as well, with OPA values ranging from 78.5 to 95.5%, across the different cut-offs (Table 4 and Fig. 3). This is also reflected in the PPA and NPA values; PPA values ranged from 14.3% (at the ≥50% cut-off) to 81.6% (at the ≥1% cut-off) and NPA values ranged from 77.1% (at the ≥1% cut-off) to 98.4% (at the ≥50% cut-off) (Table 4 and Fig. 3).

Intra-case concordance in PD-L1 classification
There was high agreement in TC PD-L1 classification between two different blocks from the same tumor; TC

Table 2 Demographics of patients who provided samples for analysis

Patient	Sample type	Sample age, years	Patient age at surgery, years	Sex	Primary diagnosis	Clinical stage
NSCLC						
1	Lung	9	79	Male	Squamous cell carcinoma	II
2	Lung	2	50	Male	Squamous cell carcinoma	IIIA
3	Lung	1	82	Male	Adenocarcinoma	IIB
4	Lung	13	70	Female	Adenocarcinoma	IB
5	Lung	13	71	Male	Squamous cell carcinoma	IIA
HNSCC						
6	Tonsil	10	64	Female	Squamous cell carcinoma	I
7	Tongue	9	71	Female	Squamous cell carcinoma	I
8	Larynx	6	55	Male	Squamous cell carcinoma	III
9	Tonsil	6	49	Female	Squamous cell carcinoma	I
10	Tongue	3	68	Male	Squamous cell carcinoma	I
UC						
11	Bladder	7	74	Female	Urothelial cell carcinoma	III
12	Bladder	4	70	Male	Urothelial cell carcinoma	II
13	Bladder	4	67	Male	Urothelial cell carcinoma	IV
14	Bladder	3	80	Female	Urothelial cell carcinoma	III
15	Bladder	3	82	Male	Urothelial cell carcinoma	III

HNSCC head and neck squamous cell carcinoma, *NSCLC* non-small cell lung cancer, *UC* urothelial carcinoma

intra-case OPA was 100% across all tumor types and at all applied cut-offs except for NSCLC at the ≥50% cut-off, where OPA was 80% (Table 5).

Intra-case PD-L1 classification in the analysis of ICs was less consistent, with OPA values ranging from 60 to 100% across all tumor types at the ≥1%, ≥5% and ≥ 10% cut-offs (Table 5). However, as with the intra-block analysis, intra-case OPA was 100% across all tumor types at

the ≥25% cut-off, again reflecting the lower levels of PD-L1 expression in ICs, compared with TCs.

Discussion

Clinical data suggest that anti-PD-1 / anti-PD-L1 treatment may be more effective in patients whose tumors have high expression of PD-L1 vs those with low/no expression of PD-L1 [4, 5, 10, 16–18]; as such, it is critical

Table 3 Intra-block concordance (OPA) in PD-L1 classification at various applied cut-offs

Applied cut-off	Concordance (OPA), %		
	NSCLC	HNSCC	UC
TC PD-L1 staining			
≥ 50%	100	100	100
≥ 25%	100	100	100
≥ 10%	100	100	100
≥ 1%	100	100	100
IC PD-L1 staining			
≥ 25%	100	100	100
≥ 10%	70	90	100
≥ 5%	90	100	80
≥ 1%	100	100	80

Fifteen NSCLC, HNSCC or UC cases; 30 blocks in total (10 blocks per indication)
HNSCC head and neck squamous cell carcinoma, *IC* tumor-infiltrating immune cell, *NSCLC* non-small cell lung cancer, *OPA* overall percentage agreement, *PD-L1* programmed cell death ligand-1, *TC* tumor cell, *UC* urothelial carcinoma

Table 4 Intra-block concordance (OPA; PPA; NPA) in PD-L1 classification of NSCLC samples at various applied cut-offs

Applied cut-off	OPA % (lower 95% CI)	PPA % (lower 95% CI)	NPA % (lower 95% CI)
TC PD-L1 staining			
≥ 50%	97.0 (94.2)	92.2 (84.3)	99.3 (96.6)
≥ 25%	98.5 (96.2)	96.7 (91.6)	100.0 (97.3)
≥ 10%	96.5 (93.5)	95.3 (90.4)	97.8 (93.4)
≥ 1%	91.0 (86.9)	96.2 (92.1)	81.4 (72.1)
IC PD-L1 staining			
≥ 50%	95.5 (92.3)	14.3 (0.7)	98.4 (96.0)
≥ 25%	86.5 (81.9)	17.9 (7.3)	97.7 (94.8)
≥ 10%	78.5 (73.2)	78.1 (71.9)	79.6 (67.8)
≥ 1%	80.5 (75.3)	81.6 (75.6)	77.1 (64.9)

200 NSCLC cases (two sections were scored for each case)
CI confidence interval, *IC* tumor-infiltrating immune cell, *NPA* negative percentage agreement, *NSCLC* non-small cell lung cancer, *OPA* overall percentage agreement, *PD-L1* programmed cell death ligand-1, *PPA* positive percentage agreement, *TC* tumor cell

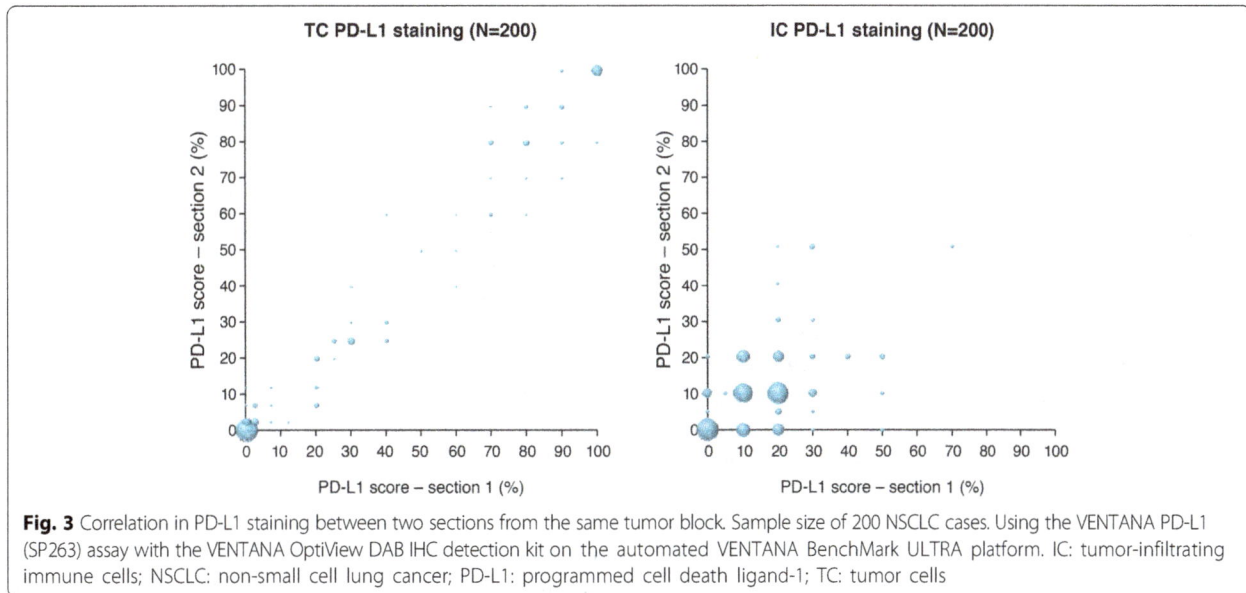

Fig. 3 Correlation in PD-L1 staining between two sections from the same tumor block. Sample size of 200 NSCLC cases. Using the VENTANA PD-L1 (SP263) assay with the VENTANA OptiView DAB IHC detection kit on the automated VENTANA BenchMark ULTRA platform. IC: tumor-infiltrating immune cells; NSCLC: non-small cell lung cancer; PD-L1: programmed cell death ligand-1; TC: tumor cells

to understand the impact of tissue sampling variability on patients' PD-L1 classification. Our study analyzed PD-L1 expression in 15 tumor samples from three indications (NSCLC, HNSCC or UC) as well as in a large, separate cohort of 200 NSCLC samples, and is the first study of PD-L1 heterogeneity using the VENTANA SP263 assay. In the analysis of TCs, we showed high intra-block and intra-case concordance in PD-L1 classification (above or below the cut-off value) across all applied cut-offs and for both sets of samples. Our findings are consistent with previously published data [24, 25], and give a high level of confidence in the reproducibility of TC scoring across the depth of the tumor.

Table 5 Intra-case concordance (OPA) in PD-L1 classification at various applied cut-offs

Applied cut-off	Concordance (OPA), %		
	NSCLC	HNSCC	UC
TC PD-L1 staining			
≥50%	80	100	100
≥25%	100	100	100
≥10%	100	100	100
≥1%	100	100	100
IC PD-L1 staining			
≥25%	100	100	100
≥10%	60	80	100
≥5%	80	100	80
≥1%	100	80	60

Fifteen NSCLC, HNSCC or UC cases (five cases per indication)
HNSCC head and neck squamous cell carcinoma, *IC* tumor-infiltrating immune cell, *NSCLC* non-small cell lung cancer, *OPA* overall percentage agreement, *PD-L1* programmed cell death ligand-1, *TC* tumor cell, *UC* urothelial carcinoma

The results from the analysis of PD-L1 expression in ICs were not as consistent as those for TCs, with a good to moderate intra-block and intra-case agreement across the applied cut-offs for the 15 NSCLC, HNSCC or UC samples. Despite this increased variability, the intra-block and intra-case OPA for ICs were 100% at the ≥25% cut-off. Whilst only one sample (a UC case) was scored above 25% for ICs, the 100% OPA reflects the fact that there were no large differences in IC scoring within or between blocks for any of the three indications. The ≥25% cut-off is the approved value for the IC component of the scoring algorithm used with the VENTANA PD-L1 (SP263) assay for identifying UC patients most likely to respond to durvalumab [4, 28] and the reproducibility in this small dataset supports the use of this cut-off. In line with these data, intra-block PD-L1 expression was also more variable in ICs than in TCs in the larger NSCLC sample set. The PPA values reported varied from 14.3 to 81.6%; however, the two lowest PPA values at the ≥50% (14.3%) and ≥ 25% (17.9%) cut-offs could be driven by the fact that very few cases were scored above these two cut-off values. The increased intra-case variability in PD-L1 expression in ICs is consistent with a recent study in NSCLC by Rehman et al., who also speculated that the low numbers of PD-L1-expressing ICs may have affected their results [23]. Moreover, the proportion of PD-L1-expressing ICs may depend on the level of infiltration of immune cells into the tumor microenvironment. This may differ between different sections of the tumor, therefore contributing to the observed heterogeneity of IC PD-L1 expression. Variability in IC scoring may also be due to a pathologist's technical ability in scoring ICs. Studies have noted that IC scoring is more variable than TC scoring when different pathologists assess identical sections [23, 37], suggesting a need for more extensive training of pathologists specifically on scoring of ICs. IC results in NSCLC should not be extrapolated to more immunogenic cancers such as UC, where there are generally higher proportions of patients with high IC PD-L1 expression (e.g. in the study by Massard et al. using the VENTANA SP263 assay, 45% of screened UC patients were found to be PD-L1-positive on the basis of IC expression, using a 25% cut-off [38]).

Our study investigated PD-L1 expression using only the VENTANA PD-L1 (SP263) assay. Similar studies have been carried out using the other approved PD-L1 assays and have been published by the US Food and Drug Administration (FDA) as part of the approval process for each assay (Table 6) [24–27]. PD-L1 expression in TCs has been assessed with the Dako PD-L1 IHC 22C3 PharmDx (intra-block and intra-case concordance: both 100% at the ≥50% cut-off, in NSCLC) [24] and the Dako PD-L1 IHC 28–8 PharmDx assay (intra-case concordance: 94% each at the ≥1%, ≥5% and ≥ 10% cut-offs, in NSCLC) [25]. PD-L1 expression has been assessed using the VENTANA PD-L1 (SP142) assay for ICs in UC (intra-block and intra-case concordance: 100 and 91%, respectively, at the ≥5% cut-off) [27] and for TCs and ICs in NSCLC (intra-block and intra-case concordance: 96 and 81%, respectively, at the ≥50% TC or ≥ 10% IC cut-offs) [26] (Table 6) [24–27]. Our data are broadly consistent with these reports, supporting the notion that a patient's TC PD-L1 classification

is unlikely to be altered under routine clinical sampling protocols. This is further supported by the Rehman et al. study, which showed minimal intra-case heterogeneity in PD-L1 staining of TCs in 35 NSCLC cases, and suggested that staining one block of a tumor should be enough to represent the entire tumor [23].

A notable strength of our study lies in the analysis of two different sections from the same tumor that were cut 7 months apart (for the 200 NSCLC cases). This mimics what might occur in the clinical setting, where an additional section may be requested from the same tissue block several months later. The high concordance observed in the analysis of TCs here gives a high level of confidence in the reliability of PD-L1 scoring in the real-life clinical situation.

Moreover, our study investigated the consistency in PD-L1 scoring of both TCs and ICs, and using a wide range of clinically relevant cut-offs. The cut-offs were chosen based on the diagnostic algorithms that have been approved or are currently being investigated for the different PD-L1 diagnostic assays and anti-PD-1 / anti-PD-L1 therapies (Table 1) [4, 8, 10–13, 17, 19–22, 30–32].

One limitation of our study is the fact that the FFPE samples used came from large tumor resections instead of biopsies, thus may not be representative of all clinical samples. This was done for practical reasons, as a large amount of tissue was required (to cut 51 sections per sample), which could not have been achieved from a small biopsy. Whether the PD-L1 status of a tumor would vary depending on the sample type (cytology vs

Table 6 Data on intra-block and intra-case concordance in PD-L1 classification, from publicly available FDA documents[a]

Assay	TC PD-L1 staining % OPA (% cut-off)	IC PD-L1 staining % OPA (% cut-off)	TC or IC PD-L1 staining % OPA (% cut-off)	n
Intra-block concordance in PD-L1 classification				
Dako 22C3				
NSCLC [24]	100% (≥50%)	–	–	20
Dako 28–8 [25]	–	–	–	
VENTANA SP142				
NSCLC [26]	–	–	96% (≥50% TC or ≥ 10% IC)	24
UC [27]	–	100% (≥5%)	–	8
Intra-case concordance in PD-L1 classification				
Dako 22C3				
NSCLC [24]	100% (≥50%)	–	–	20
Dako 28–8				
NSCLC [25]	94% (≥1%; ≥5%; ≥10%)	–	–	16
VENTANA SP142				
NSCLC [26]	–	–	81% (≥50% TC or ≥ 10% IC)	27
UC [27]	–	91% (≥5%)	–	22

[a]Summary of Safety and Effectiveness Data (SSED)
FDA Food and Drug Administration, *IC* tumor-infiltrating immune cell, *NSCLC* non-small cell lung cancer, *OPA* overall percentage agreement, *PD-L1* programmed cell death ligand-1, *TC* tumor cell, *UC* urothelial carcinoma

biopsy vs resection) is unknown. A number of studies have investigated concordance in PD-L1 expression between different types of samples using validated FDA approved PD-L1 tests [39–41]. Ilie et al. reported discordance of 19% between TC scoring in resections and biopsies, with notably higher discordance when IC scoring was also taken into account. This study used the VENTANA PD-L1 (SP142) assay, which has shown lower analytical sensitivity than SP263 [42, 43]. Skov et al. and Heymann et al. both found strong concordance between resections and small biopsies and/or cytology samples using the Dako PD-L1 IHC 22C3 PharmDx and/or PD-L1 IHC 28–8 PharmDx assays [40, 41], which have shown similar sensitivity to SP263 [29, 42].

A second limitation of our study was the small sample size of HNSCC and UC cases analyzed (only five cases of each). This may be too small a dataset to confidently draw any conclusions about these indications specifically; however, the results from the NSCLC small intra-block and intra-case study are supported by those from the much larger NSCLC dataset, giving confidence that our findings, particularly those relating to PD-L1 staining of TCs, can be applied across indications.

Thirdly, the scoring of PD-L1 expression in our study was carried out by a single pathologist. This approach was taken to allow determination of intra-block and intra-case agreement without confounding variables. However, in clinical practice samples may be scored by different pathologists, and it would, therefore, be important to establish whether inter-pathologist variability would impact the results.

Conclusions

Our study showed high intra-block and intra-case concordance in TC PD-L1 classification with the VENTANA PD-L1 (SP263) assay, at various applied cut-offs. These data provide confidence in use of this assay to determine a patient's TC PD-L1 classification, as the results were consistent across the depth of the tumor block and between resections taken from different areas of the tumor. Although more variable than TC staining, consistent IC PD-L1 classification was also observed within and between tumor blocks for most patients.

These are important data to have in hand as the value of biomarker (PD-L1) testing in immunotherapy becomes clearer, and suggest that PD-L1 classification based on the analysis of a single tumor section can be used confidently to inform treatment decisions.

Abbreviations

CI: Confidence interval; CLIA: Clinical Laboratory Improvement Amendments; FDA: Food and Drug Administration; FFPE: Formalin-fixed, paraffin-embedded; H & E: Hematoxylin and eosin; HNSCC: Head and neck squamous cell carcinoma; IC: Tumor-infiltrating immune cells; NPA: Negative percentage agreement; NSCLC: Non-small cell lung cancer; OPA: Overall percentage agreement; PD-1: Programmed cell death-1; PD-L1: Programmed cell death ligand-1; PPA: Positive percentage agreement; TC: Tumor cell; UC: Urothelial carcinoma

Acknowledgments

Pathology and PD-L1 interpretation was performed by Professor Gareth Williams (BSc MBChB PhD FRCPath FLSW; Oncologica UK Ltd., Cambridge, UK). Medical writing and editorial assistance were provided by Lietta Nicolaides, PhD, of Cirrus Communications (Ashfield Healthcare, Macclesfield, UK) and was funded by AstraZeneca.

Funding

This study was sponsored by AstraZeneca. The sponsor contributed to the design and implementation of the study, collection, analysis and interpretation of data, and writing of the report. The authors had final responsibility for the decision to submit for publication.

Authors' contributions

PS, CB and JW were involved in study design. Data acquisition was carried out by PS and NL; data analysis and interpretation was carried out by PS, MS and MJR. All authors reviewed and approved the final manuscript.

Competing interests

PS, MS, NL, CB and JW are employees of AstraZeneca and hold stocks or shares in AstraZeneca. MJR is an employee of AstraZeneca. MCR is an employee of MedImmune LLC and holds stocks or shares in AstraZeneca.

Author details

[1]Precision Medicine Laboratories, Precision Medicine and Genomics, IMED Biotech Unit, AstraZeneca, HODGKIN, C/O B310 Cambridge Science Park, Milton Road, Cambridge CB4 0WG, UK. [2]Oncology Companion Diagnostics Unit, Precision Medicine and Genomics, IMED Biotech Unit, AstraZeneca, Cambridge, UK. [3]Translational Sciences, Research, MedImmune, Gaithersburg, MD, USA.

References

1.　Zou W, Chen L. Inhibitory B7-family molecules in the tumour microenvironment. Nat Rev Immunol. 2008;8:467–77.

2. Pardoll DM. The blockade of immune checkpoints in cancer immunotherapy. Nat Rev Cancer. 2012;12:252–64.

3. Postow MA, Callahan MK, Wolchok JD. Immune checkpoint blockade in cancer therapy. J Clin Oncol. 2015;33:1974–82.

4. Powles T, O'Donnell PH, Massard C, Arkenau HT, Friedlander TW, Hoimes CJ, et al. Efficacy and safety of durvalumab in locally advanced or metastatic urothelial carcinoma: updated results from a phase 1/2 open-label study. JAMA Oncol. 2017;3:e172411.

5. Reck M, Rodriguez-Abreu D, Robinson AG, Hui R, Csoszi T, Fulop A, et al. Pembrolizumab versus chemotherapy for PD-L1-positive non-small-cell lung cancer. N Engl J Med. 2016;375:1823–33.

6. Herbst RS, Baas P, Kim DW, Felip E, Perez-Gracia JL, Han JY, et al. Pembrolizumab versus docetaxel for previously treated, PD-L1-positive, advanced non-small-cell lung cancer (KEYNOTE-010): a randomised controlled trial. Lancet. 2016;387:1540–50.

7. Larkins E, Blumenthal GM, Yuan W, He K, Sridhara R, Subramaniam S, et al. FDA approval summary: pembrolizumab for the treatment of recurrent or metastatic head and neck squamous cell carcinoma with disease progression on or after platinum-containing chemotherapy. Oncologist. 2017;22:873–8.

8. Borghaei H, Paz-Ares L, Horn L, Spigel DR, Steins M, Ready NE, et al. Nivolumab versus docetaxel in advanced nonsquamous non-small-cell lung cancer. N Engl J Med. 2015;373:1627–39.

9. Brahmer J, Reckamp KL, Baas P, Crinò L, Eberhardt WE, Poddubskaya E, et al. Nivolumab versus docetaxel in advanced squamous-cell non-small-cell lung cancer. N Engl J Med. 2015;373:123–35.

10. Ferris RL, Blumenschein G Jr, Fayette J, Guigay J, Colevas AD, Licitra L, et al. Nivolumab for recurrent squamous-cell carcinoma of the head and neck. N Engl J Med. 2016;375:1856–67.

11. Sharma P, Retz M, Siefker-Radtke A, Baron A, Necchi A, Bedke J, et al. Nivolumab in metastatic urothelial carcinoma after platinum therapy (CheckMate 275): a multicentre, single-arm, phase 2 trial. Lancet Oncol. 2017;18:312–22.

12. Rosenberg JE, Hoffman-Censits J, Powles T, van der Heijden MS, Balar AV, Necchi A, et al. Atezolizumab in patients with locally advanced and metastatic urothelial carcinoma who have progressed following treatment with platinum-based chemotherapy: a single-arm, multicentre, phase 2 trial. Lancet. 2016;387:1909–20.

13. Fehrenbacher L, Spira A, Ballinger M, Kowanetz M, Vansteenkiste J, Mazieres J, et al. Atezolizumab versus docetaxel for patients with previously treated non-small-cell lung cancer (POPLAR): a multicentre, open-label, phase 2 randomised controlled trial. Lancet. 2016;387:1837–46.

14. Rittmeyer A, Barlesi F, Waterkamp D, Park K, Ciardiello F, von Pawel J, et al. Atezolizumab versus docetaxel in patients with previously treated non-small-cell lung cancer (OAK): a phase 3, open-label, multicentre randomised controlled trial. Lancet. 2017;389:255–65.

15. Kaufman HL, Russell J, Hamid O, Bhatia S, Terheyden P, D'Angelo SP, et al. Avelumab in patients with chemotherapy-refractory metastatic Merkel cell carcinoma: a multicentre, single-group, open-label, phase 2 trial. Lancet Oncol. 2016;17:1374–85.

16. Rizvi NA, Mazières J, Planchard D, Stinchcombe TE, Dy GK, Antonia SJ, et al. Activity and safety of nivolumab, an anti-PD-1 immune checkpoint inhibitor, for patients with advanced, refractory squamous non-small-cell lung cancer (CheckMate 063): a phase 2, single-arm trial. Lancet Oncol. 2015;16:257–65.

17. Bauml J, Seiwert TY, Pfister DG, Worden F, Liu SV, Gilbert J, et al. Pembrolizumab for platinum- and cetuximab-refractory head and neck cancer: results from a single-arm, phase II study. J Clin Oncol. 2017;35:1542–9.

18. Chow LQ, Haddad R, Gupta S, Mahipal A, Mehra R, Tahara M, et al. Antitumor activity of pembrolizumab in biomarker-unselected patients with recurrent and/or metastatic head and neck squamous cell carcinoma: results from the phase Ib KEYNOTE-012 expansion cohort. J Clin Oncol. 2016;34:3838–45.

19. Ventana Medical Systems. VENTANA PD-L1 (SP263) Assay. Updated 2017. Available from: http://www.ventana.com/ventana-pd-l1-sp263-assay-2/. Accessed May 2017.

20. Dako. PD-L1 IHC 28–8 pharmDx. October 2015. Available from: http://www.accessdata.fda.gov/cdrh_docs/pdf15/P150025c.pdf. Accessed 10 Aug 2016.

21. Dako. PD-L1 IHC 22C3 pharmDx. September 2015. Available from: http://www.accessdata.fda.gov/cdrh_docs/pdf15/P150013c.pdf. Accessed 10 Aug 2016.

22. VENTANA. VENTANA PD-L1 (SP142) Assay. Updated 2016. Available from: http://www.ventana.com/product/1827?type=2357. Accessed May 2017.

23. Rehman JA, Han G, Carvajal-Hausdorf DE, Wasserman BE, Pelekanou V, Mani NL, et al. Quantitative and pathologist-read comparison of the heterogeneity of programmed death-ligand 1 (PD-L1) expression in non-small cell lung cancer. Mod Pathol. 2017;30:340–9.

24. Food and Drug Administration (FDA). Dako 22C3 summary of safety and effectiveness data. 2015. Available from: http://www.accessdata.fda.gov/cdrh_docs/pdf15/p150013b.pdf. Accessed May 2017.

25. Food and Drug Administration (FDA). Dako 28–8 summary of safety and effectiveness data. October 2015. Available from: http://www.accessdata.fda.gov/cdrh_docs/pdf15/P150025b.pdf. Accessed May 2017.

26. Food and Drug Administration (FDA). Ventana SP142 summary of safety and effectiveness data. October 2016. Available from: https://www.accessdata.fda.gov/cdrh_docs/pdf16/p160006b.pdf. Accessed May 2017.

27. Food and Drug Administration (FDA). Ventana SP142 summary of safety and effectiveness data. May 2016. Available from: http://www.accessdata.fda.gov/cdrh_docs/pdf16/P160002b.pdf. Accessed May 2017.

28. VENTANA. VENTANA PD-L1 (SP263) Assay. Updated April 2017. Available from: https://www.accessdata.fda.gov/cdrh_docs/pdf16/p160046c.pdf. Accessed Oct 2017.

29. Ratcliffe MJ, Sharpe A, Midha A, Barker C, Scott M, Scorer P, et al. Agreement between programmed cell death ligand-1 diagnostic assays across multiple protein expression cut-offs in non-small cell lung cancer. Clin Cancer Res. 2017;23:3585–91.

30. Rebelatto MC, Midha A, Mistry A, Sabalos C, Schechter N, Li X, et al. Development of a programmed cell death ligand-1 immunohistochemical assay validated for analysis of non-small cell lung cancer and head and neck squamous cell carcinoma. Diagn Pathol. 2016;11:95.

31. Merck Sharp & Dohme. Keytruda® (pembrolizumab) highlights of prescribing information. Updated May 2017. Available from: https://www.merck.com/product/usa/pi_circulars/k/keytruda/keytruda_pi.pdf. Accessed 12 May 2017.

32. Bellmunt J, de Wit R, Vaughn DJ, Fradet Y, Lee JL, Fong L, et al. Pembrolizumab as second-line therapy for advanced urothelial carcinoma. N Engl J Med. 2017;376:1015–26.

33. Cohen E, Harrington K, Le Tourneau C, Dinis J, Licitra L, Ahn M-J, et al. Pembrolizumab vs standard of care for recurrent or metastatic head and neck squamous cell carcinoma: Phase 3 KEYNOTE-040 trial. Oral presentation at the European Society for Medical Oncology (ESMO) Annual Meeting, Madrid, Spain, September 8–12, 2017 (Abstr. LBA45).

34. Food and Drug Administration (FDA). Guidance for industry and FDA staff. Statistical guidance on reporting results from studies evaluating diagnostic tests. March 13, 2007. Available from: http://www.fda.gov/downloads/MedicalDevices/DeviceRegulationandGuidance/GuidanceDocuments/ucm071287.pdf. Accessed Apr 2017.

35. Clopper CJ, Pearson ES. The use of confidence or fiducial limits illustrated in the case of the binomial. Biometrika. 1934;26:404–13.

36. Scott M, Ratcliffe MJ, Sharpe A, Barker C, Scorer P, Rebelatto M, et al. Concordance of tumor and immune cell staining with Ventana SP263, Dako 28-8, Dako 22C3 and Ventana SP142 PD-L1 immunohistochemistry assays in NSCLC patient samples. Poster presentation at the ASCO-SITC Clinical Immuno-Oncology Symposium, Orlando, FL, USA, February 23–25, 2017.

37. Scheel AH, Dietel M, Heukamp LC, Johrens K, Kirchner T, Reu S, et al. Harmonized PD-L1 immunohistochemistry for pulmonary squamous-cell and adenocarcinomas. Mod Pathol. 2016;29:1165–72.

38. Massard C, Gordon MS, Sharma S, Rafii S, Wainberg ZA, Luke J, et al. Safety and efficacy of durvalumab (MEDI4736), an anti-programmed cell death ligand-1 immune checkpoint inhibitor, in patients with advanced urothelial bladder cancer. J Clin Oncol. 2016;34:3119–25.

39. Ilie M, Long-Mira E, Bence C, Butori C, Lassalle S, Bouhlel L, et al. Comparative study of the PD-L1 status between surgically resected specimens and matched biopsies of NSCLC patients reveal major discordances: a potential issue for anti-PD-L1 therapeutic strategies. Ann Oncol. 2016;27:147–53.

40. Skov BG, Skov T. Paired comparison of PD-L1 expression on cytologic and histologic specimens from malignancies in the lung assessed with PD-L1 IHC 28-8pharmDx and PD-L1 IHC 22C3pharmDx. Appl Immunohistochem Mol Morphol. 2017;25:453–9.

41. Heymann JJ, Bulman WA, Swinarski D, Pagan CA, Crapanzano JP, Haghighi M, et al. PD-L1 expression in non-small cell lung carcinoma: comparison among cytology, small biopsy, and surgical resection specimens. Cancer. 2017;125:896–907.

42. Hirsch FR, McElhinny A, Stanforth D, Ranger-Moore J, Jansson M, Kulangara K, et al. PD-L1 immunohistochemistry assays for lung cancer: results from

phase 1 of the blueprint PD-L1 IHC assay comparison project. J Thorac Oncol. 2017;12:208–22.

43. Scott M, Ratcliffe MJ, Sharpe A, Barker C, Scorer P, Rebelatto M, et al. Concordance of tumor cell (TC) and immune cell (IC) staining with Ventana SP142, Ventana SP263, Dako 28–8 and Dako 22C3 PD-L1 IHC tests in NSCLC patient samples. J Clin Oncol. 2017;35(15_suppl):e14503.

13

Molecular profiling of lung cancer specimens and liquid biopsies using MALDI-TOF mass spectrometry

Eleonora Bonaparte[1,2], Chiara Pesenti[1,2], Laura Fontana[1], Rossella Falcone[1], Leda Paganini[1,2], Anna Marzorati[1], Stefano Ferrero[2,3], Mario Nosotti[1,4], Paolo Mendogni[4], Claudia Bareggi[5], Silvia Maria Sirchia[6], Silvia Tabano[1,2*], Silvano Bosari[1,2] and Monica Miozzo[1,2]

Abstract

Background: Identification of predictive molecular alterations in lung adenocarcinoma is essential for accurate therapeutic decisions. Although several molecular approaches are available, a number of issues, including tumor heterogeneity, frequent material scarcity, and the large number of loci to be investigated, must be taken into account in selecting the most appropriate technique. MALDI-TOF mass spectrometry (MS), which allows multiplexed genotyping, has been adopted in routine diagnostics as a sensitive, reliable, fast, and cost-effective method. Our aim was to test the reliability of this approach in detecting targetable mutations in non-small cell lung cancer (NSCLC). In addition, we also analyzed low-quality samples, such as cytologic specimens, that often, are the unique source of starting material in lung cancer cases, to test the sensitivity of the system.

Methods: We designed a MS–based assay for testing 158 mutations in the *EGFR*, *KRAS*, *BRAF*, *ALK*, *PIK3CA*, *ERBB2*, *DDR2*, *AKT*, and *MEK1* genes and applied it to 92 NSCLC specimens and 13 liquid biopsies from another subset of NSCLC patients. We also tested the sensitivity of the method to distinguish low represented mutations using serial dilutions of mutated DNA.

Results: Our panel is able to detect the most common NSCLC mutations and the frequency of the mutations observed in our cohort was comparable to literature data. The assay identifies mutated alleles at frequencies of 2.5–10%. In addition, we found that the amount of DNA template was irrelevant to efficiently uncover mutated alleles present at high frequency. However, when using less than 10 ng of DNA, the assay can detect mutations present in at least 10% of the alleles. Finally, using MS and a commercial kit for RT-PCR we tested liquid biopsy from 13 patients with identified mutations in cancers and detected the mutations in 4 (MS) and in 5 samples (RT-PCR).

Conclusions: MS is a powerful method for the routine predictive tests of lung cancer also using low quality and scant tissues. Finally, after appropriate validation and improvement, MS could represent a promising and cost-effective strategy for monitoring the presence and percentage of the mutations also in non-invasive sampling.

Keywords: Molecular diagnostics, MALDI-TOF mass spectrometry, Non-small cell lung cancer, Targeted therapy, Tumor genotyping

* Correspondence: silvia.tabano@unimi.it
[1]Department of Pathophysiology & Transplantation, Università degli Studi di Milano, Via Francesco Sforza, 35 -20122 Milan, Italy
[2]Division of Pathology, Fondazione IRCCS Ca' Granda Ospedale Maggiore Policlinico, Via Francesco Sforza, 35 –20122 Milan, Italy
Full list of author information is available at the end of the article

Background

Lung cancer is the leading cause of cancer death worldwide. Non-small cell lung cancers (NSCLCs), primarily adenocarcinoma (ADC) and squamous cell carcinoma (SCC), account for approximately 80% of lung cancer cases [1].

With the introduction of the Epidermal Growth Factor Receptor/Tyrosine Kinase inhibitors (EGFR-TKIs), which target cancer cells harboring activating *EGFR* mutations, the detection of somatic mutations became relevant to treatment choices for lung ADC [2]. Erlotinib, gefitinib, and afatinib are used to target *EGFR*-activating mutations. More recently, the new drug osimertinib was introduced. This molecule can inhibit *EGFR* kinase activity in the presence of the *EGFR* T790 M mutation, which confers resistance to the other inhibitors [3–6]. Yet another drug, crizotinib, inhibits ALK, ROS1, and MET when their kinase activities are aberrantly activated [7–10].

Ongoing clinical trials are investigating emerging agents capable of avoiding acquired tumor resistance to the common TKIs, or of targeting other activated proteins, such as PI3K, AKT1, ERBB2, MEK1, and DDR2 [10, 11].

Mutations in *KRAS* (found in 25–40% of ADC) are a negative prognostic biomarker for NSCLC, since no drugs have been developed to inhibit the mutant protein. Alternative strategies, such as inhibition of MEK, have been suggested as treatment for patients with *KRAS*-mutated cancers [12].

The most frequent activating mutations in lung ADC, other than *KRAS*, involve *EGFR* (15%), whereas *BRAF*, *ERBB2*, and *MEK1* are mutated in less than 2% of cases.

PIK3CA mutations are present in approximately 1–3% of NSCLCs, and are more common in SCCs (15%). *DDR2* mutations are present in 2% of SCCs. *ALK* and *ROS1* translocations and *MET* amplifications are typical of ADCs, representing 5%, 4%, and 2% of cases, respectively. *AKT1* mutations are found in 1% of lung cancers, more frequently in SCCs [10, 11].

A list of druggable molecular markers and pathways in lung cancer is provided in Fig. 1.

Based on the growing knowledge of inhibitors that target abnormally activated kinases and the resultant clinical inclusion of new drugs, the optimal choice of treatment of NSCLC patients relies critically on screening the tumor-related genetic alterations.

Different issues should be taken into account for the molecular characterization of NSCLC. First, NSCLC are heterogeneous and cells harboring a specific mutation may represent a minor clone in a mixture of neoplastic cells, as well as of non-neoplastic, stromal and inflammatory cells [13]. In addition, the availability and/or the quality of the specimens suitable for molecular evaluations could be scare, since formalin-fixed paraffin-embedded (FFPE) samples from small biopsies or cytology specimens could represent the only available material. [14]. Moreover, in recent years, non-invasive approaches (collectively called "liquid biopsy") have been developed to identify the molecular profile of tumor circulating cells (TCCs) or circulating tumor DNA (ctDNA) [15–18] and therefore very sensitive detection methods are required. For all of these reasons, it

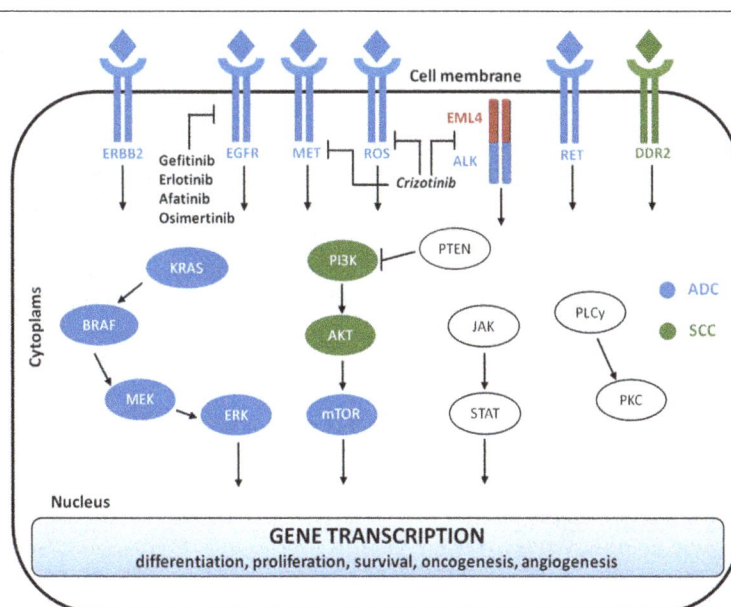

Fig. 1 Simplified schema of the most frequently altered signaling pathways in NSCLC. Blue and green ovals indicate the proteins commonly activated in ADC and SSC, respectively. Druggable TKIs and approved targeted agents are specified

is critical to use reliable and sensitive diagnostic methods capable of simultaneously detecting a wide range of mutations also in poor quality samples.

Different molecular approaches, such as Sanger sequencing, real-time PCR, pyrosequencing, MALDI-TOF mass spectrometry (MS) and next-generation sequencing (NGS) are currently available [19–22]. Among them, Sanger sequencing is the less sensitive (at least 20% of mutant alleles); MS is considered a robust approach for the genotyping of known mutations, able to combine the advantages of multiplexing, high sensitivity, and specificity with rapid turnaround, easy sample handling, and cost-effectiveness [19, 20]. Finally, although NGS is a very robust approach with the highest sensitivity [23], it is less affordable than the other approaches and poses several additional challenges, including validation and data handling for diagnostic purposes. Besides, to preserve the cost per test and avoid wasting resources, a consistent number of cases should be simultaneously analyzed.

Using the MS genotyping approach, we tested a cohort of 92 NSCLCs, investigating a wide spectrum of actionable mutations currently targeted by specific therapies or for which clinical trials are ongoing. Our aim was to verify the performance and sensitivity of the method using low levels of tumor DNA. Finally, we evaluated the performance of MS on plasma DNA from 13 lung cancer patients with *EGFR-* or *KRAS*-mutated tumors.

Methods

Patients and tumor specimens

The study group included 92 NSCLC cases collected for clinical purposes at the Fondazione IRCCS Ca' Granda, Ospedale Maggiore Policlinico di Milano (Italy), between September 2011 and December 2013. The molecular evaluation of all cases at the time of diagnosis was carried out by pyrosequencing using Ce-IVD kits (EGFR TKi response (sensitivity), EGFR TKI response (resistance), Anti-EGFR MoAb response KRAS status, Anti-EGFR MoAb response BRAF status - Diatech Pharmacogenetics s.r.l., Jesi, Italy). We included in the study the NSCLC cases for which the biologic material was available. The study was approved by the Institutional Ethic Committee (Fondazione IRCCS Ca' Granda, Ospedale Maggiore Policlinico di Milano N°526/2015).

For ctDNA analysis, peripheral blood samples were collected from additional 13 lung cancer patients at the time of biopsy/surgical procedures after informed consent. The inclusion criteria were the presence of ADC, the availability of tumor specimens and the positivity for *EGFR* or *KRAS* mutations.

Hematoxylin/eosin-stained sections (H&E) from FFPE tissues were evaluated by a pathologist for routine histopathologic classification and identification of the

tumor component. Diagnosis was performed according to the criteria of the 2015 WHO classification for lung tumors [24].

Ninety-two NSCLC specimens of primary or metastatic lung tumors, including 28 cytological and 64 histological samples, were classified as follows: 78 ADCs, 11 SCCs, and 3 NSCLCs, not classified more precisely because of the paucity of biological specimens (Table 1). All thirteen cases selected for ctDNA profiling were ADCs.

DNAs from NSCLC FFPE samples were obtained using the BiOstic FFPE Tissue DNA Isolation Kit (MO BIO Laboratories Inc., Carlsbad, CA, USA) and quantified using a NanoDrop 1000 UV spectrophotometer, software version 3.7.1 (Thermo Fisher Scientific Inc., Waltham, MA, USA).

ctDNA was extracted with the Helix Circulating Nucleic Acid kit (Diatech Pharmacogenetics, Jesi, Italy) from 3 to 5 ml of plasma obtained from about 10 ml of peripheral blood, collected in EDTA tubes. Following the manufacturer's instructions, ctDNA was finally eluted in 30 μl and not subsequently quantified.

MS genotyping assay

A panel of actionable loci was selected based on the Catalogue of Somatic Mutations in Cancer (COSMIC; http://cancer.sanger.ac.uk/cosmic), My Cancer Genome (https://www.mycancergenome.org), and relevant literature [11]. The panel comprised 158 variations affecting commonly mutated genes in NSCLC: *EGFR*, *KRAS*, *BRAF*, *ALK*, *PIK3CA*, *ERBB2*, *DDR2*, *AKT*, and *MEK1*. Reference DNA sequences were retrieved from Ensembl Genome Browser (http://www.ensembl.org/index.html).

Tissue DNAs and ctDNAs were genotyped using the single-base extension technique on a MassARRAY analyzer 4. Amplification and extension primers were designed using the Assay Designer Suite v.1.0 (Agena Bioscience, Hamburg, Germany). Amplification primers were designed with a 10mer tag sequence (lower cases) at 5′-end, to avoid their masses overlapping the range of detection of the MS assay. Primers sequences are available in Additional file 1: Table 1.

The MS panel consists of 48 assays multiplexed in eight wells, testing 158 mutations including base

Table 1 Tumor specimens and classification of the 92 NSCLCs cohort

Number of cases	ADC	SSC	NSC
Total	78	11	3
Histological specimens	57	7	0
Cytological specimens	21	4	3
Primary tumors	64	8	3
Metastases	14	3	0

substitutions, deletions, and insertions. A complete description of the mutations is provided in Additional file 2: Table 2. For PCR, SAP (shrimp alkaline phosphatase), and extension reactions, the Complete iPLEX Pro Genotyping Reagent Set (Agena Bioscience) was used. Amplification products were processed using Spectro-CHIP II Arrays and Clean Resin Kit and the MassARRAY Nanodispenser (Agena Bioscience). Analyses were performed using the MassARRAY Typer 4.0 software (Agena Bioscience).

Depending on the abundance of each sample, the amount of DNA from FFPE specimens, used as template, was 10–40 ng per well.

MS assay sensitivity

The analytical sensitivity of the MS assay was determined by verifying the lowest detectable frequency of a mutated allele using commercial reference standards HORIZON (Cambridge, UK) for the following mutations: EGFR G719A, T790 M and L861Q, KRAS Q61L, and BRAF V600E. The standards were heterozygous for the mutations, and thus contained the mutated alleles at 50% frequency. Serial dilutions containing 10%, 5%, and 2.5% of the mutated alleles were obtained by mixing standard samples with wild-type DNA from peripheral blood lymphocytes (PBLs). PCRs were performed using 50 ng of DNA from each dilution.

To determine the minimum amount of DNA needed to detect a mutation present at a low allelic frequency, we used decreasing amounts of DNA (20 ng, 10 ng and 5 ng) from four tumor samples harboring the following mutations at specific percentages: 30% KRAS G12C, 20% KRAS G12C, 10% EGFR L858R, and 9% PIK3CA H1047R. These percentages had been assessed previously using 40 ng of template DNA.

ctDNA genotyping assay

The presence of mutations in ctDNAs was verified using our MS analysis, testing only the assay specific for the mutation previously identified in the tumor sample. To compare MS with another sensitive method, we performed RT-PCR using the commercial IVD-CE kits Easy EGFR and Easy KRAS (Diatech Pharmacogenetics, Jesi, Italy) on Rotor-Gene (Qiagen, Hilden, Germany), following the manufacturer's instructions. RT-PCR results were analyzed and reported as ΔCt values (Ct sample − Ct wild-type control).

Notably, the amount of the ctDNA requested by RT-PCR and MS was 5 and 2 μl, respectively.

Results
Tumor genotyping
We tested 158 actionable mutations comprising base substitutions, insertions, and deletions of the EGFR, KRAS, BRAF, ALK, PIK3CA, ERBB2, DDR2, AKT, and MEK1 genes (Additional file 2: Table 2) in 92 NCSLCs and in plasma samples from 13 additional NSCLC patients with known somatic mutations. The mutation profiling of all cases is detailed in Additional file 3: Table 3. The overall data from the 92 NCSLCs revealed that 49 (53.3%) harbored mutations in at least at one gene. In ADCs, we identified mutations in EGFR (15.4%), KRAS (37.2%), BRAF (1.3%), ERBB2 (3.8%), and AKT (2.6%), whereas SCCs exclusively harbored PIK3CA mutations (27.3%). Mutations of ALK, DDR2, and MEK1 were never detected (Table 2). EGFR primarily contained in-frame deletions in exon 19 (6 out of 12 EGFR mutated cases). The T790 M and L858R mutations, concomitantly detected in two cases, were the only EGFR variants found simultaneously in the same tumor sample (Additional file 3: Table 3).

KRAS was predominantly mutated at codon 12, exon 2 (25 out of 30 KRAS mutated cases) (Additional file 3: Table 3).

Only KRAS variants were found concomitant with other mutated genes: AKT and ERBB2, in one case respectively (Additional file 3: Table 3).

Out of the three unclassified NSCLCs, one had KRAS G12A mutation (Additional file 3: Table 3), suggesting that it was ADCs since KRAS is most frequently mutated in this tumor subtype.

To evaluate the correlation between the mutated alleles percentages detected by MS and the amount of tumor cells at the histopathological evaluation, in two representative mutated ADCs we compared the stained slides with the corresponding MS spectra. As displayed in Additional file 4: Fig. 1, the percentages of mutated alleles are not strictly related to the amount of cancer cells in the samples. Indeed, in the first sample (left), more than 70% of cells are neoplastic, but only a subset of them (23% of the alleles) harbors the EGFR L858R mutation; conversely, in the second ADC (right), the percentage of mutated allele (49%) indicates that about

Table 2 Mutations found in 92 NSCLC FFPE samples

Classification	Total cases	Mutated cases	EGFR	KRAS	BRAF	ALK	PIK3CA	ERBB2	DDR2	AKT	MEK1
ADC	78	45 (57.7%)	12 (15.4%)	29 (37.2%)	1 (1.3%)	–	–	3 (3.8%)	–	2 (2.6%)	–
SCC	11	3 (27.3%)	–	–	–	–	3 (27.3%)	–	–	–	–
NSCLC	3	1 (33.3%)	–	1 (33.3%)	–	–	–	–	–	–	–

Table 3 MS assay sensitivity tested with reference standard DNA using decreasing percentages of mutated alleles

Reference standard	Percentages of the mutated allele			
	50%	10%	5%	2.5%
EGFR G719A (c.2156 G > C)	D	D	D	D
EGFR L861Q (c.1582 T > A)	D	D	ND	ND
EGFR T790 M (c.2369C > T)	D	D	D	D
KRAS Q61L (c.182 A > T)	D	D	ND	ND
BRAF V600E (c. 1799 T > A)	D	D	ND	ND

D: detected. ND: not detected

all tumor cells in the sample (tumor content >70%) have the KRAS G12D mutation.

Genotyping sensitivity

The MS sensitivity was assessed evaluating four common mutations in NSCLC, for which standard commercial references were available. Using 50 ng of HORIZON reference standard DNA (RSs, HORIZON) containing the mutations EGFR G719A, EGFR L861Q, EGFR T790 M, KRAS Q61L, and BRAF V600E in serial dilutions (50%, 10%, 5%, and 2.5%), we found that the sensitivity of MS assays varied depending on the specific mutation tested. For EGFR G719A and T790 M, the sensitivity of the assays was 2.5%, whereas it was 10% for EGFR L861Q, KRAS Q61L, and BRAF V600E (Table 3). These data suggest that MS can detect a mutation with frequency lower than 10%, and that the sensitivity depends on the specific mutation.

In addition, we tested the performance of MS using decreasing amounts of DNA (20 ng, 10 ng, and 5 ng) from four tumor samples harboring mutations at various allelic frequencies (previously identified using 40 ng of DNA). When the frequency of the mutated allele was lower than 10%, the amount of the template DNA influenced the efficiency of detection (Table 4, Fig. 2). Indeed, in cases with KRAS G12C and EGFR L858R at 30%, 20%, and 10% allelic frequencies, the mutations could be detected irrespective of the amount of DNA (Table 4, Fig. 2). In these cases, the frequency of the mutated alleles remained stable. Conversely, in the H1047R

Table 4 MS assay sensitivity considering various percentages of mutated alleles with serially diluted DNAs from three FFPE sample cases

Template DNA amount (ng)	KRAS G12C	EGFR L858R	PIK3CA H1047R
40	30%	20% 10%	9%
20	D	D D	D
10	D	D D	ND
5	D	D D	ND

D: detected. ND: not detected

PIK3CA sample, with an allelic frequency < 10% (mean value based on triplicate runs: 8% ± 1), the mutated allele could be clearly identified by analyzing 20 ng of DNA, whereas, at lower DNA quantities, the results were uncertain because the signal corresponding to the mass of the mutated analyte was insufficient for a positive call (Table 4, Fig. 2).

These overall data suggest that the sensitivity of MS for detection of point mutation at low levels of mosaicism should be tested for each assay, and that low levels of DNA amounts could affect the recognition of mutations present at low allelic frequencies.

ctDNA molecular profiling

During the routine molecular evaluation of additional ADCs, we selected thirteen cases harboring mutations of EGFR or KRAS and analyzed the corresponding ctDNA taken from plasma at the time of biopsy/surgery. Of the thirteen mutations identified in tumor DNA, five (Table 5: cases 1–5) were also detected in plasma DNA by real-time PCR, and four of them (Table 5: cases 1–4) were also detected by MS.

In general, the lower detection of mutations in plasma compared to FFPE samples, could be due to the sensitivity limit of the methods and/or to the tumor features (grade, dimension, vascularization, and tissue necrosis), which can affect the amount of tumor DNA released into the bloodstream [25].

The discrepancies between the two approaches were probably not related to the frequencies of mutated alleles in a tumor sample. The percentages of tumor mutated alleles of cases 1–4 were indeed comparable to those of cases 5–13, that were not detected in the plasma (t-test $p = 0.06$) (Table 5), suggesting that the ratio of the mutated alleles in the tumor specimens does not impact their detection by MS assay in plasma samples. The difference in detection rate, between ctDNA and FFPE DNA, could be due to the intrinsic heterogeneity of tumor samples, which could in turn be related to the different amounts of ctDNA released [26].

In plasma samples the range of the mutated alleles frequency detected by MS was 5–19%. RT-PCR does not allow the alleles percentages, a data that could have a clinical significance in monitoring patients.

Discussion

A large number of proteins activated in cancer and involved in the intracellular signaling pathways have been investigated as approved or potential targets for biological inhibitors. These discoveries led to a significant increase in molecular testing on tumor samples. Consequently, it becomes crucial to select a robust diagnostic method capable of identifying a wide spectrum of mutations in low-quality samples and in

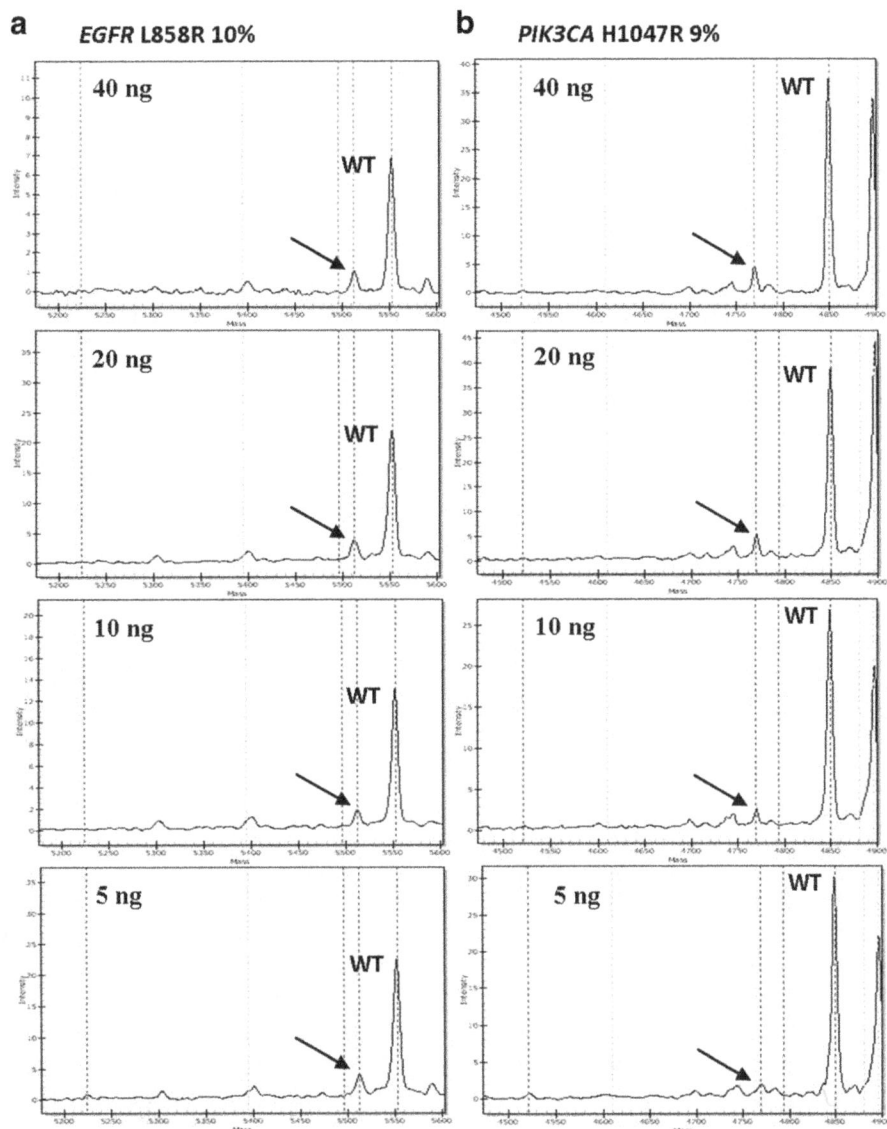

Fig. 2 Spectrograms, mass (x-axis) versus intensity (y-axis) from two histological samples (**a**, **b**) containing *EGFR* and *PIK3CA* mutations, respectively, at specific percentages of the mutated alleles (in brackets). Arrows indicate the mass peaks of the mutated alleles, using the specified decreasing amounts of DNA. The mass peaks of the wild-type alleles are also shown (WT). Using 5 ng of tumor DNA, the peak corresponding to the mutations was insufficient for a positive call for *PIK3CA* (**b**), but sufficient for EGFR

a cost-effective manner. We investigated whether MS would be reliable for this purpose, considering several challenges of tumor genotyping: the frequent paucity of available biological material, the low yield of DNA from FFPE specimens or liquid biopsy, and tumor heterogeneity, which is associated with variable frequencies of somatic mosaicism.

We found that mutations at 10% frequency could always be detected using our multiplexed genotyping panel, which covers 158 mutations in six genes. However, we confirmed that the sensitivity of MS depended on the specific assay, and genetic alterations could also be detected when the mutated allele frequency is very

low, e.g., 5% or 2.5% [19, 20]. On this basis, assuming that mutations are heterozygous, a 10% mutated allele frequency corresponds to 20% of cells carrying the mutation [27]. In turn, this implies that a minimum of 20% of tumor cells in a tissue specimen should be required to detect mutations at 10%. However, considering the tumor heterogeneity, it is also possible that a target mutation could be present only in a subset of cancer cells, and thus identifiable by MS, depending on MS performance for each mutation and the DNA quality.

Another crucial issue is the minimum amount of DNA needed for analysis. Frequently, the available amount of DNA is limited by the small sizes of biopsies or cytology

Table 5 Mutation detection in ctDNA by real-time PCR and MS approaches

Patients with *EGFR/KRAS* mutated tumors	Mutation in FFPE tumors (mutated allele percentage)	Mutation detection in ctDNA by real-time PCR (ΔCt values)	Mutation detection in ctDNA by MS (mutated allele percentage)
1	EGFR L858R (56%)	D (2.55)	EGFR L858R (7%)
2	EGFR E746_A750delELREA (27%)	D (1.44)	EGFR E746_A750delELREA (5%)
3	EGFR E746_A750delELREA (60%)	D (3.66)	EGFR E746_A750delELREA (12%)
4	EGFR E746_A750delELREA (55%)	D (3)	EGFR E746_A750delELREA (19%)
5	EGFR E746_E750delELREA (50%)	D (4.02)	ND
6	EGFR E746_A750delELREA (30%)	ND (12.61)	ND
7	EGFR E746_A750delELREA (30%)	ND (14.03)	ND
8	EGFR L858R (18%)	ND (18.99)	ND
9	KRAS G12 V (50%)	ND (27.23)	ND
10	KRAS G12 V (41%)	ND (18.78)	ND
11	KRAS G12C (17%)	ND (19.63)	ND
12	KRAS G12 V (33%)	ND (27.23)	ND
13	KRAS G12C (20%)	ND (16.95)	ND

D: detected. ND: not detected

specimens. We observed a relationship between the frequency of a mutated allele in the sample and the amount of DNA required for detection. This is partially in contrast to the findings of Magliacane et al. (2015), who reported that mutations could be detected even using very small amounts of DNA (1 ng per reaction) [28]. In particular, we observed that, in the presence of highly represented mutations (about 20%), only a very small amount of DNA (about 5 ng) was sufficient for the detection. By contrast, the quantity of DNA is crucial when identifying mutations with a frequency lower than 10%. Mutations represented at 10% and 30% were detected in all cases, but, when the mutated allele frequency was lower than 10%, the amount of template DNA influenced the performance of the MS analysis.

Taken together, these results showed that, to define the robustness of molecular profiling using MS, it is necessary to set the sensitivity of the method for each mutation to be investigated.

The validity of the mutation detection by MS was confirmed by comparison with the results reported in the literature: *KRAS* is the most frequently mutated gene in ADCs (37.2%), followed by *EGFR* (14.4%), whereas *PIK3CA* is frequently mutated in SCCs (27.3%) [10].

Three NSCLC cases were not further classified because of the paucity of specimens. Our molecular results identified the *KRAS* G12A mutation in one of them, suggesting that it could be classified as ADCs. This case confirms the importance of molecular profiling evaluation in lung cancer to complete the histopathological diagnosis, as already indicated for brain tumors [29].

In summary, MS allows the genotyping of several samples simultaneously by screening many known mutations in a single and cost effective test. It has high sensitivity, an important feature when a minority of mutant alleles must be distinguished from abundant wild-type alleles, and also allows mutations to be detected from a small amount of low-quality DNA, such as that typically obtained from poor-quality tissue specimens. Therefore, our experience emphasizes that it may not be appropriate to decline to perform molecular diagnosis on tissue specimens with a tumor component lower than 20%, or on poor biological materials.

Regarding the ctDNA evaluation, we observed concordant mutation detection between tumor tissue and plasma in four out of thirteen cases using MS, whereas, when using real-time PCR, we detected the tumor mutation in an additional case. The low sensitivity of both methods could be due to the low level of the mutated allele in the bloodstream or to tumor heterogeneity, although the small number of analyzed cases prevents us from drawing definitive conclusions. MS seems to be quite less sensitive than real-time PCR; however, MS has the advantage to screen panels of variations simultaneously. Our preliminary data suggest that, although in some cases analysis of ctDNA alone can be insufficient, MS has the potential to analyze liquid biopsy and monitor patients during treatment. Moreover, MS allows the estimation of alleles percentages, a data that could have a clinical significance in monitoring patients.

Conclusions

Our paper provides important advises for the use of MS in predictive analyses.

By analyzing 158 sequence alterations of the most frequently NSCLCs mutated genes in 92 tumor specimens, we confirmed that the method is able to detect mutated alleles present at 2,5% in the tumor specimens, and that the sensitivity can vary, depending on the mutation analyzed [19].

Interestingly, we noticed that the amount of DNA could affect the analysis. Specifically, when the mutation is present in more than 10% of alleles it is detectable even using low DNA amount (5 ng), but when the mutated alleles are less than 10%, the mutation detection can be compromised when using as low as 10 ng of DNA.

Finally, a proof-of concept investigation on liquid biopsy testing suggests that MS can be a reliable approach for this purpose even though it needs to be improved.

MS is a powerful and high throughput method for detecting known mutations, and allows to genotype scarce component of tumor cells in the tissue specimen, this has an important impact on patient clinical management.

Additional files

Additional file 1: Table S1. Amplification and extension primer sequences for MS panel. (DOCX 16 kb)

Additional file 2: Table S2. List of alterations (base substitutions, deletions, and insertions) included in the MS panel. On the left, mutations not distinguishable from one another are indicated by the same number. (DOCX 30 kb)

Additional file 3: Table S3. Molecular profile of NSCLC mutated cases. For each detected mutation, the number of positive cases and the diagnosis are reported. (DOCX 14 kb)

Additional file 4: Figure 1. H&E staining of two ADCs cases and the corresponding mutation MS spectra. **A** H&E staining of two ADCs cases. 5X zoom of the rectangular area is shown. The percentage of cancer cells is higher than 70% in both samples. **B** MS spectra of the two ADCs cases harboring EGFR L858R and KRAS G12D mutations, respectively. The mutated alleles are pointed out by black arrows and the corresponding percentages are reported in each spectrum. (TIFF 26330 kb)

Abbreviations

ADC: adenocarcinoma; AKT: AKT serine/threonine kinase 1; ALK: anaplastic lymphoma kinase; BRAF: B-Raf proto-oncogene, serine/threonine kinase;; COSMIC: catalogue of somatic mutations in cancer; ctDNA: circulating tumor DNA; DDR2: discoidin domain receptor tyrosine kinase 2; EGFR: epidermal growth factor receptor; EGFR-TKIs: epidermal growth factor receptor/tyrosine kinase inhibitors; ERBB2: human epidermal growth factor receptor 2; FFPE: formalin-fixed paraffin-embedded; H&E: (Hematoxylin & Eosin staining).; KRAS: Kirsten rat sarcoma viral oncogene homolog; MEK1: mitogen-activated protein kinase kinase 1; MET: MET proto-oncogene, receptor tyrosine kinase; MS: MALDI-TOF mass spectrometry; NGS: next-generation sequencing; NSCLC: non-small cell lung cancers; PI3K: phosphoinositide 3-kinase; PIK3CA: phosphatidylinositol-4,5-bisphosphate 3-kinase catalytic subunit alpha; ROS1: ROS proto-oncogene 1, receptor tyrosine kinase; SAP: shrimp alkaline phosphatase; SCC: squamous cell carcinoma; TCCs: tumor circulating cells

Acknowledgements
Not applicable

Fundings
Ministero della Salute, Regione Lombardia (Ricerca Finalizzata 2011–2012, RF-2011-02347106 to Monica Miozzo). IRCCS Ca' Granda – Ospedale Maggiore Policlinico di Milano (Progetto a Concorso 2014–2015 to Mario Nosotti).

Authors' contributions
EB, CP, LF, RF, LP: substantial contribution to design and acquisition of data; interpretation of the results; drafting the manuscript. AM: performing the experiments and data interpretation. SF, SB: pathological evaluation of specimens and data interpretation, revision and final approval of the manuscript. MN: funding support, patient's recruitment, revision of the manuscript and clinical evaluation; PM: patient's recruitment, revision of the manuscript and clinical evaluation; CB: patient's recruitment, revision of the manuscript and clinical evaluation; MM: funding support, planning of the experiments, data interpretation, drafting and revision of the manuscript and final approval of the version to be published. SMS: data interpretation, revision of the manuscript and final approval of the version to be published; ST: revision of the manuscript, data interpretation and final approval of the version to be published. All the authors read and approved the final version of the manuscript.

Competing interests
The authors declare that they have no financial nor ethical conflict of interest.

Author details
[1]Department of Pathophysiology & Transplantation, Università degli Studi di Milano, Via Francesco Sforza, 35 -20122 Milan, Italy. [2]Division of Pathology, Fondazione IRCCS Ca' Granda Ospedale Maggiore Policlinico, Via Francesco Sforza, 35 –20122 Milan, Italy. [3]Department of Biomedical, Surgical and Dental Sciences, Università degli Studi di Milano, Medical School, Via Francesco Sforza, 35 -20122 Milan, Italy. [4]Thoracic Surgery and Lung Transplantation Unit, Fondazione IRCCS Ca' Granda Ospedale Maggiore Policlinico, Via Francesco Sforza, 35 -20122 Milan, Italy. [5]Oncology Unit, Fondazione IRCCS Ca' Granda Ospedale Maggiore Policlinico, Via Francesco Sforza, 35 -20122 Milan, Italy. [6]Medical Genetics, Department of Health Sciences, Università degli Studi di Milano, via Antonio di Rudini, 8 –20142 Milan, Italy.

References
1. Reck M, Heigener DF, Mok T, et al. Management of non-small-cell lung cancer: recent developments. Lancet. 2013;382:709–19.
2. Keedy VL, Temin S, Somerfield MR, et al. American Society of Clinical Oncology provisional clinical opinion: epidermal growth factor receptor (EGFR) mutation testing for patients with advanced non-small-cell lung cancer considering first-line EGFR tyrosine kinase inhibitor therapy. J Clin Oncol. 2011;29:2121–7.
3. Inoue A, Kobayashi K, Maemondo M, et al. North-East Japan study group: updated overall survival results from a randomized phase III trial comparing gefitinib with carboplatin-paclitaxel for chemo-naïve non-

small cell lung cancer with sensitive EGFR gene mutations (NEJ002). Ann Oncol. 2013;24:54–9.

4.   Jänne PA, Yang JC, Kim DW, et al. AZD9291 in EGFR inhibitor-resistant non-small-cell lung cancer. N Engl J Med. 2015;372:1689–99.

5.   Rosell R, Carcereny E, Gervais R, et al. Spanish lung cancer group in collaboration with Groupe Français de Pneumo-Cancérologie and Associazione Italiana Oncologia Toracica: Erlotinib versus standard chemotherapy as first-line treatment for European patients with advanced EGFR mutation-positive non-small-cell lung cancer (EURTAC): a multicentre, open-label, randomised phase 3 trial. Lancet Oncol. 2012;13:239–2346.

6.   Sequist LV, Yang JC, Yamamoto N, et al. Phase III study of afatinib or cisplatin plus pemetrexed in patients with metastatic lung adenocarcinoma with EGFR mutations. J Clin Oncol. 2013;31:3327–34.

7.   Jorge SE, Schulman S, Freed JA, et al. Responses to the multitargeted MET/ALK/ROS1 inhibitor crizotinib and co-occurring mutations in lung adenocarcinomas with MET amplification or MET exon 14 skipping mutation. Lung Cancer. 2015;90:369–74.

8.   Shaw AT, Ou SH, Bang YJ, et al. Crizotinib in ROS1-rearranged non-small-cell lung cancer. N Engl J Med. 2014;371:1963–71.

9.   Solomon BJ, Mok T, Kim DW, et al. PROFILE 1014 investigators: first-line crizotinib versus chemotherapy in ALK-positive lung cancer. N Engl J Med. 2014;371:2167–77.

10. Chan BA, Hughes BG. Targeted therapy for non-small cell lung cancer: current standards and the promise of the future. Transl Lung Cancer Res. 2015;4:36–54.

11. Liu SV, Subramaniam D, Cyriac GC, et al. Emerging protein kinase inhibitors for non-small cell lung cancer. Expert Opin Emerg Drugs. 2014;19:51–65.

12. Jänne PA, Smith I, McWalter G, et al. Impact of KRAS codon subtypes from a randomised phase II trial of selumetinib plus docetaxel in KRAS mutant advanced non-small-cell lung cancer. Br J Cancer. 2015;113:199–203.

13. Sirchia SM, Faversani A, Rovina D, et al. Epigenetic effects of chromatin remodeling agents on organotypic cultures. Epigenomics. 2016;8:341–58.

14. Cagle PT, Allen TC, Dacic S, Beasley MB, et al. Revolution in lung cancer: new challenges for the surgical pathologist. Arch Pathol Lab Med. 2011;135:110–6.

15. Heitzer E, Ulz P, Geigl JB. Circulating tumor DNA as a liquid biopsy for cancer. Clin Chem. 2015;61:112–23.

16. Nakamura T, Sueoka-Aragane N, Iwanaga K, et al. A noninvasive system for monitoring resistance to epidermal growth factor receptor tyrosine kinase inhibitors with plasma DNA. J Thorac Oncol. 2011;6:1639–48.

17. Sorensen BS, Wu L, Wei W, et al. Monitoring of epidermal growth factor receptor tyrosine kinase inhibitor-sensitizing and resistance mutations in the plasma DNA of patients with advanced non-small cell lung cancer during treatment with erlotinib. Cancer. 2014;120:3896–901.

18. Weber B, Meldgaard P, Hager H, et al. Detection of EGFR mutations in plasma and biopsies from non-small cell lung cancer patients by allele-specific PCR assays. BMC Cancer. 2014;14:294.

19. Arcila M, Lau C, Nafa K, Ladanyi M. Detection of KRAS and BRAF mutations in colorectal carcinoma roles for high-sensitivity locked nucleic acid-PCR sequencing and broad-spectrum mass spectrometry genotyping. J Mol Diagn. 2011;13:64–73.

20. Kriegsmann M, Arens N, Endris V, et al. Detection of KRAS, NRAS and BRAF by mass spectrometry - a sensitive, reliable, fast and cost-effective technique. Diagn Pathol. 2015;10:132.

21. Ogino S, Kawasaki T, Brahmandam M, et al. Sensitive sequencing method for KRAS mutation detection by pyrosequencing. J Mol Diagn. 2005;7:413–21.

22. Young EC, Owens MM, Adebiyi I, et al. Clinical molecular genetics society (CMGS) scientific subcommittee: a comparison of methods for EGFR mutation testing in non-small cell lung cancer. Diagn Mol Pathol. 2013;22:190–5.

23. de Biase D, Visani M, Malapelle U, et al. Next-generation sequencing of lung cancer EGFR exons 18-21 allows effective molecular diagnosis of small routine samples (cytology and biopsy). PLoS One. 2013;8:e83607. https://doi.org/10.1371/journal.pone.0083607

24. Travis WD, Brambilla E, Burke AP, et al. WHO classification of Tumours of the lung, pleura, thymus and heart. Lyon: International Agency for Research on. Cancer. 2015;

25. Diaz LA Jr, Bardelli A. Liquid biopsies: genotyping circulating tumor DNA. J Clin Oncol. 2014;32(6):579–86. Review

26. Perkins G, Yap TA, Pope L, Cassidy AM, et al. Multi-purpose utility of circulating plasma DNA testing in patients with advanced cancers. PLoS One. 2012;7:e47020. https://doi.org/10.1371/journal.pone.0047020

27. Fontana L, Tabano S, Bonaparte E, et al. MGMT-Methylated Alleles Are Distributed Heterogeneously Within Glioma Samples Irrespective of IDH Status and Chromosome 10q Deletion. J Neuropathol Exp Neurol. 2016 Jun 26. pii: nlw052. [Epub ahead of print].

28. Magliacane G, Grassini G, Bartocci P, et al. Rapid targeted somatic mutation analysis of solid tumors in routine clinical diagnostics. Oncotarget. 2015;6:30592–603.

29. Louis DN, Ohgaki H, Wiestler OD, et al. World Health Organization histological classification of Tumours of the central nervous system. France: International Agency for Research on Cancer; 2016.

14

Immunohistochemical staining with non-phospho β-catenin as a diagnostic and prognostic tool of COX-2 inhibitor therapy for patients with extra-peritoneal desmoid-type fibromatosis

Tomohisa Sakai, Yoshihiro Nishida[*] (iD), Shunsuke Hamada, Hiroshi Koike, Kunihiro Ikuta, Takehiro Ota and Naoki Ishiguro

Abstract

Background: Immunohistochemical staining with conventional anti-β-catenin antibody has been applied as a diagnostic tool for desmoid-type fibromatosis (DF). This study aimed to evaluate the diagnostic and prognostic value of immunohistochemical staining with anti-non-phospho β-catenin antibody, which might more accurately reflect the aggressiveness of DF, in comparison to the conventional anti-β-catenin antibody.

Methods: Between 2003 and 2015, 40 patients with extra-peritoneal sporadic DF were prospectively treated with meloxicam or celecoxib, a COX-2 inhibitor, therapy. The efficacy of this treatment was evaluated according to Response Evaluation Criteria in Solid Tumors (RECIST). Immunohistochemical staining was performed on formalin-fixed material to evaluate the expression of β-catenin and non-phospho β-catenin, and the positivity was grouped as negative, weak, moderate, and strong. DNA was isolated from frozen tissue or formalin-fixed materials, and the *CTNNB1* mutation status was determined by direct sequencing.

Results: Of the 40 patients receiving COX-2 inhibitor treatment, there was one with complete remission, 12 with partial remission, 7 with stable disease, and 20 with progressive disease. The mutation sites in *CTNNB1* were detected in 22 (55%) of the 40 cases: T41A (17 cases), S45F (3 cases), and T41I and S45P (1 each). The positive nuclear expression of non-phospho β-catenin showed a significant correlation with positive *CTNNB1* mutation status detected by Sanger method ($p = 0.025$), and poor outcome in COX-2 inhibitor therapy ($p = 0.022$). In contrast, nuclear expression of β-catenin did not show a significant correlation with either *CTNNB1* mutation status ($p = 0.43$) or outcome of COX-2 inhibitor therapy ($p = 0.38$).

Conclusions: Nuclear expression of non-phospho β-catenin might more appropriately reflect the biological behavior of DF, and immunohistochemical staining with non-phospho β-catenin could serve as a more useful diagnostic and prognostic tool of COX-2 inhibitor therapy for patients with DF.

Keywords: Non-phospho β-catenin, Desmoid-type fibromatosis, Meloxicam, Prognosis, Diagnosis

* Correspondence: ynishida@med.nagoya-u.ac.jp
Department of Orthopaedic Surgery, Nagoya University Graduate School and School of Medicine, 65 Tsurumai, Showa, Nagoya, Aichi 466-8550, Japan

Background

Desmoid-type fibromatosis (DF), also known as aggressive fibromatosis, is characterized by benign and locally infiltrative fibroblastic tumors. Extra-peritoneal DF are at high risk of local recurrence after planned surgery even with a wide surgical margin (range 14.1–68%) [1–5], and surgical treatment occasionally leads to crucial post-operative morbidity such as amputation or serious functional impairment such as severe limitation of the range of motion of an involved joint. On the other hand, some cases of DF show stabilization or spontaneous regression of tumor without treatment [6]. Considering these enigmatic behaviors, the therapeutic approach for extra-peritoneal DF has been shifting from surgery with a wide surgical margin to conservative therapy [7, 8]. Recently, several therapeutic modalities for DF were reported including 'wait & see' only [9], COX-2 inhibitor therapy [10], hormonal therapy [11], low-dose chemotherapy [12], and tyrosine kinase inhibitors [13, 14], while few studies have investigated the prognosticators of these conservative therapies thus far.

In the tumorigenesis of DF, activation of Wnt signaling plays an important role, and aberrant nuclear accumulation of β-catenin has been utilized for pathological diagnosis to differentiate DF from other conditions [15]. Somatic mutations at exon 3 of Catenin β-1 (CTNNB1) gene have been reported in 64–85% of sporadic DF. The mutation generally occurs at codon 41 or 45, with T41A (threonine to alanine), S45F (serine to phenylalanine), or S45P (serine to proline) being the most frequent [16–18]. These mutations inhibit phosphorylation of β-catenin, which protect β-catenin from degradation by APC (adenomatous polyposis coli) complex, resulting in nuclear accumulation of β-catenin, where it binds to the TCF/LEF family of transcription factors and turns on a number of target genes [19]. Fewer patients have mutations in Adenomatous Polyposis Coli (APC) sporadically. Mutation of APC gene is implicated in the pathogenesis of familial adenomatous polyposis (FAP). Functional impairment of APC complex is induced by these mutations, and β-catenin retains its non-phosphorylated status, translocates and accumulates in the nucleus. In patients with FAP, similar activation of Wnt-β-catenin pathway will occur to that in patients with CTNNB1 mutation. The degree of β-catenin phosphorylation will differ based on the mutation type; codon 41, 45, wild type (WT), or APC gene. Together, the degree of Wnt-β-catenin pathway activation will be dependent on the mutation status of patients with DF. Recent studies have demonstrated that the mutation status of CTNNB1 can help to predict the outcome of surgical [16, 17] and conservative therapies [18, 20]. In the clinical setting, immunohistochemical evaluation has been the standard for evaluation, and CTNNB1 mutation cannot be evaluated at all institutions. A more appropriate antibody that better reflects desmoid biology is required for pathologists and physicians.

We previously reported that higher nuclear expression of β-catenin correlated with the efficacy of meloxicam treatment for patients with extra-peritoneal sporadic DF [21]. However, an increasing number of DF patients with lower nuclear β-catenin expression have proven resistant to meloxicam treatment since the previous report, prompting us to re-investigate the significance of nuclear β-catenin expression as a prognosticator for meloxicam treatment. Moreover, we hypothesized that non-phospho (active) β-catenin would reflect CTNNB1 mutation status, and help to predict the treatment outcome of patients with DF more precisely than β-catenin.

Methods

Patients and outcome evaluation

Fifty cases with extra-peritoneal DF were diagnosed in our institutions since 2003. Ten cases were excluded from this study. Five of them did not agree to treatment with COX-2 inhibitor, or had already received "wait and see" follow-up before the referral with status of stable disease. In three, biopsy specimens and formalin-fixed histological preparations were not available for the analyses, while two were excluded due to lack of adequate imaging for evaluation. Finally, this study focused on 40 patients with extra-peritoneal DF, all of whom were prospectively observed with COX-2 inhibitor therapy (meloxicam in 38 and celecoxib in 2). There were no patients with definitive FAP-related DF based on the complete history examinaton. All 40 cases were histologically evaluated and diagnosed with DF by experienced pathologists after thorough discussion. At the beginning of treatment, DF was evaluated with magnetic resonance imaging (MRI) and/or computed tomography (CT) in all cases. Patients were examined physiologically and received MRI and/or CT on an outpatient basis every 3 to 6 months. The efficacy of COX-2 inhibitor treatment was determined based on Response Evaluation Criteria in Solid Tumors (RECIST) [22] evaluated with MRI or CT at the latest follow-up or the endpoint of COX-2 inhibitor therapy as compared to that at the beginning. Patients with PD status could discontinue this therapy and select other treatment options such as low-dose methotrexate and vinblastine therapy [10] or surgery [23] with careful consideration of the tumor features, which included location and infiltrative behavior of the tumor, and individual patient's preference. Considering characteristics of DF (locally aggressive but no metastasis), SD status with no clinical symptom impairing patient's QOL is thought to reflect tumor dormancy. Patients were classified into a unfavorable group (PD) and favorable group (CR, PR, SD).

Mutation analysis of *CTNNB1*

Mutation analysis of *CTNNB1* was achieved as we previously described [18]. Briefly, DNA was extracted from frozen or formalin-fixed, paraffin-embedded (FFPE) tissue with the High Pure PCR Template Preparation Kit (Roche Molecular Diagnostics, Mannheim, Germany). DNA was amplified with polymerase chain reaction (PCR) (40 cycles, annealing temperature; 58 °C, extension temperature; 72 °C) using LightCycler 480 System (Roche). We used two pairs of primers to evaluate the presence or absence of point mutations in codons 41 or 45 of *CTNNB1* exon 3: forward 5′–GATTTGATGGAGTTGGACATGG–3′, reverse 5′- TCTTCCTCAGGATTGCCTT -3′, and forward 5′-TGGAACCAGACAGAAAAGCG-3′, reverse 5′-TCAGGATTGCCTTTACCACTC -3′. PCR products were extracted from the isolated bands after gel electrophoresis in 2% agarose, and purified. Direct sequencing was performed with the forward primers, using Applied Biosystems Big Dye Terminator V3.1, and Applied Biosystems 3730× DNA analyzer (Applied Biosystems, Foster City, CA) at FASMAC Co. Ltd. (Kanagawa, Japan). Results of the direct sequencing were evaluated using the databases of NCBI-BLAST to determine the mutation sites.

Immunohistochemistry

Tumor specimens were obtained by needle or incisional biopsy in advance of COX-2 inhibitor therapy, fixed in 10% formalin, and embedded in paraffin, and subjected to immunohistochemical study to analyze the expression of β-catenin. According to the previous report [21], the slides were treated overnight at 4 °C with anti-human β-catenin mouse monoclonal antibody (M3539; Dako, Carpinteria, CA; 1:200 dilution) and anti-human non-phospho (active) β-catenin (Ser33/37/Thr41) rabbit monoclonal antibody (8814S; Cell Signaling Technology, Danvers, MA; 1:200 dilution), counterstained with hematoxylin, dehydrated, and mounted. Non-phospho (Active) β-Catenin rabbit monoclonal antibody recognizes endogenous β-Catenin protein when residues Ser33, Ser37, and Thr41 are not phosphorylated. It does not detect β-catenin protein if tri-phosphorylated at Ser33/Ser37/Thr41. A previous report indicated that colon carcinoma was positively stained with this non-phospho β-catenin [24]. We used colon carcinoma tissues for non-phospho β-catenin staining as a positive control, and non-aggressive fibrous tumors, fibroma, was also subjected to this staining. This non-phospho β-catenin antibody was also used for western blotting using oral squamous cell carcinoma in another previous study [25]. Nuclear and cytoplasmic positivity of β-

catenin and non-phospho β-catenin were analyzed by two observers (S. H., T. S.) without the clinical information of cases, and classified into 4 groups according to definition of a previous report [21]; 0% for positively stained cells (negative; 0), 1% to 10% (weak; 1+), 11% to 50% (moderate; 2+) and 51% to 100% (strong; 3+) on 10 randomly selected high-power fields. In accordance with a previous report [16], the intensity of nuclear staining was also evaluated. If positive staining was observed partially in cytoplasmic area adjacent to the positive nuclear staining, we evaluated the case as positive for both "nuclear" and "cytoplasmic". Results of immunohistochemistry for β-catenin and non-phospho β-catenin were subjected to the association analyses between the positivity and efficacy of COX-2 inhibitor therapy or *CTNNB1* mutation status.

Statistical evaluation

Fisher exact test and Pearson chi-square test were applied to examine correlations of di- or tri-chotomous variables among the outcome of COX-2 inhibitor therapy, clinical characteristics, results of nuclear staining for β-catenin and non-phospho β-catenin by immunohistochemistry, and *CTNNB1* mutation status. Continuous variables of age and tumor size were compared between the favorable and unfavorable groups, and highly positive and lower positive group for β-catenin and non-phospho β-catenin using the Mann-Whitney U test. All statistical analyses were performed using SPSS statistics 20 (IBM Corp. Armonk, NY). $P < 0.05$ was considered significant.

Results

Clinical features and outcome of COX-2 inhibitor therapy

Of the 40 patients with extra-peritoneal DF, 16 were male and 24 were female. The mean age was 41.7 years (median, 36.0 years; range, 10–87 years). The location of the tumor was the abdominal wall in 10 patients, other sites in the trunk in 11, extremities in 15, and neck in 4. The diameter of the tumor ranged from 22.5 to 143.7 mm (mean, 76.2 mm; median, 74.5 mm). There were no patients treated with radiotherapy or other conservative treatment including anti-hormonal therapy or low-dose chemotherapy of methotrexate and vinblastine for DF prior to the COX-2 inhibitor therapy.

Mean follow up duration from the first visit to the final follow up date of meloxicam therapy was 29.6 months ranging from 2 to 104 months. Of the 40 patients evaluated with RECIST criteria, one patient was classified with CR, 12 with PR, 7 with SD, and 20 with PD. Of the 20 cases with PD, 10 received surgical treatment, and 9 low-dose methotrexate with vinblastine and/or doxorubicin-based chemotherapy, while one refused any other treatment with only continuation of meloxicam therapy.

Between the favorable (CR, PR, and SD) and unfavorable (PD) groups, no variable was associated with a significant impact on the prognosis for COX-2 inhibitor therapy, Age ($p = 0.089$) and tumor size ($p = 0.11$) had a trend and marginal impact on the prognosis, respectively. Regarding the site of involvement, all 4 cases with neck involvement were assigned to the unfavorable group (Table 1).

Mutation status of *CTNNB1*

All the 40 cases of the present study cohort received genotyping of *CTNNB1* exon 3. Point mutations existed in 22 of the 40 cases (55%) and were localized to just two codons (41 and 45). The most frequent mutation was replacement of threonine by alanine in codon 41 (T41A), which was detected in 17 cases (43%). Substitution of serine by phenylalanine in codon 45 (S45F) existed in 3 (8%), and that of threonine by isoleucine in codon 41 (T41I) and serine by proline in codon 45 (S45P) in one (3%) each. In the remaining 18 cases (45%), no mutation site was identified in the hot focus (codon 33–45) of *CTNNB1* gene (wild type) by Sanger method. Of interest all 4 cases with mutation in codon 45, including 3 cases with S45F mutation, showed progressive disease with COX-2 inhibitor therapy (Table 1).

Immunohistochemical findings

In all 40 cases, positivities and intensities of nuclear β-catenin and non-phospho β-catenin staining were evaluated. Nuclear and/or cytoplasmic staining pattern

Table 1 Patients characteristics between two prognosis group

Variables	Favorable group (n = 20)	Unfavorable group (n = 20)	p value
Gender			0.2
Female	10	14	
Male	10	6	
Mean age, years (range)	49.7 (19–87)	33.8 (10–74)	0.089
Mean size, mm (range)	70.6 (38.8–143.7)	81.8 (22.5–127.7)	0.11
Site			0.076
Abdominal wall	6	4	
Other trunk	4	7	
Extremities	10	5	
Neck	0	4	
CTNNB1 mutation			0.2
T41A	8	9	
T41I	1	0	
S45F	0	3	
S45P	0	1	
Wild type	11	7	

was observed, which was dependent on each case (Fig. 1a-d). Colon carcinoma was positive as a control (Fig. 1e). Three cases of fibroma of tendon sheath were subjected to non-phospho β-catenin staining, and all cases showed negative stainability. A representative staining was shown in Fig. 1f. With evaluation of nuclear positivities for β-catenin staining, there was no case with negative staining status. 6 cases showed weak, 22 cases showed moderate, and 12 cases showed strongly positive staining. On the other hand, with evaluation of non-phospho β-catenin staining, 4 cases showed negative staining status. 21 cases showed weak, 13 cases showed moderate and 2 cases showed strongly positive staining (Fig. 2) (Table 2). In the evaluation of positivity for cytoplasmic staining, no case showed negative staining status for either β-catenin or non-phosphop β-catenin staining. Nineteen cases showed moderate and 21 cases showed strong β-catenin staining, and 21 cases showed weak, 13 cases moderate, and 6 cases strong staining for non-phosphop β-catenin.

As a result, in non-phospho β-catenin staining, all 40 cases showed the same degree or weaker staining status compared with that of β-catenin. It could be explained that anti-non-phospho β-catenin antibody did not detect β-catenin protein if tri-phosphorylated at Ser33/Ser37/Thr41, in contrast to anti-β-catenin antibody, which could detect β-catenin protein including the tri-phosphorylated type. With respect to nuclear staining intensity for β-catenin, there were 13 cases with weak, 16 with moderate and 11 with strong intensity. For non-phospho β-catenin, there were 4 cases with negative, 14 with weak, 17 with moderate and 5 with strong intensity.

Correlation between mutation status of *CTNNB1* and immunohistochemical status of β-catenin

Positive nuclear staining of non-phospho β-catenin was significantly correlated with positive *CTNNB1* mutational status ($p = 0.025$) detected by Sanger sequencing, whereas no correlation was observed between nuclear staining of β-catenin and that of *CTNNB1* ($p = 0.43$). An interesting finding was that fewer cases ($n = 1$) showed strongly positive for non-phospho β-catenin in WT, T41A, and T41I as compared with that ($n = 9$) for β-catenin. Among cases with WT and T41A mutated cases, only 30% cases showed strong or moderate positivity for non-phospho β-catenin staining, whereas more than 80% cases showed strong or moderate for β-catenin staining. In contrast, all four cases with mutation of codon 45 (S45F and S45P) showed strong or moderate nuclear positive staining for both β-catenin and non-phospho β-catenin (Table 2).

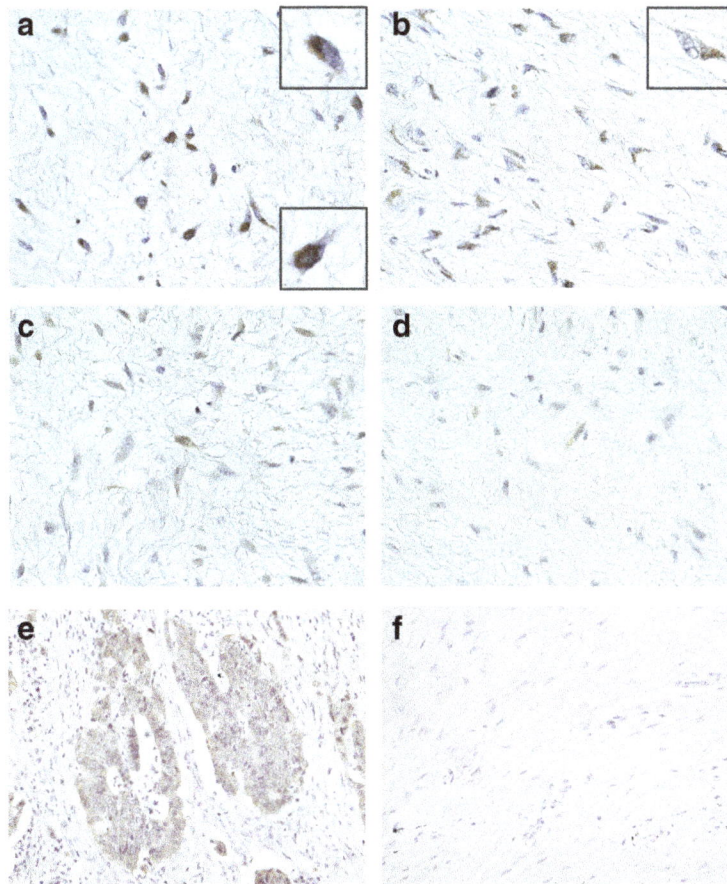

Fig. 1 Immunohistochemical staining for β-catenin and non-phospho β-cateninRepresentative images were shown with staining for β-catenin (**a** and **b**) and non-phospho β-catenin (**c** and **d**). Nuclear and cytoplasmic staining was observed in **a** and **c** (a: upper right inset; higher magnification of cytoplasmic staining, a: lower right inset; higher magnification of nuclear staining). Only cytoplasmic staining was observed in b and d (b: upper right inset; higher magnification of cytoplasmic staining). Positive staining was observed in human colon carcinoma tissue (**e**). A representative case of fibroma of tendon sheath showed negative staining (**f**). (counterstained with hematoxylin; original magnification: **a**-**d**; ×400, e-f; ×200).

Correlation between clinical outcome of COX-2 inhibitor therapy and immunohistochemical results of β-catenin

Statistical analyses with Fisher's exact test revealed that neither β-catenin nor non-phospho β-catenin significantly correlated with the clinical outcome of COX-2 inhibitor therapy (p = 0.16 and p = 0.11, respectively) (Table 3). Of the 12 cases with strong nuclear staining for β-catenin, 4 showed a favorable outcome and 8 an unfavorable one. Interestingly, both of the 2 cases with strong nuclear expression of non-phospho β-catenin were evaluated as unfavorable. These results prompted us to set the adequate cut off value for positivity of β-catenin staining. A cut off value of 10% (negative and weak vs moderate and strong) demonstrated that stronger nuclear expression of non-phospho β-catenin had a significant impact on prognosis (p = 0.022), whereas that of β-catenin expression did not (p = 0.38) (Table 4). On the other hand, cytoplasmic staining status of both β-catenin and non-phospho β-catenin staining had no significant correlation with the clinical outcome (p = 0.75 and p = 0.51, respectively). Nuclear staining intensity of β-catenin and non-phospho β-catenin had no significant correlation with clinical outcome (p = 0.91 and p = 0.67, respectively). Analyses of the relationship between staining positivity of non-phospho β-catenin and clinical variables revealed that age (p = 0.013) and tumor size (p = 0.081) had a correlation (Table 5).

Discussion

Wnt signaling plays an important role in the tumorigenesis of DF [26]. In the absence of Wnt stimulation, β-catenin is continuously phosphorylated by a multiprotein complex composed of tumor suppressor proteins APC, Axin, casein kinase 1 (CK1), and glycogen synthase kinase-3β (GSK-3β). In this process, phosphorylation starts at the S45 of N terminus encoded by exon 3 of the *CTNNB1* gene by 'priming kinase' CK1, then at T41,

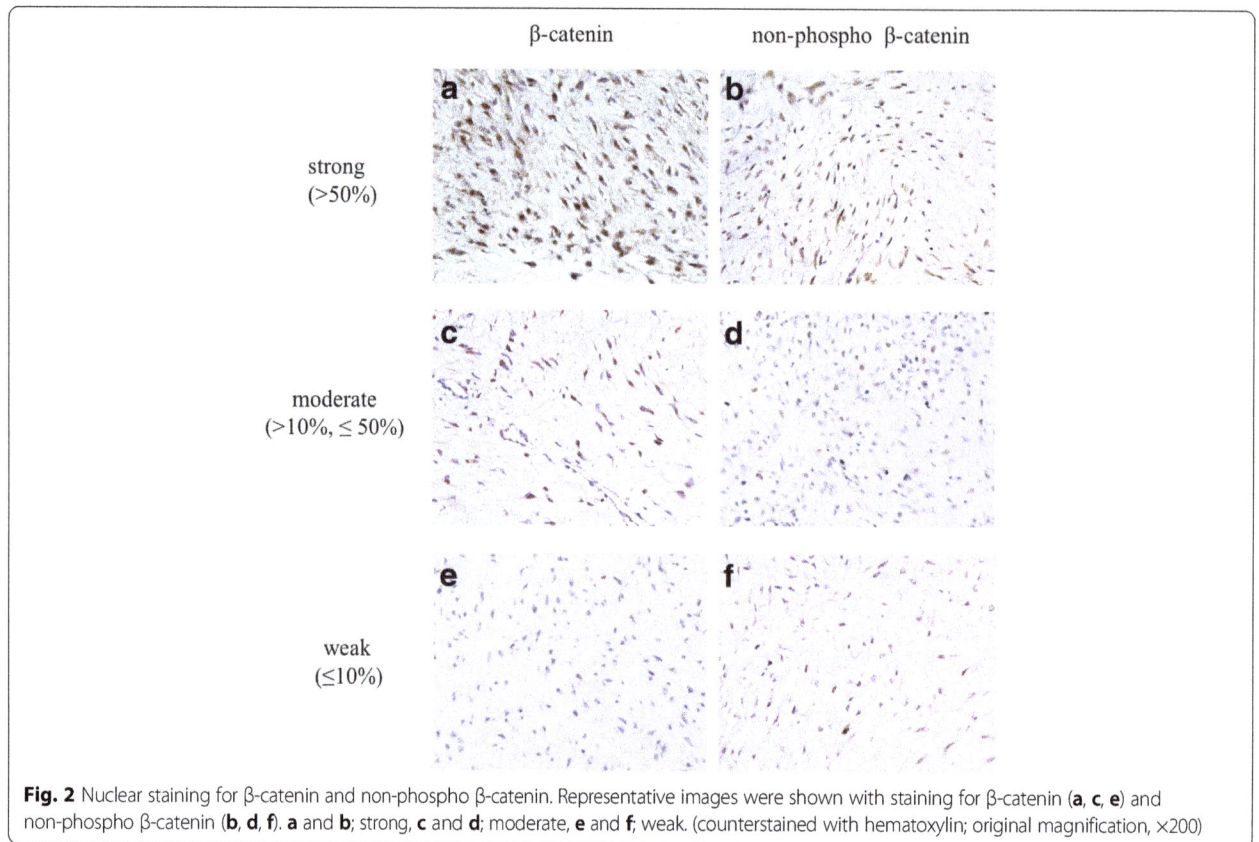

β-catenin   non-phospho β-catenin

Fig. 2 Nuclear staining for β-catenin and non-phospho β-catenin. Representative images were shown with staining for β-catenin (**a**, **c**, **e**) and non-phospho β-catenin (**b**, **d**, **f**). **a** and **b**; strong, **c** and **d**; moderate, **e** and **f**; weak. (counterstained with hematoxylin; original magnification, ×200)

S37, and S33 by GSK3β. Phosphorylation of β-catenin by the APC-axin-GSK-3β complex leads to its degradation by the ubiquitin-proteasome system. With a mutation of any one of these amino acid residues in exon 3 of the *CTNNB1* gene or the presence of Wnt stimulation, β-catenin retains non-phosphorylation status, accumulates and translocates into the nucleus, where it binds to the TCF/LEF family of transcription factors and turns on a

Table 2 Nuclear expression of β-catenin and non-phospho β-catenin. Relationship with *CTNNB1* mutation status

	Mutation status					
	WT	T41A	T41I	S45F	S45P	p value
β-catenin[a]						0.43
weak	4	2	0	0	0	
moderate	8	12	1	1	0	
strong	6	3	0	2	1	
non-phospho β-catenin						0.025
negative	3	0	1	0	0	
weak	10	11	0	0	0	
moderate	4	6	0	2	1	
strong	1	0	0	1	0	

WT wild type
[a]No cases showed negative

number of target genes [19]. In shedding light on the underlying pathogenesis of DF, evaluation for phosphorylation status can serve as a biomarker of DF aggressiveness.

Several studies have reported the correlation between nuclear expression of β-catenin by immunohistochemical examination and the prognosis of patients with DF. Gebert et al. revealed that nuclear β-catenin expression was significantly associated with an increased rate of local recurrence after surgical resection (5-year event-free survival; 0%, $P < 0.05$) [27]. They used a tissue microarray of 37 cases, although clinical follow-up data were available in only 23 cases. Our previous study reported that higher nuclear expression of β-catenin was significantly associated with a poor response ($p = 0.017$) to meloxicam therapy based on the 31 cases investigated [21]. However, in additional analyses of the cases accumulated after the previous report [21], an increased number of cases showed resistance to COX-2 inhibitor therapy. This may explain the discrepancy in the results between the previous and present studies regarding the usefulness of nuclear expression of β-catenin as a prognostic marker for COX-2 inhibitor therapy (previous report; $p = 0.017$, present study, $p = 0.38$). Lazar et al. observed nuclear β-catenin expression in 98% of

Table 3 Nuclear expression of β-catenin and non-phospho β-catenin. Relationship with clinical outcome of COX-2 inhibitor therapy

	Favorable group (n = 20)	Unfavorable group (n = 20)	p value
β-catenin[a]			0.16
weak	2	4	
moderate	14	8	
strong	4	8	
non-phospho β-catenin			0.11
negative	3	1	
weak	13	8	
moderate	4	9	
strong	0	2	

[a]No cases showed negative

Table 5 Clinical variables and nuclear positivity for non-phospho β-catenin

Variables	Nuclear non-phospho β-catenin staining		
	≤10% (n = 25)	>10% (n = 15)	p value
Gender			0.5
Female	14	10	
Male	11	5	
Mean age, years (range)	48.7 (18–87)	31.4 (10–67)	0.013
Mean size, mm (range)	70.3 (38.8–130.2)	86.0 (22.5–143.7)	0.081
Site			0.95
Abdminal wall	6	4	
Other trunk	7	4	
Extremities	9	6	
Neck	3	1	

specimens, with the percentage of positive nuclear staining cells for β-catenin not correlated with desmoid recurrence, and intensity inversely correlated with the incidence of desmoid recurrence ($p < 0.01$) [16]. The reason why decreased nuclear β-catenin intensity was associated with a higher recurrence rate of desmoid was not clarified nor speculated on in their study. The present study using non-phospho β-catenin antibody may provide more useful information based on the mechanistic aspects because non-phospho β-catenin antibody detects β-catenin only when residues S33, S37 and T41 are not phosphorylated, that is active β-catenin. There were 5 cases with "wait and see" policy, which were not included in the present study. Three cases were unfavorable course and 2 favorable. Interestingly, 2 favorable cases showed weak or negative nuclear stainability for non-phospho β-catenin, 3 unfavorable cases showed strong (1), moderate (1), or weak (1).

Recently, as the treatment algorithm for extra-peritoneal DF has been shifting from primary wide resection to conservative therapy, prognosticators for conservative therapy are also urgently needed. The correlation between

Table 4 Nuclear expression of β-catenin and non-phospho β-catenin on cut off value of 10% setting. Relationship with clinical outcome of COX-2 inhibitor therapy

	Favorable group (n = 20)	Unfavorable group (n = 20)	p value
β-catenin			0.38
≤ 10%	2	4	
> 10%	18	16	
non-phospho β-catenin			0.022
≤ 10%	16	9	
> 10%	4	11	

CTNNB1 mutation status and clinical outcome of DF has been focused on in several reports. In surgical treatment, DF with the S45F had a greater tendency for local recurrence compared to DF without S45F mutation [16, 17, 28]. A poor clinical outcome in DF patients with S45F was also reported in COX-2 inhibitor therapy with meloxicam [21]. Consistent with these studies, DF with S45F mutation were all evaluated as belonging to the unfavorable group for meloxicam therapy in the present study. However, how the mutation is implicated in the poor clinical outcome observed has not been fully analyzed and clarified. We previously reported that cultured DF cells obtained from a patient with S45F mutation showed strong nuclear expression of β-catenin immunohistochemically and higher mRNA expression levels of Wnt target genes, Axin-2 and Cyclin-D1, with RT-PCR compared with DF cells from patients without S45F mutation (T41A and wild type) [29]. These findings indicate that DF with S45F mutation shows higher upregulation of Wnt signal, which may contribute to the poor clinical outcome seen with conservative treatment as well as surgery. Because convenient means for evaluation of prognosis are preferably applied in the clinical setting, immunohistochemical evaluation using non-phospho β-catenin will be more easily utilized than mutation analysis.

Certainly mutation S45F might be a prognosticator for treatment in DF, although the proportion of DF with S45F was only 6–28% of extra-peritoneal DF [16–18, 28, 30]. Although prognostic factors other than CTNNB1 mutation have been reported such as age, size and location of the tumor [3, 15, 34, 35], a biomarker reflecting a more mechanistic property of desmoid is necessary for better evaluation of prognosis. In this study, non-phospho β-catenin staining could categorize tumors with S45F mutation detected by Sanger method as strong or moderate, and those with other mutations as strong-negative. Other factors may affect the stainability of the staining. Other than *CTNNB1* mutation, several causes of Wnt signal activation such as *APC* mutation [31], activation via TGF-β signal [32] and connective tissue growth factor (CTGF) have been reported [33].

There were several limitations in our study. First, the number of patients was small due to the rarity of DF, and thus it may have been underpowered to detect a significant difference between groups. However, the cohort of this study was prospectively treated with COX-2 inhibitor and subjected to *CTNNB1* mutation analysis. It is valuable and worth accumulating further studies. Second, non-phospho β-catenin staining could not completely predict the prognosis of patients with COX-2 inhibitor therapy. Nine of the 20 patients with an unfavorable outcome showed negative/weak nuclear non-phospho β-catenin expression, suggesting that Wnt signal activation is not the sole prognosticator in DF. Of clinical characteristics, younger age [34, 35] and larger tumor size [3, 34, 35] were reported as negative prognostic factors. In the future, a nomogram for prognosis should be established including clinical factors, *CTNNB1* mutation status, and results of immunohistochemical staining. Third, gene mutation was analyzed only in *CTNNB1* exon 3 by direct sequencing. Recently Crago et al. performed whole-exome sequence on wild type DF diagnosed with direct sequencing, and reported that 5 of 8 cases with wild type actually had the mutation in Wnt-related gene (3 in *CTNNB1*, 2 in *APC*) [36]. Similarly, our present study might also include some cases with wild type, which would harbor mutations of Wnt-related genes. Actually, mutation status is now investigated in different multi-center study using next generation sequencing, and preliminary results indicates one of the "wild type" cases in the present study has *APC* mutation despite no history of FAP. Another possible reason is that inadequate fixation time in formalin may cause low quality of extracted DNA, and the false negative results of *CTNNB1* mutation status because 22 cases were analyzed using FFPE samples. Further studies with additional molecular analyses will be required to better determine the correlation of prognosis and patient characteristics, mutation status, and immunohistochemical findings.

Conclusions

We demonstrate for the first time that nuclear non-phospho β-catenin expression could predict the treatment efficacy of with COX-2 inhibitor in patients with sporadic DF. Larger prospective clinical studies and molecular analyses are still necessary to determine the significance of this non-phospho β-catenin staining.

Abbreviations

APC: adenomatous polyposis coli; CK1: casein kinase 1; CT: computed tomography; CTGF: connective tissue growth factor; DF: desmoid-type fibromatosis; FAP: familial adenomatous polyposis; GSK-3β: glycogen synthase kinase-3β; MRI: magnetic resonance imaging; PCR: polymerase chain reaction; RECIST: response evaluation criteria in solid tumors; WT: wild type

Acknowledgements

We thank Drs. Hiroshi Urakawa, Eisuke Arai, to collect specimens. We thank Dr. Yuta Tsuyuki to provide carcinoma tissues. We thank Ms. Eri Ishihara and Naoko Takemoto for her secretarial assistance for this study. The manuscript has been carefully reviewed by Mr. John Gelblum, whose first language is English and who specializes in editing papers written by scientists.

Funding

This work was supported in part by the Ministry of Education, Culture, Sports, Science and Technology of Japan [Grant-in-Aid 26,293,334 for Scientific Research (B)] and [Grant-in-Aid 17H01585 for Scientific Research (A)], Health Labour Sciences Research Grant of Japan [201610088A].

Author's contributions

TS performed immunohistochemical staining, prepared figures and tables, and drafted the manuscript. TS, SH, KI, HK, and TO reviewed histological and immunostained sections. TS, KI and TO performed statistical analysis. YN and NI designed the study, drafted and edited the manuscript. All the authors were involved in data interpretation and approved the final manuscript.

Competing interests

The Authors declare that there is no competing interest.

References

1. Ballo MT, Zagars GK, Pollack A, Pisters PW, Pollack RA. Desmoid tumor: prognostic factors and outcome after surgery, radiation therapy, or combined surgery and radiation therapy. J Clin Oncol. 1999;17:158–67.
2. Shido Y, Nishida Y, Nakashima H, Katagiri H, Sugiura H, Yamada Y, et al. Surgical treatment for local control of extremity and trunk desmoid tumors. Arch Orthop Trauma Surg. 2009;129:929–33.
3. Gronchi A, Casali PG, Mariani L, Lo Vullo S, Colecchia M, Lozza L, Bertulli R, Fiore M, Olmi P, Santinami M, Rosai J. Quality of surgery and outcome in extra-abdominal aggressive fibromatosis: a series of patients surgically treated at a single institution. J Clin Oncol. 2003;21:1390–7.
4. Van Broekhoven DL, Verhoef C, Elias SG, Witkamp AJ, van Gorp JM, van Geel BA, Wijrdeman HK, van Dalen T. Local recurrence after surgery for primary extra-abdominal desmoid-type fibromatosis. Br J Surg. 2013;100:1214–9.
5. Rock MG, Pritchard DJ, Reiman HM, Soule EH, Brewster RC. Extra-abdominal desmoid tumors. J Bone Joint Surg Am. 1984;66:1369–74.
6. Nakayama T, Tsuboyama T, Toguchida J, Hosaka T, Nakamura T, et al. Natural course of desmoid-type fibromatosis. J Orthop Sci. 2008;13:51–5.

7. Bonvalot S, Desai A, Coppola S, Terrier P, Dômont J, Le Cesne A. The treatment of desmoid tumors: a stepwise clinical approach. Ann Oncol. 2012;23:x158–66.

8. Nishida Y, Tsukushi S, Shido Y, Urakawa H, Arai E, et al. Transition of treatment for patients with extra-abdominal desmoid tumors: Nagoya University modality. Cancers (Basel). 2012;4:88–99.

9. Briand S, Barbier O, Biau D, Bertrand-Vasseur A, Larousserie F, Anract P, Gouin F. Wait-and-see policy as a first-line management for extra-abdominal desmoid tumors. J Bone Joint Surg Am. 2014;96:631–8.

10. Nishida Y, Tsukushi S, Shido Y, Wasa J, Yamada Y, et al. Successful treatment with meloxicam, a cyclooxygenase-2 inhibitor, of patients with extra-abdominal desmoid tumors: a pilot study. J Clin Oncol. 2010;28:e107–9.

11. Fiore M, Colombo C, Radaelli S, Callegaro D, Palassini E, Barisella M, Morosi C, Baldi GG, Stacchiotti S, Casali PG, Gronchi A. Hormonal manipulation with tolemifene in sporadic desmoid-type fibromatosis. Eur J Cancer. 2015;51:2800–7.

12. Nishida Y, Tsukushi S, Urakawa H, Kozawa E, Ikuta K, Ando Y, et al. Low-dose chemotherapy with methotrexate and vinblastine for patients with desmoid tumors: relationship to CTNNB1 mutation status. Int J Clin Oncol. 2015;20:1211–7.

13. Chugh R, Wathern JK, Patel SR, Maki RG, Meyers PA, Schuetze SM, Priebat DA, Thomas DG, Jacobsen JA, Samuels BL, Benjamin RS, Baker LH. Efficacy of imatinib in aggressive fibromatosis: results of a phase II multicenter sarcoma alliance for research through collaboration (SARC) trial. Clin Cancer Res. 2010;16:4884–91.

14. Gounder MM, Lefkowitz RA, Keohan ML, D'Adamo DR, Hameed M, Antonescu CR, Singer S, Stout K, Ahn L, Maki RG. Activity of Sorafenib against desmoid tumor/deep fibromatosis. Clin Cancer Res. 2011;17:4082–90.

15. Bhattacharya B, Dilworth HP, Iacobuzio-Donahue C, Ricci F, Weber K, Furlong MA, Fisher C, Montgomery E. Nuclear beta-catenin expression distinguishes deep fibromatosis from other benign and malignant fibroblastic and myofibroblastic lesions. Am J Surg Pathol. 2005;29:653–9.

16. Lazar AJ, Tuvin D, Hajibashi S, Habeeb S, Bolshakov S, Mayordomo-Aranda E, Warneke CL, Lopez-Terrada D, Pollock RE, Lev D. Specific mutations in the beta-catenin gene (CTNNB1) correlate with local recurrence in sporadic desmoid tumors. Am J Pathol. 2008;173:1518–27.

17. Colombo C, Miceli R, Lazar AJ, Perrone F, Pollock RE, Le Cesne A, Hartgrink HH, Cleton-Jansen AM, Domont J, Bovée JV, Bonvalot S, Lev D, Gronchi A. CTNNB1 45F mutation is a molecular prognosticator of increased postoperative primary desmoid tumor recurrence: an independent, multicenter validation study. Cancer. 2013;119:3696–702.

18. Hamada S, Futamura N, Ikuta K, Urakawa H, Kozawa E, Ishiguro N, Nishida Y. CTNNB1 S45F mutation predicts poor efficacy of meloxicam treatment for desmoid tumors: a pilot study. PLoS One. 2014;9:e96391.

19. Liu C, Li Y, Semenov M, Han C, Baeg GH, Tan Y, Zhang Z, Lin X, He X. Control of beta-catenin phosphorylation/degradation by a dual-kinase mechanism. Cell. 2002;108:837–47.

20. Kasper B, Gruenwald V, Reichardt P, Bauer S, Hohenberger P, Haller F. Correlation of CTNNB1 mutation status with progression arrest rate in RECIST progressive Desmoid-type fibromatosis treated with Imatinib: translational research results from a phase 2 study of the German interdisciplinary sarcoma group (GISG-01). Ann Surg Oncol. 2016;23:1924–7.

21. Hamada S, Urakawa H, Kozawa E, Futamura N, Ikuta K, Shimoyama Y, Nakamura S, Ishiguro N, Nishida Y. Nuclear expression of β-catenin predicts the efficacy of meloxicam treatment for patients with sporadic desmoid tumors. Tumour Biol. 2014;35:4561–6.

22. Therasse P, Arbuck SG, Eisenhauer EA, Wanders J, Kaplan RS, Rubinstein L, Verweij J, van Glabbeke M, van Oosterom AT, Christian MC, Gwyther SG. New guidelines to evaluate the response to treatment in solid tumors. European Organization for Research and Treatment of cancer, National Cancer Institute of the United States, National Cancer Institute of Canada. J Natl Cancer Inst. 2000;92:205–16.

23. Nishida Y, Tsukushi S, Urakawa H, Hamada S, Kozawa E, Ikuta K, Ishiguro N. Simple resection of truncal desmoid tumors: a case series. Oncol Lett. 2016;12:1564–8.

24. Beyaz S, Mana MD, Roper J, Kedrin D, Saadatpour A, Hong SJ, Bauer-Rowe KE, Xifaras ME, Akkad A, Arias E, Pinello L, Katz Y, Shinagare S, Abu-Remaileh M, Mihaylova MM, Lamming DW, Dogum R, Guo G, Bell GW, Selig M, Nielsen GP, Gupta N, Ferrone CR, Deshpande V, Yuan GC, Orkin SH, Sabatini DM, Yilmaz OH. High-fat diet enhances stemness and tumorigenicity of intestinal progenitors. Nature. 2016;531:53–8.

25. Shiah SG, Hsiao JR, Chang WM, Chen YW, Jin YT, Wong TY, Huang JS, Tsai ST, Hsu YM, Chou ST, Yen YC, Jiang SS, Shieh YS, Chang IS, Hsiao M, Chang JY. Downregulated miR329 and miR410 promote the proliferation and invasion of oral squamous cell carcinoma by targeting Wnt-7b. Cancer Res. 2014;74:7560–72.

26. Tejpar S, Nollet F, Li C, Wunder JS, Michils G, Dal Cin P, van Cutsem E, Bapat B, van Roy F, Cassiman JJ, Alman BA. Predominance of beta-catenin mutations and beta-catenin dysregulation in sporadic aggressive fibromatosis (desmoid tumor). Oncogene. 1999;18:6615–20.

27. Gebert C, Hardes J, Kersting C, August C, Supper H, Winkelmann W, Buerger H, Gosheger G. Expression of beta-catenin and p53 are prognostic factors in deep aggressive fibromatosis. Histopathology. 2007;50:491–7.

28. Van Broekhoven DL, Verhoef C, Grünhagen DJ, van Gorp JM, den Bakker MA, Hinrichs JW, de Voijs CM, van Dalen T. Prognostic value of CTNNB1 gene mutation in primary sporadic aggressive fibromatosis. Ann Surg Oncol. 2015;22:1464–70.

29. Hamada S, Urakawa H, Kozawa E, Arai E, Ikuta K, Sakai T, Ishiguro N, Nishida Y. Characteristics of cultured desmoid cells with different CTNNB1 mutation status. Cancer Med. 2016;5:352–60.

30. Huss S, Nehles J, Binot E, Wardelmann E, Mittler J, Kleine MA, Künstlinger H, Hartmann W, Hohenberger P, Merkelbach-Bruse S, Buettner R, Schildhaus HU. β-catenin (CTNNB1) mutations and clinicopathological features of mesenteric desmoid-type fibromatosis. Histopathology. 2013;62:294–304.

31. Alman BA, Li C, Pajerski ME, Diaz-Cano S, Wolfe HJ. Increased beta-catenin protein and somatic APC mutations in sporadic aggressive fibromatoses (desmoid tumors). Am J Pathol. 1997;151:329–34.

32. Amini Nik S, Ebrahim RP, van Dam K, Cassiman JJ, Tejpar S. TGF-beta modulates beta-catenin stability and signaling in mesenchymal proliferations. Exp Cell Res. 2007;313:2887–95.

33. Varghese S, Braggio DA, Gillespie J, Toland AE, Pollock R, Mayerson J, Scharschmidt T, Iwenofu OH. TGF-β and CTGF are Mitogenic Output Mediators of Wnt/β-Catenin Signaling in Desmoid Fibromatosis. Appl Immunohistochem Mol Morphol. Epub ahead of print 18 Feb 2016. doi: https://doi.org/10.1097/PAI.0000000000000340.

34. Salas S, Dufresne A, Bui B, Blay JY, Terrier P, Ranchere-Vince D, Bonvalot S, Stoeckle E, Guillou L, Le Cesne A, Oberlin O, Brouste V, Coindre JM. Prognostic factors influencing progression-free survival determined from a series of sporadic desmoid tumors: a wait-and-see policy according to tumor presentation. J Clin Oncol. 2011;29:3553–8.

35. Crago AM, Denton B, Salas S, Dufresne A, Mezhir JJ, Hameed M, Gonen M, Singer S, Brennan MF. A prognostic nomogram for prediction of recurrence in desmoid fibromatosis. Ann Surg. 2013;258:347–53.

36. Crago AM, Chmielecki J, Rosenberg M, O'Connor R, Byrne C, Wilder FG, Thorn K, Agius P, Kuk D, Socci ND, Qin LX, Meyerson M, Hameed M, Singer S. Near universal detection of alterations in CTNNB1 and Wnt pathway regulators in desmoid-type fibromatosis by whole-exome sequencing and genomic analysis. Genes Chromosomes Cancer. 2015;54:606–15.

15

Prognostic significance of PD-L1 expression and CD8+ T cell infiltration in pulmonary neuroendocrine tumors

Haiyue Wang[1†], Zhongwu Li[1†], Bin Dong[2], Wei Sun[1], Xin Yang[1], Ruping Liu[3], Lixin Zhou[1], Xiaozheng Huang[1], Ling Jia[1] and Dongmei Lin[1*]

Abstract

Background: Recent research supports a significant role of immune checkpoint inhibitors in the treatment of solid tumors. However, relevant reports for programmed death-ligand 1 (PD-L1) and CD8+ tumor-infiltrating lymphocytes (TILs) in pulmonary neuroendocrine tumors (PNETs) have not been fully studied. Therefore, we investigated PNETs for the expression of PD-L1 and infiltration by CD8+ TILs as well as the prognostic value of both factors.

Methods: In total, 159 specimens of PNETs (35 TC, 2 AC, 28 LCNEC, 94 SCLC) were included in this study. Immunohistochemistry (IHC) was used to detect the expression of PD-L1 in these cases. Cases demonstrating ≥5% tumor cell expression or any expression (> 1%) of PD-L1 on immune cells were considered positive. CD8 + TILs both within stroma and tumor areas of invasive carcinoma were analyzed using whole-slide digital imaging. Manual regional annotation and machine cell counts were performed for each case.

Results: Positive expression of PD-L1 was observed in 72 cases (45.3%), including 9 cases (5.7%) with expression exclusively on tumor cells, 46 cases (28.9%) with expression exclusively on immune cells, and 17 cases (10.7%) with the expression on tumor cells and immune cells. PD-L1 expression was associated with necrosis ($p < 0.001$), high pathologic grade ($p < 0.001$) and histologic type ($p < 0.001$). No correlation was observed with overall survival (OS) ($p = 0.158$) or progression-free survival (PFS) ($p = 0.315$). In contrast, higher CD8+ T cell density was associated with the absence of vascular invasion ($p = 0.004$), histologic type ($p = 0.005$), negative lymph node metastasis ($p = 0.005$) and lower clinical staging ($p = 0.007$). Moreover, multivariate analysis revealed that CD8+ stromal TIL was an independent prognostic factor for improved OS ($p = 0.009$) and PFS ($p = 0.002$).

Conclusion: PD-L1 was expressed in approximately half of the PNETs. The majority of the expression was observed in immune cells. Positive expression of PD-L1 showed no correlation with OS or PFS, while higher CD8+ TILs within stroma was proved to be an independent prognostic factor for favorable OS and PFS of PNETs.

Keywords: Pulmonary neuroendocrine tumor, PD-L1, CD8+ TILs

* Correspondence: lindm100142@163.com
†Haiyue Wang and Zhongwu Li contributed equally to this work.
[1]Key Laboratory of Carcinogenesis and Translational Research (Ministry of Education), Department of Pathology, Peking University Cancer Hospital & Institute, No. 52 Fucheng Road, Haidian District, Beijing 100142, People's Republic of China
Full list of author information is available at the end of the article

Background

Neuroendocrine lung tumors represent a spectrum of low-grade typical carcinoids (TC), atypical carcinoids (AC), high-grade large cell neuroendocrine carcinoma (LCNEC) and small cell lung carcinoma (SCLC). SCLC is the most aggressive and most common of all malignant neuroendocrine tumors, with an incidence of 15–20%. LCNEC represents approximately 3% of lung tumors. TC accounts for 1–2%, while AC is the rarest of the lung neuroendocrine tumors (0.1–0.2%) [1–3]. Traditional treatments for high-grade malignancy, which include chemotherapy and radiation, have remained unchanged for decades. Prognosis remains dismal for these patients [4]. Therefore, to improve the prognosis of PNETs, a promising therapeutic strategy is urgently needed.

In the process of tumorigenesis, neoplastic transformation alters the structure of the normal tissue, leading to the activation of effector T cells, which then seeks to eliminate the transformed cells. Novel immunotherapy targeting immune checkpoint molecules such as programmed death-ligand 1 (PD-L1), based on the mechanism of cancer-immune escape, have successfully garnered increasing attention. Programmed death ligand 1 (PD-L1; also called B7-H1 or CD274) can be detected in many cancer cells and immune cells including the antigen-presenting cells (APCs) [5]. During the development of human cancer, the PD-L1 molecule is abnormally activated and overexpressed, which may suppress T cell migration, proliferation, secretion of cytotoxic mediators, and restrict cancer cell killing [6]. Therefore, monoclonal antibodies (mAbs) blocking the PD-L1 pathway or immunomodulatory agents with similar effects may improve anticancer immunity via enhancing T cell functions. Monoclonal antibodies targeting PD-L1 or PD-1 are currently being investigated in clinical trials. The results obtained to date have demonstrated remarkable clinical responses in many different types of cancer [6–10].

Cytotoxic lymphocytes (CTLs), which play a critical role in the anticancer response, are actively suppressed in the tumor microenvironment [11]. Some CTLs manage to be released into circulation, then migrate into tumor tissue through complicated interactions with adhesion receptors, at which point they are called tumor-infiltrating lymphocytes (TILs) [12]. Given that PD-L1 on tumor cells or immune cells interacts with CD8 expressed on T cells in the tumor environment, a comprehensive analysis of CD8/PD-L1 related molecules might provide important information for determining the clinical relevance to the neuroendocrine tumors of the lung. However, to the best of our knowledge, expression of PD-L1 on PNETs has not been fully studied [13].

In this study, we investigated the pattern of PD-L1 expression and the density of CD8+ TILs in PNETs. Moreover, we analyzed the clinicopathological characteristics with the expression of PD-L1 and the number of CD8+ TIL levels. We also performed a survival analysis to determine the correlation of PD-L1 expression and CD8+ TIL counts with OS and PFS.

Methods

Patient cohort

A total of 159 patients with PNETs who underwent pulmonary lobectomy or lymph node resection at Peking University Cancer Hospital (Beijing, China) from 2010 to 2015 were included in this study. Of those cases, 35 were TC, 2 were AC, 28 were LCNEC, and 94 were SCLC. All cases were reviewed by two experienced pathologists (Zhongwu Li and Bin Dong) to confirm the diagnosis based on the current WHO criteria for neuroendocrine lung tumors. The staging was undertaken according to the 8th edition AJCC tumor, lymph node, metastasis (TNM) classification. All the clinical characteristics (including age, gender, histologic type, necrosis, vascular invasion, preoperative chemotherapy, lymph node metastasis, and clinical TNM staging) were collected.

Immunohistochemistry

Serial sections with a thickness of 4 μm from the whole formalin-fixed paraffin-embedded (FFPE) samples of PNETs were cut onto glass slides, followed by IHC staining. Evaluation of PD-L1 was performed using a rabbit anti-PD-L1 monoclonal antibody (clone SP142; ZSGB-BIO, Beijing, China) at a working solution and incubated for 15 min at 37 °C on an autostainer (BOND-MAX, LEICA, Leica Biosystems Newcastle Ltd., Newcastle, UK). Cases demonstrating ≥5% tumor cell expression (membrane) or any expression (>1%) of PD-L1 on immune cells (membrane or cytoplasm) were considered positive [14]. Slides stained with CD8 were labeled by a rabbit anti-CD8 monoclonal antibody (clone SP16; ZSGB-BIO, Beijing, China) at a working solution and incubated for 36 min at 37 °C on an autostainer (BenchMark ULTRA, Roche, Ventana Medical Systems, Oro Valley, AZ, USA). For each case, manual regional annotation and machine cell counts were used to measure cell density in intratumoral as well as stromal areas of invasive carcinoma. CD8+ TIL density was analyzed by whole slide digital scanning using an Digital Pathology Scanner (Aperio VERSA, Leica Biosystems, Buffalo Grove, IL, USA), and the scoring was assessed on an Aperio Scanscope (Aperio Technologies; USA) by the method of rare event tissue test. Positive cell counts were measured in 4 peritumoral and 6 intratumoral non-overlapping fields using fixed areas of 1.44 square millimeters. The grading system was defined as two groups according to the median CD8+ T cell density in stroma and intratumor.

Statistical analysis

SPSS 17.0 version (IBM Corporation, Armonk, NY, USA) was used for all statistical analyses. Correlations between CD8+ T cell density and PD-L1 expression with the clinicopathological variables were performed using the Pearson's chi-square and Fisher's exact test. Survival analysis was performed using the univariate Kaplan-Meier method. Multivariate analysis was performed with the Cox proportional hazards model. Overall survival was calculated from the date of pathological diagnosis to time of death or last

follow-up. Progression-free survival was calculated from date of pathological diagnosis to time of last clinical evidence of recurrence, progression, or death. Two-sided p value < 0.05 was considered statistically significant.

Results

Patient clinicopathological characteristics and PD-L1 immunoreactivity

The clinicopathological features of 159 patients diagnosed as neuroendocrine tumors of lung are

Table 1 Clinical characteristics in the four subtypes

Variable	All tumors	TC	AC	LCNEC	SCLC	NA
	159 (100.0)	35 (100.0)	2 (100.0)	28 (100.0)	94 (100.0)	
Age						
$\leq$ =59.5	78 (49.1)	25 (71.4)	2 (100.0)	12 (42.9)	39 (41.5)	
> 59.5	81 (50.9)	10 (28.6)	0 (0.0)	16 (57.1)	55 (58.5)	
Gender						
Male	109 (68.6)	17 (48.6)	0 (0.0)	23 (82.1)	69 (73.4)	
Female	50 (31.4)	18 (51.4)	2 (100.0)	5 (17.9)	25 (27.6)	
Necrosis						
No	85 (53.5)	35 (100.0)	0 (0.0)	9 (32.1)	41 (43.6)	
Yes	74 (46.5)	0 (0.0)	2 (100.0)	19 (67.9)	53 (56.4)	
Vascular invasion						
No	129 (81.1)	34 (97.1)	1 (50.0)	22 (78.6)	72 (76.6)	
Yes	30 (18.9)	1 (2.9)	1 (50.0)	6 (21.4)	22 (23.4)	
Preoperative therapy						
No	150 (94.3)	35 (100.0)	2 (100.0)	27 (96.4)	86 (91.5)	
Yes	9 (5.7)	0 (0.0)	0 (0.0)	1 (3.6)	8 (8.5)	
First location						
Lung	131 (82.4)	35 (100.0)	2 (100.0)	28 (100.0)	66 (70.2)	
Lymph Node	28 (17.6)	0 (0.0)	0 (0.0)	0 (0.0)	28 (29.8)	
Lymph Node Metastasis						13 (8.2)
No	83 (52.2)	32 (97.0)	1 (50.0)	14 (60.9)	36 (40.9)	
Yes	63 (47.8)	1 (3.0)	1 (50.0)	9 (39.1)	52 (59.1)	
Clinical Staging						15 (9.4)
I	70 (48.6)	30 (90.9)	1 (50.0)	10 (43.5)	29 (33.7)	
II	27 (18.8)	2 (6.1)	0 (0.0)	9 (39.1)	16 (18.6)	
III	47 (32.6)	1 (3.0)	1 (50.0)	4 (17.4)	41 (47.7)	
Patterns of PD-L1						
Tumor[pos] stroma[neg]	9 (5.7)	3 (8.6)	0 (0.0)	5 (17.8)	1 (1.1)	
Stroma[pos]tumor[neg]	46 (28.9)	0 (0.0)	0 (0.0)	12 (42.9)	34 (36.2)	
Tumor and stroma[pos]	17 (10.7)	0 (0.0)	0 (0.0)	4 (14.3)	13 (13.8)	
Tumor and stroma[neg]	87 (54.7)	32 (91.4)	2 (100.0)	7 (25.0)	46 (48.9)	
CD8 density/mm^2 in stroma						
$\leq$ 264.6/mm^2	80 (50.3)	23 (65.7)	0 (0.0)	7 (25.0)	50 (53.2)	
> 264.6/mm^2	79 (49.7)	12 (34.3)	2 (100.0)	21 (75.0)	44 (46.8)	

Abbreviation: NA not available

presented in Table 1. The study included 109 males (68.6%) and 50 females (31.4%). Median age was 59.5 years (range, 30 to 83). A small minority of patients (5.7%) had received neoadjuvant chemotherapy before surgery, while 148 cases did not. For most cases, the primary site was in the lung ($n = 131$, 82.4%). Of the 159 samples, most tumors showed no vascular invasion ($n = 129$, 81.1%). Approximately half of the cases had tumor necrosis ($n = 74$, 46.5%). Lymph node metastasis was detected in 63 patients (47.8%). Tumors were classified as stage I ($n = 70$, 48.6%), stage II ($n = 27$, 18.8%), or stage III ($n = 47$, 32.6%).

PD-L1 was positively expressed in 72 cases (45.3%), including 9 with expression exclusively on tumor cells (5.7%), 46 with expression exclusively on immune stromal cells (28.9%), and 17 with expression both on tumor cells and immune cells (10.7%). Membranous and cytoplasmic expression of PD-L1 protein was detected in four types of PNETs, including SCLC ($n = 48$, 66.7%), LCNEC ($n = 21$, 29.2%), AC ($n = 0$, 0.0%), and TC ($n = 3$, 4.1%).

Table 2 The association between PD-L1 expression, CD8+ T cell infiltration and clinicopathologic parameters in PNETs

Variable	N(%)	PD-L1 expression			CD8+ T cell density in stroma			NA
		Positive	Negative	p	≤264.6/mm²	>264.6/mm²	p	
Total	159 (100.0)	72 (45.3)	87 (54.7)		80 (50.3)	79 (49.7)		
Age				0.241			0.578	
≤59.5	78 (49.1)	39 (54.2)	39 (44.8)		41 (51.3)	37 (46.8)		
>59.5	81 (50.9)	33 (45.8)	48 (55.2)		39 (48.7)	42 (53.2)		
Gender				0.365			0.189	
Male	109 (68.6)	52 (72.2)	57 (65.5)		51 (63.8)	58 (73.4)		
Female	50 (31.4)	20 (27.8)	30 (34.5)		29 (36.3)	21 (26.6)		
Necrosis				< 0.001*			0.096	
No	85 (53.5)	17 (23.6)	68 (78.2)		48 (60.0)	37 (46.8)		
Yes	74 (46.5)	55 (76.4)	19 (21.8)		32 (40.0)	42 (53.2)		
Vascular invasion				0.072			0.004*	
No	129 (81.1)	54 (75.0)	75 (86.2)		72 (90.0)	57 (72.2)		
Yes	30 (18.9)	18 (25.0)	12 (13.8)		8 (10.0)	22 (27.8)		
Preoperative therapy				0.538			0.113	
No	148 (93.1)	68 (94.4)	80 (92.0)		77 (96.3)	71 (89.8)		
Yes	11 (6.9)	4 (5.6)	7 (8.0)		3(3.7)	8 (10.2)		
Tumor type				< 0.001*			0.005*	
SCLC	94 (59.1)	48 (51.1)	46 (48.9)		50 (53.2)	44 (46.8)		
LCNEC	28 (17.6)	21 (75.0)	7 (25.0)		7 (25.0)	21 (75.0)		
TC	35 (22.0)	3 (8.6)	32 (91.4)		23 (65.7)	12 (34.3)		
AC	2 (1.3)	0 (0.0)	2 (100.0)		0 (0.0)	2 (100.0)		
Pathological grading				< 0.001*			0.100	
High	122 (76.7)	69 (95.8)	53 (60.9)		57 (71.2)	65 (82.3)		
Low	37 (23.3)	3 (4.2)	34 (39.1)		23 (28.8)	14 (17.7)		
Lymph node metastasis				0.170			0.005*	13 (8.2)
No	83 (56.8)	34 (50.7)	49 (62.8)		33 (45.2)	50 (68.5)		
Yes	63 (43.2)	33 (49.3)	30 (37.2)		40 (54.8)	23 (31.5)		
Clinical Staging				0.314			0.007*	15 (9.4)
I	70 (48.6)	29 (41.4)	41 (58.6)		27 (38.6)	43 (61.4)		
II	27 (18.8)	10 (37.0)	17 (63.0)		14 (51.9)	13 (48.1)		
III	47 (32.6)	25 (53.2)	22 (46.8)		32 68.1)	15 (31.9)		

Abbreviation: NA not available
*stands for the value of $p < 0.05$

Association between PD-L1 expression and clinicopathologic parameters

Associations between PD-L1 and clinical parameters in patients with PNETs are described in Table 2. The expression of PD-L1 was significantly associated with the presence of tumor necrosis ($p < 0.001$), high pathologic grade ($p < 0.001$), and histologic type (particularly for LCNEC) ($p < 0.001$). There was no significant association between PD-L1 and age ($p = 0.241$), gender ($p = 0.365$), prior neo-adjuvant therapy ($p = 0.538$), vascular invasion ($p = 0.072$), lymph node metastasis ($p = 0.170$), or clinical staging ($p = 0.314$). The pattern of PD-L1 expression was reclassified as tumor-positive and stroma-positive. Statistical correlations between tumor cell or immune cell and clinical parameters are present in Table 3. The PD-L1 positive expression in immune cells was associated with tumor

Table 3 The expression patterns of PD-L1 to clinicopathologic parameters in PNETs

	N(%)	PD-L1 expression Tumor^pos	Tumor^neg	p	Stroma^pos	Stroma^neg	p	NA
Total	159 (100.0)	26 (16.4)	133 (83.6)		63 (39.6)	96 (60.4)		
Age				0.593			0.497	
≤ 59.5	78 (49.1)	14 (53.8)	64 (48.1)		33 (52.4)	45 (46.9)		
>59.5	81 (50.9)	12 (46.2)	69 (51.9)		30 (47.6)	51 (53.1)		
Gender				0.142			0.527	
Male	109 (68.6)	21 (80.8)	88 (66.2)		45 (71.4)	64 (66.7)		
Female	50 (31.4)	5 (19.2)	45 (33.8)		18 (28.6)	32 (33.3)		
Necrosis				0.094			< 0.001*	
No	85 (53.5)	10 (38.5)	75 (56.4)		11 (17.5)	74 (77.1)		
Yes	74 (46.5)	16 (61.5)	58 (43.6)		52 (82.5)	22 (22.9)		
Vascular invasion				0.251			0.088	
No	129 (81.1)	19 (73.1)	110 (82.7)		47 (74.6)	82 (85.4)		
Yes	30 (18.9)	7 (26.9)	23 (17.3)		16 (25.4)	14 (14.6)		
Preoperative therapy				0.865			0.819	
No	148 (93.1)	24 (92.3)	124 (93.2)		59 (93.7)	89 (92.7)		
Yes	11 (6.9)	2 (7.7)	9 (6.8)		4 (6.3)	7 (7.3)		
Tumor type				0.066			< 0.001*	
SCLC	94 (59.1)	14 (14.9)	80 (85.1)		47 (50)	47 (50)		
LCNEC	28 (17.6)	9 (32.1)	19 (67.9)		16 (57.1)	12 (42.9)		
TC	35 (22.0)	3 (8.6)	32 (91.4)		0 (0.0)	35 (100.0)		
AC	2 (1.3)	0 (0.0)	2 (100.0)		0 (0.0)	2 (100.0)		
Pathological grading				0.122			< 0.001*	
High	122 (76.7)	23 (88.5)	99 (74.4)		63 (100.0)	59 (61.5)		
Low	37 (23.3)	3 (11.5)	34 (25.6)		0 (0.0)	37 (38.5)		
Lymph node metastasis				0.377			0.113	13 (8.2)
No	83 (52.2)	15 (65.2)	68 (55.3)		30 (49.2)	53 (62.4)		
Yes	63 (47.8)	8 (34.8)	55 (44.7)		31 (50.8)	32 (37.6)		
Clinical Staging				0.309			0.077	15 (9.4)
I	70 (48.6)	14 (63.6)	56 (45.9)		25 (43.1)	45 (52.3)		
II	27 (18.8)	3 (13.6)	24 (19.7)		8 (13.8)	19 (22.1)		
III	47 (32.6)	5 (22.7)	42 (34.4)		25 (43.1)	22 (25.6)		
CD8 density/mm² in stroma				0.002*			0.005*	
≤ 264.6/mm²	80 (50.3)	6 (23.1)	74 (55.6)		23 (36.5)	57 (59.4)		
>264.6/mm²	79 (49.7)	20 (76.9)	59 (44.4)		40 (63.5)	39 (40.6)		

Abbreviation: NA not available
*stands for the value of $p < 0.05$

necrosis ($p < 0.001$), high pathologic grade ($p < 0.001$), and histologic type (particularly for LCNEC) ($p < 0.001$).

Correlations among CD8+ T cell infiltration and clinicopathologic parameters

CD8+ TILs grading was subdivided into two groups based on the median CD8+ T cell density within stroma ($264.6/mm^2$) in PNETs (Table 2). Higher CD8+ T cell density ($> 264.6/mm^2$) was associated with the absence of vascular invasion ($p = 0.004$), histologic type (particularly for AC) ($p = 0.005$), negative lymph node metastasis ($p = 0.005$), and lower clinical staging ($p = 0.007$). No correlation was observed between CD8+ TILs and age, gender, necrosis or neoadjuvant therapy.

PD-L1 expression was positively correlated with CD8+ TIL expression within stroma. Figure 1 presents the patterns of PD-L1 expression and CD8+ T cell infiltration in high-grade and low-grade malignancies.

Association of PD-L1 expression and CD8+ TILs with OS and PFS

Univariate survival analysis showed a trend toward an association between positive expression of PD-L1 in patients with PNETs and decreased OS ($p = 0.158$) and PFS ($p = 0.315$). However, this trend did not reach the level of statistical significance. Similarly, expression of PD-L1 on tumor cells showed a related trend toward poorer OS ($p = 0.459$) and PFS ($p = 0.708$) (Fig. 2).

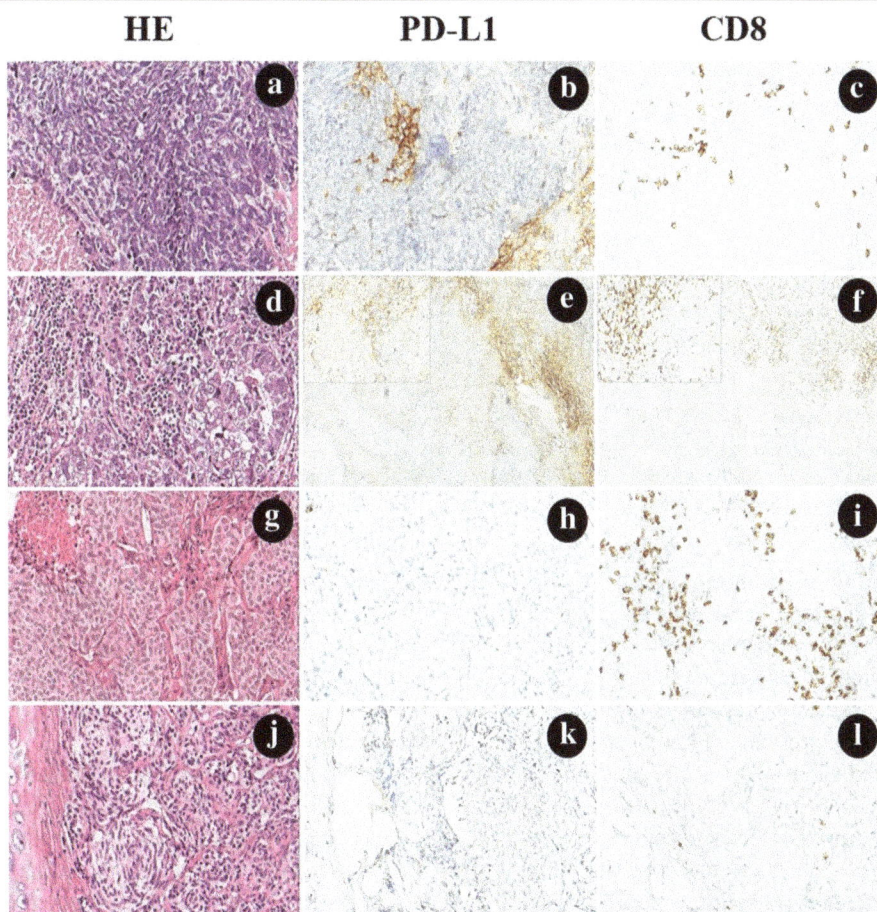

Fig. 1 Hemotoxylin and eosin (H&E), PD-L1 and CD8 stains, each performed on histologic sections of small cell lung cancer (**a-c**), large cell neuroendocrine carcinoma (**d-f**), atypical carcinoid (**g-i**) and typical carcinoid (**j-l**). **a** Small cell lung cancer was showing a scant cytoplasm, fine nuclear chromatin, absent or inconspicuous nucleoli, extensive necrosis. **b** PD-L1 was moderately expressed on the membrane of stromal immune cells in the desmoplastic stroma between clusters of tumor cells. **c** CD8+ TILs were observed in the stroma, while the intratumoral pattern of CD8 expression was not common. **d** Large cell neuroendocrine carcinoma with prominent nucleoli and abundant eosinophilic cytoplasm, necrosis was not shown. **e, f** PD-L1 was positively expressed on the membrane and cytoplasm of the immune cells, and a large number of CD8+ TILs could also be observed at the borderline (the 200× magnification for PD-L1 and CD8 was shown in the upper left, respectively). **g** Atypical carcinoid with vascularized stroma, focal necrosis and 6 mitosis/2 mm². **h, i** PD-L1 was negative expression either in tumor cells or stromal cells, while CD8+ TILs were exhibited in the interface of tumor and stroma. **j** Typical carcinoid with organoid growth pattern with intervening vascular stroma. **k, l** No PD-L1 can be detected, and only several CD8+ TILs could be found in the stroma. (The original magnification of **e-f** was 100×, magnification for remaining cases were 200×)

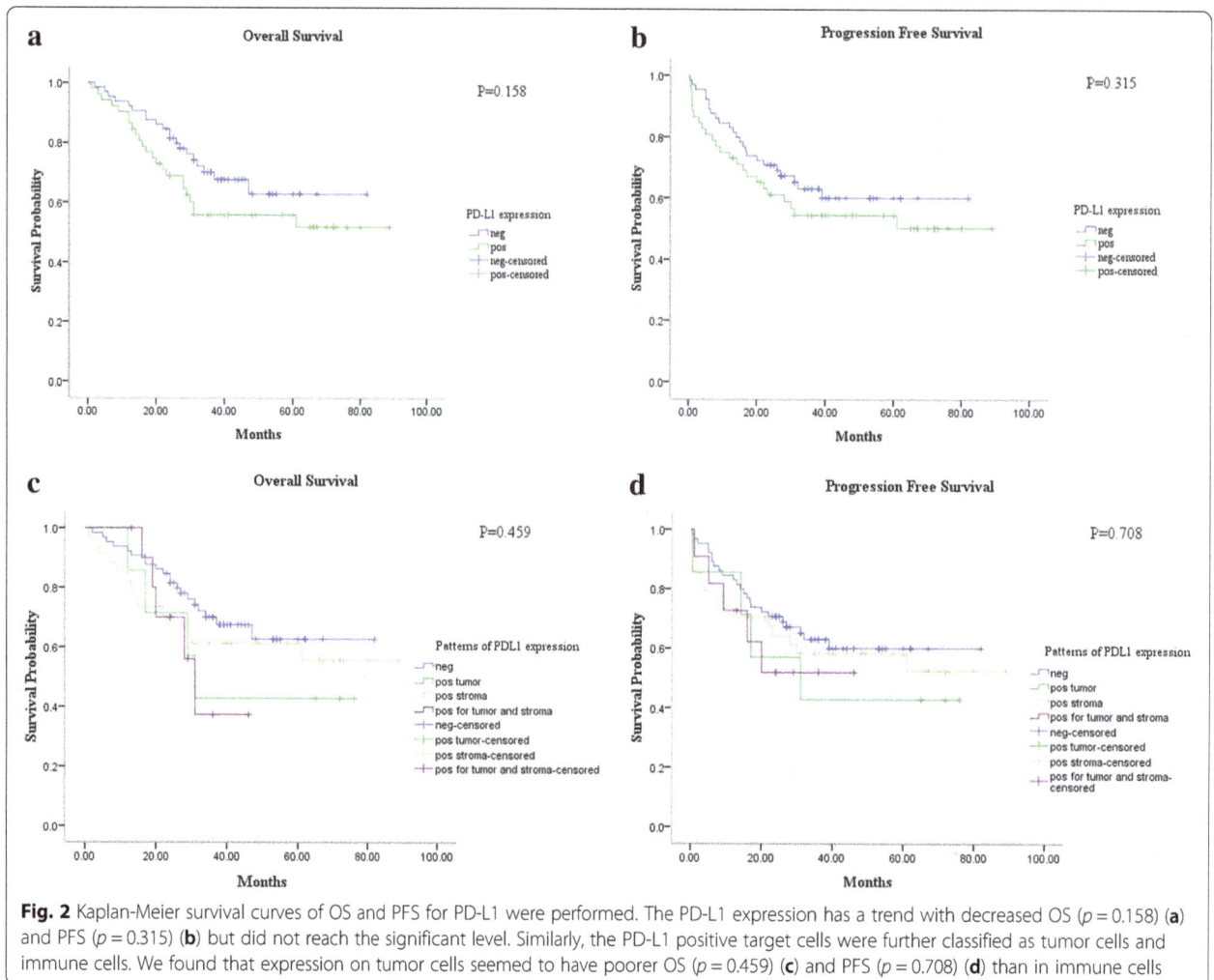

Fig. 2 Kaplan-Meier survival curves of OS and PFS for PD-L1 were performed. The PD-L1 expression has a trend with decreased OS ($p = 0.158$) (**a**) and PFS ($p = 0.315$) (**b**) but did not reach the significant level. Similarly, the PD-L1 positive target cells were further classified as tumor cells and immune cells. We found that expression on tumor cells seemed to have poorer OS ($p = 0.459$) (**c**) and PFS ($p = 0.708$) (**d**) than in immune cells

We also evaluated the relationship of CD8+ TIL density in stromal and intratumoral areas with OS and PFS. Immune stromal CD8+ T cell density was classified as low ($\leq264.6/mm^2$) or high ($>264.6/mm^2$). Intratumoral CD8+ T cell density was also subdivided as low ($\leq24.5/mm^2$) or high ($>24.5/mm^2$). The presence of high CD8+ TIL density in stroma proved to be a better prognostic factor for improved OS ($p = 0.000$) and PFS ($p = 0.000$). No correlation between intratumoral CD8+ T cell density and OS ($p = 0.417$) or PFS ($p = 0.387$) was observed (Fig. 3).

For multivariate analysis, the Cox proportional hazards model was performed and included age, gender, necrosis, vascular invasion, lymph node metastasis, clinical staging, PD-L1 expression and CD8+ TILs in the stroma. The results revealed that expression of PD-L1 was not an independent prognostic factor for OS (Hazard ratio [HR] = 0.707; 95% confidence interval [CI], 0.367–1.364; $p = 0.301$) or PFS (Hazard ratio [HR] = 0.921; 95% confidence interval [CI], 0.420–2.021; $p = 0.838$). In contrast, the presence of high CD8+ TIL density in stroma was an independent prognostic factor for improved OS (Hazard ratio

[HR] = 2.770; 95% confidence interval [CI], 1.294–5.930; $p = 0.009$) and PFS (Hazard ratio [HR] = 3.011; 95% confidence interval [CI], 1.492–6.079; $p = 0.002$).

Discussion

In this study, we investigated the associations between PD-L1 and other clinicopathologic characteristics. Our examination of PNETs showed that expression of PD-L1 was significantly associated with high pathologic grade, advanced histologic type and presence of tumor necrosis. These results reflect the increase in total mutation frequency associated with the malignancy of tumor type. High-grade SCLC and LCNEC have a higher somatic mutation rate (> 7 per million base pairs) than the lung carcinoids (0.4 per million base pairs) [15]. Thus, the high-grade carcinoma might secret stronger neoantigens to generate higher immunogenicity to recruit more cytotoxic T lymphocytes to kill non-self-components. Then, PD-L1, which is expressed by tumor cells, is increased to resist the immune protection function of CD8+ TILs.

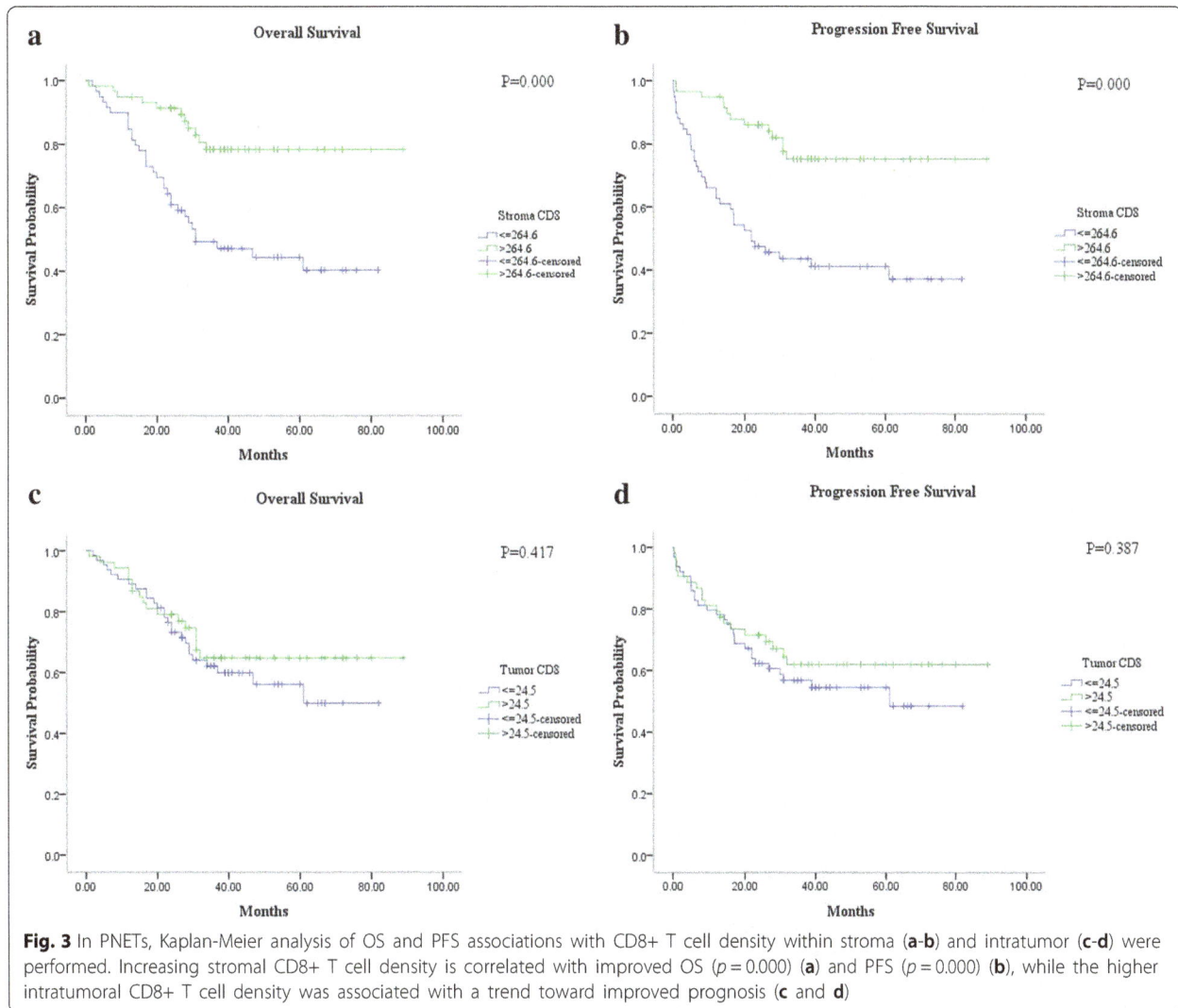

Fig. 3 In PNETs, Kaplan-Meier analysis of OS and PFS associations with CD8+ T cell density within stroma (**a**-**b**) and intratumor (**c**-**d**) were performed. Increasing stromal CD8+ T cell density is correlated with improved OS ($p = 0.000$) (**a**) and PFS ($p = 0.000$) (**b**), while the higher intratumoral CD8+ T cell density was associated with a trend toward improved prognosis (**c** and **d**)

Inflammatory cytokines, particularly interferon gamma (INF-r), can up-regulate PD-L1 expression in various cell types including tumors. In both melanoma and squamous cell carcinoma of head and neck (HNSCC), INF-r has been highlighted as a major cytokine driving PD-L1 expression [16, 17]. This indicates that PD-L1 is upregulated in tumor cells in response to secretion of INF by CD8+ T cells, as an adaptive immune-resistance mechanism that suppresses local effector T-cell function [18–20]. The results detailed above indicate that positive expression of PD-L1, especially in tumor cells, is associated with a trend toward decreased OS and PFS of PNETs. Such a trend is consistent with results previously published [21]. Moreover, we found that PD-L1 expression was predominantly present at the tumor-stroma margin, in the presence of accumulated stromal CD8+ T cells. This indicates that the PD-L1 expression manifests as a result of forces favoring tumor progression, while stromal CD8+ T cell infiltration manifests as a result of the body's efforts at immune protection [17].

We also found that the higher CD8+ T cell density, the higher it was significantly associated with the absence of vascular invasion, negative lymph node metastasis and lower clinical staging. These findings may partially explain why stromal presence of CD8+ T cell infiltration was an independent factor for favorable OS and PFS in neuroendocrine carcinomas of the lung.

Notably, we detected PD-L1 expression in 45.3% (72/159) of neuroendocrine carcinoma of the lung. Our result was inconsistent with the study conducted by Schultheis et al. [13]. In that study, they found that tumor-infiltrating macrophages (TIMs) and tumor-infiltrating lymphocytes (TILs) rather than tumor cells showed PD-L1 protein expression. Additionally, the positive rate of PD-L1 in our study was lower than the result previously reported [21]. The inconsistent results can be attributed to the different antibodies and different criteria of scoring used in different studies.

Nonetheless, our study reports several important findings that may have implications for targeting PD-L1 immunotherapy in PNETs. First, we proved that CD8+ T cell infiltration was positively correlated with PD-L1 expression, which indicates an adaptive immune resistance-type mechanism that can also be observed in PNETS. Second, while the PD-L1 expression was observed in 16.4% of the tumor cells, 39.6% cases of PNETs showed PD-L1 expression in the immune cells at the invasive stroma-tumor margin. Though it has increasingly been recognized that PD-L1 expression on immune cells at the invasive margin represents evidence of an immune resistance mechanism, in our study, the PD-L1 expression on tumor cells was of great importance to predict the prognosis [18, 22]. Third, we showed a trend toward the correlation between expression of PD-L1 and decreased OS and PFS. This may provide a theoretical basis for anti-PD-L1 immunotherapy in PNETs. Moreover, increased CD8+ TILs density in stroma was an independent prognostic factor for improved OS and PFS. When sufficient T cells present in the tumor induce an adaptive expression of PD-L1, the PD-L1+/CD8+ patients may be most likely to respond to anti-PD-1/PD-L1 therapy. Therefore, there is a need for quantitative assessment of TIL and PD-L1 presence in resected samples to produce the desired predictive information [23].

Use of traditional treatments such as chemotherapy and radiotherapy may lead to the emergence of tumor-associated antigens, which was released from the apoptotic tumor cells [24]. If the initial traditional therapy can effectively present the tumor cells as foreign tumor antigens, it is obvious that subsequent immunotherapy is possible to be a favorable endeavor [25]. Recent studies have reported that the presence of TILs may predict a positive response to neoadjuvant chemotherapy [26]. We, therefore, sought to select patients who were more available for the immunotherapy, to maximize the benefit derived from the chemotherapy/radiotherapy-immunotherapy combined strategies.

Though we believe our study illustrates the value of PD-L1 as a potential prognostic marker, there were some limitations. First, this study involved a relatively small number of patients. This small sample size may have resulted in selection bias. Second, mature survival information was limited as the follow-up duration in our study was not long enough to fully evaluate 5-year survival rates.

Conclusion

We found that PD-L1 was expressed in half of the PNETs and associated with necrosis, high pathologic grade and advanced histologic type. PD-L1 expression was observed primarily in immune stromal cells but showed no associations with OS or PFS. In contrast, higher levels of CD8+ TILs observed in stroma were associated with the absence of vascular invasion, negative lymph node metastasis,

lower clinical staging and was demonstrated to be an independent factor for improved OS and PFS. Our results may highlight a promising method for the selection of patients with PNETs who are most likely to benefit from immunotherapy in the future.

Abbreviations

AC: Atypical carcinoid; APCs: Antigen-presenting cells; CTLs: Cytotoxic lymphocytes; FFPE: Formalin-fixed paraffin-embedded; HNSCC: Squamous cell carcinoma of head and neck; IHC: Immunohistochemistry; INF-r: Inteferon gamma; LCNEC: Large cell neuroendocrine carcinoma; mAbs: Monoclonal antibodies; OS: Overall survival; PD-L1: Programmed death-ligand 1; PFS: Progression free survival; PNETs: Pulmonary neuroendocrine tumors; SCLC: Small cell lung carcinoma; TC: Typical carcinoid; TILs: Tumor-infiltrating lymphocytes; TIMs: Tumor-infiltrating macrophages

Funding

This study was supported by the Beijing Municipal Science and Technology Commission NOVA program (NO.2010 B033), the Beijing Municipal Science and Technology Commission Capital Characteristic Clinical Application Research (No.Z141107002514077), the National Nature Science Foundation of China (No.61501039), and grants from the funding of the Beijing Cancer Hospital (approval #:13-11).

Authors' contributions

DML and ZWL conceived and designed the experiments. HYW, ZWL, BD, XY, XZH and LJ performed the experiments. HYW, ZWL, BD, WS and RPL analyzed the data. BD and LXZ contributed the materials/analysis tools for the study. HYW and ZWL wrote the paper. All authors have read and approved the final manuscript.

Competing interests

The authors declare that they have no competing interests.

Author details

[1]Key Laboratory of Carcinogenesis and Translational Research (Ministry of Education), Department of Pathology, Peking University Cancer Hospital & Institute, No. 52 Fucheng Road, Haidian District, Beijing 100142, People's Republic of China. [2]Key Laboratory of Carcinogenesis and Translational Research (Ministry of Education), Department of Central Laboratory, Peking University Cancer Hospital & Institute, Beijing 100142, People's Republic of China. [3]Beijing Institute of Graphic Communication, Beijing 102600, People's Republic of China.

References

1. Travis WD. Advances in neuroendocrine lung tumors. Ann Oncol. 2010; 21(Suppl 7):vii65–71.
2. Rekhtman N. Neuroendocrine tumors of the lung: an update. Arch Pathol Lab Med. 2010;134:1628–38.
3. Bertino EM, Confer PD, Colonna JE, Ross P, Otterson GA. Pulmonary neuroendocrine/carcinoid tumors: a review article. Cancer. 2009;115: 4434–41.

4. Metro G, Duranti S, Fischer MJ, Cappuzzo F, Crino L. Emerging drugs for small cell lung cancer - an update. Expert Opin Emerg Drugs. 2012;17:31–6.
5. Ohaegbulam KC, Assal A, Lazar-Molnar E, Yao Y, Zang X. Human cancer immunotherapy with antibodies to the PD-1 and PD-L1 pathway. Trends Mol Med. 2015;21:24–33.
6. Herbst RS, Soria JC, Kowanetz M, et al. Predictive correlates of response to the anti-PD-L1 antibody MPDL3280A in cancer patients. Nature. 2014;515:563–7.
7. Khoja L, Kibiro M, Metser U, et al. Patterns of response to anti-PD-1 treatment: an exploratory comparison of four radiological response criteria and associations with overall survival in metastatic melanoma patients. Br J Cancer. 2016;115:1186–92.
8. Hamid O, Robert C, Daud A, et al. Safety and tumor responses with lambrolizumab (anti-PD-1) in melanoma. N Engl J Med. 2013;369:134–44.
9. Ramos-Esquivel A, van der Laat A, Rojas-Vigott R, Juarez M, Corrales-Rodriguez L. Anti-PD-1/anti-PD-L1 immunotherapy versus docetaxel for previously treated advanced non-small cell lung cancer: a systematic review and meta-analysis of randomised clinical trials. ESMO Open. 2017;2:e000236.
10. Powles T, Eder JP, Fine GD, et al. MPDL3280A (anti-PD-L1) treatment leads to clinical activity in metastatic bladder cancer. Nature. 2014;515:558–62.
11. Domagala-Kulawik J. The role of the immune system in non-small cell lung carcinoma and potential for therapeutic intervention. Transl Lung Cancer Res. 2015;4:177–90.
12. Aerts JG, Hegmans JP. Tumor-specific cytotoxic T cells are crucial for efficacy of immunomodulatory antibodies in patients with lung cancer. Cancer Res. 2013;73:2381–8.
13. Schultheis AM, Scheel AH, Ozretic L, et al. PD-L1 expression in small cell neuroendocrine carcinomas. Eur J Cancer. 2015;51:421–6.
14. Thompson ED, Zahurak M, Murphy A, et al. Patterns of PD-L1 expression and CD8 T cell infiltration in gastric adenocarcinomas and associated immune stroma. Gut. 2017;66:794–801.
15. Vollbrecht C, Werner R, Walter RF, et al. Mutational analysis of pulmonary tumours with neuroendocrine features using targeted massive parallel sequencing: a comparison of a neglected tumour group. Br J Cancer. 2015; 113:1704–11.
16. Lyford-Pike S, Peng S, Young GD, et al. Evidence for a role of the PD-1: PD-L1 pathway in immune resistance of HPV-associated head and neck squamous cell carcinoma. Cancer Res. 2013;73:1733–41.
17. Taube JM, Anders RA, Young GD, et al. Colocalization of inflammatory response with B7-h1 expression in human melanocytic lesions supports an adaptive resistance mechanism of immune escape. Sci Transl Med. 2012;4: 127ra137.
18. Tumeh PC, Harview CL, Yearley JH, et al. PD-1 blockade induces responses by inhibiting adaptive immune resistance. Nature. 2014;515:568–71.
19. Taube JM, Young GD, McMiller TL, et al. Differential expression of immune-regulatory genes associated with PD-L1 display in melanoma: implications for PD-1 pathway blockade. Clin Cancer Res. 2015;21:3969–76.
20. Pardoll DM. The blockade of immune checkpoints in cancer immunotherapy. Nat Rev Cancer. 2012;12:252–64.
21. Fan Y, Ma K, Wang C, et al. Prognostic value of PD-L1 and PD-1 expression in pulmonary neuroendocrine tumors. Onco Targets Ther. 2016;9:6075–82.
22. Topalian SL, Hodi FS, Brahmer JR, et al. Safety, activity, and immune correlates of anti-PD-1 antibody in cancer. N Engl J Med. 2012;366:2443–54.
23. Teng MW, Ngiow SF, Ribas A, Smyth MJ. Classifying cancers based on T-cell infiltration and PD-L1. Cancer Res. 2015;75:2139–45.
24. Twyman-Saint Victor C, Rech AJ, Maity A, et al. Radiation and dual checkpoint blockade activate non-redundant immune mechanisms in cancer. Nature. 2015;520:373–7.
25. Dushyanthen S, Beavis PA, Savas P, et al. Relevance of tumor-infiltrating lymphocytes in breast cancer. BMC Med. 2015;13:202.
26. Yamaguchi R, Tanaka M, Yano A, et al. Tumor-infiltrating lymphocytes are important pathologic predictors for neoadjuvant chemotherapy in patients with breast cancer. Hum Pathol. 2012;43:1688–94.

16

Composite intestinal adenoma-microcarcinoid in the colon and rectum: a case series and historical review

Mi-Jung Kim[1], Eun-Jung Lee[2], Do Sun Kim[2], Doo Han Lee[2], Eui Gon Youk[2] and Hyun-Jung Kim[3*]

Abstract

Background: Composite intestinal adenoma-microcarcinoid (CIAM) is a rare colorectal lesion that mostly comprises a conventional adenomatous component with a minute proportion of neuroendocrine (NE) component. Although microcarcinoids are well-recognized in the setting of chronic inflammatory disorders of the gastrointestinal tract, large intestinal microcarcinoids associated with intestinal adenoma are exceedingly rare and their clinicopathologic characteristics are yet to be elucidated. This study was performed to clarify their clinicopathologic characteristics and to review the relevant literature.

Methods: In total, 24 cases of CIAM in which tumors were excised endoscopically ($n = 22$) or surgically ($n = 2$) were retrieved from the Department of Pathology, Daehang Hospital. We analyzed their clinicopathologic characteristics and performed immunohistochemical staining for NE markers to determine their endocrine nature.

Results: CIAM usually developed in middle-aged and elderly patients, with a mean age of 62.0 years (range, 44–81 years). Thirteen patients were men and 11 were women, indicating a nearly equal sex ratio. Unlike classic carcinoid tumors, CIAMs occurred mostly in the colon (83.3% of cases), particularly in the proximal colon. Histologically, the microcarcinoid component consisted of low-grade NE cells arranged in small nests, glands or cords interspersed with glandular elements or less frequently resembled squamous morules. There was no expansile nodular or organoid growth pattern, which is typical of carcinoid tumors. The microcarcinoids were 1–20 mm in size (mean size, 4.7 mm) and were mostly situated in the basal lamina propria with no submucosal layer involvement; none showed desmoplastic reaction or increased proliferative activity. Follow-up data (mean, 23.1 months) were available for 18 patients; all patients are alive and well.

Conclusions: To the best of our knowledge, ours is the largest series of patients with CIAM in the English-language literature. Microcarcinoids found in CIAMs appear to show favorable clinical outcomes regardless of their size, likely due to the absence of submucosal extension and/or increased proliferative activity. We recommend avoiding additional radical surgeries in patients who have endoscopically undergone complete CIAM excision unless they exhibit ominous histologic features such as submucosal extension or increased proliferative activity.

Keywords: Composite intestinal adenoma, Microcarcinoid, Neuroendocrine tumor, Colorectal lesions

* Correspondence: hjkim@paik.ac.kr
[3]Department of Pathology, University of Inje College of Medicine, Sanggye
Paik hospital, Dongil-ro 1342, Nowon-gu, Seoul, Republic of Korea
Full list of author information is available at the end of the article

Background

Composite intestinal adenoma-microcarcinoid (CIAM) is a rare colorectal lesion that comprises conventional adenomatous components intermingled with smaller microcarcinoids [1]. Microcarcinoids refer to microscopic aggregates of monotonous cells with neuroendocrine (NE) features that do not form grossly evident masses; they have been well-described in the setting of chronic inflammatory disorders of the gastrointestinal tract, particularly the stomach [2, 3]. Large intestinal microcarcinoids are extremely rare compared to gastric lesions, and have been observed almost exclusively in patients with ulcerative colitis [4–6].

CIAM appears to be a much rarer condition than microcarcinoids that occur in the setting of ulcerative colitis; their NE cells are well-differentiated (WD) and are situated within the basal lamina propria [1, 7, 8]. They have been reported sporadically since they were first described by Pulitzer et al. [1, 7–9]. However, the nature and clinical behavior of CIAMs remain poorly understood. To attain a clearer understanding of this tumor type, we analyzed the clinicopathologic features of 24 new cases of CIAM and also reviewed previous reports of patients with this disease [1, 7–10].

Methods

Study sample and histologic evaluation

Twenty-four cases of CIAM were retrieved from the Department of Pathology, Daehang Hospital, between March 2011 and March 2017. Ten were retrospectively collected from pathological data files of patients treated between March 2011 and December 2013, while 14 were identified prospectively between January 2014 and March 2017. All lesions were completely excised either endoscopically (n = 22) or surgically (n = 2); 1 of the latter lesions was removed by right hemicolectomy because of the presence of a synchronous huge adenoma, and the other was removed via low anterior resection because the physician suspected a malignancy. None of the patients had any history of inflammatory bowel disease (IBD) or familial adenomatous polyposis (FAP).

All specimens were routinely processed, stained with hematoxylin and eosin, and evaluated by a gastrointestinal pathology specialist (M.J.K.). The degree of dysplasia in the epithelial component was assessed according to the architectural complexity, extent of nuclear stratification, and severity of abnormal nuclear morphology, and was classified into low-grade dysplasia (LGD) or high-grade dysplasia (HGD) [11]. Tumors exhibiting lamina propria invasion with no submucosal extension were diagnosed as intramucosal carcinomas.

The sizes of the polyps were measured by the pathologist, while the anatomical locations were identified and classified as the proximal colon (up to the splenic flexure) versus the distal colon/rectum.

The study was performed according to the Declaration of Helsinki, and was approved by the institutional review board at Daehang Hospital (approval number DH17–001). Obtaining additional informed consent for the use of patient samples was not required, as the specimens were coded to protect patient confidentiality.

Patients were assessed for clinicopathologic characteristics including age, sex, and pathology reports. Follow-up data (mean, 23.1 months) were available for 18 patients who underwent endoscopic procedures (n = 17) or surgery (n = 1) between March 2011 and May 2016. Two patients were lost to follow-up. The remaining samples (n = 6) were collected subsequently from patients who had not yet undergone routinely scheduled follow-up visits.

Immunohistochemical staining

Immunohistochemistry was manually performed by using formalin-fixed, paraffin-embedded blocks. Sections (3 μm) were cut, deparaffinized in xylene, and dehydrated in increasing concentrations of ethanol. Immunohistochemical staining was performed with anti-synaptophysin (clone Z66, 1:100 dilution; Invitrogen, Melbourne, Australia), anti-chromogranin (clone NS55, 1:100 dilution; Invitrogen), and mouse monoclonal anti-Ki-67 (clone 7B11, 1:100 dilution; Invitrogen) after routine microwave antigen retrieval. Negative control samples underwent the same procedure with the omission of the primary antibody. Slides were counterstained with Mayer's hematoxylin.

Immunoreactivity for synaptophysin and chromogranin was evaluated as positive or negative. Negative protein expression was defined as the complete absence of cytoplasmic staining in the microcarcinoid component in the presence of positive labeling in non-neoplastic internal control cells, while the opposite staining pattern was considered positive expression. Ki-67 immunostaining was performed to determine the proliferative activity and grade of the microcarcinoid NE cells. Nuclear immunostaining at known proliferative locations, such as germinal centers and the basal half of the crypt epithelium, was used as an internal positive control for each sample.

Statistical analysis

Data analyses were performed using SPSS version 21.0 (SPSS Inc., Chicago, IL, USA). Student's t-test was used to compare parametric distributions, while the χ^2 or Fisher's exact test was used for frequency distributions. A P-value <0.05 was considered statistically significant.

Results

Patient demographics and tumor characteristics

The patients' ages ranged between 44 and 81 years (mean, 62.0 years). Samples were obtained from 13 men and 11 women (the male to female ratio was 1.2:1). Among the 24 cases, the majority (n = 20; 83.3%) occurred in the colon, the remaining 4 were in the rectum. Sixteen of the 20 CIAMs occurring in the colon (80.0%) affected the proximal colon. The polyp sizes ranged from 5 to 127 mm (mean, 27.2 mm). Follow-up data were available for 18 patients, all of whom are alive and well. The results are summarized in Table 1.

Histologic findings and immunohistochemical staining results

The microcarcinoid component was most often located in the center of the polyp with no clear demarcation from the glandular component. The microcarcinoids were 1–20 mm in size (mean size, 4.7 mm) and were mostly situated in the basal lamina propria beneath the glandular component (Fig. 1a, b). Only 5 microcarcinoids were focally extended to the muscularis mucosae with no involvement of the submucosal layer, while 1 case involved both the upper and basal portions of the lamina propria.

Histologically, the NE cells within the microcarcinoid component were arranged in small nests or glands, irregular clusters, and cords with or without connections to the glandular component. Specifically 11 of 24 cases (45.8%) were connected to the glandular component (Fig. 1b). The glandular component was a conventional adenoma with LGD in most cases (86.4%) except for 2 intramucosal and 1 submucosal invasive carcinoma cases. The NE cells were sometimes scattered individually or else resembled

Table 1 Clinicopathologic features of the present study

Case	Age (yrs) / Sex	Location of polyp	Procedure	Polyp size (mm)	Histology of glandular component	Initial diagnosis	Size of micro-carcinoid (mm)	SYN	CHR
1	76/F	Ascending colon	ESD	18	IMAC, WD	IMAC, WD	2	+	+
2	68/M	Transverse colon	ESD	25	IMAC, WD	IMAC, WD	4	+	+
3	55/M	Splenic flexure	EMR	27	TA	TA with endocrine cell proliferation	3	+	+
4	65/F	Hepatic flexure	ESD	33	TA	TA	4	+	+
5	49/F	Sigmoid colon	EMR	18	TA	Composite TA and carcinoid tumor	5	+	–
6	74/F	Ascending colon	ESD	23	TVA, HGD	TVA, HGD, with microcarcinoid component	8	+	+
7	55/M	Ascending colon	EMR	10	TA	TA and microcarcinoid	2	+	+
8	47/F	Cecum	EMR	18	TVA	TVA and microcarcinoid	4	+	+
9	61/M	Hepatic flexure	RHC	17	TA	TA and microcarcinoid	2	+	+
10	68/M	Ascending colon	EMR	11	SIAC, WD	Adenocarcinoma, WD, with microcarcinoid component	5	+	+
11	59/M	Splenic flexure	Polypectomy	5	TA	TA and microcarcinoid	1	+	+
12	65/M	Rectum	ESD	20	TVA, HGD	TVA and microcarcinoid	2	+	–
13	78/M	Rectum	ESD	36	TVA, HGD	TVA and microcarcinoid	2	+	–
14	44/M	Sigmoid colon	ESD	17	TA, HGD	TA and microcarcinoid	3	+	+
15	56/F	Ascending colon	ESD	30	TA	TA and microcarcinoid	6	+	+
16	81/F	Rectosigmoid colon	EMR	11	TA	TA and microcarcinoid	2	+	–
17	57/F	Ascending colon	ESD	25	TA, HGD	TA and microcarcinoid	7	+	+
18	46/M	Ascending colon	Polypectomy	20	TVA	TVA and microcarcinoid	2	+	+
19	56/M	Hepatic flexure	Polypectomy	8	TA	TA and microcarcinoid	1	+	+
20	52/M	Rectum	ESD	127	TVA	TVA and microcarcinoid	4	+	–
21	73/M	Transverse colon	Polypectomy	12	TA	TA and microcarcinoid	4	+	+
22	78/F	Rectum	LAR	100	TVA, HGD	TVA and microcarcinoid	20	+	–
23	69/F	Ascending colon	ESD	28	TA	TA and microcarcinoid	13	+	+
24	57/F	Sigmoid colon	EMR	13	TA	TA and microcarcinoid	6	+	+

CHR chromogranin, *EMR* endoscopic mucosal resection, *ESD* endoscopic submucosal dissection, *F* female, *HGD* high-grade dysplasia, *IMAC* intramucosal adenocarcinoma, *LAR* low anterior resection, *M* male, *RHC* right hemicolectomy, *SIAC* submucosal invasive adenocarcinoma, *SYN* synaptophysin, *TA* tubular adenoma, *TVA* tubulovillous adenoma, *WD* well-differentiated

infiltrative glands or tumor budding; however, there was no desmoplastic reaction characterized by myofibroblastic proliferation (Fig. 2a, b). Expansile nodular growth patterns or interconnected trabecular and/or lobular structures were not observed in any of the cases. The NE cells had scant to abundant eosinophilic, granular cytoplasm and round central nuclei with stippled or dusty chromatin. Two cases showed endocrine cell aggregates resembling squamous morules or metaplasia (Fig. 3a, b). All microcarcinoids consisted of monotonous cells lacking significant nuclear atypia, mitotic activity, or necrosis; however, some cases showed mild nuclear atypia.

All cases were positive for synaptophysin; moreover, 18 (75.0%) expressed chromogranin-A, which was indicative of their endocrine differentiation (Figs. 1c, d, 2c, d, and 3c, d). The glandular component of the polyps did not show any generalized increase in the expression of NE markers. None of the samples exhibited an increase in the Ki-67 labeling index (all were less than 1%). The results are summarized in Table 1.

Discussion

Since first described by Pulitzer et al. in 2006, CIAMs have been recognized as a rare intestinal neoplasm consisting of intermingled adenomatous and WD NE components [1]. Unlike other mixed adenoneuroendocrine tumors of the large intestine in which the NE component occupies a substantial proportion of the tumor, the NE component of a CIAM occupies only a minute region of the polyp without disturbing the overall architecture [1, 11]. The NE component found in CIAM differs from classic colorectal neuroendocrine tumors (NETs) in that it does not form a visible nodule and is always accompanied by a glandular neoplasm occupying the majority of the polyp by definition [1]. Additionally, most microcarcinoids in CIAMs are reportedly located in the basal lamina propria, contrary to classic NETs in which the epicenters are located in the submucosa [1, 11]. Therefore, the NE component in CIAMs is always incidentally found during the pathologic examination of adenomatous polyps, while rectal NETs are discovered during routine rectal examinations or endoscopies as submucosal masses or due to the presence of clinical symptoms such as rectal bleeding, pain, or constipation [11]. The majority of colonic NETs are large, with average sizes of 4.9 cm; therefore, they are frequently symptomatic [11].

To date, reports of CIAMs have been sporadic. The largest study was conducted by Salaria et al., who investigated 11 prospectively collected cases over a 7-year period [1, 7–10]. However, their study was limited by the fact that most cases (*n* = 9, 81.8%) were obtained by external consultation; therefore, clinicopathologic data regarding polyp location, procedure type, and immunohistochemical staining results for NE markers were lacking. Another study of 7 CIAM cases by Lin et al. included 5 in the large intestine and 2 in the duodenum [7]. We excluded 2 duodenal cases from our literature review because our study includes CIAMs that occurred only in the colon and rectum. We also excluded 1 of Lin

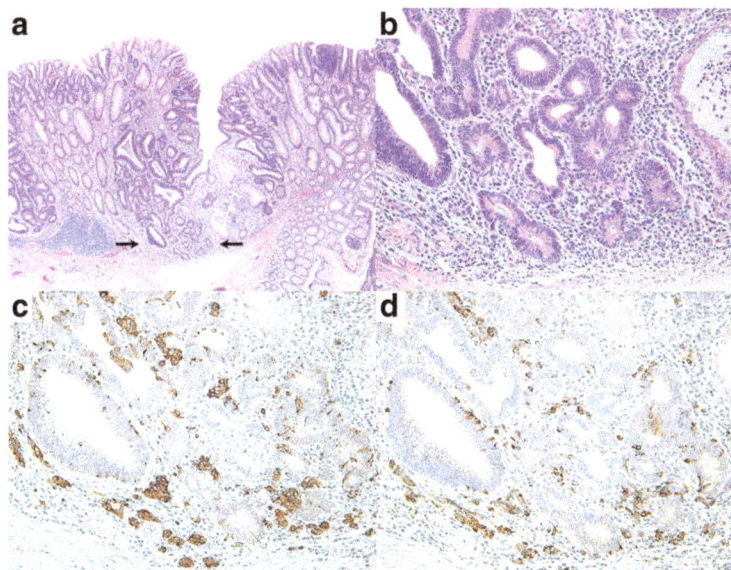

Fig. 1 Histological and immunohistochemical findings of composite intestinal adenoma-microcarcinoid. **a** Low power magnification shows adenomatous polyp with hardly recognizable microcarcinoid component (×40). Black arrows indicate microcarcinoid component. **b** High power magnification displays adenomatous glands and neuroendocrine cell nests in the lamina propria, which are connected to each other (×200). **c** Immunohistochemical staining for synaptophysin shows diffuse cytoplasmic reactivity in the microcarcinoid component (×200). **d** The microcarcinoid component is diffusely stained for chromogranin-A on immunostaining (×200)

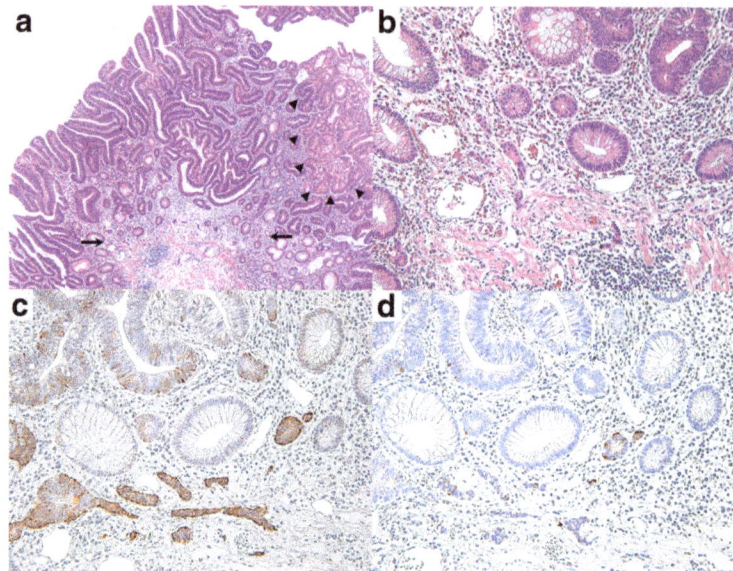

Fig. 2 Histological and immunohistochemical features of composite intestinal adenoma-microcarcinoid, mimicking invasive carcinoma. **a** Low power magnification shows adenomatous glands with minute microcarcinoid component (black arrows, ×40). Arrow heads indicate adjacent carcinomatous area. **b** High power magnification reveals endocrine cell nests with angulated shape and infiltrative growth pattern, harboring the potential for misdiagnosis as carcinoma invasion (×200). **c** Immunohistochemical staining for synaptophysin shows diffuse cytoplasmic reactivity in microcarcinoid component (×200). **d** The microcarcinoid component displays focal positivity for chromogranin-A on immunostaining (×200)

et al.'s remaining 5 cases because the lesion resembled a goblet cell carcinoid based on histologic photographs showing bland-looking glands with prominent goblet cells infiltrating the submucosa [7]. A goblet cell carcinoid is a distinct form of mixed adenoneuroendocrine tumors, which usually shows aggressive biologic behavior despite its bland-looking histology [11, 12]. We also excluded a study published by Estrella et al. because we could not clearly distinguish CIAM cases from adenoma/low-grade NETs [13]; in their study, the majority of

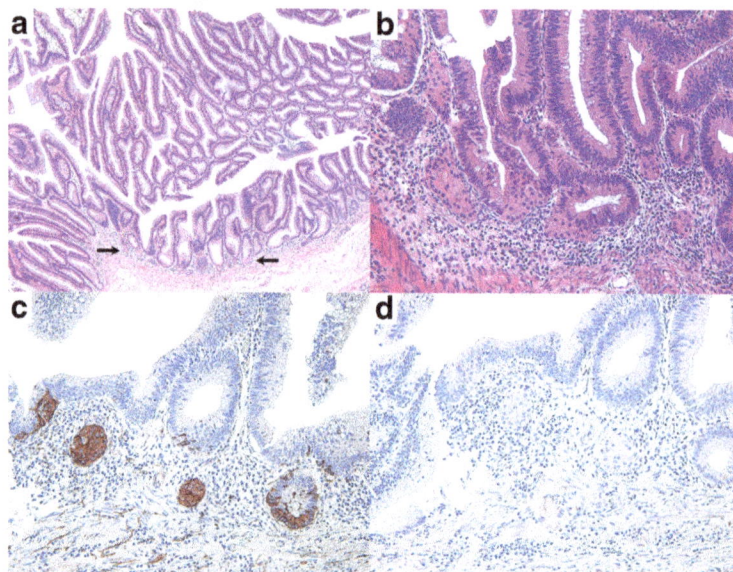

Fig. 3 Histological and immunohistochemical features of composite intestinal adenoma-microcarcinoid, mimicking adenoma with squamous metaplasia (squamous morules). **a** Low power magnification shows adenomatous glands with a few eosinophilic cell nests (black arrows) in basal lamina propria (×40). **b** High power magnification shows adenomatous glands and eosinophilic cell nests resembling squamous metaplasia (×200). **c** Immunohistochemical staining for synaptophysin shows diffuse cytoplasmic reactivity in the eosinophilic cells nests, supporting the neuroendocrine differentiation (×200). **d** The neuroendocrine component is negative for chromogranin-A on immunostaining (×200)

cases included in the adenoma/low-grade NET category are presumed to be mixed adenoma/classic NET because a substantial proportion of their cases (40%) invaded the submucosa. Additionally, the authors classified 4 cases arising from the duodenum under the same category as 19 colorectal cases, despite pre-existing evidence indicating that the anatomic site is one of the most important factors that affect the clinical behavior of NETs [11]. Four patients known to have FAP were also included in the adenoma/low-grade NET category, raising our concerns over the pathogenetic heterogeneity of their cases, which can potentially affect the analysis of clinical outcomes. After excluding the above-mentioned cases, we summarized the clinicopathologic data of 21 previously reported CIAMs in Table 2. In our present study, we enrolled and analyzed CIAM cases that only occurred in the colon and rectum, and did not include any patients with a history of IBD or FAP to minimize the genetic and pathogenetic heterogeneity of the investigated cases (Table 1).

Herein, we summarized the clinicopathologic findings of a total of 45 CIAM cases, including results from previous studies as well as our own. There were 24 men and 21 women, indicating a nearly equal sex ratio (male:female = 1.1:1). The patients' ages ranged from 28 to 82 years, with a mean age of 62.6 years. Notably, the mean age among our 24 patients (62.0 years) did not significantly differ from the 21 patients in the previous studies (63.1 years, $p = 0.767$). Approximately two-thirds ($n = 29$, 64.5%) of the microcarcinoid components were accompanied by adenoma with LGD (17 tubular, 11 tubulovillous, and 1 unspecified), 12 by adenoma with HGD (4 tubular, 8 tubulovillous), 2 by intramucosal carcinoma arising in tubulovillous adenoma, and 2 by submucosal invasive adenocarcinoma. Therefore, we suggest that the terminology of "CIAM" might be misleading because microcarcinoids can be associated with glandular lesions that exhibit various histologic degrees of dysplasia.

Contrary to classic NET, CIAMs tended to occur in the colon according to data from previous studies as well as ours, which indicated that most lesions (38 of 44, 86.4%) were located in the colon except for 6 (13.6%) that occurred in the rectum and 1 that had an unknown location. In particular, more than half of the polyps were located in the proximal colon (27 of 44 cases, 61.4%), with the most frequent site being the ascending colon (9 of 44 cases, 20.5%). The size of the polyps ranged from 5 to 127 mm, with a mean size of 23.8 mm. There was no significant difference in polyp size between our study and previous findings (27.2 mm vs. 19.6 mm, respectively; $p = 0.277$). The microcarcinoid component was confined to the mucosa with (22 of 40 cases) or without (18 of 40 cases) a connection to the glandular component. The mean size of the microcarcinoid component was 4.7 mm, and did not differ significantly in our

patients compared to those in previous studies (4.7 mm vs. 3.1 mm, respectively; $p = 0.201$).

In our study, all lesions were completely removed either by endoscopic procedures ($n = 22$) or surgical resection ($n = 2$), and no subsequent surgeries were required. This is inconsistent with the results of previous studies in which most patients underwent subsequent surgery ($n = 7$, 77.8%) because of incomplete or partial prior polypectomy ($n = 9$). Moreover, removal of the majority of samples (83.3%) by endoscopic mucosal resection (EMR, $n = 7$), endoscopic submucosal dissection (ESD, $n = 11$), and surgery ($n = 2$) in our study facilitated the procurement of well-oriented tissue sections perpendicular to the basal lamina and muscularis mucosae; this assisted us in collecting the largest series of CIAM samples. A microcarcinoid component cannot be detected in poorly-oriented tissue samples such as small polypectomy specimen because it is mainly located in the basal lamina propria. Nevertheless, the prevalence rate of CIAM appears to be extremely low based on our estimates. We prospectively collected 13 CIAM cases from among 40,939 patients who underwent endoscopic procedures including polypectomy, EMR, and ESD between January 2014 and March 2017.

So far, the natural history as well as the pathogenetic mechanism of colorectal microcarcinoids have not been fully elucidated because of their rarity, which in turn may partly be due to their under-recognition. As a result, microcarcinoids occurring in the colon and rectum have remained an ambiguous entity denoting small-sized NE lesions in many instances. According to the definition of microcarcinoid described by Pulitzer et al., most previously reported microcarcinoids occurring in ulcerative colitis patients appear to correspond to small-sized classic NETs [1]. As for the stomach, most enterochromaffin-like cell NETs arise in patients with chronic atrophic gastritis or multiple endocrine neoplasia type 1-Zollinger-Ellison syndrome through a sequence of hyperplasia-dysplasia-neoplasia, where growth patterns as well as endocrine cell sizes are known to be important for the classification of such lesions [2, 3, 11]. A gastric NE lesion is classified as a microcarcinoid when the nodule is greater than 0.5 mm but less than 5 mm in size, or if it invades the submucosa; lesions less than 0.5 mm and confined to the mucosa are designated as carcinoma in situ/dysplasia [11]. However, to our knowledge, such size-based criteria have not yet been defined in colorectal microcarcinoids. Based on our findings, the clinical outcomes of colorectal microcarcinoids appear to be quite favorable regardless of their sizes, likely because none of the patients showed submucosal invasion and/or increased proliferative activity. Considering that none of the 45 CIAM patients showed recurrence or metastasis after endoscopic or surgical treatment, even in lesions larger than or equal to 5 mm

Table 2 Clinicopathologic features of the previous studies

Case	Reference	Age (yrs) / Sex	Location of polyp	Procedure	Polyp size (mm)	Histology of glandular component	Initial diagnosis	Size of micro-carcinoid (mm)	SYN	CHR
1	Lyda et al., 1988 [10]	80/M	Ascending colon	Polypectomy followed by RHC	30	TVA, HGD	TVA and carcinoid tumor	NS	+	NS
2	Pulitzer et al., 2006 [1]	77/F	Cecum	Polypectomy followed by RHC	<10	TA, HGD	TA with HGD and endocrine neoplasia of UMP	NS	+	+
3	Pulitzer et al., 2006 [1]	77/M	Cecum	Polypectomy	13	TA	TA with squamous metaplasia	NS	+	–
4	Pulitzer et al., 2006 [1]	77/F	Cecum	Polypectomy followed by RHC	20	SIAC	TVA, HGD	NS	+	+
5	Pulitzer et al., 2006 [1]	62/F	Descending colon	Polypectomy	5	TA	TA with microcarcinoid	NS	+	+
6	Lin et al., 2012 [7]	51/M	Rectum	Polypectomy followed by proctosigmoidectomy	20	TVA	TVA with microcarcinoid	1	+	+
7	Lin et al., 2012 [7]	59/M	Rectum	Polypectomy followed by proctosigmoidectomy	13	Adenoma	Adenocarcinoma	1	+	+
8	Lin et al., 2012 [7]	66/F	Cecum	Polypectomy followed by RHC	15	TA	TA and microcarcinoid	1	NS	NS
9	Lin et al., 2012 [7]	56/M	Sigmoid colon	Polypectomy followed by transanal excision	25	TVA	TVA and microcarcinoid	1	NS	NS
10	Salaria et al., 2013 [8]	55/M	Right colon	NS	53	TA	Suspicion of invasive carcinoma	2	+	NS
11	Salaria et al., 2013 [8]	54/F	Transverse colon	NS	14	TA, HGD	TA, HGD	1	NS	NS
12	Salaria et al., 2013 [8]	81/F	Left colon	NS	12	TVA, HGD	TVA, HGD	3	+	–
13	Salaria et al., 2013 [8]	28/F	Right colon	NS	34	TVA, HGD	TVA, HGD, with squamous morules	7	+	–
14	Salaria et al., 2013 [8]	82/M	Right colon	NS	15	TVA	Suspicion of invasive carcinoma	5	+	–
15	Salaria et al., 2013 [8]	72/F	NS	NS	15	TVA	NS	5	NS	NS
16	Salaria et al., 2013 [8]	60/F	Right colon	NS	7	TVA, HGD	TVA, HGD	3	–	–
17	Salaria et al., 2013 [8]	55/M	Left colon	NS	12	TA	TA with squamous morules	7	NS	NS
18	Salaria et al., 2013 [8]	48/M	Left colon	NS	15	TVA	TVA with squamous morules	4	+	–
19	Salaria et al., 2013 [8]	62/M	Left colon	NS	25	TVA	TVA with squamous morules	4	NS	NS
20	Salaria et al., 2013 [8]	51/F	Left colon	NS	30	TVA	TVA with squamous morules	2	NS	–
21	Thosani et al., 2014 [9]	73/M	Hepatic flexure	NS	NS	TVA	NS	NS	+	–

CHR chromogranin, F female, HGD high-grade dysplasia, M male, NS not specified, RHC right hemicolectomy SIAC submucosal invasive adenocarcinoma, SYN synaptophysin, TA tubular adenoma, TVA tubulovillous adenoma, UMP uncertain malignant potential, WD well-differentiated

(8 of 39 cases, 20.5%), the 5 mm-size cutoff appears to be meaningless. Therefore, we posit that the absence of submucosal invasiveness and/or proliferative activity of the NE cells, and not their size, explain the favorable biologic behavior of microcarcinoids.

It is also worth considering whether or not colorectal microcarcinoids are neoplastic lesions and how best to define them. We suggest that it is premature to define colorectal microcarcinoids as neoplastic lesions, particularly when these lesions are confined to the mucosa with no obvious signs of proliferative activity. Indeed, 7 of 9 patients (77.8%) in previous studies underwent additional surgery after polypectomy for fear of residual lesions and possible ominous outcome. We suggest that intramucosal WD NE lesions in the colorectum should be distinguished from classic small-sized or microscopic NETs.

From a pathologist's perspective of view, awareness of microcarcinoids is critical; however, it is also important to avoid over-interpretation while not overlooking or under-recognizing such lesions. Pathologists can misinterpret microcarcinoids as high-grade lesions such as invasive components of associated glandular lesions, particularly when microcarcinoids show infiltrative or single-cell patterns, or else can consider them small-sized classic NET. In the former case, identifying desmoplastic reactions that appear as myofibroblastic proliferation as well as checking for NE differentiation are important. According to our analysis, the most common mistake was to overlook the microcarcinoid component (7 of 43 cases, 16.3%), followed by misdiagnosis of the microcarcinoid as a squamous metaplasia (squamous morules) (6 cases, 14.0%) or invasive glandular component (3 cases, 7.0%) [1, 7, 8]. To that point, a CIAM reported by Lyda et al. was diagnosed as a composite adenoma-carcinoid tumor [10].

Conclusions

To our knowledge, we have reported the largest series of colorectal CIAM. Clinically, CIAM tends to develop in middle-aged to elderly patients and manifests as a colorectal polyp that is usually located in the proximal colon. Microcarcinoids found in CIAM exhibits 2 histologic patterns: they are more commonly observed as WD NE cells arranged in small clusters, glands, or cords interspersed with glandular elements; and are less commonly observed as cell aggregates resembling squamous morules. Microcarcinoids found in CIAMs appear to have favorable clinical outcomes, likely because they are not accompanied by submucosal extension and/or increased proliferative activity. We recommend avoiding further radical surgeries in patients with CIAM that was completely removed endoscopically unless they show submucosal extension or increased proliferative activity.

Abbreviations
CIAM: Composite intestinal adenoma-microcarcinoid; EMR: Endoscopic mucosal resection; ESD: Endoscopic submucosal dissection; FAP: Familial adenomatous polyposis; HGD: High-grade dysplasia; IBD: Inflammatory bowel disease; LAR: Low anterior resection; LGD: Low-grade dysplasia; NE: Neuroendocrine; NET: Neuroendocrine tumor; TA: Tubular adenoma; TVA: Tubulovillous adenoma; WD: Well-differentiated

Acknowledgements
Not applicable.

Funding
This study was supported by a grant-in-aid for Scientific Research from Inje University Research Foundation (20100557) to Hyun-Jung Kim.

Authors' contributions
MJK performed histopathological evaluations and drafted the manuscript. EJL, DSK, DHL, and EGY were responsible for the clinical data. HJK conceived the study and revised the manuscript. All authors read and approved the final manuscript.

Competing interests
The authors declare that they have no competing interests.

Author details
Department of Pathology, Daehang hospital, 481-10 BangBae3-dong, Seocho-gu, 137-820 Seoul, Republic of Korea. [2]Department of Surgery, Daehang hospital, 481-10 BangBae3-dong, Seocho-gu, 137-820 Seoul, Republic of Korea. [3]Department of Pathology, University of Inje College of Medicine, Sanggye Paik hospital, Dongil-ro 1342, Nowon-gu, Seoul, Republic of Korea.

References
1. Pulitzer M, Xu R, Suriawinata AA, Waye JD, Harpaz N. Microcarcinoids in large intestinal adenomas. Am J Surg Pathol. 2006;30:1531–6.
2. Solcia E, Bordi C, Creutzfeldt W, Dayal Y, Dayan AD, Falkmer S, et al. Histopathological classification of nonantral gastric endocrine growths in man. Digestion. 1988;41:185–200.
3. Reinecke P, Borchard F. Pattern of gastric endocrine cells in microcarcinoidosis–an immunohistochemical study of 14 gastric biopsies. Virchows Arch. 1996;428:237–41.
4. Nascimbeni R, Villanacci V, Di Fabio F, Gavazzi E, Fellegara G, Rindi G. Solitary microcarcinoid of the rectal stump in ulcerative colitis. Neuroendocrinology. 2005;81:400–4.
5. Stewart CJ, Matsumoto T, Jo Y, Mibu R, Hirahashi M, Yao T, et al. Multifocal microcarcinoid tumours in ulcerative colitis. J Clin Pathol. 2005;58:111–2. author reply 1112
6. Haidar A, Dixon MF. Solitary microcarcinoid in ulcerative colitis. Histopathology. 1992;21:487–8.
7. Lin J, Goldblum JR, Bennett AE, Bronner MP, Liu X. Composite intestinal adenoma-microcarcinoid. Am J Surg Pathol. 2012;36:292–5.

8. Salaria SN, Abu Alfa AK, Alsaigh NY, Montgomery E, Arnold CA. Composite intestinal adenoma-microcarcinoid clues to diagnosing an under-recognised mimic of invasive adenocarcinoma. J Clin Pathol. 2013;66:302–6.

9. Thosani N, Rao B, Ertan A, Guha S. Wide spectrum of neuroendocrine differentiation in identical appearing colon polyps: a report of 2 mixed endocrine-glandular polyps. Turk J Gastroenterol. 2014;25(Suppl 1):242–3.

10. Lyda MH, Fenoglio-Preiser CM. Adenoma-carcinoid tumors of the colon. Arch Pathol Lab Med. 1998;122:262–5.

11. Bosman FT, Carneiro F, Hruban RH, Theise ND. World Health Organization classification of Tumours of the digestive system. 4th ed. Lyon: IARC Press; 2010. p. 160–5.

12. Tang LH, Shia J, Soslow RA, Dhall D, Wong WD, O'Reilly E, et al. Pathologic classification and clinical behavior of the spectrum of goblet cell carcinoid tumors of the appendix. Am J Surg Pathol. 2008;32:1429–43.

13. Estrella JS, Taggart MW, Rashid A, Abraham SC. Low-grade neuroendocrine tumors arising in intestinal adenomas: evidence for alterations in the adenomatous polyposis coli/β-catenin pathway. Hum Pathol. 2014;45:2051–8.

17

Ki 67 assessment in breast cancer in an Egyptian population: a comparative study between manual assessment on optical microscopy and digital quantitative assessment

Essam Ayad[1]*[iD], Ahmed Soliman[1], Shady Elia Anis[1], Amira Ben Salem[1], Pengchao Hu[2] and Youhong Dong[2]

Abstract

Background: Breast cancer is by far the most frequent cancer among women. The proliferative index, Ki-67, is more and more taken into consideration for treatment decisions. However, the reliability of the established Ki-67 scoring is limited. Digital pathology is currently suggested to be a potential solution to Ki 67 assessment problems.

Methods: This is a retrospective and prospective study including 100 patients diagnosed with invasive breast cancer. Three senior pathologists have been asked to estimate the Ki-67 proliferative index for each of the 100 cases by examining the whole glass slides on optical microscope and providing a continuous score then a categorical score ('high' and 'low' Ki 67 index) using once 14%, once 20% as threshold indicative of high Ki67 status. Finally, a digital quantitative assessment of Ki67 was performed.

Results: A high inter-observer agreement was found when using optical microscopy for Ki 67 assessment, with correlation coefficient (CC) estimated at 0.878 (p value < 0.01). The overall agreement between manual and automated evaluation of Ki 67 was only substantial (CC estimated at 0.745 (p value < 0.01)). When using categorical scores, the inter-observers concordance was substantial using both cutoff points with kappa value estimated at 0.796 ([0.696–0.925] while using 14% as a cut off point and at 0.766 ([0.672–0.938] while using 20% as a cutoff point (p value < 0). The inter-observers agreement was better while using 14% as cutoff point. Agreement between manual and automated assessment of Ki 67 indices using both cutoff points was only substantial (Kappa estimated at 0.623, p value < 0.01). In comparison to automated assessment of Ki 67 index, while using 14% as a cutoff point, the overall tendency of all observers was to overestimate the Ki 67 values but to underestimate the proliferation index while using 20% as a cutoff point.

Conclusion: Automated assessment of Ki 67 value would appear to be comparable to visual Ki 67 assessment on optical microscopy. Such study would help define the role of digital pathology as a potential easy-to use tool for a robust and standardized fully automated Ki 67 scoring.

Keywords: Breast, Cancer, Ki67, Manual, Automated, Assessment

* Correspondence: essamayad@yahoo.com; essamayad@kasralainy.edu.eg
Preliminary results from this study were presented at the 28th European Congress of Pathology, held in Cologne, Germany from 25 - 29 September 2016
[1]Department of Pathology, Cairo University, Cairo, Egypt
Full list of author information is available at the end of the article

And Published in the **Virchows Arch (2016) 469 (Suppl 1):S1–S346:**

E. Ayad; "Evaluation of Ki-67 Index in invasive breast cancer: Comparison between visual and automated digital assessment" *Virchows Arch (2016) 469 (Suppl 1):S191. DOI 10.1007/s00428-016-1997-7* [1].

Background

Breast cancer is the most common malignancy affecting women in both developed and developing countries. It represents about 25% of all new cancer cases diagnosed in women per year. Fifty three percent of the newly reported cases are in developing countries, which represent about 82% of the world population [2].

Currently ER, PR and HER2 are recognized as prognostic and predictive factors [3, 4]. Ki-67 expression is more and more taken into consideration and has become a key factor for treatment decisions [5, 6].

Since 2011, the Saint Gallen guidelines stated that Ki 67 assessment allows for the segregation of the two types of luminal tumors (A and B) taking into account the value of the proliferation index. The application of chemotherapy is commonly recommended for patients with a high Ki-67 value [7, 8].

The 2011 Saint Gallen Consensus Meeting defined tumors with a Ki67 index of 14% or less as tumors with "low proliferation". This cut-off was established by comparison with PAM50 intrinsic multigene molecular test classification of breast cancers [7, 9]. Then, during the 2013 Saint Gallen Conference, the majority of panelists voted for a threshold of 20% as indicative of "high" Ki67 status on the basis of many studies concluding that 20% is a significant factor for OS (overal survival) in the Luminal B subtype [8, 10].

However, during the Saint Gallen consensus meeting in 2015, the minimum value of Ki 67 required for the definition of luminal B subtype was for the majority of the panel ranging between 20 and 29% as many studies showed that patients with tumor with Ki67 > 20% showed the poorest prognosis [11, 12].

Because of the persistant intra and inter observers and laboratories variabilities, the panel of experts proposed finally that each laboratory define and use a median Ki67 value providing the best intra-laboratory inter-observer agreement as the cut-off distinguishing different subgroups [12].

Due to this dilemma about the cut off levels for Ki-67 suggested to distinguish prognostic subgroups, as well as the lack of standardization concerning preanalytical, analytical and methods used for interpretation and assessment of the Ki-67 score, this marker has not been implemented for routine clinical use in many pathological centers [5]. However during the last Saint Gallen meeting in 2017, the majority of the panelists agreed that the distinction between luminal A and luminal B subtypes by immunohistochemistry (IHC) approximate multigene testing results and 80% agreed that these two categories should be used for therapy decisions [13]. So an agreement on standardized method for Ki 67 evaluation is mandatory for proper management of breast cancer cases.

Digital pathology is an emerging field that is becoming more commonplace in routine pathology practice [14, 15].

Currently, there is interest in automating the assessment of Ki-67 labeling index with possible benefits in handling increased workload, with improved accuracy and precision.

Aim of the study

To present and validate an easy-to-use, standardized and accurate Ki-67 scoring method in breast cancer by comparing observer's performance on assessment of Ki-67 index on optical microscopy, then, by comparing the concordance between the results of the visual manual method and those of the automated Ki-67 assessment.

Methods

Patient's cohort

We analyzed 100 cases of invasive breast cancer collected for the study from the pathology laboratory of Cairo university hospital during a period of 2 months (June–July 2015). Histological sections were obtained from paraffin blocks of 100 specimens (62 surgical specimens and 38 cores biopsies). Patient's age ranges between 26 and 88 years old. Patients diagnosed with only ductal or lobular carcinoma in situ were excluded from the study.

Immunohistochemistry for Ki 67

4 μm thick sections were cut from paraffin-blocks which contained formalin fixed tumor tissue. During the whole staining procedure the slides were treated with the fully automated Benchmark Staining System (Ventana Medical Systems) using the primary antibody (rabbit monoclonal anti Ki – 67 human clone 30–09 Ventana Medical System). Then all the Ki 67 stained slides were scanned by iScan device [Produced by BioImagene (New Roche-Ventana)] present in the Digital Pathology Unit, Faculty of Medicine, Cairo University.

Study design

Three different pathologists were asked to estimate the Ki-67 proliferative index for each of the 100 cases by examining the whole glass slide using *optical microscope* and to provide Ki-67 results using:

- **Continuous score**: a score in the range of 0 to 100 corresponding to the percentage of positive tumors cells.
- **Categorical scores**: The results provided by different observers were then classified into 2 categories using 2 different cutoff points;
- *First*: Cutoff point = 14%: patients were considered to have a 'High Ki 67' status if the observer judged that 14% of cells or more were positive for Ki-67 expression and 'low Ki 67' status otherwise.
- *Second*: Cutoff point = 20%: patients were considered to have a 'High Ki 67' status if the observer judged that 20% of cells or more were positive for Ki-67 expression and 'low Ki 67' status otherwise.

Stained nuclei were considered positive regardless of the intensity of staining. A whole slide average score, including hot spot areas, was the method used to estimate the Ki 67 value in all cases.

All the pathologists performed Ki 67 assessment independently and were blinded to patient outcome as well as other observer's results.

Quantitative digital analysis of Ki67

The whole scanned slide was examined then; multiple snapshots were captured with a ($\times$ 40) objective covering almost the whole scanned slide (15–50 snapshots per case). Areas rich in tumor cells were preferably chosen. Areas showing necrosis or significant lymphocytic infiltrate were avoided to minimize false positive results. Finally, a digital quantitative analysis of Ki 67 proliferative index was performed corresponding to the digital quantitative assessment of the percentage of the positive tumour cells for Ki67 using **ImmunoRatio website** [including the algorithm needed for nuclear counting of both positive & negative nuclei]. The program made a primary step of pseudo-color image showing staining component followed by image analysis according to the scale selected for the analysis. For each case, the software was able to identify stained and unstained nuclei (regardless of the intensity of staining) and to provide a percentage of positive nuclei for each snapshot. Then the final value of Ki 67 index of the case was calculated taking the arithmetic mean of all Ki 67 index values for each image individually.

Statistical analysis

Inter-observers agreement was analyzed for each case, using categorical scores (with the two different cutoffs) and continuous scores. A study of agreement between Ki 67 assessment results provided using optical microscopy in comparison to the digital quantitative assessment of Ki 67 was also done.

Statistical tests used for data management

Data was tabulated and analyzed using the computer program SPSS (Statistical package for social science) version 16. In the statistical comparison between the different groups, the significance of difference was tested using one of the following tests:

1) Kappa (κ): The interobserver agreement for each pair of observers was estimated then a mean of the kappa values was calculated. Kappa was interpreted as following: 0.0–0.20: Slight agreement, 0.21–0.40: Fair agreement, 0.41–0.60: Moderate agreement, 0.61–0.80: Substantial agreement, 0.81–1.00: Almost perfect agreement [16].
2) Correlation coefficient (CC): The inter-observer agreement for each pair of observers was estimated then a mean of the CC values was calculated.

There is no universally accepted standard criteria for the CC, the following criteria, similar to the kappa coefficient were used here to aid interpretation: 0.00–0.20 was interpreted as "slight correlation"; 0.21–0.40 as "fair correlation"; 0.41–0.60 as "moderate correlation"; 0.61–0.80 as "substantial correlation"; and > 0.80 as "almost perfect correlation" [17].

A 'p' value < 0.05 was considered statistically significant (*) while > 0.05 statistically insignificant 'p' value < 0.01 was considered highly significant (**) in all analyses.

Results

One hundred cases of invasive breast carcinoma were included in this study. The patients were 99 women and one man and ranged in age from 26 to 88 years old with a mean age of 55.46 years old.

The majority of cases were diagnosed as invasive duct carcinoma, with only one case of invasive lobular carcinoma. Invasive tumors were classified as grade 1 in 4% of cases, as grade 2 in 73% of cases and as grade 3 in 13% of cases. Regarding the hormonal receptors and HER 2 profile, 79% of cases were ER and/or PR positives, 14% of cases were triple negatives and 7% of cases were only Her 2 positives.

Inter-observer variability on optical microscopy using continuous scores (Fig. 1)

The correlation coefficient (CC) runs to determine the relationship between Ki 67 assessment performed by the 3 observers showed an almost perfect agreement (CC: 0.878, p value < 0.01).

The main groups with highest variable Ki 67 index values were the groups with Ki 67 value varying between 11 and 35%, and for some pairs of observers the most discordant values were within the group with Ki 67 index between 15 and 25%.

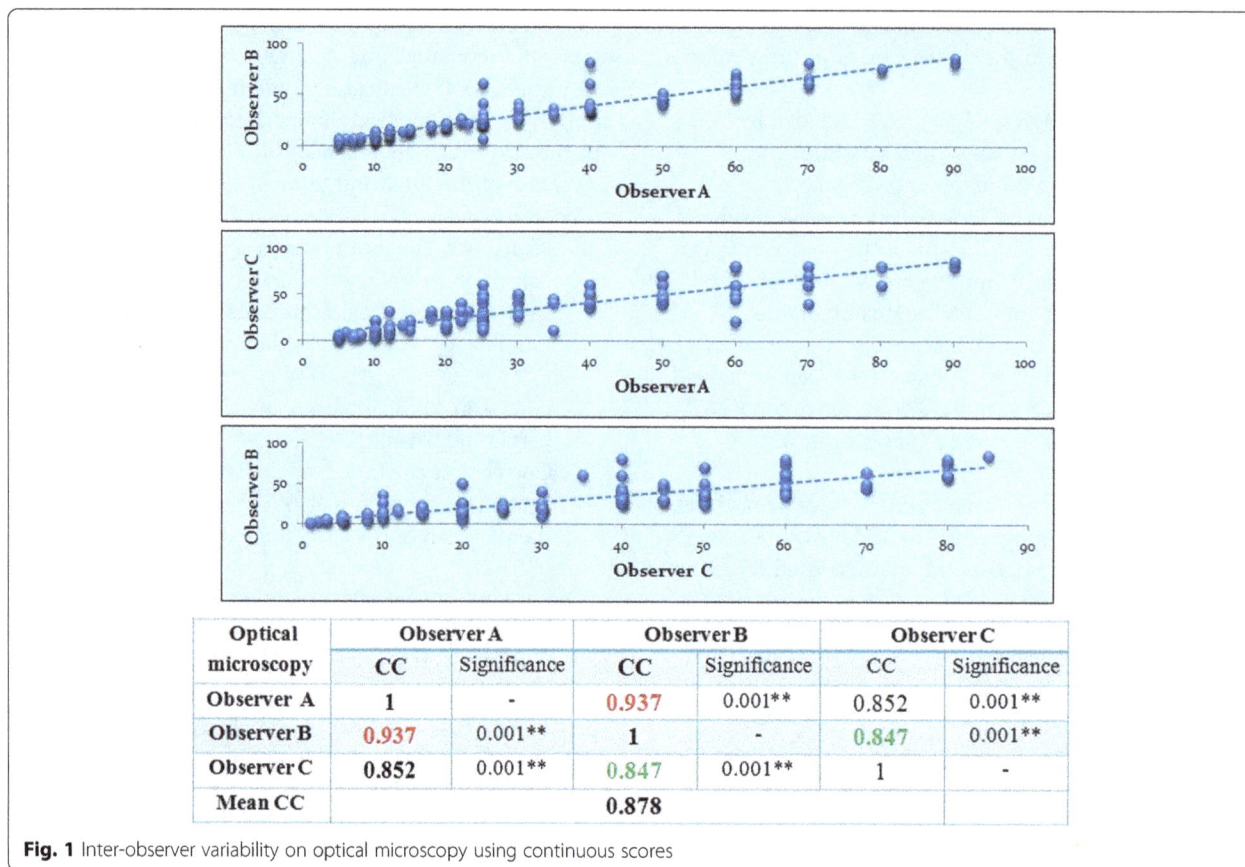

Optical microscopy	Observer A		Observer B		Observer C	
	CC	Significance	CC	Significance	CC	Significance
Observer A	1	-	0.937	0.001**	0.852	0.001**
Observer B	0.937	0.001**	1	-	0.847	0.001**
Observer C	0.852	0.001**	0.847	0.001**	1	-
Mean CC	0.878					

Fig. 1 Inter-observer variability on optical microscopy using continuous scores

Inter-observer variability on optical microscopy using categorical scores (Fig. 2)

While using 14% as a cutoff indicative of 'High Ki 67' status: 67% to 71% of cases were classified as having high Ki 67 index and 21% to 26% were classified as having low Ki 67 index at least by 2 observers. However 3% to 12% of cases were variably classified by the observers. The Kappa coefficient used to evaluate the inter-observers variability showed a substantial agreement between the 3 observers (kappa: 0.796, *p* value< 0.01).

While using 20% as a cutoff indicative of 'High Ki 67' status: 50% to 57% of cases were classified as having high Ki 67 index and 33% to 40% were classified as having low Ki 67 index at least by 2 observers. However 3% to 16% of cases were variably classified by the observers. The inter-observers agreement was substantial with kappa value, slightly lower than the kappa value found with the cut off 14%. (Kappa: 0.766, *p* value< 0.01).

Comparison of Ki 67 assessment results on optical microscopy and automated quantitative analysis results using continuous scores (Fig. 3)

The overall agreement between the manual and automated evaluation of Ki 67 was substantial with CC estimated at 0.745 (*p* value < 0.01).

Comparison of Ki 67 assessment results on optical microscopy and automated quantitative analysis results using categorical scores

While using 14% as a cutoff point, 88.2% to 90.8% of the cases classified as having high Ki 67 index by quantitative analysis were classified as such by the 3 observers on optical microscopy and 75% to 79.2% of the cases classified as having low Ki 67 index by quantitative analysis were classified as such by the 3 observers on optical microscopy.

However, in 20.8% to 25% of cases the Ki 67 index was overestimated by the observers in comparison to automated assessment results and in 9.2% to 11.8% of cases the Ki 67 value was underestimated.

So, while using 14% as a cutoff point, the overall tendency was to overestimate the Ki 67 index using manual Ki 67 assessment in comparison to the automated method.

The overall agreement between manual and automated assessment of Ki 67 indices was only substantial (Kappa: 0.623, *p* < 0.01).

While using 20% as a cutoff point, 76.1% to 80.9% of cases classified as having high Ki 67 index by quantitative analysis were classified as such by the 3 observers on optical microscopy and 84.4% to 87.5% of cases classified as having low Ki 67 index by quantitative analysis

Inter-observer variability on optical microscopy using 14% as cutoff indicative of 'High Ki 67' status:

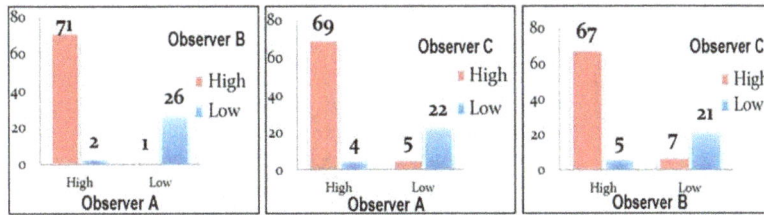

Cut off 14%	Observer A		Observer B		Observer C	
	Kappa	Significance	**Kappa**	Significance	**Kappa**	Significance
Observer A	1	-	0.925	0.001**	0.769	0.001**
Observer B	0.925	0.001**	1	-	0.696	0.001**
Observer C	0.769	0.001**	0.696	0.001**	1	-
Mean	0.796					

Inter-observer variability on optical microscopy using 20% as cutoff indicative of 'High Ki 67' status:

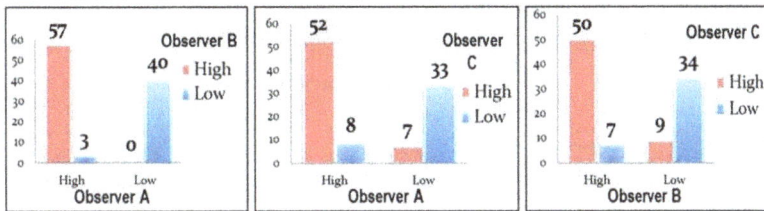

Cut off 20%	Observer A		Observer B		Observer C	
	Kappa	Significance	**Kappa**	Significance	**Kappa**	Significance
Observer A	1	-	0.938	0.001**	0.689	0.001**
Observer B	0.938	0.001**	1	-	0.672	0.001**
Observer C	0.689	0.001**	0.672	0.001**	1	-
Mean	0.766					

Fig. 2 Inter-observer variability on optical microscopy using categorical scores

were classified as such by the 3 observers on optical microscopy. However, in 12.5% to 15.6% of cases the Ki 67 index was overestimated by 3 observers in comparison to automated assessment results and in 19.1% to 23.9% of cases the Ki 67 value was underestimated.

So, while using 20% as a cutoff point, the overall tendency was to underestimate the Ki 67 index using optical microscopy in comparison to the automated method.

The overall agreement between visual assessment using optical microscopy and automated assessment of Ki 67 indices was also only substantial, but with Kappa value slightly lower than the kappa value found with the cut off 14 (Kappa: 0.602, $p < 0.01$).

Discussion

Numerous studies have investigated the potential role of Ki67 as a prognostic marker as well as its role in predicting response to adjuvant and neo-adjuvant therapy. Although multiple meta-analyses showed that high Ki 67 index is associated with a higher risk of relapse and a worse survival in patients with early breast cancer [18, 19] and with a good response to neo-adjuvant chemotherapy

[20], this marker is still not universally used in clinical routine. This is mainly due in one hand to the large inter-observer variability in assessment of the percentage of this marker, and in the other hand to the fact that clinical decision-making regarding treatment options in breast cancer often relies on the application of a Ki 67 cutoff to classify patients into "Ki67 high" or "Ki67 low" risk groups, however widely varying cutoff values (ranging from 0 to 28.6%) have been used to define the group with high Ki 67 [21, 22]. Also, several works reported that the lowest reproducibility of Ki67 results is mainly observed in the subset of cancers with intermediate proliferation activity (between 15 and 30%), the range in which most cutoffs are located for making clinical decisions [23–25], this further impede the clinical utility of Kin67 and make it difficult to compare Ki67 data across different studies.

Our study was designed to compare two different Ki 67 assessment modalities: visual estimation on optical microscopy and quantitative automated analysis. It also aimed to assess the reproducibility of both Ki 67 cutoffs proposed by the Saint Gallen Consensus Meetings in

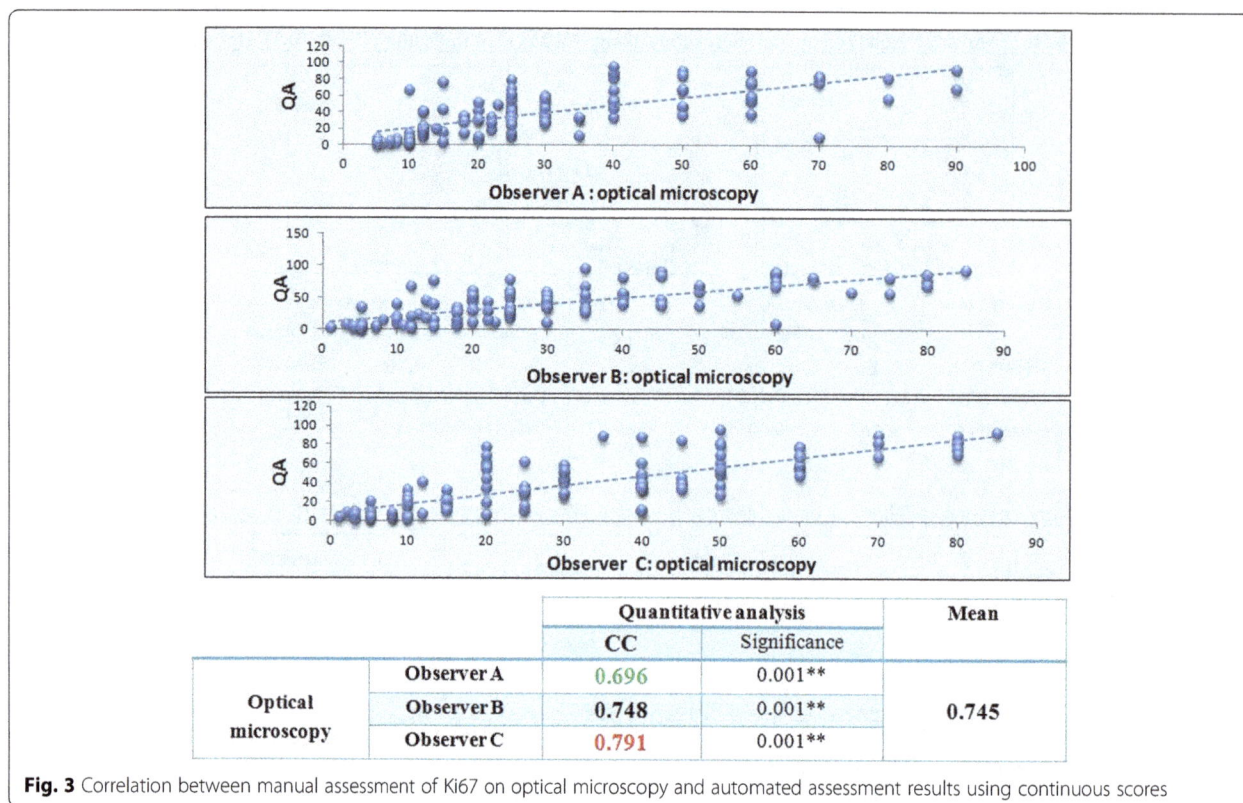

Fig. 3 Correlation between manual assessment of Ki67 on optical microscopy and automated assessment results using continuous scores

| | | Quantitative analysis | | Mean |
		CC	Significance	
Optical microscopy	Observer A	0.696	0.001**	0.745
	Observer B	0.748	0.001**	
	Observer C	0.791	0.001**	

2011 and 2013 to classify the tumors as having 'high' or 'low' Ki 67 index.

In contrast to many studies showing that inter-observer reproducibility of routine Ki-67 assessment in breast cancer on optical microscopy is poor to moderate especially in the grade 2 breast cancer group [26–28], the inter-observer agreement in our study was almost perfect agreement (CC: 0.878, p value < 0.01). However while comparing the results of Ki 67 assessment performed by different observers we found, as many studies showed [23–25], that the main group with highest variable Ki 67 index values was the group with Ki67 value varying between 11 and 35%, and for some pairs of observers the most discordant values were within the group with Ki 67 index between 15 and 25% (Fig. 1).

When we used the 2 cut off values (14% and 20%) to classify the cases as having "low Ki 67" or "high Ki 67" status, the inter-observer agreement on optical microscopy was only substantial using both cutoff points with kappa value when using 14% as cut off point, slightly higher than the kappa value found while using the cutoff 20% (Fig. 2).

A similar result was found by Varga Z et al. who showed higher inter-observer agreement while using the cutoff 14% in comparison to 20% but with lower kappa values than those found in our study with only slight to moderate agreement while using the 2 cutoff points (Kappa values 0.58 with cutoff 14% and 0.48 while using the cutoff 20%) [29].

According to these studies results, the inter-observer agreement was better using 14% as cutoff point although, according to other studies, 20% seems to be better reflecting the patient's prognosis [30].

However, without standardization of the methodology, these cutoffs have limited value outside of the studies from which they were derived and the centers that performed them.

That is why researches have been conducted in order to develop other methods to ameliorate the inter-observer agreement and allow the reliable use of Ki 67 assessment as an additive factor for proper and consistent therapeutic decision.

Digital pathology is now a new approach used in many tasks [31, 32]. Many studies are now proposing the automated digital image analysis (DIA) as a potential efficient method of Ki67 index assessment, with benefits of increased precision and accuracy in comparison with visual evaluation or manual counting especially that it is tedious and labor intensive to count at least 1000 tumor cells, which has often been recommended for proper evaluation of Ki67 index [4].

A high correlation between manual and automated Ki 67 assessment have been showed by many studies which concluded that visual assessment and DIA both could be used for Ki67 assessment in clinical practice [33–35].

However, in our study, the overall agreement between the manual and automated evaluation of Ki 67 was only

Ki 67 assessment in breast cancer in an Egyptian population: a comparative study between manual...

155

substantial with CC estimated at 0.745 (p value < 0.01) meaning that the correlation between manual and automated assessment methods is not always perfect.

So why to choose the automated Ki 67 index assessment?

In fact, recent studies showed that automated assessment of Ki 67 correlates better with clinical and pathological characteristics of breast cancer as well as the prognostic factors [36]. Gudlaugsson et al. concluded that Ki67 index assessment by DIA, but not subjective counts, was reproducible and prognostically strong [37].

Also, Stålhammar G et al. showed that all automated Ki 67 assessment methods are far better than the most meticulous manual assessment in terms of sensitivity and specificity, especially for the most diagnostic controversial subtype, the Luminal B subtype. Moreover, the level of agreement between the automated Ki 67 assessment results and the PAM50 gene expression assays was higher than that between the latter and the manual methods [38].

In our study, the overall agreement between manual and automated assessment of Ki 67 indices using 14% as well as 20% as cutoff points was only substantial.

The best kappa values reflecting the best consistency with quantitative analysis results were found while using 14% as a cutoff point. So for our laboratory, 14% seems to be a better reproducible cutoff point, with better inter-observer and inter-modalities agreement.

However, In comparison to automated assessment of Ki 67 index, the overall tendency of all observers was to overestimate the Ki 67 values while using 14% as a cutoff point but to underestimate the Ki 67 values while using the cutoff point 20%. That means that the results of Ki 67 assessment for the group with Ki 67 indices varying between14 and 20%, the group in which most controversial cutoffs are located for making clinical decisions, were highly discordant between the 3 observers and quantitative analysis (Fig. 4).

Zhong F et al. study demonstrated similar results. For cases with high Ki 67 index (> 30%), DIA and visual assessment results were highly concordant. However, in

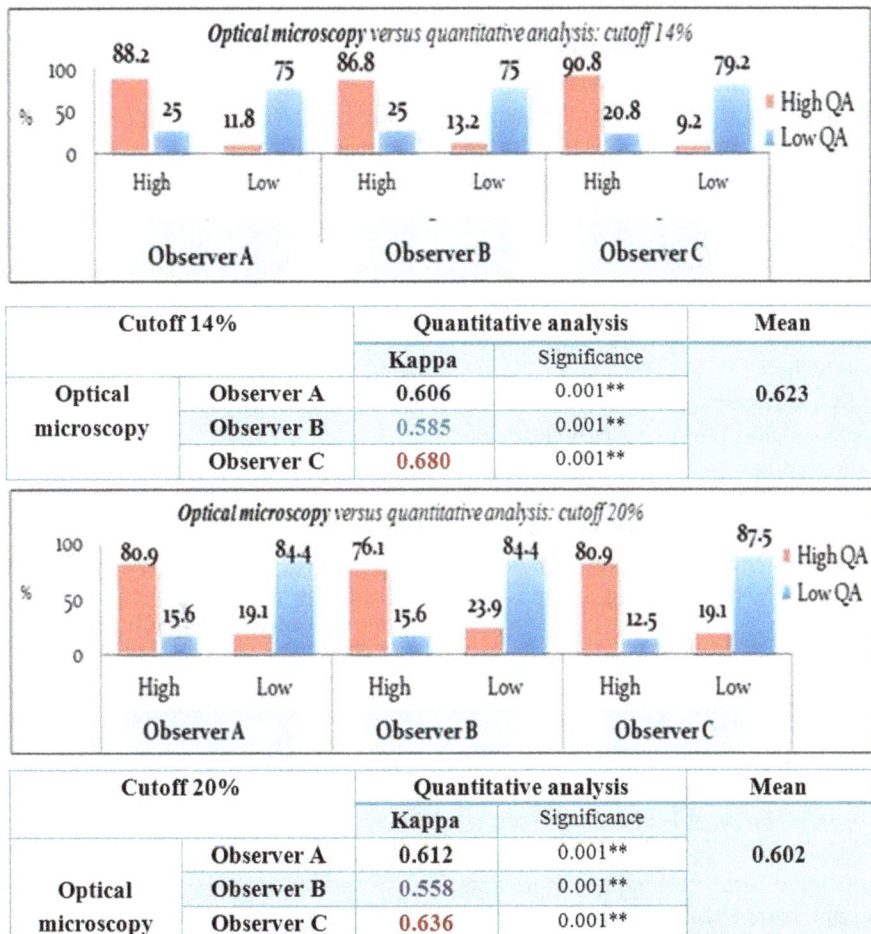

Cutoff 14%		Quantitative analysis		Mean
		Kappa	Significance	
Optical microscopy	Observer A	0.606	0.001**	0.623
	Observer B	0.585	0.001**	
	Observer C	0.680	0.001**	

Cutoff 20%		Quantitative analysis		Mean
		Kappa	Significance	
Optical microscopy	Observer A	0.612	0.001**	0.602
	Observer B	0.558	0.001**	
	Observer C	0.636	0.001**	

Fig. 4 Correlation between manual assessment of Ki67 on optical microscopy and automated assessment results using categorical scores

cases showing intermediate Ki 67 index (11–30%), the agreement between both methods was only substantial to perfect [34].

By summarizing all these data, it seems that the computer-assisted quantitative analysis can improve the accuracy and inter-observer reproducibility of Ki 67 assessment and be a potential easy-to use tool for standardized fully automated Ki 67 scoring replacing the widely criticized current manual evaluation. This could prevent a wide proportion of patients from either receiving potentially harmful treatment such as cytotoxic chemotherapy without benefit or from being excluded from the beneficial treatment that a better diagnostic method would indicate.

However, DIA has some disadvantages. Some studies showed that automated assessment methods are less accurate than the visual ones in tumor cells identification, especially in tumors rich in lymphocytes, where some Ki67-positive lymphocytes may be identified as tumor cells. This will lead to Ki67 index value overestimation [34].

To overcome this problem, some authors proposed a method with semi-automated evaluation of Ki 67 index which allows for the determination of the exact proliferation index value by marking the immunostained tumor cells and the negative tumor cells manually then the cells are automatically counted and the ratio between immunomarked and negative cells gives the Ki 67 value [36, 39].

In our study, while choosing the areas to capture snapshots for automated quantitative analysis, we tried to avoid areas with significant lymphocytic infiltration to minimize the risk of over or underestimation of Ki 67 index.

It should be mentioned that the findings of this study might not be generalized due to the large KI67 inter-laboratory variability.

Newly developed DIA softwares tend also to overcome this problem by tissue classification using virtual double staining. For example, the same section will be stained for both cytokeratin and Ki67 markers; tumor cells are recognized by positive cytokeratin expression, and only cells that co-express both markers are automatically counted as positive tumor cells excluding any positive lymphocytes [38].

Conclusion

Manual methods of Ki 67 assessment using optical microscopy lack perfect accuracy especially in cases with Ki 67 index ranging between 10 and 35% leading to improper distinction between Luminal A and B subtypes of breast cancer.

Further studies providing better techniques improving the accuracy of the automated Ki 67 assessment, especially identifying and detecting the tumor cells only, as well as trying to reduce the cost of this technique and make it more available, could help to consider automated assessment of Ki 67 as the most accurate and standard method and then could allow the universal agreement on a standard cut off that better distinguish the prognostic subgroups and concord with the molecular classification.

Abbreviations
CC: Correlation coefficient; DIA: Digital image analysis; ER: Estrogen Receptor; HER2: Human epidermal growth factor receptor 2; IHC: Immunohistochemistry; PR: Progesteron Receptor

Acknowledgements
We thank the Pathology Department, Faculty of Medicine, Cairo University.

Authors' contributions
Conceived and designed the experiments: EA, AS, SEA & ABS, Performed the experiments: EA, AS, SEA & ABS. Analyzed the data: EA, PH, YD. Wrote the paper: EA, SEA & ABS. All authors read and approved the final manuscript.

Competing interests
The authors declare that they have no competing interests.

Author details
[1]Department of Pathology, Cairo University, Cairo, Egypt. [2]Department of Oncology, XiangYang No.1 People's Hospital Affiliated to Hubei University of Medicine, Xiangyang, Hubei 441000, People's Republic of China.

References
1. Ayad E. Evaluation of Ki-67 Index in invasive breast cancer: Comparison between visual and automated digital assessment. Virchows Arch. 2016; 469(Suppl 1):S191. https://doi.org/10.1007/s00428-016-1997-7.
2. American Cancer Society. Global Cancer Facts & Figures. 3rd ed. Atlanta: American Cancer Society; 2015. p. 37.
3. Montemurro F, Di Cosimo S, Arpino G. Human epidermal growth factor receptor 2 (HER2)-positive and hormone receptor-positive breast cancer: new insights into molecular interactions and clinical implications. Ann Oncol. 2013;24(11):2715–24.
4. Purdie CA, Quinlan P, Jordan LB, Ashfield A, Ogston S, Dewar JA, et al. Progesterone receptor expression is an independent prognostic variable in early breast cancer: a population-based study. Br J Cancer. 2014;110(3):565–72.
5. Dowsett M, Nielsen TO, A'Hern R, Bartlett J, Coombes RC, Cuzick J, et al. Assessment of Ki67 in breast cancer: recommendations from the international Ki67 in breast Cancer working group. J Natl Cancer Inst. 2011; 103(22):1656–64.
6. Luporsi E, André F, Spyratos F, Martin PM, Jacquemier J, Penault-Llorca F, et al. Ki-67: level of evidence and methodological considerations for its role

in the clinical management of breast cancer: analytical and critical review. Breast Cancer Res Treat. 2012;132:895–915.

7. Goldhirsch A, Wood WC, Coates AS, Gelber RD, Thurlimann B, Senn HJ, et al. Strategies for subtypes—dealing with the diversity of breast Cancer: highlights of the St. Gallen international expert consensus on the primary therapy of early breast Cancer 2011. Ann Oncol. 2011;22:1736–47.

8. Goldhirsch A, Winer EP, Coates AS, Gelber RD, Piccart-Gebhart M, Thürlimann B, et al. Personalizing the treatment of women with early breast cancer: highlights of the St. Gallen international expert consensus on the primary therapy of early breast Cancer 2013. Ann Oncol. 2013;24:2206–23.

9. Cheang MC, Chia SK, Voduc D, Gao D, Leung S, Snider J, et al. Ki67 index, HER2 status, and prognosis of patients with luminal B breast cancer. J Natl Cancer Inst. 2009;101:736–50.

10. Tashima R, Nishimura R, Osako T, Nishiyama Y, Okumura Y, Nakano M, et al. Evaluation of an Optimal Cut-Off Point for the Ki-67 Index as a Prognostic Factor in Primary Breast Cancer: A Retrospective Study. PLoS One. 2015; 10(7):e0119565.

11. Maisonneuve P, Disalvatore D, Rotmensz N, Curigliano G, Colleoni M, Dellapasqua S, et al. Proposed new clinicopathological surrogate definitions of luminal a and luminal B (HER2-negative) intrinsic breast cancer subtypes. Breast Cancer Res. 2014;16:R65.

12. Coates AS, Winer EP, Goldhirsch A, Gelber RD, Gnant M, Piccart-Gebhart M. Tailoring therapies-improving the management of early breast cancer: St Gallen international expert consensus on the primary therapy of early breast Cancer. Ann Oncol. 2015;26:1533–46.

13. Gnanta M, Harbeckb N, Thomssen C. St. Gallen/Vienna 2017: a brief summary of the consensus discussion about escalation and De-escalation of primary breast Cancer treatment. Breast Care. 2017;12:102–7.

14. Weinstein RS, Graham AR, Richter LC, Barker GP, Krupinski EA, Lopez AM, et al. Overview of telepathology, virtual microscopy, and whole slide imaging: prospects for the future. Hum Pathol. 2009;40(8):1057–69.

15. Al-Janabi S, Huisman A, Van Diest PJ. Digital pathology: current status and future perspectives. Histopathology. 2012;61(1):1–9.

16. Landis JR, Koch GG. The measurement of observer agreement for categorical data. Biometrics. 1977;33:159–74.

17. Fleiss JL, Cohen J. The equivalence of weighted kappa and the intraclass correlation coefficient as measures of reliability. Educ Psychol Meas. 1973; 33(3):613–9.

18. Nishimura R, Osako T, Nishiyama Y, Tashima R, Nakano M. Fujisue1 M. Prognostic significance of Ki-67 index value at the primary breast tumor in recurrent breast cancer. Mol Clin Oncol. 2014;2:1062–8.

19. Pathmanathan N, Balleine RL, Jayasinghe UW, Bilinski KL, Provan PJ, Byth K. The prognostic value of Ki67 in systemically untreated patients with node-negative breast cancer. J Clin Pathol. 2014;67:222–8.

20. Tan QX, Qin QH, Yang WP, Mo QG, Wei CY. Prognostic value of Ki67 expression in HR-negative breast cancer before and after neoadjuvantchemotherapy. Int J Clin Exp Pathol. 2014;7(10):6862–70.

21. Urruticoechea A, Smith IE, Dowsett M. Proliferation marker Ki-67 in early breast cancer. J Clin Oncol. 2005;23(28):7212–20.

22. Stuart-Harris R, Caldas C, Pinder SE, Pharoah P. Proliferation markers and survival in early breast cancer: a systematic review and meta-analysis of 85 studies in 32,825 patients. Breast. 2008;17(4):323–34.

23. Varga Z, Diebold J, Dommann-Scherrer C, Frick H, Kaup D, Noske A, et al. How reliable is Ki-67 immunohistochemistry in grade 2 breast carcinomas? A QA study of the Swiss Working Group of Breast- and Gynecopathologists. PLoS One. 2012;7:e3737.

24. Polley MYC, Leung SCY, McShane LM, Gao D, Hugh JC. Mastropasqua MG et al. An international Ki67 reproducibility study on behalf of the international Ki67 in breast Cancer working group of the breast international group and north American breast Cancer group. J Natl Cancer Inst. 2013;105(24):1897–906.

25. Shui R, Yu B, Bi R, Yang F, Yang W. An Interobserver reproducibility analysis of Ki67 visual assessment in breast Cancer. PLoS One. 2015;10(5):e0125131.

26. Trihia H, Murray S, Price K, Gelber RD, Golouh R, Goldhirsch A, et al. Ki-67 expression in breast carcinoma: its association with grading systems, clinical parameters, and other prognostic factors–a surrogate marker? Cancer. 2003; 97(5):1321–31.

27. Dowsett M, Ebbs SR, Dixon JM, Skene A, Griffith C, Boeddinghaus I, et al. Biomarker changes during neoadjuvant Anastrozole, tamoxifen, or the combination: influence of hormonal status and HER-2 in breast Cancer—a study from the IMPACT Trialists. J Clin Oncol. 2005;23(11):2477–92.

28. Ellis MJ, Suman VJ, Hoog J, Lin L, Snider J, Prat A, et al. Randomized phase II neoadjuvant comparison between Letrozole, Anastrozole, and Exemestane for postmenopausal women with estrogen receptor-rich stage 2 to 3 breast Cancer: clinical and biomarker outcomes and predictive value of the baseline PAM50-based intrinsic subtype- ACOSOG Z1031. J Clin Oncol. 2011; 29(17):2342–9.

29. Varga Z, Cassoly E, Li Q, Oehlschlegel C, Tapia C, Lehr HA, et al. Standardization for Ki- 67 Assessment in Moderately Differentiated Breast Cancer. A Retrospective Analysis of the SAKK 28/12 Study. PLoS ONE. 2015; 10(4):e0123435.

30. Bustreo S, Osella-Abate S, Cassoni P, Donadio M, Airoldi M, Pedani F, et al. Optimal Ki67 cut-off for luminal breast cancer prognostic evaluation: a large case series study with a long-term follow-up. Breast Cancer Res Treat. 2016; 157(2):363–71.

31. Soenksen D. Digital pathology at the crossroads of major health care trends: corporate innovation as an engine for change. Arch Pathol Lab Med. 2009; 133:555–9.

32. Kayser K, Borkenfeld S, Kayser G. How to introduce virtual microscopy (VM) in routine diagnostic pathology: constraints, ideas, and solutions. Anal Cell Pathol. 2012;35:3–10.

33. Mohammed ZMA, McMillan DC, Elsberger B, Going JJ, Orange C, Mallon E, et al. Comparison of Visual and automated assessment of Ki-67 proliferative activity and their impact on outcome in primary operable invasive ductal breast cancer. Br J Cancer. 2012;106(2):383–8.

34. Zhong F, Bi R, Yu B, Yang F, Yang W, Shui R. A comparison of visual assessment and automated digital image analysis of Ki67 labeling index in breast Cancer. PLoS One. 2016;11(2):e0150505.

35. Fasanella S, Leonardi E, Cantaloni C, Eccher C, Bazzanella I, Aldovini D, et al. Proliferative activity in human breast cancer: Ki-67 automated evaluation and the influence of different Ki-67 equivalent antibodies. Diagn Pathol. 2011;6(1):S7.

36. Abubakar M, Orr N, Daley F, Coulson P, Ali HR, Blows F. Prognostic value of automated KI67 scoring in breast cancer: a centralised evaluation of 8088 patients from 10 study groups. Breast Cancer Res. 2016;18:104.

37. Gudlaugsson E, Skaland I, Janssen EA, Smaaland R, Shao Z, Malpica A, et al. Comparison of the effect of different techniques for measurement of Ki67 proliferation on reproducibility and prognosis prediction accuracy in breast cancer. Histopathology. 2012;61:1134–44.

38. Stålhammar G, Martinez NF, Lippert M, Tobin NP, Mølholm I, Kis L, et al. Digital image analysis outperforms manual biomarker assessment in breast cancer. Mod Pathol. 2016;29:318–29.

39. Suciu C, Muresan A, Cornea R, Suciu O, Dema A, Raica M. Semi-automated evaluation of Ki-67 index in invasive ductal carcinoma of the breast. Oncol Lett. 2014;7(1):107–14.

18

Robustness of biomarker determination in breast cancer by RT-qPCR: impact of tumor cell content, DCIS and non-neoplastic breast tissue

Kerstin Hartmann[1][*][†], Kornelia Schlombs[1][†], Mark Laible[1], Claudia Gürtler[1], Marcus Schmidt[2], Ugur Sahin[3] and Hans-Anton Lehr[4]

Abstract

Background: Tissue heterogeneity in formalin-fixed paraffin-embedded (FFPE) breast cancer specimens may affect the accuracy of reverse transcription quantitative real-time PCR (RT-qPCR). Herein, we tested the impact of tissue heterogeneity of breast cancer specimen on the RT-qPCR-based gene expression assay MammaTyper®.

Methods: MammaTyper® quantifies the mRNA expression of the four biomarkers *ERBB2*, *ESR1*, *PGR*, and *MKI67*. Based on pre-defined cut-off values, this molecular in vitro diagnostic assay permits binary marker classification and determination of breast cancer subtypes as defined by St Gallen 2013. In this study, we compared data from whole FFPE sections with data obtained in paired RNA samples after enrichment for invasive carcinoma via macro- or laser-capture micro-dissection.

Results: Compared to whole sections, removal of surrounding adipose tissue by macrodissection generated mean absolute 40-ddCq differences of 0.28–0.32 cycles for all four markers, with ≥90% concordant binary classifications. The mean raw marker Cq values in the adipose tissue were delayed by 6 to 7 cycles compared with the tumor-enriched sections, adding a trivial linear fold change of 1.0078 to 1.0156. Comparison of specimens enriched for invasive tumor with whole sections with as few as 20% tumor cell content resulted in mean absolute differences that remained on average below 0.59 Cq. The mean absolute difference between whole sections containing up to 60% ductal carcinoma in situ (DCIS) and specimens after dissection of DCIS was only 0.16–0.25 cycles, although there was a tendency for higher gene expression in DCIS. Observed variations were related to small size of samples and proximity of values to the limit of detection.

Conclusion: Expression of *ESR1*, *PGR*, *ERBB2* and *MKI67* by MammaTyper® is robust in clinical FFPE samples. Assay performance was unaffected by adipose tissue and was stable in samples with as few as 20% tumor cell content and up to 60% DCIS.

Keywords: Breast cancer, MammaTyper, RT-qPCR, DCIS, Tumor cell content, Non-neoplastic tissue, Tissue heterogeneity

* Correspondence: kerstin.hartmann@biontech.de
†Kerstin Hartmann and Kornelia Schlombs contributed equally to this work.
[1]BioNTech Diagnostics GmbH, An der Goldgrube 12, 55131 Mainz, Germany
Full list of author information is available at the end of the article

Background

Heterogeneity is an intrinsic property of formalin-fixed paraffin-embedded (FFPE) tumor material from core needle biopsies or resection specimens of breast carcinomas. On hematoxylin and eosin (H&E) stained histological slides, invasive tumor cells are seen in close proximity to other neoplastic or non-neoplastic microanatomical structures such as in situ carcinoma, atypical ductal hyperplasia, non-neoplastic ductulo-lobular structures, and stromal cells, including adipocytes, blood vessels, and other cells of the tumor microenvironment. These morphologically distinct cell types have unique biological and molecular fingerprints [1–4].

During the diagnostic work-up of breast carcinomas, immunohistochemistry (IHC) is the standard method for assessing the expression of estrogen- (ER) and progesterone-receptors (PR), human epidermal growth factor receptor 2 (HER2) as well as of Ki-67 as a marker of tumor cell proliferation. Biomarker studies are routinely performed in order to classify breast carcinomas into prognostic and therapeutic categories [5]. The fact that tissue morphology is preserved on IHC-stained slides makes it possible to assess biomarker expression specifically in the invasive tumor compartment, regardless of heterogeneity. However, IHC requires interpretation of the chromogen signal and semi-quantitative scoring of intensity or proportion of staining, procedures that are both subject to intra- and inter-observer variability and will hence result in discordance rates [6–9].

Quantification of gene expression by reverse transcription-quantitative real-time PCR (RT-qPCR) precludes such subjective interpretation. However, contrary to IHC, RT-qPCR uses RNA extracted from FFPE sections, containing both invasive tumor as well as non-tumorous cells of the tumor microenvironment. Therefore, gene expression data may thus be affected by the presence of heterogeneous cell types whose expression patterns can differ substantially from the invasive tumor [3, 4, 10, 11]. With the advent of molecular subtyping of breast cancer and the clinical endorsement of RNA-based genomic risk scores tissue heterogeneity has to be considered a potential confounder and is usually addressed by assay-specific requirements for "minimum tumor content" [12]. Macrodissection or the more time-consuming microdissection is usually applied to increase tumor cell content (TCC) in the diagnostic setting.

The MammaTyper® is an RT-qPCR-based, CE-marked molecular in vitro diagnostic assay used for categorizing tumor resection specimens and pre-operative core needle biopsies of breast carcinomas into five subtypes (*luminal A-like*, *luminal B-like* (HER2-positive), *luminal B-like* (HER2-negative), *HER2-positive* (non-luminal) and *triple negative* (ductal)) as defined by the 2013 St Gallen consensus [13]. The assay quantifies the mRNA expression of four genes *ERBB2* (HER2), *ESR1* (ER), *PGR* (PR) and *MKI67* (marker of proliferation Ki-67) relative to the mean expression of two reference genes and generates a dichotomous result (positive or negative) based on predefined cut-off values [14].

MammaTyper® may evolve as a valid alternative to IHC. This is supported by the substantial correlation that exists between protein and mRNA expression in general [15] and for breast cancer biomarkers in particular [16–18] and by the desire to increase the reproducibility of biomarker testing, in particular for the assessment of proliferative activity (i.e.Ki-67) [19]. MammaTyper® has shown excellent analytical performance, promising clinical validity both in the adjuvant and neoadjuvant setting, with concordance to IHC documented in more than 800 clinical samples [20–22].

During the assay's technical validation, we have previously studied the robustness of the gene expression assay in the face of tissue heterogeneity [14]. In the present work, we aimed to further examine the impact of tissue heterogeneity on MammaTyper® gene expression by investigating "contamination" at both ends of the histological spectrum. It is commonly assumed that non-neoplastic RNA may solely "dilute" the RT-qPCR signal, whereas in situ carcinoma (i.e.DCIS) may affect results in more complex ways due to its unique transcriptional profiles that differ from that of the invasive tumor [4, 23]. We therefore designed 3 independent experiments to assess the impact of non-neoplastic surrounding tissue on gene expression, in particular adipose tissue and DCIS as well as variations in TCC.

Methods
Sample selection and tissue handling
The study consisted of 49 FFPE resection specimens of invasive breast carcinoma. Thirteen cases were from the Institute of Molecular Gynecological Oncology, Mainz, Germany. The use of archived samples was approved by the ethics committee of the Landesärztekammer Rheinland-Pfalz (837.139.05 (4797)). Thirty one cases were obtained from PATH Biobank (Patients' Tumour Bank of Hope), Munich, Germany [24]. Patients provided individual, written informed consent for the storage of samples and data, follow-up contact, and further use of samples and data for research purposes. The processes of PATH Biobank have been approved by the ethics committee of the medical faculty of the University of Bonn (255/06). Five additional cases were purchased from commercial vendors (Asterand Biosciences, Detroit, USA MI; Proteogenex, Culver City, USA CA).

Histological review was performed on H&E slides by an experienced pathologist who identified and evaluated the percentage of the various tissue components (non-neoplastic tissue, invasive tumor and DCIS). The effect of adipose tissue, tumor cell content (TCC) and DCIS on the results of MammaTyper® for each individual breast cancer marker was investigated in different experiments (Fig. 1). TCC was defined as the planimetric ratio of areas covered by invasive carcinoma in relation to the area covered by DCIS and by non-neoplastic tissue (including connective and necrotic tissue). Because of its paucicellular nature, scar and adipose tissue were not considered as non-neoplastic tissue. The size of the tumor area (mm^2) was calculated using the ZEN2 (blue edition) software from Carl Zeiss Microscopy GmbH 2011.

To study the effect of adipose tissue on gene expression, we selected 10 FFPE samples with surrounding adipose tissue which accounted for at least 50% of the whole section. To exclude effects of other tissue components such as non-neoplastic tissue, only samples with 80 to 100% tumor cell content were used. Furthermore, in order to minimize effects of DCIS on assay results, only samples with less than 10% DCIS content were selected for these experiments (8 samples: 0% DCIS; 2 samples: ≤10% DCIS). In addition to a 10 μm curl representing the whole section, three consecutive 5 μm sections were mounted on glass slides and the invasive tumor area of each slide as well as the adipose tissue were macrodissected and transferred into separate RNase-free tubes for subsequent RNA isolation (Fig. 1, upper panel). Relative expression of the four genes ERBB2, ESR1, PGR and MKI67 in the whole sections was compared with relative gene expression in the dissected invasive tumor and the adipose tissue.

To study the impact of TCC, two 8 μm sections were cut from 15 clinical breast cancer cases with TCC ranging from 20 to 39% ($n = 7$), 40–59% ($n = 5$) and 60–79% ($n = 3$). Like in the experiments on adipose tissue contamination, effects of DCIS on assay results were minimized by selecting only samples with less than 10% DCIS content (9 samples: 0% DCIS; 6 samples: ≤10% DCIS). Sections were mounted on polyethylene naphthalate (PEN) membrane slides, stained with Cresyl violet and enriched up to almost 100% by laser microdissection with a Leica LMD DFC 7000 T (Leica Microsystems) or macrodissection (Fig. 1, middle panel). Sections were then transferred into RNase-free test tubes for subsequent RNA isolation and gene expression studies.

The effect of DCIS on the MammaTyper® results was assessed on 24 FFPE breast cancer samples with DCIS-covered areas ranging from 10 to 60%. The DCIS content was morphologically distinguished from invasive carcinoma via the preservation of the myoepithelial-cell layer, visible by standard H&E staining [25]. From each FFPE sample, three 8 μm sections were prepared for laser microdissection. Circled areas of DCIS from two slides were quantitatively microdissected and combined into an RNase-free tube for RNA isolation. Tissue sections without the microdissected DCIS were transferred in duplicates into RNase-free tubes (Fig. 1, lower panel). Relative expression of the four genes ERBB2, ESR1, PGR and MKI67 were compared between whole sections, whole sections lacking DCIS and microdissected DCIS. Moreover, 3 μm sctions of these same breast cancer samples were immunostained with an anti-Her2/neu antibody (Clone EP3 Epitomics (Quartett, Berlin, Germany, using DAB as

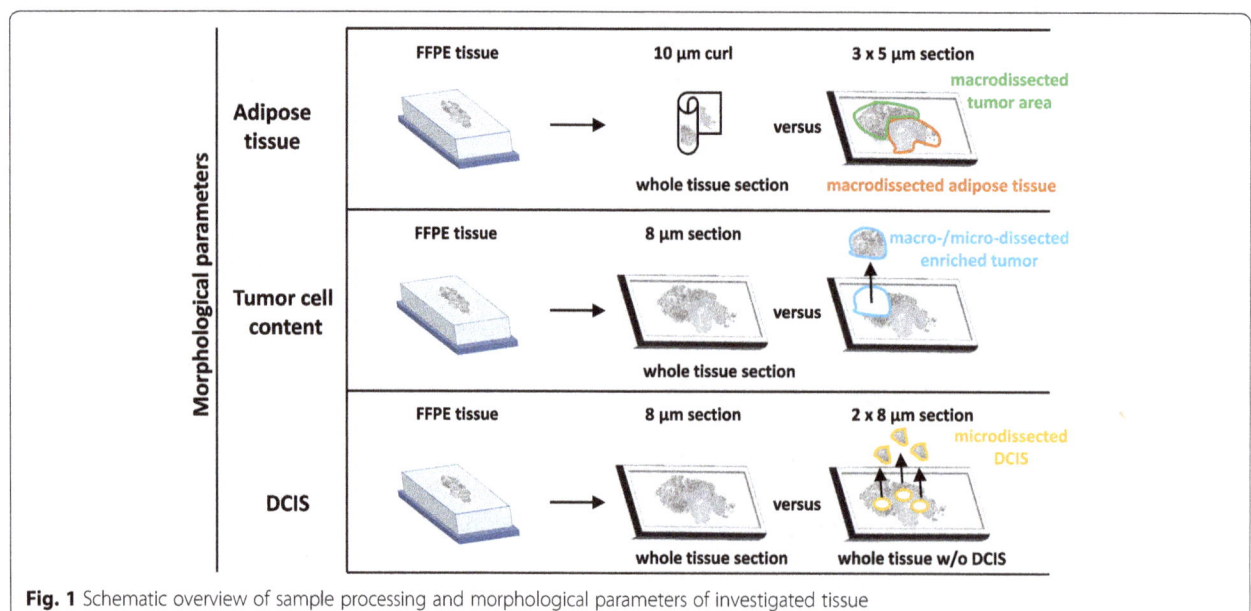

Fig. 1 Schematic overview of sample processing and morphological parameters of investigated tissue

RNA isolation and mRNA quantification via RT-qPCR

Extraction of total RNA from FFPE samples was performed using a CE-marked paramagnetic bead-based method (RNXtract®, BioNTech Diagnostics, Mainz, Germany) according to the manufacturers' instructions. RNA was eluted in 100 µl, 60 µl or 50 µl depending on the amount of input material. The median gene expression levels of both reference genes measured within the MammaTyper® test were used as a quality measure for determining the adequacy of the amount of RNA present in the sample.

The expression levels of *ERBB2*, *ESR1*, *PGR* and *MKI67* were determined by reverse transcription-quantitative real-time PCR (RT-qPCR) using the CE-marked Mamma-Typer® IVD kit (BioNTech Diagnostics, Mainz, Germany) on the LightCycler® 480 II qPCR platform (Roche Diagnostics) according to the manufacturer's instructions (160301–90020-EN Rev. 3.1). Calculations were carried out as described previously [14]. MammaTyper® results are expressed as 40-ddCq values for each marker which represent the gene expression level in the sample relative to the amount of RNA starting material as determined by the reference genes beta-2-microglobulin (*B2M*) and calmodulin 2 (*CALM2*). In addition, each individual marker was scored positive or negative according to clinically validated marker specific cutoffs [20–22]. The following cut-offs were used: *ERBB2* 41.10, *ESR1* 38.00, *PGR* 35.50, *MKI67* 35.90.

Results

Effect of adipose tissue on gene expression studies

Due to the high ratio of cytoplasm over nuclei in adipose tissue, and therefore low cellularity, the differences of 40-ddCq values across the tested pairs of whole sections and samples obtained after removing the surrounding adipose tissue were low. The mean absolute difference (and min/max observed value) was 0.28 cycles for *ERBB2* (0.00–0.64), 0.31 for *ESR1* (0.05–0.70), 0.32 for *PGR* (0.02–0.94), and 0.29 for *MKI67* (0.09–0.59) (Fig. 2, Additional file 1). On average, the difference was even smaller than the typical intra-run variation of 0.5 cycles observed in qPCR experiments (corresponding to a standard deviation (SD) of 0.35 cycles) [26]. The expected SD of Cq values is even higher (0.4 cycles) in the region of the limit of detection (LOD) of a qPCR [27]. The concordance of the binary categories was 100% for *ERBB2*, *ESR1* and *PGR* and 90% for *MKI67* caused by one single case where the initial value was very close to the cut-off (Additional file 1, sample 3). The highest difference (0.94 cycles) was detected in a single case with *PGR* gene expression close to the limit of detection in the dissected (tumor-enriched) sample (Additional file 1, sample 10).

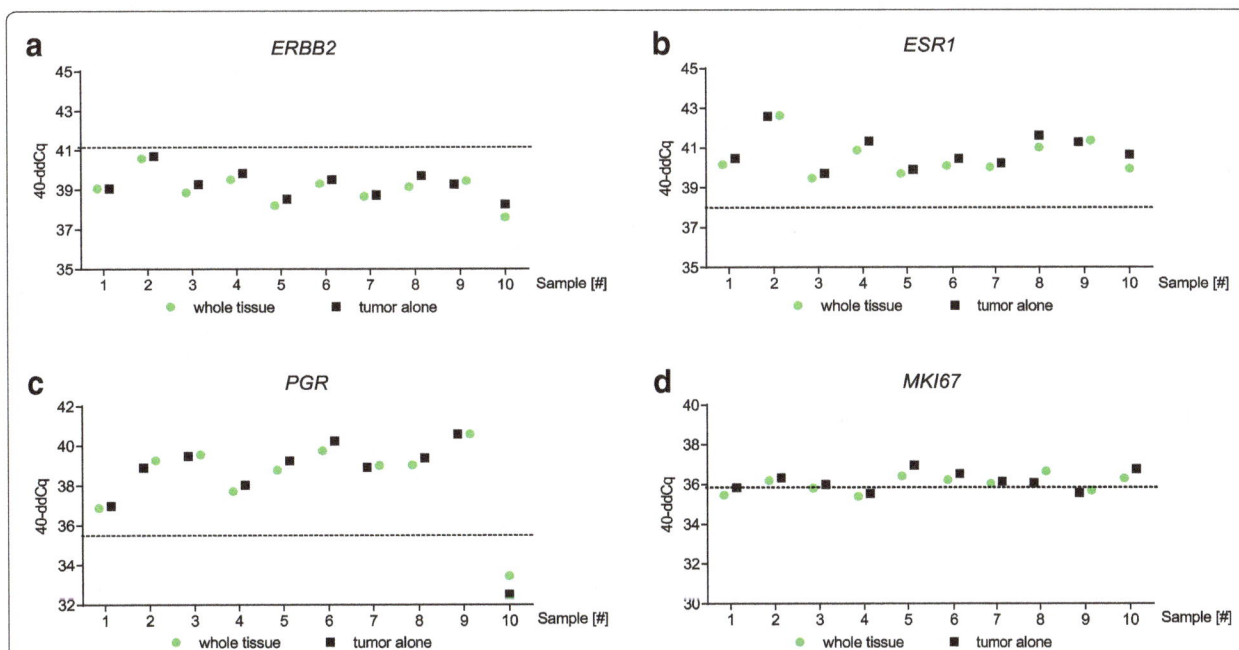

Fig. 2 Effect of adipose tissue on relative gene expression. Shown in the graph are gene expression data of *n* = 10 breast cancer specimen for *ERBB2*(**a**), *ESR1* (**b**), *PGR* (**c**) and *MKI67* (**d**) in whole sections (over 50% adipose tissue content, green circles) versus tumor-enriched sections (blue squares). Dotted lines represent the respective cut-off for the four marker genes (*ERBB2*: 41.10; *ESR1*: 38.00; *PGR*: 35.50; *MKI67*: 35.90)

Table 1 Differences in MammaTyper® relative gene expression between pairs of whole tissue and tumor-enriched specimens

Tumor cell content	Mean (min, max) absolute difference of 40-ddCq of paired measurements			
	ERBB2	ESR1	PGR	MKI67
20–39%	0.49 (0.04 to 0.86)	0.34 (0.01 to 0.80)	0.39 (0.15 to 0.72)	0.58 (0.17 to 1.46)
40–59%	0.38 (0.11 to 0.65)	0.53 (0.08 to 1.15)	0.49 (0.28 to 0.68)	0.58 (0.33 to 1.28)
60–79%	0.24 (0.15 to 0.30)	0.40 (0.22 to 0.50)	0.16 (0.04 to 0.23)	0.09 (0.01 to 0.23)

Four out of 10 macrodissected adipose-enriched tissue samples had invalid MammaTyper® results, because the RNA yield was poor, as evidenced by the very low expression levels of the reference genes. In the remaining 6 samples, the results were valid but borderline, with reference Cq values close to the limit of detection. The signal of the reference genes in the pooled adipose tissue was detected on average 4 cycles later than the signal from the invasive tumor area. Regarding the marker genes, the mean raw Cq values in the adipose tissue pools were delayed by 6 to 7 cycles compared with the tumor-enriched tissue, corresponding to a 2^{-6} to 2^{-7} change adding a linear fold change of 1.0156 or 1.0078, respectively. This results in a negligible Cq change of −0.011 to −0.022 (Additional file 2).

Effect of tumor cell content on gene expression studies

The mean absolute difference in relative gene expression between samples before and after enrichment for invasive tumor was low (< 0.59 Cq) (Table 1 and Fig. 3). In 7 out of 60 measurements (11.7%) the single marker results showed an absolute difference which was higher than 0.70 Cq, the typical intra-run variation (2x SD of 0.35 cycles) observed in experiments with qPCR [26]. These deviations were particularly observed in 4 very small samples with a tumor area less than or equal to 25 mm^2 (Additional file 3) and showed raw Cq values close to the LOD for some markers.

The binary categories were discordant in 3 MKI67 cases, having 40-ddCq values adjacent to the cut-off (Additional file 3, sample 5, 8 and 9). As a consequence,

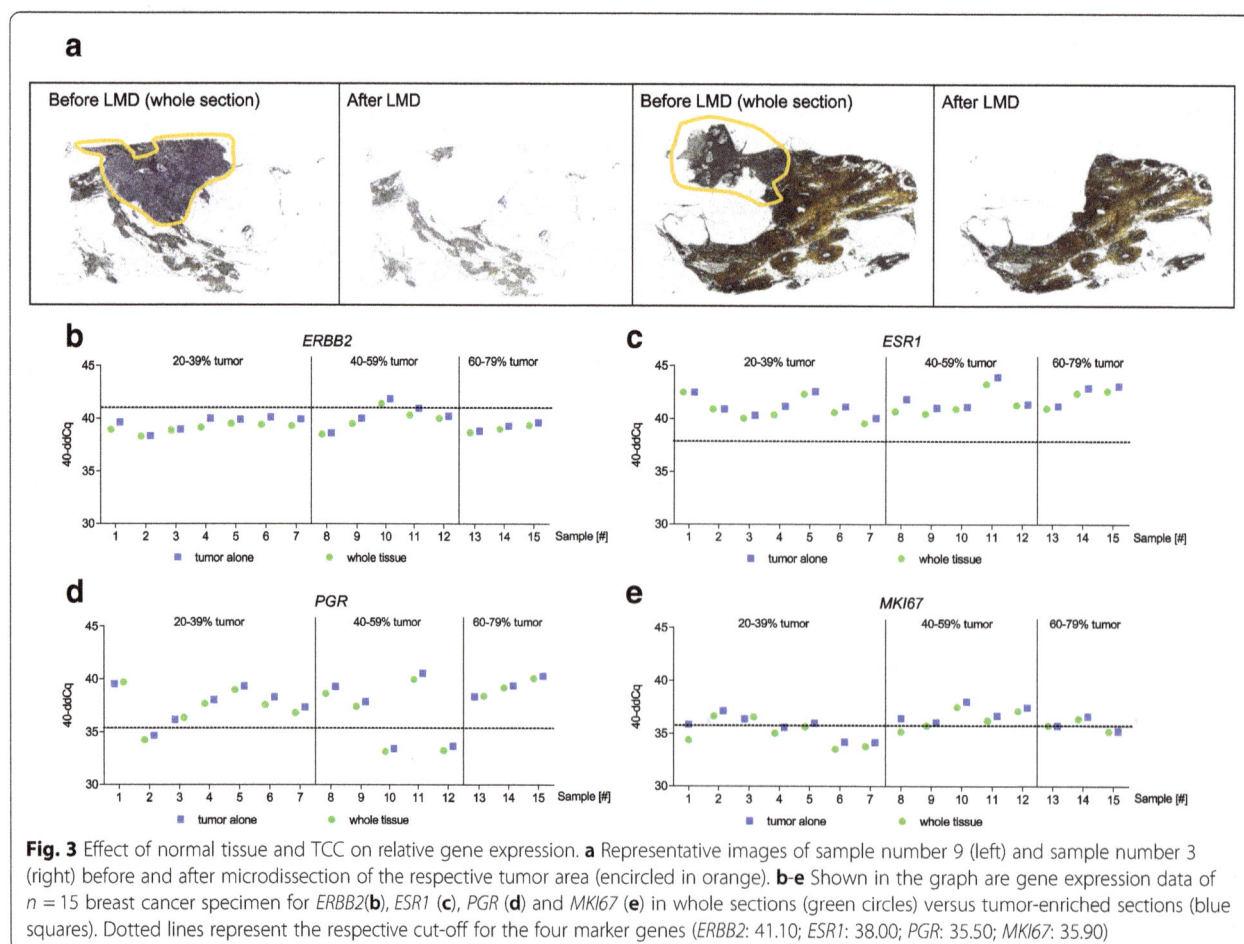

Fig. 3 Effect of normal tissue and TCC on relative gene expression. **a** Representative images of sample number 9 (left) and sample number 3 (right) before and after microdissection of the respective tumor area (encircled in orange). **b-e** Shown in the graph are gene expression data of n = 15 breast cancer specimen for ERBB2(**b**), ESR1 (**c**), PGR (**d**) and MKI67 (**e**) in whole sections (green circles) versus tumor-enriched sections (blue squares). Dotted lines represent the respective cut-off for the four marker genes (ERBB2: 41.10; ESR1: 38.00; PGR: 35.50; MKI67: 35.90)

Table 2 Characteristics of tissue samples used for the analysis of DCIS on relative gene expression

Sample #	Tumor cell content [%]	DCIS content [%]	HER2 status (IHC)	
			invasive tumor	DCIS
1	40–59	**10–19**	3+	3+
2	60–79		3+	3+
3	80–100		3+	3+
4	80–100		n.a.	n.a.
5	20–39		2+	2+
6	60–79		**2+**	**3+**
7	60–79	**20–29**	0	0
8	60–79		0	0
9	40–59		**0**	**1+**
10	40–59		0	0
11	20–39		1+	1+
12	40–59		1+	1+
13	40–59		**1+**	**2+**
14	40–59		0	0
15	60–79		n.a.	n.a.
16	60–79		1+	1+
17	20–39	**30–39**	**0**	**1+**
18	20–39		**2+**	**3+**
19	20–39		0	0
20	20–39		**1+**	**2+**
21	40–59	**40–49**	1+	1+
22	20–39	**50–60**	**1+**	**2+**
23	20–39		**1+**	**2+**
24	40–59		1+	1+

Different scores of HER2 protein expression in DCIS and corresponding invasive tumor are shown in bold

3 *Luminal A-like* samples, one with 20–39% TCC and 2 with a TCC of 40–59% were re-classified as *Luminal B-like* (*HER2-negative*) after tumor enrichment. The pairs of dissected and non-dissected samples for the other markers showed a concordance rate of 100%.

Effect of variable extent of DCIS on gene expression studies

Sample characteristics used for this gene expression study are summarized in Table 2.

40-ddCq differences across the tested pairs of whole tissue and microdissected tumor samples without DCIS were low for all four genes (Fig. 4). The mean absolute difference was 0.16 Cq for *ERBB2* (0.00 to 0.79 Cq), 0.25 for *ESR1* (0.00 to 0.61 Cq), 0.18 for *PGR* (0.01 to 0.80) and 0.24 for *MKI67* (0.03 to 0.63 Cq) (Additional file 4). When DCIS-only samples were separately analyzed, expression profiles tended to be higher (compared to

invasive tumor), exceeding the generally accepted intra-run variation of 0.70 cycles in 18/22 cases for *ERBB2* (81.8%), in 19/22 cases for *ESR1* (86.4%), in 14/22 cases for *PGR* (63.6%) and in 11/22 cases for *MKI67* (50.0%). In four cases (Table 2, samples 6, 9, 17 and 18), HER2 protein expression by immunohistochemistry showed a similar trend towards higher scores in DCIS as the one observed for gene expression studies (Fig. 4b and Table 2). This trend can be especially seen in cases that turn from 2+ (invasive tumor) to 3+ (DCIS) and from 0 (invasive tumor) to 1+ (DCIS). In 2 of 24 DCIS-only samples, gene expression studies were invalid due to insufficient RNA yield.

Discussion

The gene expression profiles of prognostic and predictive biomarkers in breast cancer likely differ between invasive carcinoma, non-invasive carcinoma (e.g. DCIS), non-neoplastic ductulo-lobular units, and adjacent or intervening stroma. Whole FFPE sections of breast cancinomas contain variable amounts of such tissue "contaminants". In this study, we investigated the robustness of MammaTyper®, an RT-qPCR-based gene-expression assay for *ERBB2*, *ESR1*, *PGR* and *MKI67* against heterogeneity due to various tissue types. We first focused on the surrounding adipose tissue, which can easily be removed by macrodissection. By measuring the expression of reference genes we showed that the total RNA obtained from adipose tissue was on average more than 10-fold lower (3.5 Cqs) than the RNA isolated from equal volumes of invasive tumor tissue, frequently falling below the limit of detection. Even when adipose tissue occupied more than 50% of the slide area, deviations of gene expression between whole sections and sections lacking the surrounding tissue fell in the range of intra-run variance.

The observation that adipose tissue contains far less RNA than similarly sized tumor tissue is explained by the fact that adipocytes have very small nucleocytoplasmic ratios (small nuclei, voluminous cytoplasm) [28]. By contrast, cancer cells tend to exhibit a particularly high nucleocytoplasmic ratio due to their increased DNA content and reduced specialized cytoplasmic organelles. Hence, invasive tumor areas have significantly more nuclei per mm^2 than surrounding non-malignant breast tissue and thus considerably larger amounts of nucleic acids. Our experiments indicate that this phenomenon is so pronounced as to trivialize the impact of RNA derived from adipose tissue on the total RNA yield of the non-dissected whole sections. The fact that RNA yields from normal breast tissue which consists largely of adipose and paucicellular fibrous tissue are often insufficient is well known and poses a challenge for studies requiring adequate non-neoplastic control material [4, 29].

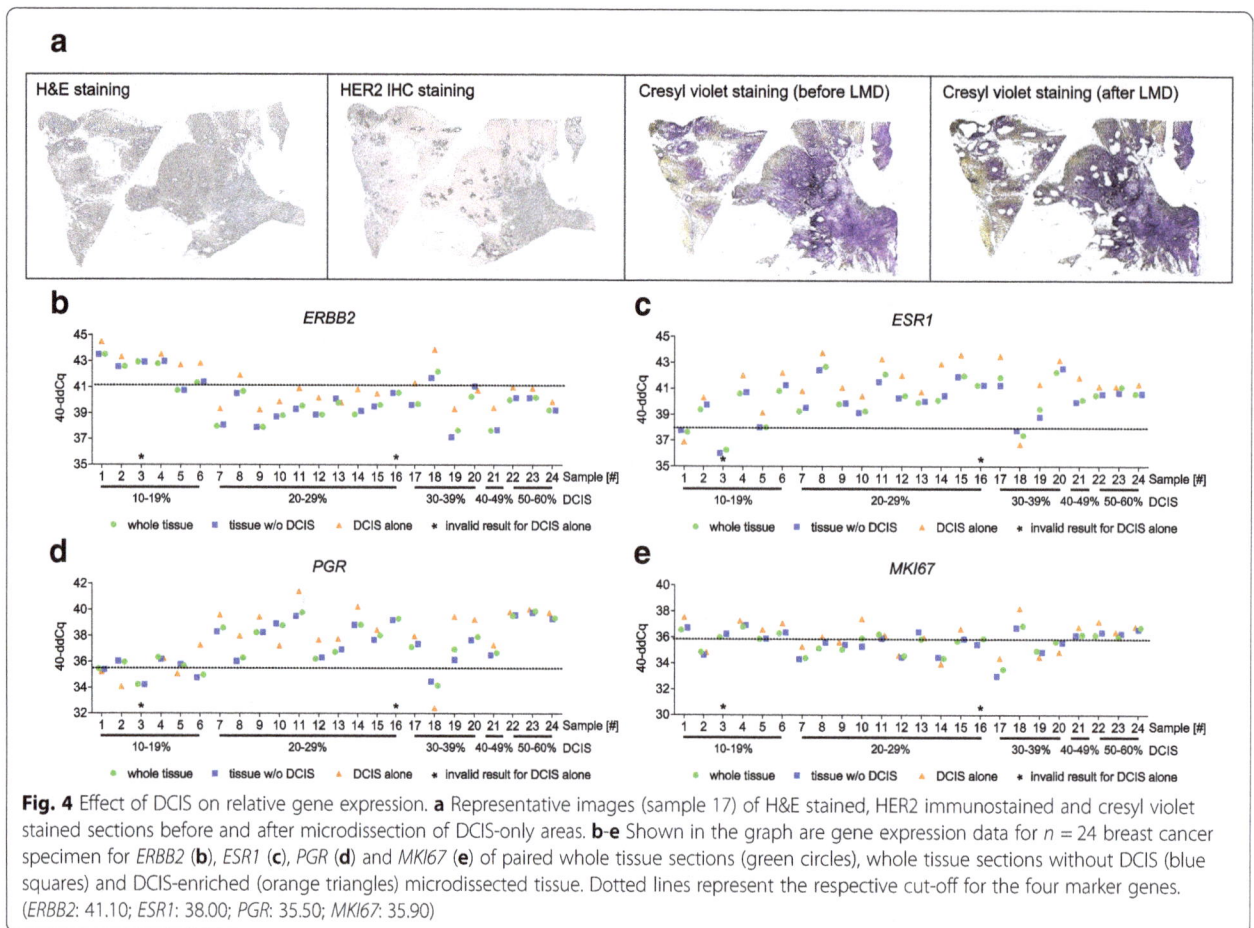

Fig. 4 Effect of DCIS on relative gene expression. **a** Representative images (sample 17) of H&E stained, HER2 immunostained and cresyl violet stained sections before and after microdissection of DCIS-only areas. **b-e** Shown in the graph are gene expression data for n = 24 breast cancer specimen for ERBB2 (**b**), ESR1 (**c**), PGR (**d**) and MKI67 (**e**) of paired whole tissue sections (green circles), whole tissue sections without DCIS (blue squares) and DCIS-enriched (orange triangles) microdissected tissue. Dotted lines represent the respective cut-off for the four marker genes. (ERBB2: 41.10; ESR1: 38.00; PGR: 35.50; MKI67: 35.90)

Due to the negligible influence of adipose tissue on gene expression for ERBB2, ESR1, PGR and MKI67, this component was disregarded for the calculations of the TCC. In the respective experiments, we found that changes in the relative gene expression were insignificant down to 20–39% TCC. This is in agreement with data reported by Tramm and coworkers, who showed an excellent agreement between gene expression data for ESR1, PGR and ERBB2 from whole tissue and from macrodissected extracts [30]. Likewise, macrodissection did not affect the prognostic significance of RNA expression of cancer-associated genes in primary breast tumor samples [12]. Moreover, Viale and coworkers showed that discordances between RNA microarray readouts and IHC/FISH for ER, PGR and HER2 in the MINDACT trial could not be explained by intratumoral heterogeneity or the presence of either DCIS or normal tissue [31]. In line with that, other breast cancer assays, like the GeneXpert Breast Cancer STRAT4 assay from Cepheid, that also measures the expression levels of ERBB2, ESR1, PGR and MKI67, found that macrodissection of whole tissue sections is not required for accurate assessment of these genes by RT-qPCR [32].

Contrary to the findings from studies looking at the effect of TCC on the expression of individual genes,

Elloumi and coworkers found that multi-gene genomic scores were susceptible to contamination of RNA eluates by normal breast tissue [33]. However, specimen volume was not normalized, which may explain why the impact of non-tumor tissue on the expression levels of the genes of interest may have been overestimated in their study. Along the same line of reasoning, first results for the Prosigna® gene signature were unstable if samples contained more than 60–70% surrounding non-tumor tissue [34]. The question whether multigene risk predictors are sensitive or not to variations of TCC is hence related to factors like test design and gene-specific ratios of tumor-vs-normal expression.

Data from studies with complex multigene predictors may not adequately address the impact of TCC on gene expression, as they depend on specificities of different genes and their particular mode of expression in different tissue compartments. For example, the outcome estimations based on MMP7, a gene which encodes for an enzyme that degrades extracellular proteins, were discordant before and after macrodissection [2], most likely because RNA expression of MMP7 is higher in stroma compared to tumor cells [35]. Conversely, ERa, the clinically relevant isoform of the estrogen receptor is confined to epithelial cells of the breast and is not expressed in mammary fibroblasts [36]. Thus, the impact of TCC on RNA relative quantification is gene-specific and as far as MammaTyper® genes *ERBB2, ESR1, PGR* and *MKI67* are concerned the bias introduced by the inclusion of tissue surrounding the invasive tumor appears to be non-critical.

The present study underscores the fact that caution must be applied when analyzing samples that are critically small in size and hence yield only low amounts of RNA. Depending on how close the respective value lies to the limit of detection, gene expression may be affected by tumor cell enrichment.

It is well documented that gene expression patterns and molecular breast cancer subtypes may vary considerably between invasive tumor and DCIS [4, 23]. In keeping with diagnostic anatomo-pathological experience, the relative expression of *ERBB2, ESR1, PGR* and *MKI67* in our study was often higher in DCIS samples than in samples enriched for invasive carcinomas. Why DCIS is nevertheless only a weak contaminant may be explained by the reduced cellularity of DCIS vs. invasive carcinomas due to cribriform and clinging architecture as well as central necrosis. Others have previously shown that the mean RNA recovery from DCIS was substantially lower than that of invasive tumor of similar volume [1-4]. Thus, it appears that DCIS does not bias gene expression of *ERBB2, ESR1, PGR* and *MKI67* because the contributory gene expression of DCIS is diluted.

Compared to previous work exploring the significance of TCC on the stability of gene expression assays, our present study has the advantage of addressing biological diversity of whole sections which underlies the apparent histological heterogeneity. Eventually, whether surrounding adipose tissue, normal tissue adjacent to tumor or admixed DCIS, the RT-qPCR signal is dominated by the invasive tumor component, allowing for consistent calculations in whole sections with up to 60% DCIS and in a TCC range of 20–100%. This TCC range remains sufficient even if the tissue area excluding adipose tissue occupies less than 50% of the whole section, indicating that macrodissection of surrounding adipose tissue is not required. Moreover, by using archived material from actual patient cases, our data are meaningful for use in a real-life routine pathology diagnostic setting.

Conclusion

Our data indicate that MammaTyper® is capable of tolerating low-purity input material with a minimum TCC of 20%. Based on these thresholds, the assay can be used for the robust quantification of *ERBB2, ESR1, PGR* and *MKI67* on whole sections of FFPE samples during routine histopathological work-up of breast carcinoma.

Additional files

Additional file 1: MammaTyper® relative gene expression and Δ40-ddCq values are shown for the effect of adipose tissue.

Additional file 2: MammaTyper® Median Cq values are shown for the effect of adipose tissue.

Additional file 3: MammaTyper® relative gene expression and Δ40-ddCq values are shown for the effect of TCC.

Additional file 4: MammaTyper® relative gene expression and Δ40-ddCq values are shown for the effect of DCIS. Tumor cell content, DCIS content, HER2 immunohistochemical score of the invasive tumor and the DCIS, as well as relative expression of the mRNA markers *ERBB2, ESR1, PGR* and *MKI67* and absolute Δ40-ddCq values are shown.

Abbreviations
B2M: beta-2-microglobulin; CALM2: calmodulin 2; Cq: quantification cycle; DCIS: ductal carcinoma in situ; ER: estrogen receptor; ERBB2: human epidermal growth factor receptor 2; ESR1: estrogen receptor 1; FFPE: formalin-fixed paraffin-embedded; H&E: hematoxylin and eosin; HER2: human epidermal growth factor receptor 2; IHC: immunohistochemistry; IVD: in vitro diagnostic; LMD: laser microdissection; MKI67: marker of proliferation Ki-67; mRNA: messenger RNA; PEN: polyethylene naphthalate; PGR: progesterone receptor; PR: progesterone receptor; RT-qPCR: reverse transcription-quantitative real time PCR; TCC: tumor cell content

Acknowledgements
We gratefully acknowledge Dr. Jeanette Reimann-Kreft for support with the tumor cell content evaluation and residual tissue classification of the breast cancer samples and Susanne Gebhardt (University clinic Mainz, Germany) for kind selection of tissue samples from breast cancer patients. We thank Sotirios Lakis for critical review and improvement of the manuscript. In addition, we thank Lukas Krimmer, Katharina Kaiser and Daniela Weiser (BioNTech Diagnostics GmbH, Mainz, Germany), as well as Regina Dorin (Friedrichshafen) for excellent technical assistance.

Funding
Not applicable.

Authors' contributions
KH reviewed the histomorphologic and immunohistochemical data and helped draft the manuscript. KS analyzed the MammaTyper® data and KS, ML, CG, US helped draft the manuscript. KH, ML collected the tissue samples. MS reviewed the manuscript and provided tissue samples. HAL conceived, designed, and coordinated the study, analyzed the Her2 immunohistochemical data and helped draft the manuscript. All authors read and approved the final manuscript.

Ethics approval and consent to participate
The study consisted of 49 human FFPE invasive breast carcinoma samples. Thirteen cases were derived from the Institute of Molecular Gynecological Oncology, Mainz, Germany. The use of archived samples was approved by the ethics committee of the Landesärztekammer Rheinland-Pfalz (837.139.05 (4797)). Thirty one cases were obtained from PATH Biobank (Patients' Tumour Bank of Hope), Munich, Germany [24]. Patients provided individual, written informed consent for the storage of samples and data, follow-up contact, and further use of samples and data for research purposes. The processes of PATH Biobank have been approved by the ethics committee of the medical faculty of the University of Bonn (255/06). Five additional cases were purchased from commercial vendors (Asterand Biosciences, Detroit, USA MI; Proteogenex, Culver City, USA CA).

Competing interests

US is founder and CEO of BioNTech Diagnostics GmbH. KH, KS, ML and CG are employees of BioNTech Diagnostics GmbH. MS and HAL declare that they have no competing interests.

Author details

[1]BioNTech Diagnostics GmbH, An der Goldgrube 12, 55131 Mainz, Germany. [2]Department of Obstetrics and Gynecology, Johannes Gutenberg University, Langenbeckstraße 1, 55131 Mainz, Germany. [3]BioNTech AG, An der Goldgrube 12, 55131 Mainz, Germany. [4]Institute of Pathology, Medizin Campus Bodensee, Röntgenstraße 2, 88048 Friedrichshafen, Germany.

References

1. Finak G, Bertos N, Pepin F, Sadekova S, Souleimanova M, Zhao H, et al. Stromal gene expression predicts clinical outcome in breast cancer. Nat Med. 2008;14:518–27. https://doi.org/10.1038/nm1764 .

2. Kotoula V, Kalogeras KT, Kouvatseas G, Televantou D, Kronenwett R, Wirtz RM, et al. Sample parameters affecting the clinical relevance of RNA biomarkers in translational breast cancer research. Virchows Arch. 2012;462: 141–54. https://doi.org/10.1007/s00428-012-1357-1 .

3. Ma X-J, Dahiya S, Richardson E, Erlander M, Sgroi DC. Gene expression profiling of the tumor microenvironment during breast cancer progression. Breast Cancer Res. 2009;11. https://doi.org/10.1186/bcr2222 .

4. Schobesberger M, Baltzer A, Oberli A, Kappeler A, Gugger M, Burger H, et al. Gene expression variation between distinct areas of breast cancer measured from paraffin-embedded tissue cores. BMC Cancer. 2008;8. https://doi.org/10.1186/1471-2407-8-343 .

5. Hagemann IS. Molecular testing in breast Cancer: a guide to current practices. Arch Pathol Lab Med. 2016;140:815–24. https://doi.org/10.5858/arpa.2016-0051-RA .

6. Hammond ME, Hayes DF, Dowsett M, Allred DC, Hagerty KL, Badve S, et al. American Society of Clinical Oncology/College of American Pathologists guideline recommendations for immunohistochemical testing of estrogen and progesterone receptors in breast cancer. Arch Pathol Lab Med. 2010; 134:907–22. https://doi.org/10.1043/1543-2165-134.6.907 .

7. Polley MY, Leung SC, McShane LM, Gao D, Hugh JC, Mastropasqua MG, et al. An international Ki67 reproducibility study. J Natl Cancer Inst. 2013;105: 1897–906. https://doi.org/10.1093/jnci/djt306 .

8. Rakha EA, Pinder SE, Bartlett JM, Ibrahim M, Starczynski J, Carder PJ, et al. Updated UK recommendations for HER2 assessment in breast cancer. J Clin Pathol. 2015;68:93–9. https://doi.org/10.1136/jclinpath-2014-202571 .

9. Varga Z, Diebold J, Dommann-Scherrer C, Frick H, Kaup D, Noske A, et al. How reliable is Ki-67 immunohistochemistry in grade 2 breast carcinomas? A QA study of the Swiss working Group of Breast- and Gynecopathologists. PLoS One. 2012;7:e37379. https://doi.org/10.1371/journal.pone.0037379 .

10. Graham K, Ge X, de las Morenas A, Tripathi A, Rosenberg CL. Gene expression profiles of estrogen receptor-positive and estrogen receptor-negative breast cancers are detectable in histologically Normal breast epithelium. Clin Cancer Res. 2010;17:236–46. https://doi.org/10.1158/1078-0432.ccr-10-1369 .

11. Ma XJ, Salunga R, Tuggle JT, Gaudet J, Enright E, McQuary P, et al. Gene expression profiles of human breast cancer progression. Proc Natl Acad Sci. 2003;100:5974–9. https://doi.org/10.1073/pnas.0931261100 .

12. Poremba C, Uhlendorff J, Pfitzner BM, Hennig G, Bohmann K, Bojar H, et al. Preanalytical variables and performance of diagnostic RNA-based gene expression analysis in breast cancer. Virchows Arch. 2014;465:409–17. https://doi.org/10.1007/s00428-014-1652-0 .

13. Goldhirsch A, Winer EP, Coates AS, Gelber RD, Piccart-Gebhart M, Thurlimann B, et al. Personalizing the treatment of women with early breast cancer: highlights of the St Gallen international expert consensus on the primary therapy of early breast Cancer 2013. Ann Oncol. 2013;24:2206–23. https://doi.org/10.1093/annonc/mdt303 .

14. Laible M, Schlombs K, Kaiser K, Veltrup E, Herlein S, Lakis S, et al. Technical validation of an RT-qPCR in vitro diagnostic test system for the determination of breast cancer molecular subtypes by quantification of ERBB2, ESR1, PGR and MKI67 mRNA levels from formalin-fixed paraffin-embedded breast tumor specimens. BMC Cancer. 2016;16. https://doi.org/10.1186/s12885-016-2476-x .

15. Schwanhäusser B, Busse D, Li N, Dittmar G, Schuchhardt J, Wolf J, et al. Global quantification of mammalian gene expression control. Nature. 2011; 473:337–42. https://doi.org/10.1038/nature10098 .

16. Fountzilas G, Christodoulou C, Bobos M, Kotoula V, Eleftheraki AG, Xanthakis I, et al. Topoisomerase II alpha gene amplification is a favorable prognostic factor in patients with HER2-positive metastatic breast cancer treated with trastuzumab. J Transl Med. 2012;10:212. https://doi.org/10.1186/1479-5876-10-212 .

17. Schleifman EB, Desai R, Spoerke JM, Xiao Y, Wong C, Abbas I, et al. Targeted biomarker profiling of matched primary and metastatic estrogen receptor positive breast cancers. PLoS One. 2014;9:e88401. https://doi.org/10.1371/journal.pone.0088401 .

18. Wilson TR, Xiao Y, Spoerke JM, Fridlyand J, Koeppen H, Fuentes E, et al. Development of a robust RNA-based classifier to accurately determine ER, PR, and HER2 status in breast cancer clinical samples. Breast Cancer Res Treat. 2014;148:315–25. https://doi.org/10.1007/s10549-014-3163-8 .

19. Duffy MJ, Harbeck N, Nap M, Molina R, Nicolini A, Senkus E, et al. Clinical use of biomarkers in breast cancer: updated guidelines from the European group on tumor markers (EGTM). Eur J Cancer. 2017;75:284–98. https://doi.org/10.1016/j.ejca.2017.01.017 .

20. Sinn H-P, Schneeweiss A, Keller M, Schlombs K, Laible M, Seitz J, et al. Comparison of immunohistochemistry with PCR for assessment of ER, PR, and Ki-67 and prediction of pathological complete response in breast cancer. BMC Cancer. 2017;17. https://doi.org/10.1186/s12885-017-3111-1 .

21. Varga Z, Lebeau A, Bu H, Hartmann A, Penault-Llorca F, Guerini-Rocco E, et al. An international reproducibility study validating quantitative determination of ERBB2, ESR1, PGR, and MKI67 mRNA in breast cancer using MammaTyper®. Breast Cancer Res. 2017;19. https://doi.org/10.1186/s13058-017-0848-z .

22. Wirtz RM, Sihto H, Isola J, Heikkilä P, Kellokumpu-Lehtinen P-L, Auvinen P, et al. Biological subtyping of early breast cancer: a study comparing RT-qPCR with immunohistochemistry. Breast Cancer Res Treat. 2016;157:437–46. https://doi.org/10.1007/s10549-016-3835-7 .

23. Tamimi RM, Baer HJ, Marotti J, Galan M, Galaburda L, Fu Y, et al. Comparison of molecular phenotypes of ductal carcinoma in situand invasive breast cancer. Breast Cancer Res. 2008;10. https://doi.org/10.1186/bcr2128 .

24. Waldmann A, Anzeneder T, Katalinic A. Patients and methods of the PATH biobank - a resource for breast Cancer research. Geburtshilfe Frauenheilkd. 2014;74:361–9. https://doi.org/10.1055/s-0033-1360263 .

25. Pandey PR. Role of myoepithelial cells in breast tumor progression. Front Biosci. 2010;15:226. https://doi.org/10.2741/3617 .

26. Kennedy S, Oswald N. PCR troubleshooting and optimization : the essential guide. Norfolk, UK: Caister Academic Press; 2011. vii, 235 p, 4 p. of plates p.

27. Stahlberg A, Kubista M. The workflow of single-cell expression profiling using quantitative real-time PCR. Expert Rev Mol Diagn. 2014;14:323–31. https://doi.org/10.1586/14737159.2014.901154 .

28. LCUa J, Carneiro J. Basic histology. 11th ed. New York, USA: McGraw Hill; 2005. p. 123–7.

29. Mee BC, Carroll P, Donatello S, Connolly E, Griffin M, Dunne B, et al. Maintaining breast Cancer specimen integrity and individual or simultaneous extraction of quality DNA, RNA, and proteins from Allprotect-stabilized and nonstabilized tissue samples. Biopreservation and Biobanking. 2011;9:389–98. https://doi.org/10.1089/bio.2011.0034 .

30. Tramm T, Hennig G, Kyndi M, Alsner J, Sørensen FB, Myhre S, et al. Reliable PCR quantitation of estrogen, progesterone and ERBB2 receptor mRNA from formalin-fixed, paraffin-embedded tissue is independent of prior macro-dissection. Virchows Arch. 2013;463:775–86. https://doi.org/10.1007/s00428-013-1486-1 .

31. Viale G, Slaets L, De Snoo F, van 't Veer LJ, Rutgers EJ, Bogaerts J, et al. Comparison of molecular (BluePrint and MammaPrint) and pathological subtypes for breast cancer among the first 800 patients from the EORTC 10041/BIG 3-04 (MINDACT) trial. J Clin Oncol. 2012;30:32. https://doi.org/10.1200/jco.2012.30.27_suppl.32 .

32. Elloumi F, Hu Z, Li Y, Parker JS, Gulley ML, Amos KD, et al. Systematic Bias in genomic classification due to contaminating non-neoplastic tissue in breast tumor samples. BMC Med Genet. 2011;4. https://doi.org/10.1186/1755-8794-4-54 .

33. Gupta S, Mani NR, Carvajal-Hausdorf DE, Bossuyt V, Ho K, Weidler J, et al. Macrodissection prior to closed system RT-qPCR is not necessary for estrogen receptor and HER2 concordance with IHC/FISH in breast cancer. Lab Investig. 2018. https://doi.org/10.1038/s41374-018-0064-1 .

34. Nielsen T, Wallden B, Schaper C, Ferree S, Liu S, Gao D, et al. Analytical validation of the PAM50-based Prosigna breast Cancer prognostic gene signature assay and nCounter analysis system using formalin-fixed paraffin-embedded breast tumor specimens. BMC Cancer. 2014;14. https://doi.org/10.1186/1471-2407-14-177 .

35. Kohrmann A, Kammerer U, Kapp M, Dietl J, Anacker J. Expression of matrix metalloproteinases (MMPs) in primary human breast cancer and breast cancer cell lines: new findings and review of the literature. BMC Cancer. 2009;9:188. https://doi.org/10.1186/1471-2407-9-188 .

36. Palmieri C, Saji S, Sakaguchi H, Cheng G, Sunters A, O'Hare MJ, et al. The expression of oestrogen receptor (ER)-beta and its variants, but not ERalpha, in adult human mammary fibroblasts. J Mol Endocrinol. 2004;33:35–50 https://www.ncbi.nlm.nih.gov/pubmed/15291741.

19

Automatic evaluation of tumor budding in immunohistochemically stained colorectal carcinomas and correlation to clinical outcome

Cleo-Aron Weis[1*], Jakob Nikolas Kather[2], Susanne Melchers[3], Hanaa Al-ahmdi[1], Marion J. Pollheimer[4], Cord Langner[4] and Timo Gaiser[1]

Abstract

Background: Tumor budding, meaning a detachment of tumor cells at the invasion front of colorectal carcinoma (CRC) into single cells or clusters (<=5 tumor cells), has been shown to correlate to an inferior clinical outcome by several independent studies. Therefore, it has been discussed as a complementary prognostic factor to the TNM staging system, and it is already included in national guidelines as an additional prognostic parameter. However, its application by manual evaluation in routine pathology is hampered due to the use of several slightly different assessment systems, a time-consuming manual counting process and a high inter-observer variability. Hence, we established and validated an automatic image processing approach to reliably quantify tumor budding in immunohistochemically (IHC) stained sections of CRC samples.

Methods: This approach combines classical segmentation methods (like morphological operations) and machine learning techniques (k-means and hierarchical clustering, convolutional neural networks) to reliably detect tumor buds in colorectal carcinoma samples immunohistochemically stained for pan-cytokeratin. As a possible application, we tested it on whole-slide images as well as on tissue microarrays (TMA) from a clinically well-annotated CRC cohort.

Results: Our automatic tumor budding evaluation tool detected the absolute number of tumor buds per image with a very good correlation to the manually segmented ground truth (R2 value of 0.86).
Furthermore the automatic evaluation of whole-slide images from 20 CRC-patients, we found that neither the detected number of tumor buds at the invasion front nor the number in hotspots was associated with the nodal status. However, the number of spatial clusters of tumor buds (budding hotspots) significantly correlated to the nodal status (p-value = 0.003 for N0 vs. N1/N2). TMAs were not feasible for tumor budding evaluation, as the spatial relationship of tumor buds (especially hotspots) was not preserved.

Conclusions: Automatic image processing is a feasible and valid assessment tool for tumor budding in CRC on whole-slide images. Interestingly, only the spatial clustering of the tumor buds in hotspots (and especially the number of hotspots) and not the absolute number of tumor buds showed a clinically relevant correlation with patient outcome in our data.

Keywords: Colorectal carcinoma, Digital pathology, Tumor budding, Image processing, Convolutional neural network

* Correspondence: cleo-aron.weis@medma.uni-heidelberg.de
[1]Institute of Pathology, University Medical Centre Mannheim, University of Heidelberg, 68167 Mannheim, Germany
Full list of author information is available at the end of the article

Declaration of presentation of findings at a conference

This study was presented in part at the 101st annual meeting of the German Society of Pathology (DGP) in Berlin, Germany in May 2018 and will be presented at the 30th European Congress of Pathology in Bilbao, Spain, in September 2018.

Background

Tumor budding as an additional prognostic parameter in colorectal cancer

The most commonly applied clinicopathological staging system for colorectal cancer (CRC), which is one of the most frequent solid tumors worldwide [1], is the T (tumor) N (lymph nodes) M (metastases) staging system, which classifies tumors based on primary tumor extension, regional nodal involvement and the absence or presence of metastases [2, 3].

Despite this complex and multivariate staging system, there is still room for improvement. On one hand, cases with a low T or N stage sometimes show distant metastasis, while on the other hand, high T or N stage tumors can exhibit an uneventful clinical course [4–6]. For cases classified as intermediate according to TNM, prognostic statements are nearly impossible. It is therefore generally agreed that new features or molecular markers allowing a better stratification are necessary [6].

One morphological feature that is discussed to close this gap is the concept of tumor budding, which goes back to the 1950s, when Imai postulated the existence and biological relevance of detachment of tumor cells at the invasion front [7]. For this feature—despite the different concepts around how to define tumor budding, the problem of how to evaluate budding and the huge inter-observer variance—many studies in general, and in particular for CRC [8], have been able to show a correlation to clinical outcome and to the likelihood of nodal positivity [9, 10].

Different tumor budding definitions and assessment approaches

The morphological feature "tumor budding" was first described in the 1950s and showed a correlation to clinical outcome in many studies with different analytical approaches (e.g., visual assessment vs. image processing) [4, 5, 7, 9–13], especially in colorectal carcinoma. This is notable since the definition of tumor buds is not trivial and there have been many discussions about how to assess budding.

Most research projects on tumor budding in CRC defined a tumor bud as a cluster of a few (in most studies less than 5 neighboring cells) poorly or dedifferentiated tumor cells in the desmoplastic stroma that are detached from larger tumor islands. This more or less arbitrary

definition goes back to works from Gabbert et al. [14] and Hase et al. [8]. They defined tumor buds as clusters of tumor cells with a distinct morphology that could be described as epithelial-mesenchymal transition or focal dedifferentiation [14, 15]. Obviously, this has led to confusion with dedifferentiated morphology in the sense of the WHO grading and is also difficult to discriminate from a diffuse infiltration pattern [1, 8, 16].

Concerning the assessment of tumor budding, there are different approaches throughout the literature. Most approaches include focusing on hotspots, without explicitly defining them, and subsequent evaluation of the numbers of tumor buds. For instance, the German S3 guidelines from 2017, which included tumor budding as an additional risk factor for nodal positivity in early colorectal cancer, gives the following recommendations [17–21]: 1) the invasion front should be scanned at low magnification for the area of the highest tumor budding ("hottest spot") [17, 21]; 2) in this area, the absolute number of tumor buds should be counted [17, 21]; 3) the tumor should be graded based on the number of buds (grade 1 with 0–4 buds, grade 2 with 5–9 buds and grade 3 with < 9 buds) [17, 21].

Study aims

Although tumor budding evaluation is a painstaking counting task, there are only a few works focusing on automatization. In the context of CRC, there is only one work from Caie et al. on automatic tumor budding quantification [12]. The vast majority of works rely on human evaluation with the abovementioned problems of low inter-observer correlation. Additionally, this is very time consuming and requires intensive training.

Against this background, we here establish an automatic image processing approach to reliably quantify tumor budding in immunohistochemically (IHC) stained sections of CRC samples. By publicly sharing all source codes, we hope to enable others to reproduce our results and apply it in their own scientific work or on routine histology sections. We also tested our tool on whole-slide images (WSI) with clinical annotations, investigating whether there is a correlation with clinical outcome, which has been shown for this patient cohort previously by manual counting [9, 10]. Furthermore, we also tested our approach on tissue microarrays (TMAs) to check whether this could be used for the assessment of tumor budding.

Methods

Patient specimens and raw data generation

Specimen and data management

Whole-slide tissue specimens of formalin-fixed paraffin-embedded tumor tissue (n = 20 whole tissue slides) and TMAs of tumor tissue were retrieved from the pathology archive of the Institute of Pathology (Medical University of Graz, Austria). These cases belong to a previously published patient cohort of 381 patients (166 males, 215 females; median age 70.1 years) used and described by Harbaum et al. [9]. All procedures were carried out in accordance with the Declaration of Helsinki and in accordance with the local ethics committee (decision 18–199 ex 06/07).

All cases have been included in the study in a completely anonymized way with unique identifier for case (e.g., "GraMa001"), sample (which corresponds to tissue type) (e.g., "Samp001") and TMA core (e.g., "Core0001"). In the end, every measurement has one complete unique composite identifier, such as "GraMa001-Samp001-Core0001". The clinical information includes age, gender, TNM stage, number of infiltrated lymph nodes, grading and recurrence time.

Staining and digitalization

The tissue blocks underwent routine histochemical (HE) and immunohistochemical staining for pan-cytokeratin (cytokeratin, clone AE1/AE3, M3515, Dako/Agilent, Santa Clara, CA, USA) [22, 23]. The resulting sequential sections were digitalized as whole-slide images (WSI) using a digital microscope and M8 scanner (PreciPoint GmbH, Freising) and saved after conversion as svs files on a local Omero server [24].

Image processing in general

Image processing was performed in MATLAB (R2017a) on a desktop PC (Windows 7 Enterprise, Intel Core i7–4790, 32GB RAM, NVIDIA GeForce GT 630).

MATLAB-coding was carried out in accordance with style guidelines proposed by Johnson to increase the readability [25, 26]. Furthermore, object-oriented programming was applied [27], and speed up guidelines by Altman were followed [28].

In summary, all images underwent image modifying processing steps as part of the analysis, which are mentioned within the text and the legends in accordance with Digital Image Ethics [29].

Convolutional neural network training and application in general

To decide whether a tile (a tumor bud proposal) contained a single tumor bud or not, we used MatConvNet by Vedaldi et al. as CNN-toolbox in MATLAB [30]. For this classification task, we constructed an 8-layer CNN (see Additional file 1: Table S1). It was trained on a data set of 6292 images (100 × 100 pixel). These data set had been manually labeled by a pathologist (CAW). The dataset is available on HeiData.

The training was performed for 10,000 epochs with a constant learning rate of 10–5 on the BwUniCluster (state of Baden-Württemberg, bwHPC).

Tissue microarray (TMA) image processing

The MATLAB code of the method described below is available on GitHub (DOI: https://doi.org/10.5281/zenodo.1300211). It comprises tools tested for a scientific approach.

Data access and image registration

On the basis of the MATLAB Omero toolbox [24, 31], thumbnails from two WSIs (HE- and IHC-stained) were loaded into MATLAB's workspace (Additional file 2: Figure S3).

By using color thresholding, the TMA cores were separated from the background, the images were converted to binary images and the objects were automatically counted and named per image (Additional file 3: Pseudocode 1).

Subsequently, the thumbnails were registered by the MATLAB built-in SURF-based registration. These registration results were visually checked and in the case of an obviously wrong registration, a manual control-point-based registration was applied. By doing so, the corresponding core pairs could be consolidated for their numbers and positions in both images (Additional file 3: Pseudocode 2).

Download of the TMA cores

On the basis of the consolidated core pairs, every single core could be loaded from the Omero server in full resolution and locally saved as TMA core object (containing the slide ID, the core ID, the core position and an HE and IHC image of the core).

Core analysis

The pan-cytokeratin-stained cores were analyzed by a custom-written MATLAB tool to detect tumor buds, defined as small, independent clusters of 1–5 poorly or undifferentiated tumor cells:

(i) A custom-written implementation of color deconvolution was applied to separate the background and foreground staining [32, 33].

(ii) The intensity information for the brown component was thresholded by k-means clustering for back- and foreground and thus converted into a binary image (Additional file 3: Pseudocode 3).

(iii) The detected objects in the binary image underwent two steps of clustering. First, objects with near coordinates and equal morphology (area, perimeter) were combined. Thereby, huge tumor areas with unequal staining were recombined. Second, objects were clustered in regard to their border distance and area. By doing so, small tumor fragments that were in close proximity to a huge tumor mass were included with that mass (Additional file 3: Pseudocode 4).

(iv) Then, objects were classified in regard to their size; if they were too small or too big to be a tumor bud, they were discarded. Next, they were classified by a custom-trained convolutional neural network (CNN; MatConvNet by Vedaldi et al. [30]) to discard objects that did not show the expected morphology. The (completely anonymous) training and validation data is available on heiDATA.

(v) Finally, for the resulting labeled images, the number, size, shape, etc. of the objects could be calculated by MATLAB built-in functions [34]. Furthermore, the spatial distribution and the distances of all objects to their neighbors were calculated on the basis of Delaunay triangulation [34]. In contrast to other works on automatic tumor bud detection, we relied only on pan-cytokeratin-positive area and size [12].

Whole-slide image (WSI) image processing
Tumor and tumor border region of interest generation
On the pan-cytokeratin-stained WSI ($n = 20$) a region of interest (ROI) for the complete tumor and the border zone tumor-surrounding tissue was manually drawn in a local Omero client [24]. The corresponding ROI data were loaded by the Omero-MATLAB-toolbox [31] into the local MATLAB workspace.

Generation of virtual TMA (vTMA) cores
A grid with a grid point distance of half the mean TMA core diameter (1800 pixel) was drawn on the WSI (compare Fig. 3). Thereby, every grid point corresponded to the center of one virtual TMA (vTMA) core. Subsequently, all grid points within the above specified ROI were loaded on the basis of the Omero-MATLAB-toolbox and saved as a TMA core object (containing the slide ID, the core name and position, and an IHC image of the core).

vTMA core analysis
Due to different times of staining (TMA slides were stained in 2016, whole-slide cases were stained in 2017) there were staining differences between the two batches (initial TMA slides and whole tissue slides). To overcome this, Rheinard stain normalization was applied in a MATLAB implementation by Manohar P. Kuse [35–37]. However, best results were obtained with k-means clustering of the colors and CNN evaluation without color adaption.

Subsequently, the virtual cores underwent the same image processing workup as described above for the TMA cores (section "Convolutional neural network training and application in general").

Data management
As described above, image processing was performed in the MATLAB environment. The results were saved in Excel spreadsheets (Microsoft Excel 2010, Microsoft Corporation, Redmond, WA, USA).

The clinical information and the TMA slide information (link between TMA core position and patient ID) were also saved in Excel spreadsheets. For the latter, we manually combined the automatic MATLAB generated core numbers (referred to as MATLAB core IDs) with the real-world IDs on a schematic illustration of the TMAs in a (humorously Rosetta Stone-like) Excel spreadsheet.

The information was gathered in different R databases [38]: one database for the patient level and one database for the core level. Statistical analyses were performed in R version 3.2.4 [38].

Major parts of the image processing data are also freely available on heiDATA.

Monte Carlo simulation
To determine what sample size, how many randomly distributed cores per case were needed to reassemble the cases' characteristics, we ran a Monte Carlo-like analysis. Therefore, (i) from every case, a predefined number of vTMAs were randomly (10 times per case and sample size) selected and then the median number of buds, the median budding score and the normalized Shannon entropy were calculated [39–45]; (ii) then the number of random samples ($n = [2:1:200]$) was changed and step i was repeated.

By doing so, we obtained a range of expected values for every sample size or relative sample size (normalized to the total number of slides per case).

Results
Is there a correlation between the human estimation-based budding score and clinical parameters within the analyzed patient cohort?
As previously published by Harbaum et al. [9] and Max et al. [10] on the herein analyzed patient database, there was a correlation between a high budding score based on visual estimation on whole-tissue slides to clinical parameters such as positive nodal status and inferior regression free survival. By using their data and sample set, we could independently confirm the previously published correlation between nodal status and budding score (Fig. 1a) ($p < 0.05$), as well as the correlation between the budding score and regression-free survival (Fig. 1b). As a new analytical feature, we could also find a correlation between the budding score and morphologic tumor grading within these datasets (Fig. 1c) [8].

Can we define a reliable and reproducible automatic image processing approach?
There is no common generally valid definition of tumor budding in the literature. We decided to use the definition established by Satoh et al. [13], in

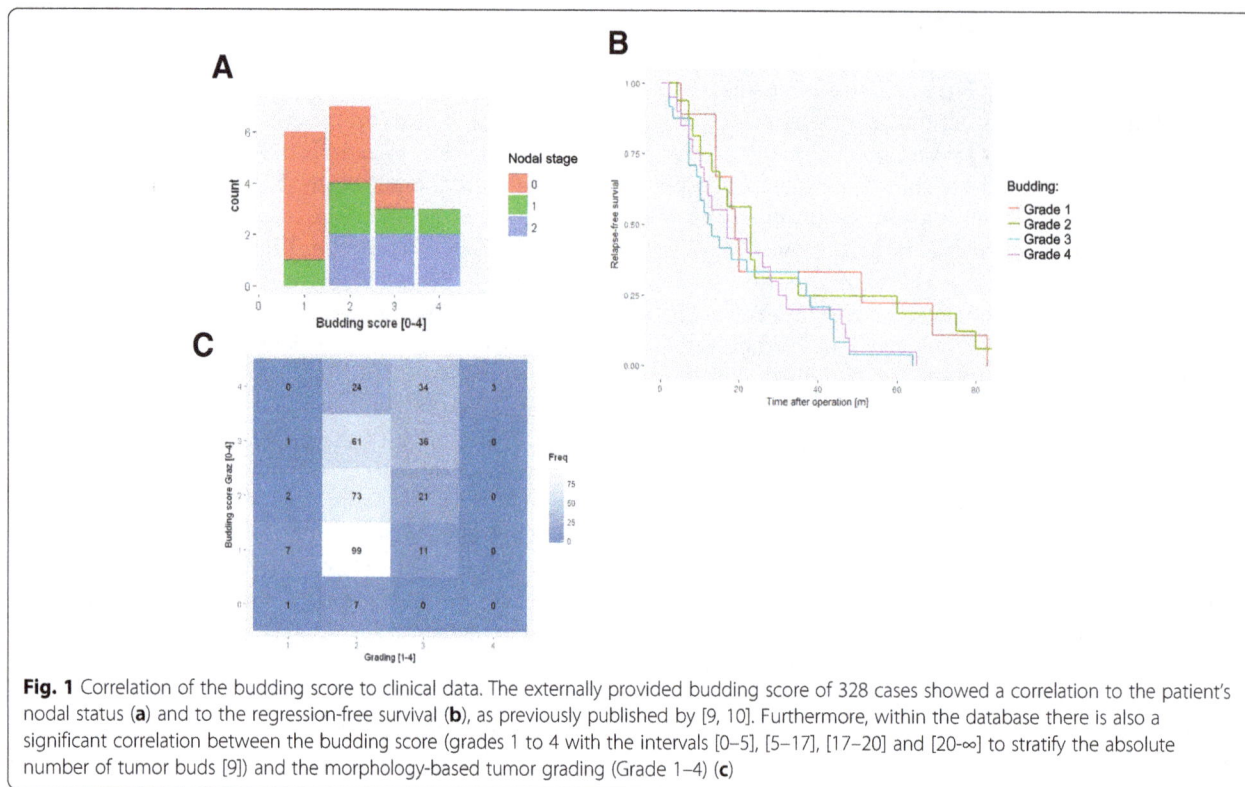

Fig. 1 Correlation of the budding score to clinical data. The externally provided budding score of 328 cases showed a correlation to the patient's nodal status (**a**) and to the regression-free survival (**b**), as previously published by [9, 10]. Furthermore, within the database there is also a significant correlation between the budding score (grades 1 to 4 with the intervals [0–5], [5–17], [17–20] and [20–∞] to stratify the absolute number of tumor buds [9]) and the morphology-based tumor grading (Grade 1–4) (**c**)

which they defined tumor budding as "cancer cell nests of fewer than five cells in the interstitium" with subsequent grouping of budding in an interval of 5 grades (grade 0 with 0 buds, grade 1 with 1–5 buds, grade 2 with 6–10 buds, grade 3 with 10–19 buds and grade 4 with ≥20 buds). This work was chosen because of its linear grading intervals for stratification of tumor buds.

Transferred to our image processing approach, this corresponds to a stained/brown area of 72–750 μm^2 (300–3125 pixels) as a threshold for tumor buds (compare red circle in Fig. 2 A and histograms of the area of tumor objects in Fig. 2b). On the basis of this definition, potential tumor buds could be separated from other small tumor aggregates, which we referred to as tumor islets and which are larger in size. Since this area-based

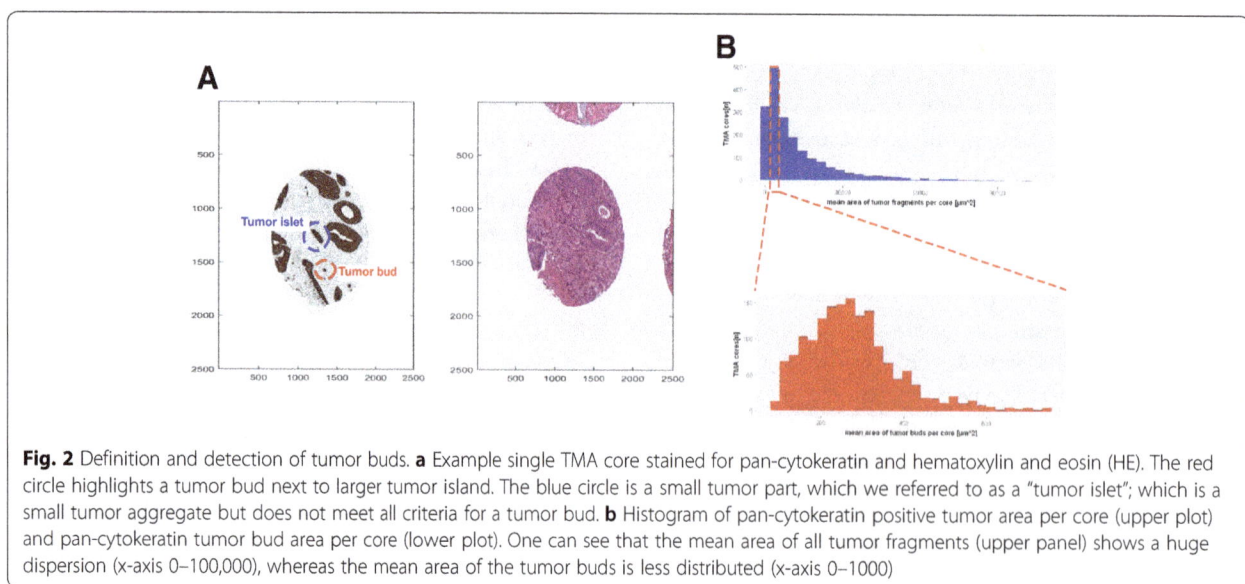

Fig. 2 Definition and detection of tumor buds. **a** Example single TMA core stained for pan-cytokeratin and hematoxylin and eosin (HE). The red circle highlights a tumor bud next to larger tumor island. The blue circle is a small tumor part, which we referred to as a "tumor islet"; which is a small tumor aggregate but does not meet all criteria for a tumor bud. **b** Histogram of pan-cytokeratin positive tumor area per core (upper plot) and pan-cytokeratin tumor bud area per core (lower plot). One can see that the mean area of all tumor fragments (upper panel) shows a huge dispersion (x-axis 0–100,000), whereas the mean area of the tumor buds is less distributed (x-axis 0–1000)

definition is prone to size variation (e.g., clusters of more than 5 very small tumor cells or stained area without nuclei) or staining variations (e.g., big structures are unequally stained leading to several stained spots in one structure), further validation steps were applied.

The detected tumor buds underwent further evaluation by cluster analysis (in regard to size, shape and border distance) and by a convolutional neural network (custom-trained MatConvNet [30]) to reduce the false positive rate. By doing so, small islets of positive staining within whole tumor mass were no longer recognized as tumor buds.

Our detection method (details in section "Tissue microarray (TMA) image processing") was optimized and validated on 20 test cores (10 real TMA cores (rTMA) and 10 virtual TMA cores (see section "Is there a correlation between the number of tumor buds and the budding score to the nodal status in virtual TMA-cores?")). We initially marked tumor buds manually on images of these cores ("ground truth") and compared these findings to the automatic segmentation; regarding the absolute number of tumor buds per core, there were more discrepancies, especially for cores with high numbers of tumor buds, but still an R^2-value of 0.86 was achieved. With one exception (budding score 3 instead of 2), we achieved an R^2-value of 0.96 (perfect correlation) for manual vs. automatic evaluation.

vTMA as a method to represent whole slide image analysis

Is there a correlation between the number of tumor buds and the budding score to the nodal status in virtual TMA-cores?

We randomly selected 20 cases from our cohort (pN0 ($n = 9$), pN1 ($n = 5$), pN2 ($n = 6$)) and digitalized pan cytokeratin-stained whole slides, with manually delineated tumor areas ("ROI tumor") and tumor invasion fronts ("ROI tumor border"). These regions were used to create virtual TMA (vTMA), which were TMA core sized tiles cropped from the whole-slide image (Fig. 3 A and section "Tissue microarray (TMA) image processing").

Comparing image processing results with human estimation-based data from previous publications [9, 10] for these 20 cases showed only a weak correlation for median budding (data not shown). Furthermore, there was no significant correlation for the median number of tumor buds in the ROI border or for the 10 hottest spots within the ROI border. The latter (10 hottest spots) was implemented according to Koelzer et al., who proposed to focus on the 10 hottest spots with the highest budding activity. There is also no correlation between our automatically obtained budding score and the median number of tumor buds (Fig. 4a). Furthermore, we found no correlation between the obtained budding score and the nodal status (Fig. 4b).

Is there a difference regarding hotspots for pN1/2 cases vs. pN0 by vTMA?

Dealing with spatial data, we plotted our measurements per vTMA in relation to their coordinates on the slide and interpolated between the measurement points. To carve out significant hotspots, we calculated the Z-score for every measurement with the formula $(x - \mu)/\sigma$, where x is the local value, μ is the mean value and σ is the standard deviation. Then, we plotted the Z-score values against the coordinates (heat maps in Additional file 4: Figure S2) and finally defined hotspots as areas with a Z-score > 1.67 (in parallel to our previous work on angiogenic hotspots in CRC [33]).

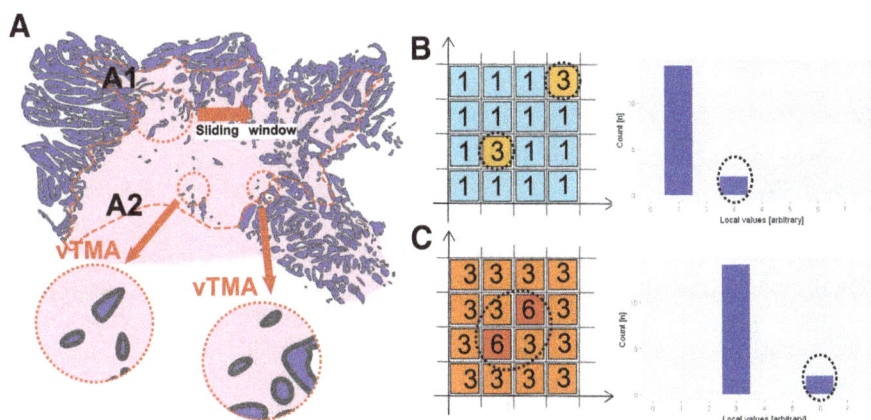

Fig. 3 Sketch of the analysis. A) ROI tumor (not shown) and the ROI border (dashed red line) were manually delineated by a pathologist (CW). A1: **a** sliding window moved over the ROI border and cropped every half TMA diameter in the underlying, TMA core-sized image. A2: The resulting tile (exactly the size of one TMA core) was then defined as a virtual TMA (vTMA). **b, c** This procedure leads to a value (number of tumor buds or budding score) per vTMA. This spatial data could be plotted as a heat map (example heat maps with arbitrary values in the left part) or as a histogram (right part of the figure)

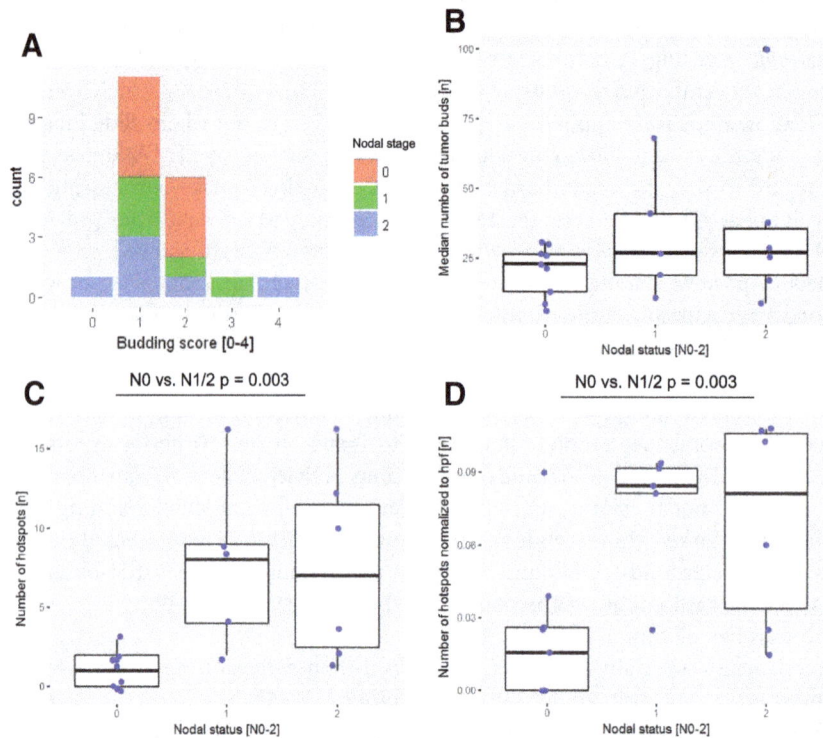

Fig. 4 Analysis of vTMAs from 20 cases. From 20 selected cases (pN0 ($n = 9$), pN1 ($n = 5$), pN2 ($n = 6$)) one pan-cytokeratin-stained slide was digitalized and disassembled into virtual, overlapping vTMA cores ($n = 290 \pm 152$). **a** No significant correlation was detected between the resulting budding score and the nodal status and **b** the median number of tumor buds within the 10 hottest spots and the nodal status for the complete ROI border. **c, d** Significant positive correlation between the nodal status and the absolute number of significant budding hotspots and the normalized number of significant budding hotspots. The latter is done to compensate for a trend toward higher tumor areas on the WSI for pN1 and pN2 cases

By doing so, the number of significant budding hotspots (areas where the number of tumor buds is significantly different in regard to the overall distribution of that case) could be calculated per slide. The number of budding hotspots normalized to the analyzed area significantly correlated with the nodal status (Wilcoxon rank sum test p-value = 0.031) (Fig. 4c-d). Modeling the nodal infiltration (present or absent) by logistic regression led to good fit with an area under the curve (AUC) of 0.838.

Is there spatial heterogeneity for budding and nodal status in whole-slide images by vTMA?

The above described data indicates that the number of budding hotspots (calculated in comparison to the underlying distribution) and not the underlying values themselves show a correlation to the nodal status; for example, in the sketch in Fig. 3b, the heat map has a mean value of 1.25 and the two tiles with an arbitrary value of 3 are significant hotspots in relation to their background. The heat map in Fig. 3c has a mean value of 3.75 and the tiles with an arbitrary value of 6 are significant hotspots. Thus, the absolute value per tile does not define our approach a hotspot, but the relation of the tile value to the rest. In addition, these hotspots are

defined by the distance of the tiles. For example, both heat maps in Fig. 3b-c had two significantly different tiles, but only in Fig. 3b are they spatially separated and therefore forming two hotspots and not one as in Fig. 3c. The histograms for both example heat maps have equal statistical distributions. In conclusion, it seems to be a problem of spatial heterogeneity.

Since the spatial information is lacking for the later rTMA analysis in sections, we checked whether features describing the heterogeneity, calculated on the basis of the histogram, were able to predict the nodal outcome. First, we separated the histogram on the basis of the Z-score into measurements within and outside the normal distribution of the cases (histograms in Additional file 4: Figure S2) and then analyzed the values outside the normal distribution; no correlation to the nodal status was found for the resulting number of significant vTMAs normalized to the overall number of vTMAs per slide ($n = 0.07 \pm 0.02$, $n = 0.07 \pm 0.01$ and $n = 0.07 \pm 0.01$), the median number of tumor buds per vTMA ($n = 19.50 \pm 7.46$, $n = 26.40 \pm 17.60$ and $n = 31.67 \pm 31.50$), or the maximum number of tumor buds per vTMA ($n = 26.44 \pm 10.57$, $n = 45.20 \pm 33.32$ and $n = 46.50 \pm 36.74$). The latter, interestingly, is in contrast to the work by

Koelzer et al. [11] proposing to focus on hotspots. Similarly, comparing the median and maximum budding score for these vTMAs outside the normal distribution showed no correlation.

Second, we calculated the histological Shannon's entropy [40, 41] as proposed by Kayser et al. [42–45] and as previously applied by us to describe the spatial heterogeneity in thymus specimens [39]. The entropy normalized to the sample size (Fig. 5a and c) showed a no significant trend towards higher entropy for pN1 and lower entropy for pN2 (pN0 0.83 ± 0.13 bit, pN1 0.86 ± 0.11 bit and pN2 0.78 ± 0.17 bit).

Summary of vTMA analysis

In summary, within the subcohort of 20 cases, there were no significant correlations among the absolute number of tumor buds, the budding score and their statistical derivates (e.g., median values). Accordingly, by means of our established tumor bud detection, we could not reproduce for whole-slide images the previously published results that were based on human evaluation [9, 10].

However, we could show a significant correlation between the number of significant budding hotspots and the nodal status for that subcohort. Since a hotspot definition based on histogram analysis only failed to show a significant correlation, we defined hotspots on the basis of spatial statistics by taking the relation of a local value to the remaining analyzed field (histogram analysis) and by taking the position of measurement values (spatial information) into account.

Analysis of real TMA (rTMA)

What is a reasonable number of TMA cores per case to reproduce whole-slide analyses?

Regarding rTMA data, we tested how many TMA cores per slide were needed to reassemble the cases' characteristics, especially in regard to their heterogeneity. Therefore, we ran a Monte Carlo-like simulation on the basis of our vTMA data from the tumor border (compare section "rTMA: Correlation between ground truth and TMA-based budding score").

As expected, the simulation showed that the results for normalized entropy (Fig. 5b) and for the median number of buds per core (Fig. 5d) align to the overall results (Fig. 5a and c) with increasing relative sample size.

rTMA: Correlation between ground truth and TMA-based budding score

As mentioned above, in previous works, the budding score was evaluated by a pathologist for this patient cohort [9, 10]. Therefore, we defined this budding score as ground truth for our work.

In our rTMA data, the number of cores from the tumor region with $n = 4 \pm 2$ was rather constant (Fig. 6a). However, in regard to the results of the Monte Carlo simulation, where the values began to close on the overall values for sample sizes > 100, these numbers are far too small to be representative.

Consequently, comparing to this human estimation-based ground truth, the median (accuracy = 0.208) and the maximum rTMA-based budding score (accuracy = 0.239) showed only a weak correlation. Furthermore,

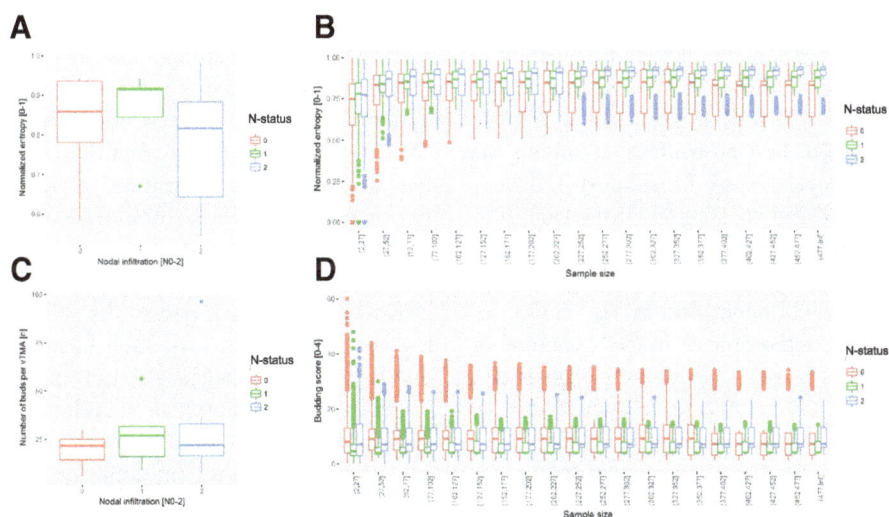

Fig. 5 Monte Carlo-like simulation. From every case (of the 20 cases with 290 ± 152 vTMAs from the tumor border) repetitively a predefined number of vTMAs were chosen at random, and subsequently the median number of buds, the median budding score and the normalized entropy were calculated. This process was repeated several times (*n* = 10) with different sample sizes (from *n* = 2 to *n* = 200). **a** and **c** show the normalized entropy and the median number of tumor buds in relation to the sample size, respectively. **b** and **d** show the normalized entropy and the median number of tumor buds for the complete tumor border, respectively

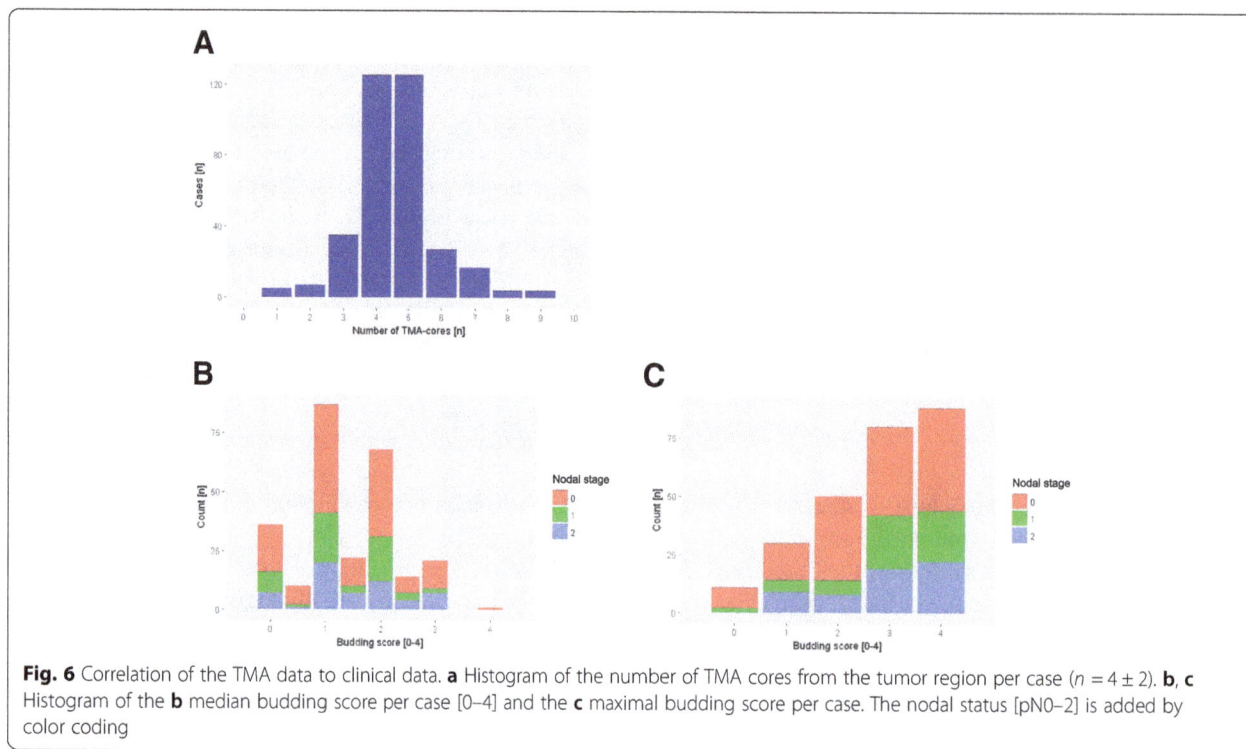

Fig. 6 Correlation of the TMA data to clinical data. **a** Histogram of the number of TMA cores from the tumor region per case ($n = 4 \pm 2$). **b**, **c** Histogram of the **b** median budding score per case [0–4] and the **c** maximal budding score per case. The nodal status [pN0–2] is added by color coding

stratifying the median (Fig. 6b) or maximum (Fig. 6c) rTMA-based budding score to clinical data such as nodal status did not reveal any correlation.

Against this background, with more or less randomly sampled TMA cores without spatial information, calculating the number of significant budding hotspots (as previously described in section "Is there a difference regarding hotspots for pN1/2 cases vs. pN0 by vTMA?") is not possible. Calculating the entropy on the basis of the number of cores per case and the obtained probabilities does not show significant differences in regard to the nodal status (pN0 0.57 ± 0.20 bit, pN1 0.60 ± 0.22 bit and pN2 0.57 ± 0.24 bit). In this context, changing the number of intervals and the cut-off criteria of the budding score also did not lead to a better distinction. The above-described algorithms were tested on a set of new tiles ($n = 16$) from different tissue blocks, staining and processing rounds after manual annotation in Fiji. These images had not been used in the process of CNN-training or method development. To avoid overlap and edge issues, these images contained only complete cells and the edge zones were blackened (compare black area in Fig. 3a).

For these 16 tiles, the results of the manual segmentation (as ground truth) were compared to the results of the automatic, CNN cascade-based detection on the basis of calculating the bounding box overlap (as described above). By doing so, the correct positive rate (0.87 ± 0.03), false positive rate (0.11 ± 0.04), false negative rate (0.11 ± 0.04), double detection rate (0.04 ± 0.01)

and precision (0.88 ± 0.03) were calculated (compare Fig. 3c for tile #5).

Discussion

Comparison of the tumor budding definition and assessment in the literature with our approach

In literature, tumor budding is most often defined as (i) clusters of 1–5 poorly or dedifferentiated tumor cells at the invasive front of tumors, next to larger, circumscribed tumor formations [14, 15]; (ii) and needs to be strictly discriminated from a diffuse infiltrative growth pattern [1, 8, 16]. Our image processing approach is consistent with the abovementioned definition. It takes the size and the localization in relation to the main tumor masses into account and considers the tumor bud morphology through a convolutional neural network. Furthermore, it covers the problematic area of diffuse growth or infiltration pattern by the hierarchical clustering step, which sums up such formations as one object due to the shape and localization of its subparts (step iii in section "Convolutional neural network training and application in general".3). Several works from different groups address tumor budding for CRC and its related role as a prognostic factor, in particular in regard to nodal status [8, 10, 16, 46–48]. Thereby, a plethora of different tumor budding assessments have been applied. For example, some groups have counted tumor buds in absolute numbers (e.g., Ueno et al. [48], Prall et al. [16]), others have stratified the absolute number into different grades (e.g., Max et al. [10]), and still others just defined high- and low-grade budding activity on the basis of the absolute numbers (Hase et al. [8]). Our approach primarily counted the number of tumor buds per high power field (one high-power field had approximately the size of a single TMA core). These numbers were then stratified into five budding grades (from grade 0 with no budding to grade 4 with extensive budding) in reference to previous works by Koelzer et al. and Satoh et al. [11, 13]. Of note, the findings of Koelzer and Satoh were mainly established based on HE staining, and their transferability to more sensitive IHC-based estimations is problematic. The higher sensitivity of the latter method could lead to higher grades [49].

In comparison to the results of a manually defined ground truth (blinded annotation by a trained pathologist, CAW), the automatic evaluation showed a very good accordance for the budding score and a good accordance for the overall number of tumor buds for whole-slide analysis (section "Tissue microarray (TMA) image processing" and Additional file 5: Figure S1), which opens the possibility of analyzing entire sections in a reliable and reproducible fashion.

One spatial statistics derived definition of clinically significant budding hotspots

For a subcohort of 20 cases, we focused on the manually delineated infiltrative border in accordance with Caie et al., who also focused on infiltrative border and showed a correlation of immunofluorescence-based image processing-based tumor budding assessment with manual budding analyses and clinical parameters [12]. Surprisingly, for our data, we could not show a correlation between the median or maximum number of tumor buds and the nodal status. Additionally, we found no correlation between budding score and nodal status. Even focusing budding analyses on hotspots (as proposed by many researchers) did not lead to a significant stratification of cases in regard to the nodal status.

By applying methods of spatial statistics [50–53] to describe the spatial heterogeneity (as recently published for vessels in CRC [33], for lymphatic hyperplasia in the thymus [54] or for lymphatic infiltrates in the bone marrow [55]), we found significant accumulations of tumor budding foci independent of the overall frequency of tumor budding, which we called budding hotspots. The number of these budding hotspots and not their budding metrics (e.g., median budding score in the hotspots) did correlate with the nodal status. This leads obviously to the conclusion that TMAs are not suitable for analyzing tumor budding.

Pros and cons of our automatic image processing and the ground truth

In addition to the nonnegligible hassle of counting tumor buds in a section, the reproducibility of human-based results and/or the training efforts to ensure such reproducibility are major limitations and hamper routine estimation of budding. Studies showed inter-observer variations in the range of kappa = 0.61–0.83 [56, 57]. However, a different human-based evaluation method using 10 high power fields (hpf) in the region with the highest density of peri-tumoral budding showed a slightly better reproducibility (kappa-values in the range 0.5–0.87) [11, 58].

Our image processing approach has been validated in terms of absolute budding number and budding score with good to very good accordance compared to manually drawn "ground truth" (Additional file 5: Figure S1). This offers the option for reproducible, time-saving whole-slide analysis and the resulting possibility of applying spatial statistics.

Interestingly, mimicking the strategies of the human evaluation (considering only the hottest spot or the 10 hottest spots) with our automatized method did not lead to significant results. Only the number of hotspots defined by spatial statistics correlated with nodal status.

Conclusions

Tumor budding in CRC is a complex phenomenon for which the visual assessment by a surgical pathologist cannot be easily reproduced by automatic image processing. On the basis of a combination of image processing and machine learning, we found that not the absolute number of tumor formations classified as "tumor buds" within the infiltrative region but rather their spatial arrangement in significant hotspots and especially the number of such hotspots is clinically meaningful. Consequently, the advice for the surgical pathologist is to focus more on the spatial distribution (as kind of pattern diagnosis), rather than on the absolute number, of tumor buds.

Additional files

Additional file 1: Table S1. Architecture of the applied CNN. The 8-layer CNN has been designed to classify (100x100x3 pixel) images to the classes "tumor bud" and "no tumor" bud. It consists of two block of a combination of convolutional, rectifier and pooling layers and a fully connected layer.

Additional file 2: Figure S3. Finding the corresponding core on two separate TMA-slides. Thumbnail of an HE-stained (A) and a pan-cytokeratin-stained (B) TMA-slide. The green circle highlights the same core on both slides, which has due morphological variations different numbers by the image processing based automatic counting.

Additional file 3: Pseudocode 1 create TMA-map. Pseudocode 2 combine TMA-maps of different staining. Pseudocode 3 image analysis part I. Pseudocode 4 image analysis part II.

Additional file 4: Figure S2. Dealing with spatial heterogeneity by different means. Histogram: On basis of the Z-score the vTMAs with values outside the underlying normal distribution could be identified. By doing so the histogram for the number of tumor buds per vTMA could be binarized into vTMA within and outside. Overlay WIS and heatmap for the ROI border: Furthermore by plotting the Z-score values against the coordinates on the WSI, a heatmap with the hotspot-probability could be obtained. In this map values > 1.67 are regarded as significant.

Additional file 5: Figure S1. Validation of the detection method on 20 test cores. In 10 real TMA cores (rTMA) and 10 virtual TMA-cores (vTMA) every tumor bud has been manually segmented in Fiji [23] as ground truth.

Abbreviations
CNN: Convolutional neural network; CRC: Colorectal carcinoma; rTMA: real TMA; TMA: Tissue micro array; vTMA: virtual TMA

Acknowledgements
The authors acknowledge support by the state of Baden-Württemberg through bwHPC.
The authors also thank the IT department staff of Medical Faculty Mannheim and especially Mr. Bohne-Lang for the supervision of the computer administration and infrastructure.
Finally, we want to thank Katrin Wolk for expert technical assistance.

Funding
C.-A.Weis is supported by a SEED fellowship of the Medical Faculty Mannheim, Heidelberg University, and by the TraPS-Program, Heinrich Lanz Center, Ministry of Science and Art, Baden-Wuerttemberg and Medical Faculty Mannheim, Heidelberg University.
JN Kather is supported by the "Heidelberg School of Oncology" (NCT-HSO) and by the "German Consortium for Translational Cancer Research" (DKTK) fellowship program.

Authors' contributions
CAW designed the study and Matlab tool, trained and validated it and wrote the manuscript. JNK and SM contributed to the study design, data management and prepared the datasets analysed. HA prepared datasets and validation data. MJP and CL manged the patient cohort and contributed to the study design. TG designed the study and contributed to the manuscript drafting. All authors have read and approved the final manuscript.

Competing interests
The authors declare that they have no competing interests.

Author details
[1]Institute of Pathology, University Medical Centre Mannheim, University of Heidelberg, 68167 Mannheim, Germany. [2]Department of Medical Oncology and Internal Medicine VI, National Center for Tumor Diseases, University Hospital Heidelberg, Heidelberg University, Heidelberg, Germany. [3]Department of Dermatology, Venereology and Allergology, University Medical Center Mannheim, Heidelberg University, Mannheim, Germany. [4]Institute of Pathology, Medical University Graz, Graz, Austria.

References
1. WHO. Classification of Tumors of the Digestive System. 4th ed; 2010.
2. Wittekind C. TNM: Klassifikation maligner Tumoren: Wiley; 2017.
3. Gospodarowicz MK, Brierley JD, Wittekind C. TNM classification of malignant tumors: Wiley; 2017.
4. Park KJ, Choi HJ, Roh MS, Kwon HC, Kim C. Intensity of tumor budding and its prognostic implications in invasive colon carcinoma. Dis Colon Rectum. 2005;48:1597–602.
5. Mitrovic B, Schaeffer DF, Riddell RH, Kirsch R. Tumor budding in colorectal carcinoma: time to take notice. Mod Pathol. 2012;25:1315–25.
6. Puppa G, Sonzogni A, Colombari R, Pelosi G. TNM staging system of colorectal carcinoma: a critical appraisal of challenging issues. Arch Pathol Lab Med. 2010;134:837–52.
7. Imai T. The growth of human carcinoma: a morphological analysis. Fukuoka Igaku Zasshi. 1954;45:102.
8. Hase K, Shatney C, Johnson D, Trollope M, Vierra M. Prognostic value of tumor "budding" in patients with colorectal cancer. Dis Colon Rectum. 1993; 36:627–35.
9. Harbaum L, Pollheimer MJ, Kornprat P, Lindtner RA, Bokemeyer C, Langner C. Peritumoral eosinophils predict recurrence in colorectal cancer. Mod Pathol. 2015;28:403–13.
10. Max N, Harbaum L, Pollheimer MJ, Lindtner RA, Kornprat P, Langner C. Tumor budding with and without admixed inflammation: two different sides of the same coin? Br J Cancer. 2016;114:368–71.
11. Koelzer VH, Zlobec I, Lugli A. Tumor budding in colorectal cancer--ready for diagnostic practice? Hum Pathol. 2016;47:4–19.
12. Caie PD, Turnbull AK, Farrington SM, Oniscu A, Harrison DJ. Quantification of tumor budding, lymphatic vessel density and invasion through image analysis in colorectal cancer. J Transl Med. 2014;12:156.
13. Satoh K, Nimura S, Aoki M, Hamasaki M, Koga K, Iwasaki H, Yamashita Y, Kataoka H, Nabeshima K. Tumor budding in colorectal carcinoma assessed by cytokeratin immunostaining and budding areas: possible involvement of c-Met. Cancer Sci. 2014;105:1487–95.
14. Gabbert H, Wagner R, Moll R, Gerharz CD. Tumor dedifferentiation: an important step in tumor invasion. Clin Exp Metastasis. 1985;3:257–79.
15. Prall F. Tumor budding in colorectal carcinoma. Histopathology. 2007; 50:151–62.
16. Prall F, Nizze H, Barten M. Tumor budding as prognostic factor in stage I/II colorectal carcinoma. Histopathology. 2005;47:17–24.
17. Leitlinienprogramm Onkologie (Deutsche Krebsgesellschaft, Deutsche Krebshilfe, AWMF): S3-Leitlinie Kolorektales Karzinom, Langversion 2.0, 2017. vol. AWMF Registrierungsnummer: 021/007OL: Arbeitsgemeinschaft der Wissenschaftlichen Medizinischen Fachgesellschaften e. V. Deutschen Krebsgesellschaft e.V. Deutschen Krebshilfe; 2017.
18. Glasgow SC, Bleier JI, Burgart LJ, Finne CO, Lowry AC. Meta-analysis of histopathological features of primary colorectal cancers that predict lymph node metastasis. J Gastrointest Surg. 2012;16:1019–28.
19. Mou S, Soetikno R, Shimoda T, Rouse R, Kaltenbach T. Pathologic predictive factors for lymph node metastasis in submucosal invasive (T1) colorectal cancer: a systematic review and meta-analysis. Surg Endosc. 2013;27:2692–703.
20. Wada H, Shiozawa M, Katayama K, Okamoto N, Miyagi Y, Rino Y, Masuda M, Akaike M. Systematic review and meta-analysis of histopathological predictive factors for lymph node metastasis in T1 colorectal cancer. J Gastroenterol. 2015;50:727–34.
21. Kawachi H, Eishi Y, Ueno H, Nemoto T, Fujimori T, Iwashita A, Ajioka Y, Ochiai A, Ishiguro S, Shimoda T, et al. A three-tier classification system based on the depth of submucosal invasion and budding/sprouting can improve the treatment strategy for T1 colorectal cancer: a retrospective multicenter study. Mod Pathol. 2015;28:872–9.
22. Welsch U, Mulisch M. Romeis Mikroskopische Technik: Spektrum Akademischer Verlag; 2010.
23. Taylor CR, Rudbeck L. Immunohistochemical staining methods: Dako; 2013.
24. OMERO [https://www.openmicroscopy.org/site].

25. Johnson R. Matlab programming style guidelines. USA Datatool Version. 2002;1
26. Johnson R. MATLAV Style Guidelines 2.0. In: Datatool; 2014.
27. MATLAB Object-Oriented Programming. The MathWorks, Inc.; 2015.
28. Altman YM. Accelerating MATLAB performance: 1001 tips to speed up MATLAB programs: CRC Press; 2014.
29. Cromey DW. Avoiding twisted pixels: ethical guidelines for the appropriate use and manipulation of scientific digital images. Sci Eng Ethics. 2010;16:639–67.
30. MatConvNet: CNNs for MATLAB [http://www.vlfeat.org/matconvnet/].
31. OMERO.matlab toolbox [https://www.openmicroscopy.org/omero/downloads/].
32. Ruifrok AC, Johnston DA. Quantification of histochemical staining by color deconvolution. Anal Quant Cytol Histol. 2001;23:291–9.
33. Kather JN, Marx A, Reyes-Aldasoro CC, Schad LR, Zöllner FG, Weis C-A. Continuous representation of tumor microvessel density and detection of angiogenic hotspots in histological whole-slide images. Oncotarget. 2015;6:19163–76.
34. Gonzalez RC, Woods RE, Eddins SL. Digital image processing using MATLAB: McGraw Hill Education; 2013.
35. Reinhard Stain Normalization [https://de.mathworks.com/matlabcentral/fileexchange/42580-reinhard-stain-normalization].
36. Magee D, Treanor D, Crellin D, Shires M, Smith K, Mohee K, Quirke P. Colour normalisation in digital histopathology images. In: Elson D, editor. Proc Optical Tissue Image analysis in Microscopy, Histopathology and Endoscopy (MICCAI Workshop); 2009.
37. Reinhard E, Adhikhmin M, Gooch B, Shirley P. Color transfer between images. IEEE Comput Graph Appl. 2001;21:34–41.
38. R Project [http://www.r-project.org].
39. Weis CA, Aban IB, Cutter G, Kaminski HJ, Scharff C, Grießmann BW, Deligianni M, Kayser K, Wolfe GI, Ströbel P, Marx A. Histopathology of thymectomy specimens from the MGTX-trial: Entropy analysis as strategy to quantify spatial heterogeneity of lymphoid follicle and fat distribution. PLoS One. 2018;13(6):e0197435. https://doi.org/10.1371/journal.pone.0197435. eCollection 2018. PMCID: PMC5999223. PMID: 29897907.
40. Shannon CE. A mathematical theory of communication. Bell Syst Tech J. 1948;27:379–423.
41. Shannon CE. A mathematical theory of communication. SIGMOBILE Mob Comput Commun Rev. 2001;5:3–55.
42. Pincus SM. Approximate entropy as a measure of system complexity. Proc Natl Acad Sci U S A. 1991;88:2297–301.
43. Kayser K, Schultz H, Goldmann T, Gortler J, Kayser G, Vollmer E. Theory of sampling and its application in tissue based diagnosis. Diagn Pathol. 2009;4:6.
44. Kayser K, Kayser G, Metze K. The concept of structural entropy in tissue-based diagnosis. Anal Quant Cytol Histol. 2007;29:296–308.
45. Kayser K, Gabius HJ. Graph theory and the entropy concept in histochemistry. Theoretical considerations, application in histopathology and the combination with receptor-specific approaches. Prog Histochem Cytochem. 1997;32:1–106.
46. Nakamura T, Mitomi H, Kikuchi S, Ohtani Y, Sato K. Evaluation of the usefulness of tumor budding on the prediction of metastasis to the lung and liver after curative excision of colorectal cancer. Hepatogastroenterology. 2005;52:1432–5.
47. Okuyama T, Nakamura T, Yamaguchi M. Budding is useful to select high-risk patients in stage II well-differentiated or moderately differentiated colon adenocarcinoma. Dis Colon Rectum. 2003;46:1400–6.
48. Ueno H, Murphy J, Jass JR, Mochizuki H, Talbot IC. Tumor 'budding' as an index to estimate the potential of aggressiveness in rectal cancer. Histopathology. 2002;40:127–32.
49. Koelzer VH, Zlobec I, Berger MD, Cathomas G, Dawson H, Dirschmid K, Hadrich M, Inderbitzin D, Offner F, Puppa G, et al. Tumor budding in colorectal cancer revisited: results of a multicenter interobserver study. Virchows Arch. 2015;466:485–93.
50. Hengl T. A Practical Guide to Geostatistical Mapping: BPR Publishers; 2011.
51. Trauth MH, Gebbers R, Marwan N. MATLAB® recipes for earth sciences: Springer; 2007.
52. Wainwright J, Mulligan M. Environmental modelling: finding simplicity in complexity: Wiley; 2013.
53. Mahajan S, Mead CA. Street-fighting mathematics: the art of educated guessing and opportunistic problem solving: MIT Press; 2010.
54. Weis CA, Aban IB, Cutter GR, Kaminski HJ, Scharff C, Grießmann BW, Deligianni M, Kayser K, Ströbel P, Marx A: Histopathology of thymectomy specimens from the MGTX-trial: strategies to reveal spatial heterogeneity of lymphoid follicle and fat distribution. 2017. manuscript submitted.
55. Weis C-A, Grießmann BW, Scharff C, Detzner C, Pfister E, Marx A, Zoellner FG. On the representation of cells in bone marrow pathology by a scalar field: propagation through serial sections, co-localization and spatial interaction analysis. Diagn Pathol. 2015;10:151.
56. Graham RP, Vierkant RA, Tillmans LS, Wang AH, Laird PW, Weisenberger DJ, Lynch CF, French AJ, Slager SL, Raissian Y, et al. Tumor budding in colorectal carcinoma: confirmation of prognostic significance and histologic cutoff in a population-based cohort. Am J Surg Pathol. 2015;39:1340–6.
57. Koelzer VH, Assarzadegan N, Dawson H, Mitrovic B, Grin A, Messenger DE, Kirsch R, Riddell RH, Lugli A, Zlobec I. Cytokeratin-based assessment of tumor budding in colorectal cancer: analysis in stage II patients and prospective diagnostic experience. J Pathol Clin Res. 2017;3:171–8.
58. Karamitopoulou E, Zlobec I, Kolzer V, Kondi-Pafiti A, Patsouris ES, Gennatas K, Lugli A. Proposal for a 10-high-power-fields scoring method for the assessment of tumor budding in colorectal cancer. Mod Pathol. 2013;26:295–301.

20

Predictive value of tumor-infiltrating lymphocytes to pathological complete response in neoadjuvant treated triple-negative breast cancers

Miao Ruan[1,2†], Tian Tian[1,2†], Jia Rao[1,2], Xiaoli Xu[1,2], Baohua Yu[1,2], Wentao Yang[1,2] and Ruohong Shui[1,2*]

Abstract

Background: Triple-negative breast cancers (TNBCs) are a group of heterogeneous diseases with various morphology, prognosis, and treatment response. Therefore, it is important to identify valuable biomarkers to predict the therapeutic response and prognosis for TNBCs. Tumor-infiltrating lymphocytes (TILs) may have predictive value to pathological complete response (pCR) in neoadjuvant treated TNBCs. However, absence of standardized methodologies for TILs measurement has limited its evaluation and application in practice. In 2014, the International TILs Working Group formulated the recommendations of pathologic evaluation for TILs in breast cancers.

Methods: To evaluate the predictive value of TILs scored by methods recommended by International TILs Working Group 2014, we performed a retrospective study of TILs in 166 core needle biopsy specimens of primary invasive TNBCs with neoadjuvant chemotherapy (NAC) in a Chinese population. Intratumoral TILs (iTILs) and stromal TILs (sTILs) were scored respectively. The associations between TILs and pCR were analyzed.

Results: Both sTILs ($p = 0.0001$) and iTILs ($P = 0.001$) were associated with pCR in univariate logistic regression analysis. Multivariate logistic regression analysis indicated that both sTILs ($P = 0.006$) and iTILs ($P = 0.04$) were independent predictors for pCR. Receiver operating characteristics (ROC) curve analysis was used to identify the optimal thresholds of TILs. TNBCs with more than 20% sTILs ($P = 0.001$) or with more than 10% iTILs ($P = 0.003$) were associated with higher pCR rates in univariate analysis. Multivariate analysis showed that a 20% threshold of sTILs ($P = 0.005$) was an independent predictive factor for pCR.

Conclusions: Our study indicated that TILs scored by recommendations of International TILs Working Group 2014 in pre-NAC core needle biopsy specimens was significantly correlated with pCR in TNBCs, higher TILs scores predicting higher pCR rate. Both sTILs and iTILs were independent predictors for pCR in TNBCs. A 20% threshold for sTILs may be feasible to predict pCR to NAC in TNBCs.

Keywords: Tumor-infiltrating lymphocytes, Breast cancer, Triple-negative, Pathological complete response, Predictive factor

* Correspondence: shuiruohong2014@163.com
†Miao Ruan and Tian Tian contributed equally to this work.
[1]Department of Pathology, Fudan University Shanghai Cancer Center, Shanghai, China
[2]Department of Oncology, Shanghai Medical College, Fudan University, Shanghai, China

Background

Triple-negative breast cancers (TNBCs) are defined as a group of breast cancer characterized by lacking of estrogen receptor (ER), progesterone receptor (PgR) and human epidermal growth factor receptor 2 (HER2) protein expression [1]. Most of TNBCs have higher risk of early distant recurrence, mortality and more aggressive clinical behavior compared with other subtypes of breast cancers [2, 3]. Owing to the absence of effective targeted therapy, chemotherapy is the only recommended systemic treatment for TNBCs at present stage [4]. However, various therapeutic strategies have been explored, among which immunotherapy may have potential benefits to treat TNBCs [5, 6]. Therefore, several studies have been carried out to evaluate the predictive and prognostic values of tumor-infiltrating lymphocytes (TILs) in TNBCs, which have indicated that high levels of TILs may be associated with a better clinical outcome and a better response to chemotherapy in TNBCs [7–9].

It has been demonstrated that patients gaining pathological complete response (pCR) to neoadjuvant chemotherapy (NAC) may experience prolonged disease-free survival, especially in TNBCs [3, 7, 8]. Many biomarkers to predict pCR for NAC in TNBCs have been analyzed, such as immune-related gene signatures and clinicopathologic factors. Several studies have indicated that TILs in pre-NAC samples may be used to predict pCR in TNBCs [9–12]. However, methodologies of TILs evaluation in these studies were not standardized, which has hindered its application in clinical practice.

Lymphocyte-predominant breast cancer (LPBC), firstly proposed by Denkert et al., was defined as tumors with a particularly strong lymphocytic infiltration whether in tumor stroma or cell nests [9]. The LPBC-cutoff was generally 50% or 60% in previous literatures [9, 13]. However, owing to the relatively low proportion of LPBC in routine practice, it may be unreasonable to define 50–60% as the threshold for LPBC.

In this study, we conducted a retrospective analysis of TILs in 166 core needle biopsy specimens of TNBCs with NAC in a Chinese population. Stromal TILs (sTILs) and intratumoral TILs (iTILs) in pre-NAC specimens were scored using the method recommended by the International TILs Working Group 2014 [14], and the correlation between TILs and neoadjuvant chemotherapy response was analyzed. The optimal thresholds of TILs to predict pCR in TNBCs were explored. The aim of our study was to examine the predictive value of TILs to pCR in neoadjuvant treated TNBCs, and to evaluate the feasibility of the scoring methods in clinical practice.

Methods

Patients and samples

166 consecutive core needle biopsy specimens of primary invasive TNBCs diagnosed and treated with NAC following up operation between 2011 and 2016 were extracted from the pathology database of Fudan University Shanghai Cancer Center. The inclusion criteria were as follows: primary invasive TNBCs; neoadjuvant therapy before surgical operation; available complete clinicopathologic data (age, tumor size, tumor grade, histological type, lymphovascular invasion, lymph node status, Miller-Payne grade, ER, PgR, HER2 and Ki-67 index). All specimens were fixed with 10% neutral phosphate-buffered formalin and paraffin-embedded. 4 μm-thick slices of representative tumor blocks were stained with hematoxylin and eosin (H& E). Tumors were defined as triple negative as following: < 1% of ER and PgR immunoreactivity, and absence of HER2 protein overexpression or gene amplification [15, 16].

Pathologic evaluation

All core needle biopsy specimens and surgical slices were reviewed by two experienced breast pathologists (R.S. and W.Y.) to confirm the histological type, according to 2012 World Health Organization (WHO) Classification of Tumours of the Breast [17]. Histological grade of tumor was evaluated in pre-NAC core needle biopsy specimens by the Nottingham grading system [18, 19]. Miller-Payne grading system was used to evaluate the pathological response in surgical specimens [20]. The pCR of chemotherapeutic response was the endpoint of our study, which was defined as the absence of invasive carcinoma in the breast tissue and axillary lymph nodes in surgical specimens.

Evaluation of TILs on core needle biopsy specimens was performed by two breast pathologists (M.R. and T.T.). The two observers were trained by the evaluation criteria recommended by the International TILs Working Group 2014, and scored each case independently in a blind manner. The mean values of two observers were obtained as final scores for each case. STILs were defined as the percentage of tumor stroma containing infiltrating lymphocytes and plasma cells, which should exclude polymorphonuclear leukocytes (Fig. 1a, b). ITILs were defined as the percentage of lymphocytes and plasma cells within tumor cell nests or in direct contact with the tumor cells (Fig. 1a, c). Areas of in situ carcinomas, normal lobules, necrosis, hyalinization and crush artifacts were not included [14]. The TILs were scored in an average value throughout full sections rather than hotspots. The results were scored in increments of 10; 0 was defined as < 5%; 10 was defined as 5% to 10%; 20 was defined as 11% to 20% and all other scores were rounded up to the next highest decile (Fig. 1d-1g).

Statistical analysis

Two types of variables were used to test: one was continuous variables (per 10% increment); the other was binary variables categorized by 20% score cutoff (sTILs) and 10% score cutoff (iTILs). The associations between

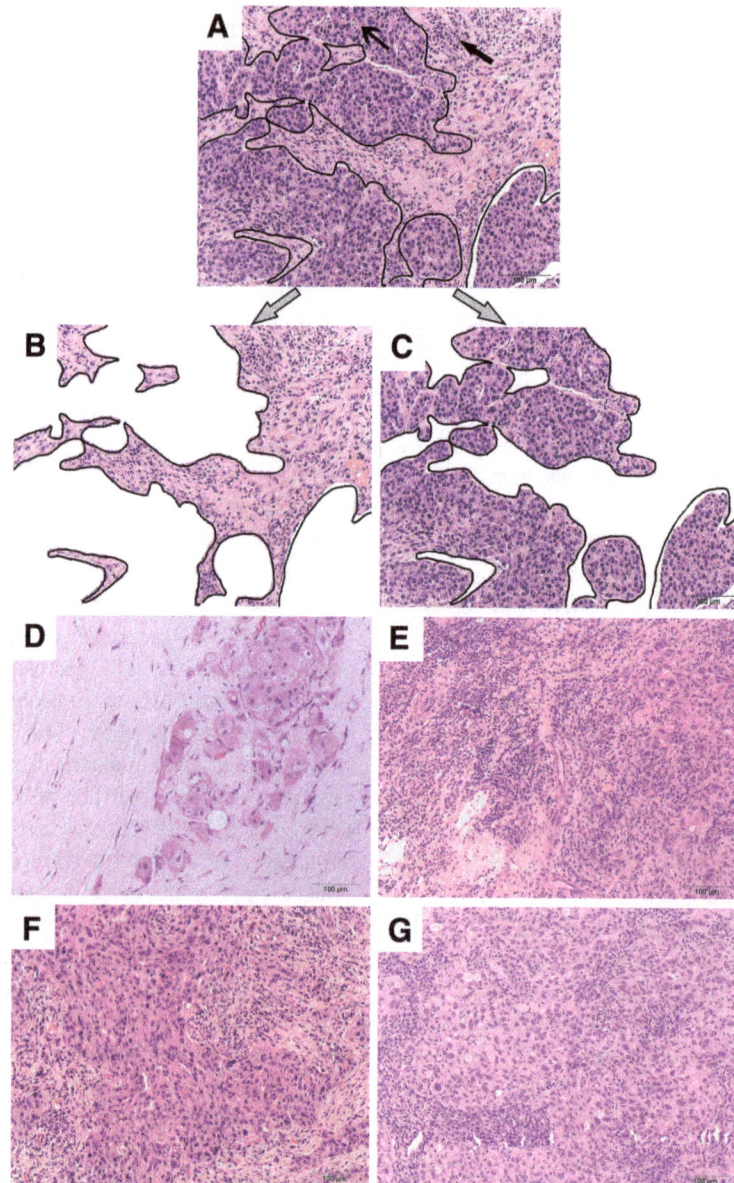

Fig. 1 Histopathologic evaluation of TILs and different scores of TILs in TNBCs. **a**: The areas of sTILs and iTILs evaluation were distinguished by black lines (bold black arrow pointed to plasma cells and lymphocytes, Fine black arrow pointed to polymorphonuclear leukocytes which should be excluded in TILs evaluation). **b**: The area of sTILs evaluation: 20%; **c**: The area of iTILs evaluation: 0%. **d**: sTILs: 0%. **e**: sTILs: 50%. **f**: iTILs: 10%. **g**: iTILs: 20% (All × 200 magnification)

TILs and clinicopathologic characteristics including patients' age (≤ 50 years versus > 50 years), tumor size (≤ 2 cm, 2–5 cm versus > 5 cm), tumor grade (1, 2 versus 3), lymph node status (negative versus positive), histological type (IDC versus special type), LVI (negative versus positive), Ki-67 index, Miller-Payne grade (1–5) and neoadjuvant chemotherapy regiments were analyzed. The correlations of TILs as continuous variables with polytomous variables were evaluated with Kruskal-Wallis test. Mann-Whitney test was performed to identify the associations between TILs and binary variables. The associations between TILs and continuous variables (Ki-67 index and Miller-Payne grade) were evaluated with Spearman's rank correlation analysis (r). The intraclass correlation coefficient analysis was used to evaluate the interobserver agreement of sTILs and iTILs scores. The correlation between pCR after NAC and TILs was analyzed by univariate logistic regression analysis. Multivariate logistic regression analysis was used to identify the independent predictors for chemotherapeutic response. Stratified analysis was used to investigate the correlation between TILs and pCR across different clinicopathologic subgroups.

Evaluation of heterogeneity effects and test for trend were performed by chi-squared test. Receiver operating characteristics (ROC) curve was conducted to detect the optimal thresholds of TILs and the predictive model to predict pCR. The maximum Youden's Index (J = sensitivity + specificity - 1) was calculated to define the optimal thresholds, then univariate and multivariate regression analysis were used to evaluate the predictive value of TILs as binary variables for pCR. A two-side p-value < 0.05 was considered statistically significant. All statistical analyses were performed using the SPSS version 20.0 (SPSS Inc., Chicago, IL) and STATA version 13.1 (Stata Corporation, College Station, TX, USA).

Results

Clinicopathologic characteristics

The clinicopathologic characteristics of 166 TNBCs were listed in Table 1. The age of patients ranged from 25 to 77 years with a mean age of 50 years. All patients were female. The pre-NAC tumor size was assessed according to radiology findings. The tumor grade was estimated in the pre-NAC specimens of core needle biopsy. In core needle biopsy, 164 (98.8%) cases were diagnosed as invasive ductal carcinoma of no special type (IDC) and only 2 (1.2%) cases were invasive carcinoma with special subtypes (carcinoma with apocrine differentiation in 2 cases). Lymph nodes involvement was found in 113 (68.1%) cases by fine needle aspiration (FNA) before neoadjuvant treatment. Patients underwent NAC based on the combination treatment regimen of anthracycline and paclitaxel (136/166, 81.9%), or paclitaxel and platinum (30/166, 18.1%). All patients received surgical operation after eight cycles of NAC. 141 (84.9%) patients underwent mastectomy, and breast-conserving surgery was performed in 25 (15.1%) patients. Lymphovascular invasion (LVI) was observed in the postoperative slices of 36 (21.7%) cases. 67 (40.4%) cases obtained pCR, and non-pCR were observed in 99 (59.6%) cases.

Correlations between TILs and clinicopathologic parameters

The distribution of TILs in 166 core needle biopsy specimens was summarized in Table 2. The average score of sTILs was 15% (range: 0–60%), and the average score of iTILs was 5% (range: 0–30%). STILs score was positively associated with iTILs ($r = 0.65$, p < 0.001) by Spearman correlation analysis. Using the intraclass correlation coefficient (ICC) analysis, the interobserver agreement of sTILs and iTILs assessment both were excellent (sTILs: ICC 0.91, 95% CI 0.88–0.93, $P = 0.001$; iTILs: ICC 0.83, 95% CI 0.77–0.88, $P = 0.001$).

The correlations between clinicopathologic characteristics and TILs were analyzed in Table 1. Mann-Whitney test showed that both sTILs ($P = 0.004$) and iTILs ($P =$ 0.03) were positively associated with histological grade (Fig. 2a, b), tumors with grade 3 having more lymphocytic infiltration than grade 2. ITILs were positively correlated with negative lymphovascular invasion ($P = 0.03$, Fig. 2c). Spearman's rank correlation analysis revealed that sTILs were positively correlated with Miller-Payne grade, higher sTILs scores in pre-NAC specimens having higher Miller-Payne grade after operation ($r = 0.263$, $P = 0.001$, Fig. 2d). Spearman's rank correlation analysis showed that both higher scores of sTILs ($r = 0.236$, $P = 0.002$) and iTILs ($r = 0.346$, $P = 0.001$) were positively related with higher Ki-67 index in TNBCs (Fig. 2e, f). There was no significant association of TILs with patients' age, tumor size, lymph node status, histological type and neoadjuvant chemotherapy regimens.

Correlations between TILs and pCR

The relationship between TILs and pCR was analyzed by logistic regression analysis (Table 3). TILs were scored as continuous variables (per 10% increment). Univariate analysis showed that both sTILs (per 10% sTILs: OR 1.07, 95% CI 1.03–1.10, $P = 0.0001$) and iTILs (per 10% iTILs: OR 1.10, 95% CI 1.04–1.16, $P = 0.001$) were significantly correlated with pCR. Higher TILs scores indicated higher pCR rate. Multivariate analysis demonstrated that both sTILs (per 10% sTILs: OR 1.05, 95% CI 1.02–1.09, $P = 0.006$) and iTILs (per 10% iTILs: OR 1.06, 95% CI 1.00–1.12, $P = 0.04$) were independent predictors for pCR, irrespective of other clinicopathologic factors.

Stratified analysis was used to investigate whether the predictive value of TILs might be different in every subgroup of clinicopathologic characteristics (Table 4). The chi-squared test showed that there was no significant difference for TILs predicting the rate of pCR in each subgroup ($p > 0.05$).

The optimal thresholds of TILs to predict pCR

Receiver operating characteristics (ROC) curve analysis was used to identify the optimal thresholds of TILs distinguishing pCR from non-pCR cases (Fig. 3). It was revealed that the area under the curve (AUC) of sTILs level was 0.645 (95% CI 0.575–0.747, $P = 0.0001$) and the best cutoff value of sTILs to predict pCR was 15%. The AUC of iTILs level was 0.612 (95% CI 0.542–0.717, $P = 0.005$) and the best cutoff value of iTILs was 5%. Because TILs was scored in 10% increments in our study, all cases were categorized into two groups respectively according to the results of ROC curve: TNBCs with sTILs ≥20% and TNBCs with sTILs < 20%; TNBCs with iTILs ≥10% and TNBCs with iTILs < 10%. The sensitivity, specificity, positive predictive value (PPV), negative predictive value (NPV), accuracy and Youden's Index of the 20% threshold for sTILs and the 10% for iTILs to predict pCR were showed in Table 5.

Table 1 Correlations between TILs and clinicopathologic characteristics in TNBCs

Characteristics	No. of patients (%)	P-value of sTILs	P-value of iTILs
Age (years)			
< 50	80 (48.2)	0.87[a]	0.79[a]
≥ 50	86 (51.8)		
Tumor size (cm)			
≤ 2	22 (13.2)	0.88[b]	0.16[b]
2–5	115 (69.3)		
> 5	29 (17.5)		
Lymph node status			
Negative	53 (31.9)	0.78[a]	0.23[a]
Positive	113 (68.1)		
Histological type			
IDC	164 (98.8)	0.58[a]	0.33[a]
Special type	2 (1.2)		
Histological grade			
2	31 (18.7)	0.004[a+]	0.03[a+]
3	135 (81.3)		
LVI			
Negative	130 (78.3)	0.17[a]	0.03[a+]
Positive	36 (21.7)		
Miller-Payne grade			
1	17 (10.2)	0.001[b+]	0.06[b]
2	26 (15.7)		
3	32 (19.3)		
4	24 (14.4)		
5	67 (40.4)		
NAC			
Anthracycline + paclitaxel	136 (81.9)	0.98[a]	0.99[a]
Paclitaxel + platinum	30 (18.1)		

Abbreviations: *TNBCs* triple-negative breast cancers, *sTILs* stromal tumor-infiltrating lymphocytes, *iTILs* intratumoral tumor-infiltrating lymphocytes, *IDC* invasive ductal carcinoma of no special type, *LVI* lymphovascular invasion, *NAC* neoadjuvant chemotherapy
[a]Mann-Whitney test
[b]Kruskal-Wallis test
[+]The p value is significant

Meanwhile, 20% threshold of sTILs was compared with 50% and 60% thresholds. The sensitivity, specificity, PPV, NPV, accuracy and Youden's Index of these thresholds for sTILs were summarized in Table 5. It was shown that 41.6% of patients had a level of sTILs more than 20%, and the sensitivity and specificity were higher than other thresholds. 10% threshold of iTILs was also compared with 20% and 30% thresholds (Table 5). 42.8% of patients had a level of iTILs more than 10%, and the sensitivity and specificity were higher than other thresholds. Therefore, our study indicated that 20% threshold

Table 2 The distribution of TILs scores in TNBCs

Score (%)	Cancer with sTILs No. (%)	Cancer with iTILs No. (%)
0	17 (10.2)	95 (57.2)
10	80 (48.2)	64 (38.6)
20	41 (24.7)	5 (3)
30	21 (12.7)	2 (1.2)
40	0	0
50	4 (2.4)	0
60	3 (1.8)	0
70	0	0
80	0	0
90	0	0
100	0	0

Abbreviations: *TNBCs* triple-negative breast cancers, *sTILs* stromal tumor-infiltrating lymphocytes, *iTILs* intratumoral tumor-infiltrating lymphocytes

of sTILs and 10% threshold of iTILs may be optimal to predict pCR in TNBCs.

Predictive value of the optimal thresholds of TILs

Logistic regression analysis was performed to evaluate the predictive value of the optimal thresholds in our study. As shown in Table 6, TNBCs with more than 20% sTILs (OR 2.87, 95% CI 1.51–5.47, $P = 0.001$) or more than 10% iTILs (OR 2.62, 95% CI 1.38–4.97, $P = 0.003$) both were significantly associated with higher pCR rate in univariate analysis. Multivariate analysis confirmed that a 20% threshold of sTILs (OR 2.85, 95% CI 1.38–5.90, $P = 0.005$) was an independent predictive factor for pCR, while a 10% threshold of iTILs wasn't an independent predictive factor for pCR ($P > 0.05$).

In view of the relatively low sensitivity and specificity of the 20% threshold for sTILs to independently predict pCR (56.7% and 68.7%, respectively), a predictive model for response to NAC was performed by combining sTILs with clinicopathologic parameters which had a significant association with the rate of pCR in univariate analysis (including patients' age, histological grade, LVI and Ki-67 index) (Table 6). ROC curve analysis demonstrated that the AUC for the combination of these five variables was 0.785 (95% CI 0.714–0.856, $P = 0.0001$), and the sensitivity and specificity to predict pCR were 77.6% and 72.7%, respectively. And it's indicated that the combined predictive model may be more optimal to predict pCR than these clinicopathologic parameters alone in TNBCs (Fig. 4).

Discussion

TNBCs are a group of heterogeneous diseases with various morphology, prognosis, and treatment response. Therefore, it is important to identify valuable biomarkers to predict the therapeutic response and prognosis for TNBCs. Several studies have demonstrated the prognosis

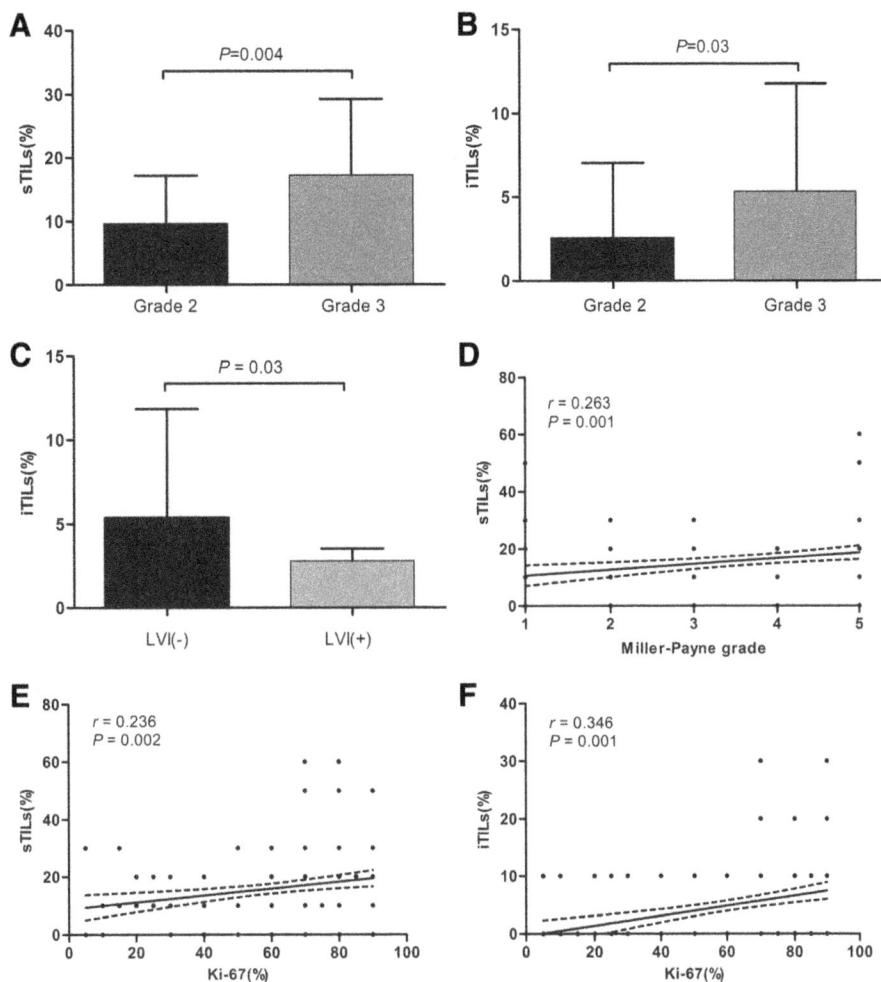

Fig. 2 The correlations of TILs with histological grade, LVI, Miller-Payne grade and Ki-67 index in TNBCs. Y axis represented the scores of TILs; X axis represented histological grade (2 or 3), LVI (−/+), Miller-Payne grade (1–5) or Ki-67 index (%). **a** and **b**: Both sTILs and iTILs were positively associated with histological grade (sTILs: $P = 0.004$; iTILs: $P = 0.03$). **c**: iTILs were positively correlated with negative lymphovascular invasion ($P = 0.03$). Dots corresponded to the scores of TILs and whiskers corresponded to its Standard Error. Red line corresponded to the mean scores of TILs. **d**: STILs was positively correlated with Miller-Payne grade ($r = 0.263$, $P = 0.001$). **e** and **f**: STILs and iTILs scores were positively associated with Ki-67 index (sTILs: $r = 0.236$, $P = 0.002$; iTILs: $r = 0.346$, $P = 0.001$). LVI: lymphovascular invasion

and the predictive values of TILs in TNBCs [12, 21–24]. However, absence of standardized methodologies for TILs measurement has limited its evaluation and application in practice. In 2014, the International TILs Working Group formulated the recommendations of pathologic evaluation for TILs in breast cancers. The recommendations need to be further validated in multiple laboratories before application in routine practice. The study of Pruneri et al. supported the validity of TILs evaluation recommendations in the clinical practice, indicating that each 10% increase in TILs strongly predicted better survival in TNBCs [25]. However, Park et al.'s study showed that TILs scored by the recommendations may not be useful for predicting survival outcomes in early TNBCs [26]. In our previous study, we carried out a retrospective analysis of TILs in 425 primary invasive TNBCs using the recommendations, indicating

that TILs scored by the recommendations could be associated with the prognosis of TNBCs [27]. In this study, we performed a retrospective analysis of TILs in 166 core needle biopsy specimens of TNBCs with NAC, aimed to evaluate the predictive value of TILs scored by the recommendations to pCR. Our study indicated that TILs scored by the recommendations in pre-NAC core needle biopsy of TNBCs were significantly correlated with pCR, higher TILs score strongly predicting higher pCR rate, and TILs score was an independent predictor for pCR. Another issue which should be evaluated is the reproducibility of the recommendations. Swisher et al. evaluated the interobserver agreement of TILs scored by recommendations among four observers, and showed an acceptable agreement in TILs evaluation [28]. In our study, an excellent interobserver agreement between two observers was

Table 3 Correlations between TILs and pCR in neoadjuvant treated TNBCs

Variables	Univariate analysis			Multivariate analysis		
	OR	95% CI	*P*-value	OR	95% CI	*P*-value
ITILs (per 10%)	1.10	1.04–1.16	0.001*	1.06	1.00-1.12	0.04*
STILs (per 10%)	1.07	1.03–1.10	0.0001*	1.05	1.02-1.09	0.006*
Age (years) (< 50 vs. ≥50)	0.51	0.27–0.95	0.04*	0.65	0.31-1.35	0.25
Histological grade (2 vs. 3)	2.74	1.11–6.80	0.03*	1.02	0.34-3.08	0.98
Tumor size (cm) (≤2 vs. 2–5 vs. > 5)	1.30	0.74–2.29	0.37	1.30	0.68-2.47	0.43
Nodal status (negative vs. positive)	0.93	0.48–1.81	0.84	1.52	0.72–3.22	0.28
LVI (negative vs. positive)	0.06	0.01–0.26	0.0001*	0.07	0.02-0.29	0.0001*
Ki-67 index	1.03	1.01–1.04	0.001*	1.02	1.006-1.04	0.009*
NAC (Anthracycline + paclitaxel vs. paclitaxel + platinum)	0.83	0.37–1.87	0.65	1.10	0.41-2.94	0.85

Abbreviations: *pCR* pathological complete response, *TNBCs* triple-negative breast cancers, *sTILs* stromal tumor-infiltrating lymphocytes, *iTILs* intratumoral tumor-infiltrating lymphocytes, *LVI* lymphovascular invasion, *NAC* neoadjuvant chemotherapy, *OR* odds ratio, *95% CI* 95% confidence interval
*The P value is significant

demonstrated in TILs evaluation. However, large-scale investigation should be performed to assess the intra- and inter-observer reproducibility of TILs evaluation before the application of TILs assessment in clinical practice.

Several studies have evaluated the predictive value of sTILs and iTILs for pCR in neoadjuvant treated TNBCs [12, 21, 29–32]. Khoury et al. found that both sTILs and iTILs were independent predictors for pCR in TNBCs

[33]. Denkert et al's study revealed that iTILs was a significant independent parameter for pCR in breast cancers in both training and validation cohorts, while sTILs was a strong predictor for pCR just in validation cohort [9]. The study of Issa-Nummer et al. showed that, in HER2-negative breast cancer, sTILs was a significant independent predictor for pCR in multivariate analysis, while iTILs was significant for pCR only in univariate

Table 4 Correlations between TILs and pCR in clinicopathologic subgroups

Variable	No. of patients	Per 10% sTILs increase			Per 10% iTILs increase		
		Adjusted OR	95% CI	*P*-value*	Adjusted OR	95% CI	*P*-value*
Age (years)							
< 50	80	1.06	1.01–1.11	0.78	1.09	1.01–1.18	0.64
≥ 50	86	1.07	1.02–1.12		1.12	1.03–1.22	
Tumor size (cm)							
≤ 2	22	1.05	0.99–1.12	0.68	1.07	0.92–1.25	0.72
2–5	115	1.06	1.02–1.10		1.09	1.02–1.16	
> 5	29	1.11	1.00–1.24		1.16	1.00–1.35	
Lymph node status							
Negative	53	1.07	1.00–1.14	0.81	1.07	0.96–1.18	0.56
Positive	113	1.06	1.02–1.10		1.11	1.04–1.19	
Grade							
2	31	1.01	0.90–1.13	0.34	1.02	0.84–1.23	0.46
3	135	1.07	1.03–1.10		1.11	1.04–1.17	
LVI							
Negative	130	1.06	1.02–1.10	0.49	1.08	1.02–1.15	0.84
Positive	36	1.14	0.93–1.39		1.11	0.83–1.48	
NAC							
Anthracycline + paclitaxel	136	1.07	1.03–1.12	0.23	1.12	1.06–1.20	0.14
Paclitaxel + platinum	30	1.01	0.93–1.10		1.00	0.87–1.14	

Abbreviations: *pCR* pathological complete response, *sTILs* stromal tumor-infiltrating lymphocytes, *iTILs* intratumoral tumor-infiltrating lymphocytes, *LVI* lymphovascular invasion, *NAC* neoadjuvant chemotherapy, *OR* odds ratio, *95% CI* 95% confidence interval
*The chi-squared test

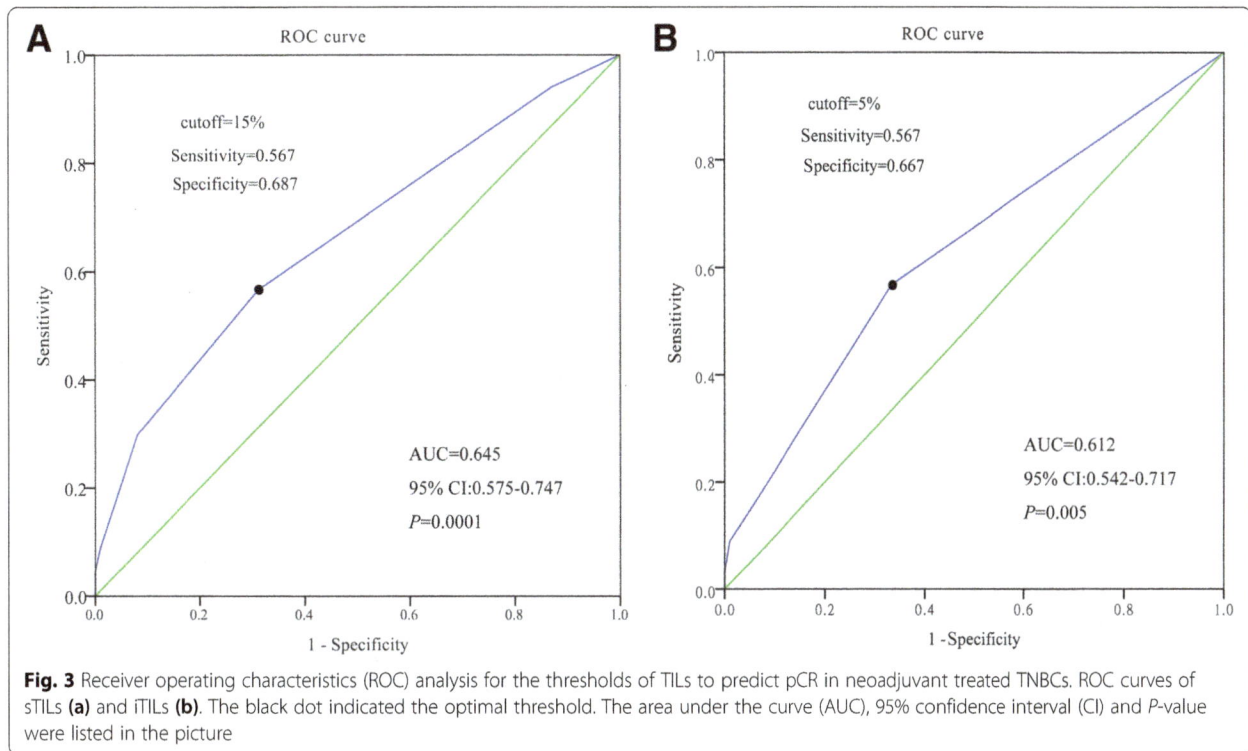

Fig. 3 Receiver operating characteristics (ROC) analysis for the thresholds of TILs to predict pCR in neoadjuvant treated TNBCs. ROC curves of sTILs (**a**) and iTILs (**b**). The black dot indicated the optimal threshold. The area under the curve (AUC), 95% confidence interval (CI) and *P*-value were listed in the picture

but not in multivariate analysis [34]. Our study indicated that both higher sTILs and iTILs score strongly predicted higher pCR rate in univariate analysis, and both sTILs and iTILs score were independent predictors for pCR in multivariate analysis in TNBCs.

The cutoff value of TILs to predict therapeutic response has been analyzed in previous studies. Some studies found that lymphocyte-predominant breast cancer (LPBC, defined as involving ≥50% or ≥ 60% lymphocytic infiltration of either tumor stroma or cell nests) was an independent predictor of pCR for neoadjuvant treated triple-negative and HER2-positive breast cancers [22, 34–36]. However, the 2014 International TILs Working Group recommendations suggested that it was

arbitrary to define 50–60% as the threshold for LPBC, because of the relatively low proportion of these cases in breast cancers [14]. In our previous study, only 3.5% of TNBCs had more than 50% lymphocytes [27]. In this study, only 7 of 166 TNBCs (4.2%) had more than 50% lymphocyte infiltration in core needle biopsy specimens. It was unsuitable to define a cutoff value of 50% as LPBC to predict pCR because of the limited clinical implication caused by the low proportion of these cases. In our study, ROC curve analysis revealed that 20% threshold of sTILs and 10% threshold of iTILs may be more optimal to predict pCR compared with other cutoff values. TNBCs with more than 20% sTILs or with more than 10% iTILs were associated with higher pCR rate in

Table 5 Comparisons between different thresholds of sTILs and iTILs

Threshold (%)	No. of patients (%)	Sensitivity (%)	Specificity (%)	PPV (%)[a]	NPV (%)	Accuracy (%)	Youden's Index
STILs							
20	41.6	56.7	68.7	55.1	70.1	63.9	0.254
50	4.2	9.0	99.0	85.7	61.6	62.7	0.08
60	1.8	4.5	100.0	100.0	60.7	61.4	0.045
ITILs							
10	42.8	56.7	66.7	53.5	69.5	62.7	0.234
20	4.2	8.9	98.9	85.7	61.6	62.7	0.078
30	1.2	2.9	100.0	100.0	60.4	60.8	0.029

Abbreviations: *sTILs* stromal tumor-infiltrating lymphocytes, *iTILs* intratumoral tumor-infiltrating lymphocytes, *PPV* positive predictive value, *NPV* negative predictive value, Youden's Index = sensitivity + specificity - 1

[a]PPV = pCR rate

Table 6 Correlations between the optimal thresholds of TILs and pCR in neoadjuvant treated TNBCs

Variables	Univariate analysis			Multivariate analysis		
	OR	95% CI	P-value	OR	95% CI	P-value
ITILs (< 10% vs. ≥10%)	2.62	1.38–4.97	0.003*	1.97	0.98-3.98	0.06
STILs (< 20% vs. ≥20%)	2.87	1.51–5.47	0.001*	2.85	1.38-5.90	0.005*
Age(years) (< 50 vs. ≥50)	0.51	0.27–0.95	0.04*	0.70	0.33-1.45	0.33
Histological grade (2 vs. 3)	2.74	1.11–6.80	0.03*	1.02	0.34-3.10	0.97
Tumor size (cm) (≤2 vs. 2–5 vs. > 5)	1.30	0.74–2.29	0.37	1.12	0.58–2.14	0.74
Nodal status (positive vs. negative)	0.93	0.48–1.81	0.84	1.76	0.82–3.79	0.15
LVI (positive vs. negative)	0.06	0.01–0.26	0.0001*	0.05	0.01-0.25	0.0001*
Ki-67 index	2.47	1.17–5.24	0.02*	1.03	1.01-1.04	0.004*
NAC (Anthracycline + paclitaxel vs. paclitaxel + platinum)	0.83	0.37–1.87	0.65	0.99	0.49–2.00	0.97

Abbreviations: *pCR* pathological complete response, *TNBCs* triple-negative breast cancers, *sTILs* stromal tumor-infiltrating lymphocytes, *iTILs* intratumoral tumor-infiltrating lymphocytes, *LVI* lymphovascular invasion, *NAC* neoadjuvant chemotherapy, *OR* odds ratio, *95% CI* 95% confidence interval
*The P value is significant

univariate analysis. A 20% threshold of sTILs was an independent predictor for pCR in multivariate analysis. However, a 10% threshold of iTILs wasn't an independent predictor for pCR in multivariate analysis, which may due to the relatively low score of iTILs in our study. In addition, our study performed a predictive model for therapeutic response by the combination of sTILs score, patients' age, histological grade, LVI and Ki-67 index in TNBCs. It was shown that the combined five variables had relatively high sensitivity and specificity. Therefore, the predictive model might have potential value to predict NAC treated response in TNBCs in practice.

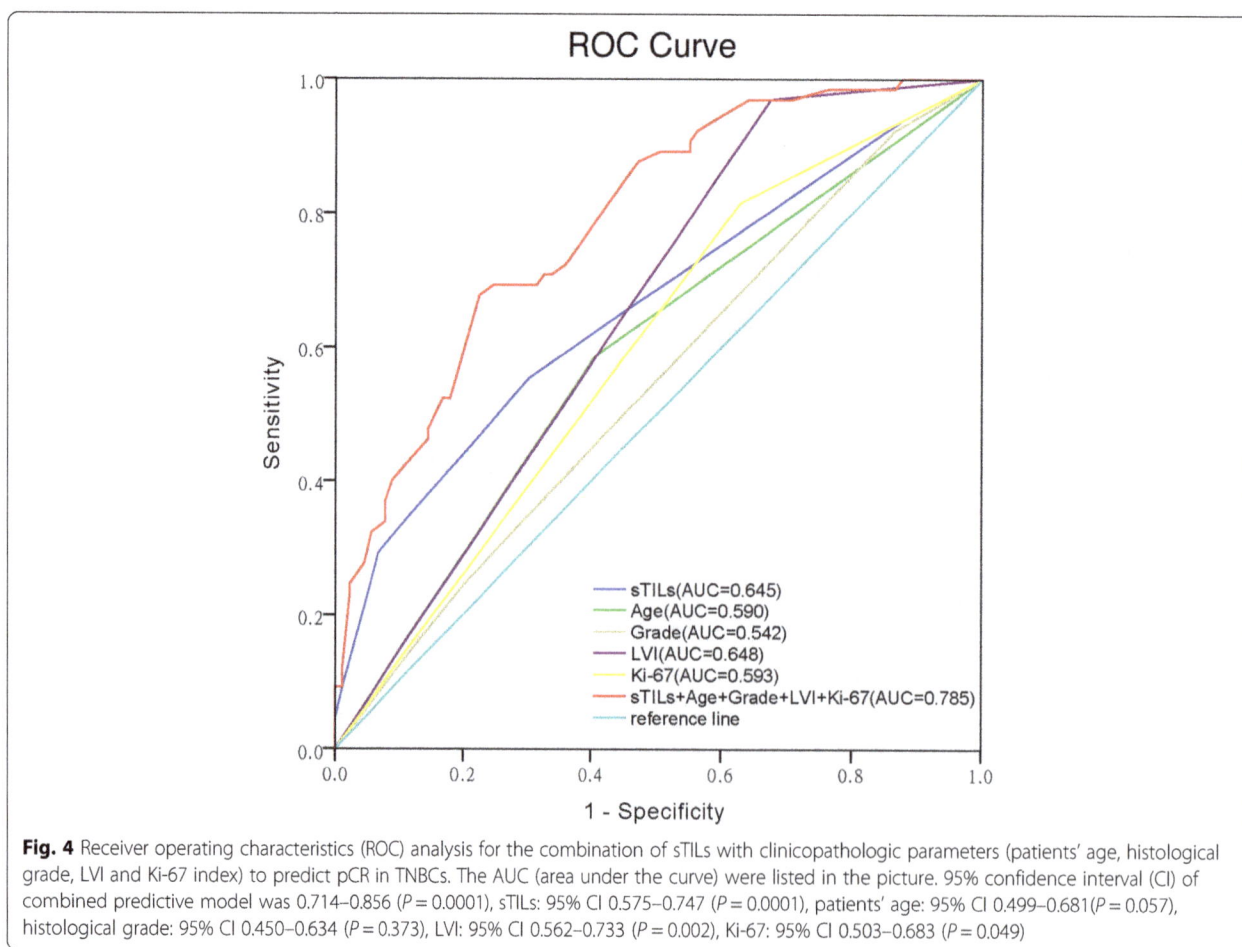

Fig. 4 Receiver operating characteristics (ROC) analysis for the combination of sTILs with clinicopathologic parameters (patients' age, histological grade, LVI and Ki-67 index) to predict pCR in TNBCs. The AUC (area under the curve) were listed in the picture. 95% confidence interval (CI) of combined predictive model was 0.714–0.856 (P = 0.0001), sTILs: 95% CI 0.575–0.747 (P = 0.0001), patients' age: 95% CI 0.499–0.681(P = 0.057), histological grade: 95% CI 0.450–0.634 (P = 0.373), LVI: 95% CI 0.562–0.733 (P = 0.002), Ki-67: 95% CI 0.503–0.683 (P = 0.049)

The relationships between clinicopathologic parameters and TILs were also analyzed in our study. It was revealed that both higher scores of sTILs and iTILs were related with higher Ki-67 index and higher histological grade, and higher iTILs scores were positively correlated with negative LVI in TNBCs. Krishnamurti et al. found that TILs was significantly associated with histologic grade 3 in TNBCs [37]. The study of Chung et al. showed that infiltration of CD4+, CD8+, and FOXP3+ TILs was significantly higher in tumors with high Ki-67 index [38]. Pan et al.'s study revealed that the percentage of sTILs and density of CD8+ T-lymphocytes were positively correlated with Ki-67 in TNBCs [39]. Lee et al. found that TNBCs with higher levels of TILs showed lower LVI [40]. However, the relationships between clinicopathologic characteristics and TILs still need to be further explored.

The relationship between TILs subpopulations and therapeutic response has been studied in breast cancers in recent years. Garcia-Martinez et al. and Castaneda et al. found that higher ratio of CD8+/CD4+ was associated with higher pCR rate in pre-NAC breast cancers [11, 12]. The study of Seo et al. revealed that CD8+ TILs was an independent predictor for pCR irrespective of breast cancer subtypes [41]. The research of Asano et al. showed that the pCR rate was significantly higher in the high CD8+/FOXP3+ TIL ratio (CFR) group, and high-CFR status was an independent predictor of a favorable prognosis for TNBC and HER2+ breast cancer [42]. However, the scoring methods of subgroup evaluation were not standardized in these studies, the clinical application of TILs subpopulations still needs more available evidence.

Conclusions

In summary, our study indicated that TILs scored by methods recommended by International TILs Working Group 2014 in pre-NAC core needle biopsy specimens was significantly correlated with pCR in TNBCs, higher TILs scores predicting higher pCR rate. Both sTILs and iTILs were independent predictors for pCR in TNBCs. A 20% threshold for sTILs may be feasible to predict pCR to NAC in TNBCs. The combination of sTILs and other clinicopathologic variables might have potential value to predict NAC treated response in TNBCs in practice.

Abbreviations

ER: estrogen receptor; HER2: human epidermal growth factor receptor 2; LPBC: lymphocyte-predominant breast cancer; pCR: pathological complete response; PgR: progesterone receptor; TILs: tumor-infiltrating lymphocytes; TNBCs: triple-negative breast cancers

Funding

This work was supported by grants from Research Project of the Science and Technology Commission of Shanghai Municipality (Project No: 15411965100, for Ruohong Shui).

Authors' contributions

Work design (all authors). Data Collection and Drafting the article (M.R). Data statistics and analysis (T.T). Revision of the article (R.S). All authors read and approved the final manuscript.

Competing interests

The author declares that they have no competing interests.

References

1. Podo F, Buydens LM, Degani H, Hilhorst R, Klipp E, Gribbestad IS, et al. Triple-negative breast cancer: present challenges and new perspectives. Mol Oncol. 2010;4:209–29.
2. Dent R, Trudeau M, Pritchard KI, Hanna WM, Kahn HK, Sawka CA, et al. Triple-negative breast cancer: clinical features and patterns of recurrence. Clin Cancer Res. 2007;13:4429–34.
3. Liedtke C, Mazouni C, Hess KR, Andre F, Tordai A, Mejia JA, et al. Response to neoadjuvant therapy and long-term survival in patients with triple-negative breast cancer. J Clin Oncol. 2008;26:1275–81.
4. Kumar P, Aggarwal R. An overview of triple-negative breast cancer. Arch Gynecol Obstet. 2016;293:247–69.
5. Stagg J, Allard B. Immunotherapeutic approaches in triple-negative breast cancer: latest research and clinical prospects. Ther Adv Med Oncol. 2013;5: 169–81.
6. van Rooijen JM, Stutvoet TS, Schroder CP, de Vries EG. Immunotherapeutic options on the horizon in breast cancer treatment. Pharmacol Ther. 2015; 156:90–101.
7. Fisher CS, Ma CX, Gillanders WE, Aft RL, Eberlein TJ, Gao F, et al. Neoadjuvant chemotherapy is associated with improved survival compared with adjuvant chemotherapy in patients with triple-negative breast cancer only after complete pathologic response. Ann Surg Oncol. 2012;19:253–8.
8. Kong X, Moran MS, Zhang N, Haffty B, Yang Q. Meta-analysis confirms achieving pathological complete response after neoadjuvant chemotherapy predicts favourable prognosis for breast cancer patients. Eur J Cancer. 2011; 47:2084–90.
9. Denkert C, Loibl S, Noske A, Roller M, Muller BM, Komor M, et al. Tumor-associated lymphocytes as an independent predictor of response to neoadjuvant chemotherapy in breast cancer. J Clin Oncol. 2010;28:105–13.
10. Jung YY, Hyun CL, Jin MS, Park IA, Chung YR, Shim B, et al. Histomorphological factors predicting the response to neoadjuvant chemotherapy in triple-negative breast Cancer. J Breast Cancer. 2016;19:261–7.
11. Garcia-Martinez E, Gil GL, Benito AC, Gonzalez-Billalabeitia E, Conesa MA, Garcia Garcia T, et al. Tumor-infiltrating immune cell profiles and their change after neoadjuvant chemotherapy predict response and prognosis of breast cancer. Breast Cancer Res. 2014;16:488.
12. Castaneda CA, Mittendorf E, Casavilca S, Wu Y, Castillo M, Arboleda P, et al. Tumor infiltrating lymphocytes in triple negative breast cancer receiving neoadjuvant chemotherapy. World J Clin Oncol. 2016;7:387–94.
13. Loi S, Sirtaine N, Piette F, Salgado R, Viale G, Van Eenoo F, et al. Prognostic and predictive value of tumor-infiltrating lymphocytes in a phase III randomized adjuvant breast cancer trial in node-positive breast cancer comparing the addition of docetaxel to doxorubicin with doxorubicin-based chemotherapy: BIG 02-98. J Clin Oncol. 2013;31:860–7.

14. Salgado R, Denkert C, Demaria S, Sirtaine N, Klauschen F, Pruneri G, et al. The evaluation of tumor-infiltrating lymphocytes (TILs) in breast cancer: recommendations by an international TILs working group 2014. Ann Oncol. 2015;26:259–71.

15. Wolff AC, Hammond ME, Schwartz JN, Hagerty KL, Allred DC, Cote RJ, et al. American Society of Clinical Oncology/College of American Pathologists guideline recommendations for human epidermal growth factor receptor 2 testing in breast cancer. J Clin Oncol. 2007;25:118–45.

16. Hammond ME, Hayes DF, Wolff AC, Mangu PB, Temin S. American society of clinical oncology/college of american pathologists guideline recommendations for immunohistochemical testing of estrogen and progesterone receptors in breast cancer. J Oncol Pract. 2010;6:195–7.

17. Lakhani SR, Ellis IO, Schnitt SJ, Tan PH, van de Vijver MJ. WHO Classification of Tumours of the Breast. Lyon: IARC. 2012;4.

18. Bloom HJ, Richardson WW. Histological grading and prognosis in breast cancer; a study of 1409 cases of which 359 have been followed for 15 years. Br J Cancer. 1957;11:359–77.

19. Elston CW, Ellis IO. Pathological prognostic factors in breast cancer. I. The value of histological grade in breast cancer: experience from a large study with long-term follow-up. Histopathology. 1991;19:403–10.

20. Ogston KN, Miller ID, Payne S, Hutcheon AW, Sarkar TK, Smith I, et al. A new histological grading system to assess response of breast cancers to primary chemotherapy: prognostic significance and survival. Breast (Edinburgh, Scotland). 2003;12:320–7.

21. Ono M, Tsuda H, Shimizu C, Yamamoto S, Shibata T, Yamamoto H, et al. Tumor-infiltrating lymphocytes are correlated with response to neoadjuvant chemotherapy in triple-negative breast cancer. Breast Cancer Res Treat. 2012;132:793–805.

22. Denkert C, Loibl S, Salat C, Sinn B, Schem C, Endris V, et al. Abstract S1-06: Increased tumor-associated lymphocytes predict benefit from addition of carboplatin to neoadjuvant therapy for triple-negative and HER2-positive early breast cancer in the GeparSixto trial (GBG 66). Cancer Res. 2013;73:S1-06–S01-06.

23. Loi S, Michiels S, Salgado R, Sirtaine N, Jose V, Fumagalli D, et al. Tumor infiltrating lymphocytes are prognostic in triple negative breast cancer and predictive for trastuzumab benefit in early breast cancer: results from the FinHER trial. Ann Oncol. 2014;25:1544–50.

24. Adams S, Gray RJ, Demaria S, Goldstein L, Perez EA, Shulman LN, et al. Prognostic value of tumor-infiltrating lymphocytes in triple-negative breast cancers from two phase III randomized adjuvant breast cancer trials: ECOG 2197 and ECOG 1199. J Clin Oncol. 2014;32:2959–66.

25. Pruneri G, Vingiani A, Bagnardi V, Rotmensz N, De Rose A, Palazzo A, et al. Clinical validity of tumor-infiltrating lymphocytes analysis in patients with triple-negative breast cancer. Ann Oncol. 2016;27:249–56.

26. Park HS, Heo I, Kim JY, Kim S, Nam S, Park S, et al. No effect of tumor-infiltrating lymphocytes (TILs) on prognosis in patients with early triple-negative breast cancer: validation of recommendations by the international TILs working group 2014. J Surg Oncol. 2016;114:17–21.

27. Tian T, Ruan M, Yang W, Shui R. Evaluation of the prognostic value of tumor-infiltrating lymphocytes in triple-negative breast cancers. Oncotarget. 2016;7:44395–405.

28. Swisher SK, Wu Y, Castaneda CA, Lyons GR, Yang F, Tapia C, et al. Interobserver agreement between pathologists assessing tumor-infiltrating lymphocytes (TILs) in breast Cancer using methodology proposed by the international TILs working group. Ann Surg Oncol. 2016;23:2242–8.

29. Mao Y, Qu Q, Zhang Y, Liu J, Chen X, Shen K. The value of tumor infiltrating lymphocytes (TILs) for predicting response to neoadjuvant chemotherapy in breast cancer: a systematic review and meta-analysis. PLoS One. 2014;9:e115103.

30. Wang K, Xu J, Zhang T, Xue D. Tumor-infiltrating lymphocytes in breast cancer predict the response to chemotherapy and survival outcome: a meta-analysis. Oncotarget. 2016;7:44288–98.

31. Li XB, Krishnamurti U, Bhattarai S, Klimov S, Reid MD, O'Regan R, et al. Biomarkers predicting pathologic complete response to neoadjuvant chemotherapy in breast Cancer. Am J Clin Pathol. 2016;145:871–8.

32. Hida AI, Sagara Y, Yotsumoto D, Kanemitsu S, Kawano J, Baba S, et al. Prognostic and predictive impacts of tumor-infiltrating lymphocytes differ between triple-negative and HER2-positive breast cancers treated with standard systemic therapies. Breast Cancer Res Treat. 2016;158:1–9.

33. Khoury T, Nagrale V, Opyrchal M, Peng X, Wang D, Yao S. Prognostic significance of stromal versus Intratumoral infiltrating lymphocytes in different subtypes of breast Cancer treated with cytotoxic neoadjuvant chemotherapy: Applied immunohistochemistry & molecular morphology : AIMM; 2017:1.

34. Issa-Nummer Y, Darb-Esfahani S, Loibl S, Kunz G, Nekljudova V, Schrader I, et al. Prospective validation of immunological infiltrate for prediction of response to neoadjuvant chemotherapy in HER2-negative breast cancer—a substudy of the neoadjuvant GeparQuinto trial. PLoS One. 2013;8:e79775.

35. Denkert C, von Minckwitz G, Brase JC, Sinn BV, Gade S, Kronenwett R, et al. Tumor-infiltrating lymphocytes and response to neoadjuvant chemotherapy with or without carboplatin in human epidermal growth factor receptor 2-positive and triple-negative primary breast cancers. J Clin Oncol. 2015;33:983–91.

36. Ingold Heppner B, Untch M, Denkert C, Pfitzner BM, Lederer B, Schmitt W, et al. Tumor-infiltrating lymphocytes: a predictive and prognostic biomarker in neoadjuvant-treated HER2-positive breast Cancer. Clin Cancer Res. 2016; 22:5747–54.

37. Krishnamurti U, Wetherilt CS, Yang J, Peng L, Li X. Tumor-infiltrating lymphocytes are significantly associated with better overall survival and disease-free survival in triple-negative but not estrogen receptor-positive breast cancers. Hum Pathol. 2017;64:7–12.

38. Chung YR, Kim HJ, Jang MH, Park SY. Prognostic value of tumor infiltrating lymphocyte subsets in breast cancer depends on hormone receptor status. Breast Cancer Res Treat. 2017;161:409–20.

39. Pan BJ, Ping GQ, Zhang WM, Wang C, Li HX, Zhang ZH. CD8 and FOXP3 expression in stromal tumor-infiltrating lymphocytes of triple-negative breast carcinomas: a clinicopathologic study. Zhonghua bing li xue za zhi. 2016;45:540–4.

40. Lee HJ, Park IA, Song IH, Shin SJ, Kim JY, Yu JH, et al. Tertiary lymphoid structures: prognostic significance and relationship with tumour-infiltrating lymphocytes in triple-negative breast cancer. J Clin Pathol. 2016;69:422–30.

41. Seo AN, Lee HJ, Kim EJ, Kim HJ, Jang MH, Lee HE, et al. Tumour-infiltrating CD8+ lymphocytes as an independent predictive factor for pathological complete response to primary systemic therapy in breast cancer. Br J Cancer. 2013;109:2705–13.

42. Asano Y, Kashiwagi S, Goto W, Kurata K, Noda S, Takashima T, et al. Tumour-infiltrating CD8 to FOXP3 lymphocyte ratio in predicting treatment responses to neoadjuvant chemotherapy of aggressive breast cancer. Br J Surg. 2016;103:845–54.

21

Detection of specific gene rearrangements by fluorescence *in situ* hybridization in 16 cases of clear cell sarcoma of soft tissue and 6 cases of clear cell sarcoma-like gastrointestinal tumor

Keiko Segawa[1], Shintaro Sugita[1*], Tomoyuki Aoyama[1], Terufumi Kubo[2], Hiroko Asanuma[1], Taro Sugawara[1], Yumika Ito[1], Mitsuhiro Tsujiwaki[1], Hiromi Fujita[1], Makoto Emori[3] and Tadashi Hasegawa[1]

Abstract

Background: Clear cell sarcoma of soft tissue (CCSST) and clear cell sarcoma-like gastrointestinal tumor (CCSLGT) are malignant mesenchymal tumors that share some pathological features, but they also have several different characteristics. They are well known to express chimeric fusions of Ewing sarcoma breakpoint region 1 (*EWSR1*) and cAMP response element-binding protein (*CREB*) family members; namely, *EWSR1*-activating transcription factor 1 (*ATF1*) and *EWSR1-CREB1*. In addition, recent studies have suggested the presence of other fusions.

Methods: We used fluorescence *in situ* hybridization to detect specific rearrangements including *EWSR1*, *ATF1*, *CREB1*, and cAMP response element modulator (*CREM*) in 16 CCSST and 6 CCSLGT cases. We also used reverse transcription polymerase chain reaction (RT-PCR) to detect specific chimeric fusions of *EWSR1-ATF1* and *EWSR1-CREB1* using fresh tumor samples in available cases.

Results: A total of 15 of 16 CCSST cases (93.8%) had *EWSR1* rearrangement, of which 11 (68.8%) also had *ATF1* rearrangement, suggestive of the presence of *EWSR1-ATF1* fusions. One CCSST case (6.3%) was found to have *EWSR1* and *CREM* rearrangements, and 4 of 6 CCSLGT cases (66.7%) had *EWSR1* rearrangement, of which 2 (33.3%) showed *ATF1* rearrangement and the other 2 cases (33.3%) showed *CREB1* rearrangement. These cases most likely had *EWSR1-ATF1* and *EWSR1-CREB1* fusions, respectively. RT-PCR was performed in 8 available cases, including 6 CCSSTs and 2 CCSLGTs. All CCSSTs showed *EWSR1-ATF1* fusions. Among the 2 CCSLGT cases, one had *EWSR1-ATF1* fusion and the other had *EWSR1-CREB1* fusion.

Conclusions: Rearrangements of *EWSR1* and *ATF1* or *EWSR1-ATF1* fusion were predominantly found in CCSST, whereas those of *EWSR1* and *CREB1* or *EWSR1-CREB1* tended to be detected in CCSLGT. A novel *CREM* fusion was also detected in a few cases of CCSST and CCSLGT. The cases in which *EWSR1* rearrangement was detected without definitive partner genes should be considered for the presence of *CREM* rearrangement.

Keywords: Clear cell sarcoma of soft tissue (CCSST), Clear cell sarcoma-like gastrointestinal tumor (CCSLGT), *EWSR1-ATF1*, *EWSR1-CREB1*, *EWSR1-CREM*

* Correspondence: ssugita@sapmed.ac.jp
[1]Department of Surgical Pathology, Sapporo Medical University, School of Medicine, Sapporo, Hokkaido 060-8543, Japan
Full list of author information is available at the end of the article

Background

Clear cell sarcoma of soft tissue (CCSST) is a malignant mesenchymal tumor that mostly affects young adults and tends to affect the lower extremities, close to the tendon and aponeuroses [1]. Histologically, CCSSTs have epithelioid tumor nests accompanied by some spindling areas, and wreath-like multinucleated giant cells. CCSSTs present with a melanocytic differentiation and often express melanocytic markers including S-100 protein, melanoma antigen (Melan-A), human melanoma black 45 (HMB45), microphthalmia-associated transcription factor (MITF), and SRY-Box 10 (SOX-10) on immunohistochemistry (IHC). Ultrastructurally, CCSST has premelanosomes in the cytoplasm of tumor cells and shares some characteristic features with malignant melanomas (MMs). MMs genetically have BRAF mutations, although CCSST lacks this mutation. Clear cell sarcoma-like gastrointestinal tumor (CCSLGT) is also a malignant mesenchymal tumor that shares some pathological features with CCSST and arises from the gastrointestinal tract, such as the small and large intestine, and stomach. CCSLGT was originally reported to be an "osteoclast-rich tumor of the gastrointestinal tract with features resembling clear cell sarcoma of the soft parts" [2] and the first case of CCSLGT was reported by Alpers et al. [3] as a "malignant neuroendocrine tumor of the jejunum with osteoclast-like giant cells" in 1985. Subsequently, the term CCSLGT was first used by Kosemehmetoglu et al. [4] in their review, which included 13 CCSLGT cases. However, some authors have proposed using the term "malignant gastrointestinal neuroectodermal tumor," because CCSLGTs lack melanocytic differentiation on IHC and ultrastructural examination and appear to have poorer prognosis [5]. Although CCSLGT has a similar histology to CCSST in some respects, such as a clear cytoplasm and epithelioid cells, there are some differing characteristics. CCSLGT has a pseudo-papillary growth pattern and many osteoclast-type giant cells, and the tumor cells tend to be positive for S-100 protein but show less expression of melanocytic markers on IHC [6]. Genetically, CCSST and CCSLGT usually have characteristic chimeric fusions of Ewing sarcoma breakpoint region 1 (*EWSR1*) with cAMP response element-binding protein (*CREB*) gene family members, *EWSR1*-activating transcription factor 1 (*ATF1*) and *EWSR1-CREB1*, which were derived from each translocation of t(12;22)(q13;q12) and t(2;22)(q34;q12), respectively [7–10]. *EWSR1-ATF1* fusion is much more frequent than *EWSR1-CREB1* fusion, but *EWSR1-CREB1* fusion of CCSLGT is comparatively often observed.

In this study, we used fluorescence *in situ* hybridization (FISH) and reverse transcription polymerase chain reaction (RT-PCR) to perform genetic analyses of 22 cases of CCSSTs and CCSLGTs, and compared their different chimeric fusion types.

Methods

Case selection

The study protocol for the collection of tumor samples and clinical information were approved by the Institutional Review Board of Sapporo Medical University Hospital (Sapporo, Japan; No. 292–3012). We selected 22 cases of clear cell sarcoma (CCS) including 16 CCSST and 6 CCSLGT cases from the clinicopathological archive at the Department of Surgical Pathology, Sapporo Medical University Hospital. We reviewed all hematoxylin and eosin-stained sections and confirmed that each case fulfilled the histologic criteria of CCSST and CCSLGT.

Immunohistochemistry

We evaluated previously reported IHC findings of melanocytic markers, including S-100 protein, Melan-A, HMB45, and SOX-10, and assessed their positivity. We also performed additional IHC using representative sections from formalin-fixed and paraffin-embedded tissues in some cases. These tissues were sliced into 3-mm-thick sections and examined with an automated IHC system at Sapporo Medical University Hospital. All slides were loaded into a PT Link module (Agilent Technologies, Santa Clara, CA) and subjected to a heat-induced antigen-retrieval protocol with EnVision FLEX Target Retrieval Solution (Agilent Technologies) before being transferred to the Autostainer Link 48 instrument (Agilent Technologies) and Dako Omnis (Agilent Technologies). We used antibodies against the following antigens: S-100 protein (polyclonal; Agilent Technologies), Melan-A (A103; Agilent Technologies), HMB45 (HMB45; Agilent Technologies), and SOX-10 (N-20; Santa Cruz Biotechnology, Santa Cruz, CA).

Fluorescence *in situ* hybridization

We performed FISH using the specimens obtained from tumor materials and 4 µm slices on glass slides. First, we selected an area showing representative histology and marked a 5-mm-diameter circle with a marker on the glass slides for FISH analyses. We performed FISH using dual color break apart probe for EWSR1 (Abbott, Abbott Park, IL), ATF1 (Empire Genomics, Buffalo, NY), CREB1 (Empire Genomics), and CREM (Empire Genomics). FISH was conducted as previously described [11], with the following modifications: baking (1 h at 60 °C), deparaffinization, target gene activation (20 min with 0.2 M HCl followed by 30 min with pretreatment solution at 80 °C), enzyme treatment (60 min with protease solution at 37 °C), re-fixation (10 min in 10% formalin neutral buffer solution), denaturation (5 min with denaturation solution at 72 °C), washing and dehydration (1 min each in 70%, 85%, and 100% ethanol), hybridization with 10 mL DNA probe solution (5 min at 90 °C followed by 48 h at 37 °C), and washing with post-hybridization wash buffer (2 min at 72 °C). As a counterstain, 10 μL 4,6-diamidino-2-phenylindole was added. Slides were coverslipped for viewing under a fluorescence microscope.

To detect the presence of *EWSR1, ATF1, CREB1*, and *CREM* rearrangements, we counted 50 nuclei in tumor cells that showed a pair of fused and split signals, and calculated the percentage of split signals. The signals were considered split when the distance between the red and green signals was at least twice the estimated signal diameter. We did not evaluate any truncated and overlapping cells in FISH analysis. We considered the specimen to be "split positive" if split signals were observed in more than 10% of tumor cells [12].

Reverse transcription-polymerase chain reaction

We detected chimeric fusions by RT-PCR using fresh tumor samples in several available cases. RT-PCR analysis was performed for *EWSR1-ATF1* and *EWSR1--CREB1* fusions. For RT-PCR detection of the *EWSR1-ATF1* and *EWSR1-CREB1* fusions, we used the forward primer EWSex7-F1 with either the CREB1ex7-RevA primer (binds both *CREB1* and *ATF1*; sequence: TCCA TCAGTGGTCTGTGCATACTG) or the CREB1ex7-Re vC primer (specific for *CREB1*; sequence: GTACCCCAT CGGTACCATTGT) [1, 7, 13].

Results
Clinical findings

This study involved 8 male and 14 female patients with a mean age of 40 years (range, 8–78 years). Mean tumor size was 4.6 cm (range, 2–10). The anatomical locations were deep soft tissue of the upper ($n = 6$) and lower ($n = 8$) extremities, esophagus ($n = 1$), small intestine ($n = 5$), abdominal wall (n = 1), and skin (n = 1). The primary site in Case 13 was the upper extremity, but a specimen was not available, so we used lymph node specimens of metastatic lesions. Mean follow-up duration was 38 months (range, 3–249 months; Table 1).

Histological and IHC findings

Histologically, the majority of CCSSTs showed sheet-like and nested growth patterns of epithelioid and/or spindle tumor cells that had round to mildly irregularly shaped nuclei with conspicuous nucleoli and clear to pale eosinophilic or amphophilic cytoplasm (Fig. 1a, and b). Among the 16 CCSSTs, 13 cases showed predominant epithelioid cytology and 3 cases exhibited predominant spindle cytology. Multinucleated giant cells were sparsely found in 14 cases. Visible melanocytic differentiation (melanin pigmentation) was observed in 4 cases. The predominant architecture was sheet-like and nested in 12 cases, fascicular in 3 cases, and pseudo-papillary in 1 case. Nucleolar prominence was found in 14 cases. Case 13, which had both *EWSR1* and *CREM* rearrangements

(metastatic lesions in lymph nodes), showed sheet-like and fascicular proliferation of epithelioid and spindle tumor cells that had round nuclei with conspicuous nucleoli and abundant pale eosinophilic cytoplasm (Fig. 2a, and b); no myxoid change was found. On the other hand, CCSLGTs often exhibited pseudo-papillary patterns of epithelioid tumor cells, with round to irregular-shaped nuclei showing a coarse chromatin pattern and having a slightly eosinophilic to less clear cytoplasm (Fig. 3a, and b). All 6 CCSLGT cases showed predominant epithelioid cytology and did not exhibit visible melanocytic differentiation. The predominant architecture was pseudo-papillary in 3 cases and sheet-like in 3 cases. Nucleoli were less conspicuous than those from CCSSTs (Fig. 3c), and nucleolar prominence was observed in 2 cases. Osteoclast-type giant cells were scattered in 5 cases (Fig. 3d). Case 18, which had *CREM* rearrangement, showed pseudo-papillary proliferation of epithelioid cells that had round nuclei without conspicuous nucleoli and pale eosinophilic cytoplasm. There were no histologic patterns indicating any correlation between *ATF1* and *CREB1* or indicating cases with *CREM* rearrangement.

We performed IHC of melanocytic markers, including S-100 protein, Melan-A, HMB45, and SOX-10, and assessed their positivity (Table 1). In Cases 8 and 16, CCS of the deep soft tissue and skin showed no reactivity with Melan-A and HMB45 and Case 13 with both *EWSR1* and *CREM* rearrangements was negative for Melan-A, but almost all of the CCSST cases were positive for all melanocytic markers. In contrast, CCSLGTs showed no reactivity with any melanocytic markers and were positive for only S-100 and SOX-10. All of the IHC results were compatible with the pathological diagnosis of CCSST and CCSLGT.

Fluorescence *in situ* hybridization

As shown in Table 1, 15 of the 16 CCSST cases (93.8%) had *EWSR1* rearrangement, of which 11 (68.8%) also showed *ATF1* rearrangement (Fig. 1c, and d), suggestive of the presence of *EWSR1-ATF1* fusion. One CCSST (Case 13) (6.3%) exhibited *EWSR1* and *CREM* rearrangements (Fig. 2c, and d), indicating *EWSR1-CREM* fusion although no fusion gene was proven by RT-PCR using formalin-fixed, paraffin-embedded materials (data not shown). Two CCSSTs with *EWSR1* rearrangement had no partner genes: one (Case 8) showed no rearrangement of *ATF1, CREB1*, or *CREM*, and one (Case 2) did not exhibit any rearrangement. Four of 6 CCSLGT cases (66.7%) exhibited *EWSR1* rearrangement: 2 (33.3%) showed *ATF1* rearrangement and the other 2 (33.3%) showed *CREB1* rearrangement (Fig. 3e, and f), suggestive of the presence of *EWSR1-ATF1* and *EWSR1-CREB1* fusions, respectively. One case (Case 18) was positive for split

Table 1 Summary of clinical, immunohistochemical, and genetic findings of CCSST and CCSLGT cases

No.	Age (years) /Sex	Location	Tumor size (cm)	Outcome (months)	Immunohistochemistry			Fluorescence in situ hybridization (%)				Expected fusion genes by FISH	RT-PCR findings
					S-100 protein	Melan-A and/or HMB45	SOX-10	EWSR1	ATF1	CREB1	CREM		
1	29/F	Leg	5	DOD (73)	+	+	NP	72	48	2	NP	EWSR1-ATF1	NP
2	41/M	Leg	4	DOD (62)	+	+	NP	68	ND	ND	NP	EWSR1- (unknown partner)	NP
3	25/M	Leg	8	DOD (29)	+	+	NP	50	32	4	NP	EWSR1-ATF1	EWSR1 exon 8-ATF1 exon 4
4	62/F	Leg	2	NED (6)	+	+	NP	8	6	0	NP	Unknown	EWSR1 exon 8-ATF1 exon 4
5	33/M	Leg	2.5	DOD (8)	+	+	NP	16	0	0	NP	EWSR1- (unknown partner)	EWSR1 exon 10-ATF1 exon 5
6	34/F	Leg	NA	AWD (16)	+	+	NP	62	32	0	NP	EWSR1-ATF1	NP
7	34/M	Leg	6	AWD (9)	+	+	NP	76	66	6	NP	EWSR1-ATF1	NP
8	12/F	Leg	2	NED (96)	+	–	–	36	0	2	2	EWSR1-(unknown partner)	NP
9	39/F	Arm	3	DOD (10)	+	+	NP	74	54	ND	NP	EWSR1-ATF1	NP
10	69/F	Arm	2	DOD (26)	+	+	NP	50	58	0	NP	EWSR1-ATF1	EWSR1 exon 8-ATF1 exon 4
11	41/M	Arm	2.5	AWD (11)	+	+	NP	58	58	2	NP	EWSR1-ATF1	EWSR1 exon 10-ATF1 exon 5
12	40/M	Arm	5.5	AWD (23)	+	+	NP	70	36	8	NP	EWSR1-ATF1	EWSR1 exon 8-ATF1 exon 5
13	49/F	Arm	4	AWD (24)	+	+	NP	70	8	4	36	EWSR1-CREM	*
14	56/F	Arm	3.9	AWD (3)	+	+	NP	80	86	2	0	EWSR1-ATF1	NP
15	8/F	Abdominal wall	9.5	DOD (249)	+	+	NP	50	36	0	NP	EWSR1-ATF1	NP
16	43/M	Skin	3	NED (29)	+	–	NP	84	76	0	NP	EWSR1-ATF1	NP
17	41/F	Ileum	4	NED (28)	+	–	NP	72	58	2	NP	EWSR1-ATF1	NP
18	78/F	Ileum	9	NED (48)	+	–	+	2	2	0	12	(unknown partner)-CREM	NP
19	38/F	Small intestine	10	DOD (17)	+	–	NP	56	6	42	NP	EWSR1-CREB1	NP
20	20/F	Ileum	4	NED (7)	+	–	+	80	94	4	NP	EWSR1-ATF1	EWSR1 exon 8-ATF1 exon 4
21	47/F	Ileum	4.5	AWD (34)	+	–	+	74	0	62	NP	EWSR1-CREB1	EWSR1 exon 7-CREB1 exon 7
22	57/M	Esophagus	3	NED (18)	+	–	+	2	2	0	8	Unknown	NP

+ Positive, – Negative, *AWD* Alive with disease, *NED* No evidence of disease, *DOD* Died of disease, *NA* Not available, *ND* Not detected, *NP* Not performed, *FISH* Fluorescence in situ hybridization, *RT-PCR* Reverse transcription PCR; *, fusion gene was not detected by RT-PCR in formalin-fixed, paraffin-embedded materials

CREM signals, although no partner genes were detected. One case (Case 22) showed no rearrangement of *EWSR1*, *ATF1*, *CREB1*, or *CREM*.

Reverse transcription-polymerase chain reaction

RT-PCR was performed in 8 available cases including 6 CCSSTs and 2 CCSLGTs (Table 1). All 6 CCSST cases showed *EWSR1-ATF1* fusion between *EWSR1* exon 8 and *ATF1* exon 4, *EWSR1* exon 10 and *ATF1* exon 5, or *EWSR1* exon 8 and *ATF1* exon 5. Although *EWSR1-ATF1* fusion

was confirmed by RT-PCR in 2 cases (Cases 4 and 5), adequate *EWSR1* or *ATF1* split signals were not detected by FISH. Among the 2 CCSLGT cases, one had *EWSR1-ATF1* fusion between *EWSR1* exon 8 and *ATF1* exon 4, and the other had *EWSR1-CREB1* fusion between *EWSR1* exon 7 and *CREB1* exon 7.

Discussion

Although CCSST and CCSLGT share similar pathological findings, there are apparent morphological and

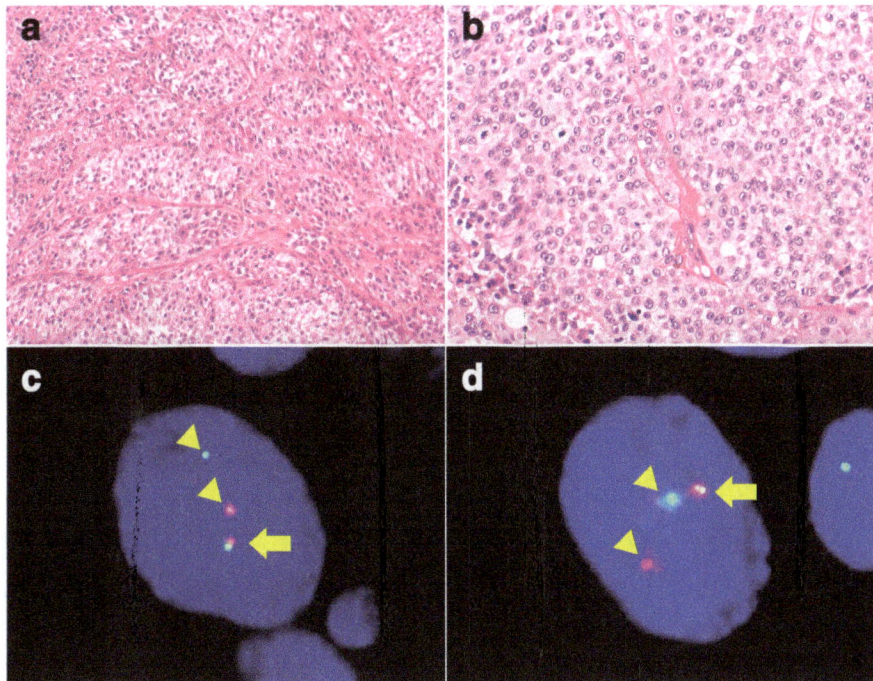

Fig. 1 Pathological findings of CCSST with *EWSR1* and *ATF1* rearrangements. **a** CCSSTs showed sheet-like and nested growth patterns of polyhedral tumor cells (200×). **b** Tumor cells had round nuclei with conspicuous nucleoli and clear to pale eosinophilic cytoplasm (400×). **c** FISH of *EWSR1* split signals. Tumor cells showed *EWSR1* split signal with a pair of fused (arrow) and split (arrow head) patterns (1000×). **d** FISH of *ATF1* split signals. Tumor cells showed *EWSR1* split signal with a pair of fused (arrow) and split (arrow head) patterns (1000×)

immunohistochemical differences between the two tumor types. We confirmed the differences in histology and IHC results in our cohort cases. Histologically, the cytological findings of tumor cells and architectural proliferation pattern differed. The tumor cells of CCSST were polyhedral to epithelioid, and spindle-shaped with round to mildly irregular-shaped nuclei and conspicuous nucleoli. In contrast, the tumor cells of CCSLGT had epithelioid tumor cells with irregular-shaped nuclei showing a coarse chromatin pattern and more eosinophilic cytoplasm. Nucleoli were not remarkable in CCSLGT compared to CCSST. CCSST exhibited sheet-like, solid, and nested tumor cell proliferation. In contrast, CCSLGT additionally showed a pseudo-papillary growth pattern. The existence of scattered osteoclast-type giant cells was also characteristic of CCSLGT. CCSSTs were positive for Melan-A and/or HMB45 melanocytic markers in addition to S-100 protein, as determined by IHC. On the other hand, CCSLGTs were not reactive for any melanocytic markers, with the exception of S-100 protein and SOX-10. As in previously reported studies, *EWSR1-CREB1* fusion tended to be detected in CCSLGTs. This genetic tendency might reflect the morphological and immunohistochemical differences between the two tumor types.

The novel finding of the study was that we discovered *CREM* rearrangement in a few CCSs. Kao et al. [14–16] stated that an *EWSR1-CREM* fusion was previously detected by RNA sequencing in 2 melanoma cell lines (CHL-1 and COLO 699) and proposed that these cell lines may have originated from CCS because of the histological and immunohistochemical overlap between malignant melanoma and CCS. On the other hand, *EWSR1-CREM* fusion was found in a unique myxoid mesenchymal tumor that was recently described as a new entity [14, 17]. This myxoid tumor is thought to have an intracranial location, and 8 cases have previously been reported, of which 7 occurred in intracranial lesions like meninges, brain tumors, and ventricles, and one case arose in the pelvic/perirectal region. A genetic study revealed *EWSR1* fusions with *CREB* family genes in all of these tumors. Among the 8 tumors, 3 had *EWSR1-CREM* fusion, 4 had *EWSR1-CREB1* fusion, and one tumor showed *EWSR1-ATF1* fusion. However, histological and immunohistochemical findings completely differed between this particular myxoid mesenchymal tumor and CCSST/CCSLGT, and interestingly, these genetic results corresponded to those of CCSST and CCSLGT.

CCSLGT was originally reported as an "osteoclast-rich tumor of the gastrointestinal tract with features

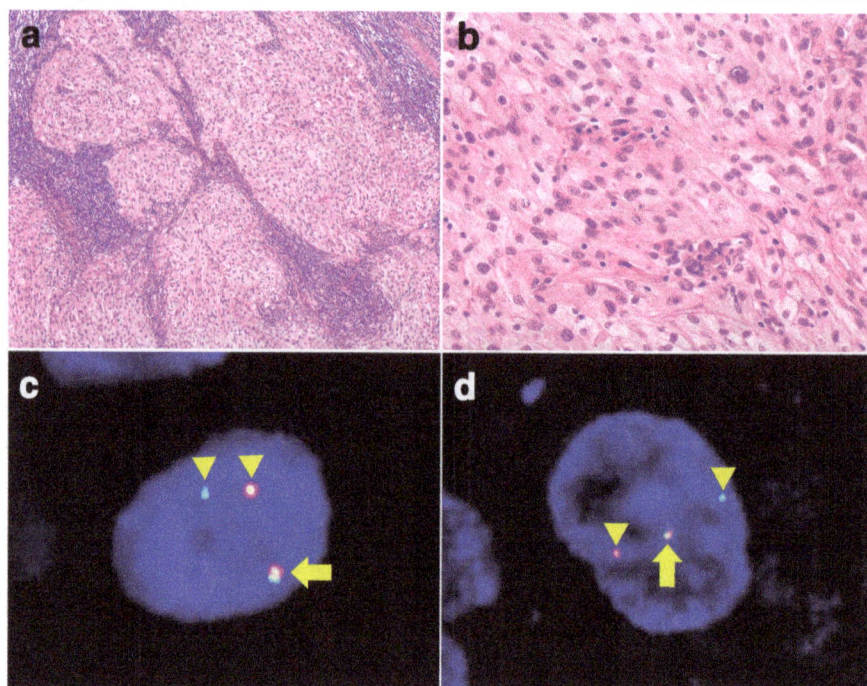

Fig. 2 Pathological findings of CCSST with *EWSR1* and *CREM* rearrangements. **a** Metastatic CCSST of the lymph nodes (100×). **b** Tumor cells were polyhedral to spindle-shaped and had oval to round nuclei with pale to clear and eosinophilic cytoplasm (400×). **c** FISH of *EWSR1* split signals. Tumor cells showed *EWSR1* split signal with a pair of fused (arrow) and split (arrow head) patterns (1000×). **d** FISH of *CREM* split signals. Tumor cells showed *CREM* split signal with a pair of fused (arrow) and split (arrow head) patterns (1000×)

resembling clear cell sarcoma of the soft parts" [2]. However, some authors prefer to refer to CCSLGT as a "malignant gastrointestinal neuroectodermal tumor" (GNET), because these tumors lack evidence of melanocytic differentiation [5]. A recent review discussed the relationship between clear cell sarcoma of the gastrointestinal tract (CCS-GIT) with GNET. There were differences in morphology and IHC findings between CCS-GIT and GNET. GNET tended to show a wider spectrum of growth patterns, including a pseudo-papillary growth pattern, and exhibited no evidence of melanocytic differentiation. Clinically, CCS-GIT affected males more often than females, and GNET occurred in younger patients although no significant differences existed in their biological behaviors [18]. It has been reported that GNET has poorer prognosis than CCS-GIT [5], but additional studies are needed to clarify the relationship between the two entities.

While a previous study revealed that *EWSR1-ATF1* fusion was identified by RT-PCR in 91% of CCSST cases [1], we detected *EWSR1-ATF1* fusion in 13 of 16 CCSST (81.3%) both by FISH and RT-PCR. Moreover, after excluding 1 case of *EWSR1-CREM* fusion, 13 of 15 CCSST cases (86.7%) had *EWSR1-ATF1* fusion. The percentage of positive cases in the present

study nearly reached that of the previous study. CCSLGT has been identified as having *EWSR1-ATF1* or *EWSR1-CREB1* fusion, with CCSLGT more frequently having *EWSR1-CREB1* fusion. These fusions have also been detected in angiomatoid fibrous histiocytoma and primary pulmonary myxoid sarcoma despite the morphological and immunohistochemical differences between CCSST/CCSLGT and these tumors. To detect specific fusions, FISH is an effective and useful tool using formalin-fixed, paraffin-embedded sections in routine pathological work. In this study, we successfully detected *EWSR1*, *ATF1*, *CREB1*, and *CREM* rearrangements by FISH in the majority of cases. Some cases showed only one specific rearrangement and did not reveal any rearrangement of partner genes. In such cases, it is expected that certain unknown partner genes can form some novel chimeric genes, and that powerful analytic tools such as next-generation sequencing will be useful for detecting these novel fusions.

Conclusions

Rearrangements of *EWSR1* and *ATF1* or *EWSR1-ATF1* fusion were predominantly found in CCSST, whereas those of *EWSR1* and *CREB1* or *EWSR1-CREB1* tended to be detected in CCSLGT. We detected a novel

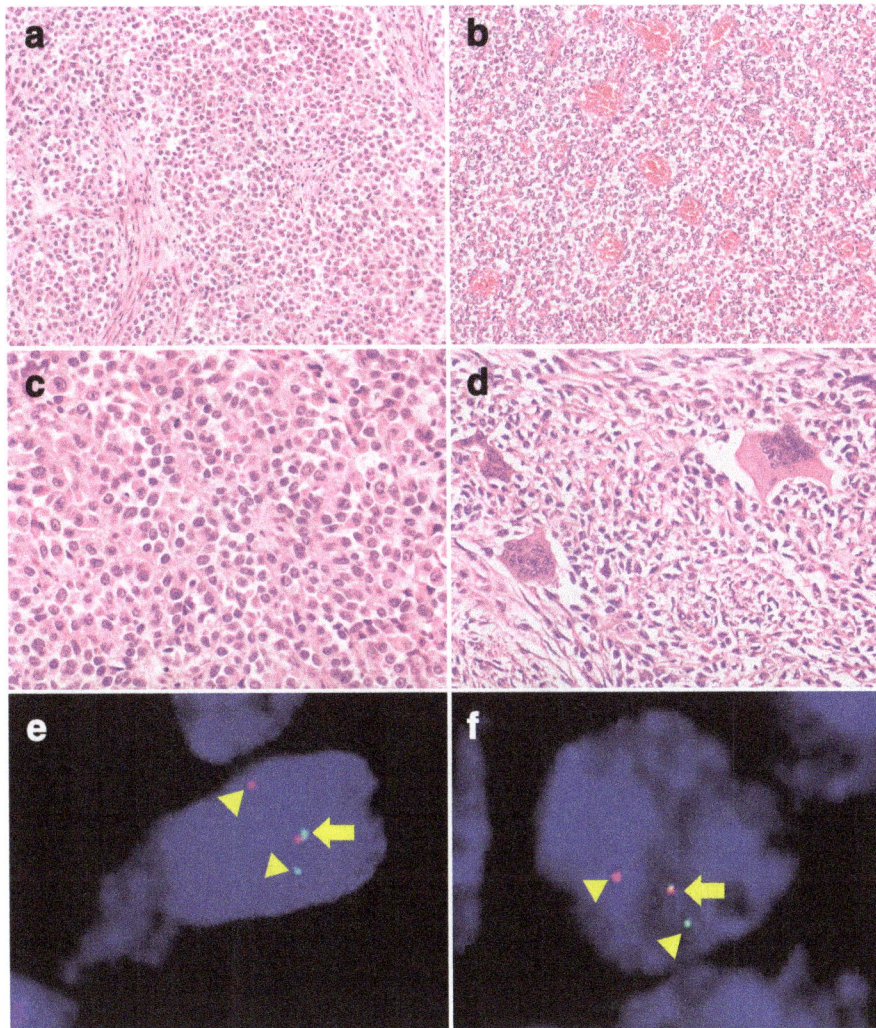

Fig. 3 Pathological findings of CCSLGT with *EWSR1* and *CREB1* rearrangements. **a** CCSLGTs often exhibited sheet-like proliferation of polyhedral and epithelioid tumor cells (200×). **b** Areas of pseudo-papillary growth pattern around the vasculatures were also observed (200×). **c** Tumor cells had mildly irregular-shaped round nuclei showing a coarse chromatin pattern and lightly eosinophilic to less frequently clear cytoplasm. Nucleoli were inconspicuous (400×). **d** Osteoclast-type giant cells were scattered in the tumor (400×). **e**. FISH of *EWSR1* split signals. Tumor cells showed *EWSR1* split signal with a pair of fused (arrow) and split (arrow head) patterns (1000×). **f**. FISH of *CREB1* split signals. Tumor cells showed *CREB1* split signal with a pair of fused (arrow) and split (arrow head) patterns (1000×)

CREM rearrangement in surgical CCSST specimens by FISH. Although this novel rearrangement occurred in a minority of CCSST cases, further studies are needed to elucidate its pathological significance.

Abbreviations
CCS: Clear cell sarcoma; CCSLGT: Clear cell sarcoma-like gastrointestinal tumor; CCSST: Clear cell sarcoma of soft tissue; FISH: Fluorescence *in situ* hybridization; IHC: Immunohistochemistry

Acknowledgements
The authors thank the following pathologists for kindly contributing case materials and clinical follow-up information: Akiko Tonooka, Department of Pathology, Tokyo Metropolitan Cancer and Infectious Diseases Center Komagome Hospital, Tokyo, Japan; Misa Ishihara and Kimio Hashimoto, Department of Pathology, Nishi-Kobe Medical Center, Hyogo, Japan; Shigeo Hara, Department of Diagnostic Pathology, Kobe City Medical Center General Hospital, Hyogo, Japan; Koki Moriyoshi, Division of Clinical Pathology, National Hospital Organization Kyoto Medical Center, Kyoto, Japan; Shin Ichihara, Department of Surgical Pathology, Sapporo Kosei General Hospital, Hokkaido, Japan; Yukio Morishita, Department of Pathology, Tokyo Medical University Ibaraki Medical Center, Ibaraki, Japan; and Atsushi Uchida, Department of Pathology, Tsukuba Medical Center Hospital, Ibaraki, Japan.

Authors' contributions
KS participated in the design of the study, performed the pathological analysis, and drafted the manuscript. SS, TH, TS, YI, MT, and HF helped with the pathological analysis. TA and HA conducted the fluorescence *in situ* hybridization. TK performed genetic analysis using available surgical materials. ME examined the clinical data of cases. SS conceived the study, participated in its design and coordination, and helped draft the manuscript. All authors read and approved the final manuscript.

Competing interests

The authors declare that they have no competing interests.

Author details

[1]Department of Surgical Pathology, Sapporo Medical University, School of Medicine, Sapporo, Hokkaido 060-8543, Japan. [2]Department of Pathology, Sapporo Medical University, School of Medicine, Sapporo, Hokkaido 060-8556, Japan. [3]Department of Orthopedic Surgery, Sapporo Medical University, School of Medicine, Sapporo, Hokkaido 060-8543, Japan.

References

1. Antonescu CR, Tschernyavsky SJ, Woodruff JM, Jungbluth AA, Brennan MF, Ladanyi M. Molecular diagnosis of clear cell sarcoma: detection of EWS-ATF1 and MITF-M transcripts and histopathological and ultrastructural analysis of 12 cases. J Mol Diagn. 2002;4:44–52.
2. Zambrano E, Reyes-Mugica M, Franchi A, Rosai J. An osteoclast-rich tumor of the gastrointestinal tract with features resembling clear cell sarcoma of soft parts: reports of 6 cases of a GIST simulator. Int J Surg Pathol. 2003;11:75–81.
3. Alpers CE, Beckstead JH. Malignant neuroendocrine tumor of the jejunum with osteoclast-like giant cells. Enzyme histochemistry distinguishes tumor cells from giant cells. Am J Surg Pathol. 1985;9:57–64.
4. Kosemehmetoglu K, Folpe AL. Clear cell sarcoma of tendons and aponeuroses, and osteoclast-rich tumour of the gastrointestinal tract with features resembling clear cell sarcoma of soft parts: a review and update. J Clin Pathol. 2010;63:416–23.
5. Stockman DL, Miettinen M, Suster S, Spagnolo D, Dominguez-Malagon H, Hornick JL, et al. Malignant gastrointestinal neuroectodermal tumor: clinicopathologic, immunohistochemical, ultrastructural, and molecular analysis of 16 cases with a reappraisal of clear cell sarcoma-like tumors of the gastrointestinal tract. Am J Surg Pathol. 2012;36:857–68.
6. Wang J, Thway K. Clear cell sarcoma-like tumor of the gastrointestinal tract: an evolving entity. Arch Pathol Lab Med. 2015;139:407–12.
7. Antonescu CR, Nafa K, Segal NH, Dal Cin P, Ladanyi M. EWS-CREB1: a recurrent variant fusion in clear cell sarcoma-association with gastrointestinal location and absence of melanocytic differentiation. Clin Cancer Res. 2006;12:5356–62.
8. Wang WL, Mayordomo E, Zhang W, Hernandez VS, Tuvin D, Garcia L, et al. Detection and characterization of EWSR1/ATF1 and EWSR1/CREB1 chimeric transcripts in clear cell sarcoma (melanoma of soft parts). Mod Pathol. 2009; 22:1201–9.
9. Hantschke M, Mentzel T, Rütten A, Palmedo G, Calonje E, Lazar AJ, et al. Cutaneous clear cell sarcoma: a clinicopathologic, immunohistochemical, and molecular analysis of 12 cases emphasizing its distinction from dermal melanoma. Am J Surg Pathol. 2010;34:216–22.
10. Washimi K, Takagi M, Hisaoka M, Kawachi K, Takeyama M, Hiruma T, et al. Clear cell sarcoma-like tumor of the gastrointestinal tract: a clinicopathological review. Pathol Int. 2017;67:534–6.
11. Miura Y, Keira Y, Ogino J, Nakanishi K, Noguchi H, Inoue T, et al. Detection of specific genetic abnormalities by fluorescence *in situ* hybridization in soft tissue tumors. Pathol Int. 2012;62:16–27.
12. Sugita S, Asanuma H, Hasegawa T. Diagnostic use of fluorescence *in situ* hybridization in expert review in a phase 2 study of trabectedin monotherapy in patients with advanced, translocation-related sarcoma. Diagn Pathol. 2016;11:37.
13. Kato T, Ichihara S, Gotoda H, Muraoka S, Kubo T, Sugita S, et al. Imprint cytology of clear cell sarcoma-like tumor of the gastrointestinal tract in the small intestine: a case report. Diagn Cytopathol. 2017;45:1137–41.
14. Kao YC, Sung YS, Zhang L, Chen CL, Vaiyapuri S, Rosenblum MK, et al. EWSR1 fusions with CREB family transcription factors define a novel Myxoid mesenchymal tumor with predilection for intracranial location. Am J Surg Pathol. 2017;41:482–90.
15. Klijn C, Durinck S, Stawiski EW, Haverty PM, Jiang Z, Liu H, et al. A comprehensive transcriptional portrait of human cancer cell lines. Nat Biotechnol. 2015;33:306–12.
16. Giacomini CP, Sun S, Varma S, Shain AH, Giacomini MM, Balagtas J, et al. Breakpoint analysis of transcriptional and genomic profiles uncovers novel gene fusions spanning multiple human cancer types. PLoS Genet. 2013;9(4):e1003464.
17. Bale TA, Oviedo A, Kozakewich H, Giannini C, Daviveni PK, Ligon K, et al. Intracranial myxoid mesenchymal tumors with EWSR1-CREB family gene fusions: myxoid variant of angiomatoid fibrous histiocytoma or novel entity? Brain Pathol. 2018;28:183–91.
18. Green C, Spagnolo DV, Robbins PD, Fermoyle S, Wong DD. Clear cell sarcoma of the gastrointestinal tract and malignant gastrointestinal neuroectodermal tumour: distinct or related entities? A review. Pathology. 2018;50:490–8.

22

Levels of uPA and PAI-1 in breast cancer and its correlation to Ki67-index and results of a 21-multigene-array

Hans-Ullrich Völker[1], Michael Weigel[2], Annette Strehl[1] and Lea Frey[3]* (iD)

Abstract

Background: Conventional parameters including Ki67, hormone receptor and Her2/neu status are used for risk stratification for breast cancer. The serine protease urokinase plasminogen activator (uPA) and the plasminogen activator inhibitor type-1 (PAI-1) play an important role in tumour invasion and metastasis. Increased concentrations in tumour tissue are associated with more aggressive potential of the disease. Multigene tests provide detailed insights into tumour biology by simultaneously testing several prognostically relevant genes. With OncotypeDX®, a panel of 21 genes is tested by means of quantitative real-time polymerase chain reaction.

The purpose of this pilot study was to analyse whether a combination of Ki67 and uPA/PAI-1 supplies indications of the result of the multigene test.

Methods: The results of Ki67, uPA/PAI-1 and OncotypeDX® were analysed in 25 breast carcinomas (luminal type, pT1/2, max pN1a, G2). A statistical and descriptive analysis was performed.

Results: With a proliferation index Ki67 of < 14%, the recurrence score (RS) from the multigene test was on average in the *low risk* range, with an intermediate RS usually resulting if Ki67 was > 14%. Not elevated values of uPA and PAI-1 showed a lower rate of proliferation (average 8.5%) than carcinomas with an increase of uPA and/or PAI-1 (average 13.9%); $p = 0.054$, Student's t-test. When Ki67 was > 14% and uPA and/or PAI-1 was raised, an intermediate RS resulted. These differences were significant when compared to cases with Ki67 < 14% with non-raised uPA/PAI-1 ($p < 0.03$, Student's t-test). Without taking into account the proliferative activity, an intermediate RS was also verifiable if both uPA and PAI-1 showed raised values.

Conclusion: A combination of the values Ki67 and uPA/PAI-1 tended to depict the RS to be expected. From this it can be deduced that an appropriate analysis of this parameter combination may be undertaken before the multigene test in routine clinical practice. The increasing cost pressure makes it necessary to base the implementation of a multigene test on ancillary variables and to potentially leave it out if not required in the event of a certain constellation of results (Ki67 raised, uPA and PAI-1 raised).

Keywords: Breast cancer, uPA, PAI-1, Multigene-array, OncotypeDX®

* Correspondence: lea.frey@uni-wuerzburg.de
[3]Institute for Pathology, University of Wuerzburg, Josef-Schneider-Str. 2, D-97080 Wuerzburg, Germany
Full list of author information is available at the end of the article

Background

The risk stratification for breast carcinoma takes into account conventional parameters such as age at onset, menopausal status, tumour size and extension, histological grading and subtype, the assessment of vascular or lymphatic invasion, lympho-nodal status, resection margins and distant metastasis. The determination of the proliferative activity (Ki67) and of the hormone receptor and Her2/neu status are indispensable for prognosis and prediction.

Supplementary analyses of tumour tissue can make the classification more precise. This is especially important in the case of node-negative or minimally positive (max. pN1a) luminal-type carcinomas, because it is in this tumour group that difficulties arise most frequently in making the decision for or against adjuvant chemotherapy.

The serine protease urokinase plasminogen activator (uPA) and the plasminogen activator inhibitor type-1 (PAI-1), as elements of the urokinase plasminogen activator system, are part of the fibrinolytic system [1]. The zymogen plasminogen is converted by uPA into its active, protein-activating and proteolytic form (plasmin) [2]. PAI-1 plays a role in the regulation of the proteolytic activity of uPA [3]. It does not only act as an inhibitor, but also participates in numerous other processes such as cell adhesion and migration, angioneogenesis, signal transduction and apoptosis [4, 5]. uPA and PAI-1 thus play an important role in tumour invasion and metastasis through an interaction with components of the basal membrane, the extracellular matrix and by local proteolysis [6–9].

Increased concentrations of uPA and/or PAI-1 in the tumour tissue of breast carcinomas are associated with a more aggressive progression of the disease, an increased risk of relapse and lower survival rates [10, 11]. Several studies have proved a prognostic significance independent of clinical and histopathological criteria [12–14]. uPA/PAI-1 testing has achieved the level of evidence 1a and has been incorporated into the recommendations of the German Working Group for Gynaecological Oncology (http://www.ago-online.de/de/infothek-fuer-aerzte/leitlinie nempfehlungen/mamma; accessed June 4th 2018). This examination is recommended for lymphonodal non-metastasized and Her2/neu-negative breast carcinoma of intermediate grade (G2). In the case of a high protein level of uPA and/or PAI-1 patients could benefit from adjuvant chemotherapy [11].

Various established multigene tests (e.g. OncotypeDX®, Mammaprint®, EndoPredict®, Prosigna®-Assay) supply detailed insights into tumour biology by simultaneously testing several genes that are relevant to prognosis. OncotypeDX® is a 21-gene assay available in Europe since 2009. The standardized and quality-controlled analysis is carried out in a central laboratory in the USA using quantitative real-time polymerase chain reaction

(qRT-PCR). A panel of 21 genes is examined, 16 of which are cancer-associated genes as well as five reference genes. The result is used to calculate the numerical recurrence score (RS), which reflects a defined risk of relapse within 10 years from the point of diagnosis. Three risk groups exist for clinical validation: *low risk* (RS < 18), *intermediate risk* (RS 18–30) and *high risk* (RS ≥ 31). The prognostic importance of these groups has been shown by various studies [15–19]. For patients with *high risk* tumours adjuvant chemotherapy has been proven to be useful [20].

However, additional tests also increase the costs of the diagnostic process considerably, and these charges are then not always assumed by German health insurance schemes. The increasing cost pressure represents a substantial problem in clinical practice; responsibilities towards the patient on the one hand and towards the cost bearers on the other hand are often irreconcilable.

Although the prognostic value of common testing procedures is well described in current literature, a correlation of the individual tests amongst each other with an assessment of costs and benefits has not to our knowledge been examined in the researchable literature.

In this initial pilot study, derived from routine clinical work, the intention is to analyse whether the ELISA test for the protein levels of uPA and PAI-1, carried out in addition to conventional histopathological parameters, is similarly suitable for the assessment of prognosis as a multigene test, for which OncotypeDX® has here been selected as an example.

Methods

Between 2013 and 2016, 954 breast carcinomas were presented and discussed in the interdisciplinary tumour conference of the Breast Cancer Centre at Leopoldina Krankenhaus der Stadt Schweinfurt GmbH (Leopoldina Hospital of the City of Schweinfurt). Male breast carcinomas were excluded. All epidemiological and clinical data of the patients were available as well as the complete postoperative histopathological tumour diagnostics (especially stage, hormone receptor status, Her2/neu status, Ki67). The data set was completely anonymized so that connections to individual cases, particularly patient names and core data, are no longer possible.

Immunohistochemical parameters were determined in a fully-automated device (BondMax, Leica) with a standardized test-kit (Leica).

The commercially available antibody clone 1D5 was used for the oestrogen receptor stain (ER), and the clone *PgR63* (both DAKO®) for the progesterone receptor stain (PR). The immunoreactive score (IRS) was calculated using the method according to Remmele and Stegner, in order to determine the hormone receptor status. This consists of the percentage of positively stained tumour cells and the stain intensity. A score of 0 counts as negative, 1–3 as weakly positive, 4–6 as moderately positive and 8–12 as strongly positive. The Pathology Department of the Leopoldina Krankenhaus Schweinfurt successfully passed the relevant yearly external quality assurance tests (QuIP®) each year within the survey period.

The test for Her2/neu was performed immunohistochemically (clone c-erbB-2, DAKO), and supplemented with a FISH analysis where the result was not clear. The immunohistochemical stains were evaluated in adherence to guidelines with the threshold for a positive result set at 10% tumour cells with a circumferential membranous stain. Here too, the Pathology Department took part successfully in the relevant external quality assurance tests (QuIP®). *The Her2/neu scoring was performed following the current ASCO/CAP-guidelines in accordance with the recently published recommendations [21].*

The Ki67 stain (clone MIB-1, DAKO) was also carried out in a standardized fashion according to protocol. The percentage of tumour cells with immunohistochemical evidence of MIB-1 protein expression was stated as the Ki-67 proliferation index. Here too there had been successful participation in the relevant external quality assurance test (QuIP®).

For 25 carcinomas with primarily surgical treatment (*all of no special type NST, G2, Elston-Ellis grading*), a sample of native tumour tissue was collected to determine the concentrations of uPA and PAI-1. *Because the information from this laboratory test was only relevant for G2 tumors without nodal metastasis in the clinical routine, no carcinomas of other grade or stage (G1 or G3, lymphonodal metastasized) were includable in this study.* From the surgical specimen a sample of frozen tissue was promptly sent to Limbach Laboratory, D-69126 Heidelberg, for an ELISA test. This procedure requires a certain minimum size of tumour (at least 1.3 cm diameter), because on the one hand a tissue sample of around 0.125cm³ is required for ELISA testing and on the other hand enough material must be retained to guarantee a complete histopathological analysis despite the removal of tumour tissue. The cut-off value for uPA concentrations which are associated with an increased risk of relapse is ≥3 ng/mg total protein, and that for PAI-1 is ≥14 ng/mg total protein. The results of the external test were available after 5 days on average.

OncotypeDX® testing was also arranged in these cases. For this purpose, a paraffin block containing tumour tissue from the routine appraisal of the surgical specimen was dispatched; the tissue had previously been fixated in 4% buffered formalin. The shipment took place via a specified logistics service provider to a central pathology laboratory (Optipath®) in D-60487 Frankfurt/Main chosen by the provider of the test. From there shipping to the central laboratory in the USA and the reporting back of the test results was

organised. On average, the result was available 8 days after the sample was sent.

The analysis was statistically descriptive. *Because most of the evaluated cases showed identical including criteria (G2, N0) no multivariate analysis was performed. The nuclear grade (intermediate or high) and the mitotic count (without exception low) were also highly similar in the 25 cases, so that we found no indication for a separate analysis.*

Results

For 25 tumours (only luminal-type carcinomas, hormone receptor positive, Her2/neu-negative, G2, pT1 or pT2, not or only minimally nodal metastasized, max. pN1a), the concentrations of uPA and PAI-1 were determined and in addition a multigene test OncotypeDX® was performed. The data for this collective is shown in Table 1.

The protein levels of uPA/PAI-1 and the numerical recurrence score (RS) from the multigene test in the groups with the other histopathological parameters (pT1, pT2, lymphatic invasion, and proliferation Ki67 < 14% or Ki67 > 14%) are presented in Table 2.

No reliable deduction of the results to be expected from additional molecular tests could be made from the conventional parameters tumour stage or lymphatic invasion. For example, pT2 carcinomas showed a substantially lower RS than pT1 carcinomas. The uPA/PAI-1 protein levels tended to be higher with pT1 tumours when compared to pT2 tumours. Factors such as tumour diameter and age at onset did not correlate with any other of the other parameters (values between $r = -0.09$ and $r = -0.13$).

The proliferation index (Ki67 < 14% and > 14%) and RS showed an interdependency. Here on average a *low risk* RS was found with Ki67 < 14% and an intermediate RS

Table 1 Data of the cohort

$n = 25$	
Age	average 52; median 50 (28–71)
pT1	$n = 12$
pT2	$n = 13$
Diameter of tumor	average 2.1 cm; median 2.0 (1.1–5.0)
pN0	$n = 23$
pN1a	$n = 2$ (1/6sn) and (2/24), metastases with max. 0.5 cm diameter
L0	$n = 15$
L1	$n = 10$
V0	$n = 25$
G2	$n = 25$
Hormone receptors for estrogen and/or progesterone	$n = 25$ positive
Her2/neu	$n = 25$ negative (Score 0: $n = 6$, Score 1+: $n = 18$, Score 2 + with negative result in FISH: $n = 1$)

Table 2 Protein levels for uPA/PAI-1 (ng/ml) and Recurrence Score (RS) from multigenetest in different variables

	Average	Median	+/− deviation
uPA pT1 (ng/ml)	4.5	3.6	2.5
uPA pT2 (ng/ml)	2.4	2.4	1.7
PAI-1 pT1 (ng/ml)	20.8	17.0	11.5
PAI-1 pT2 (ng/ml)	18.4	15.0	11.5
RS pT1	19.1	17.0	8.7
RS pT2	13.1	11.0	6.5
uPA L0 (ng/ml)	3.4	2.9	2.8
uPA L1 (ng/ml)	3.6	3.1	1.7
PAI-1 L0 (ng/ml)	22.0	20.0	11.8
PAI-1 L1 (ng/ml)	15.3	11.0	9.5
RS L0	16.9	16.0	9.2
RS L1	14.6	14.0	6.2
uPA Ki < 14 (ng/ml)	3.2	3.5	2.0
uPA Ki > 14 (ng/ml)	3.6	2.8	3.0
PAI-1 Ki < 14 (ng/ml)	18.9	17.0	11.2
PAI-1 Ki > 14 (ng/ml)	20.9	16.0	12.1
RS Ki < 14	14.5	13.0	5.7
RS Ki > 14	18.1	16.0	11.4

RS recurrence score, L0/L1 - without/with lymphangioinvasion

with Ki67 > 14% (Table 2). For individual values of uPA or PAI-1 there were no differences in the groups with lower and higher proliferation. In comparison of breast carcinomas with regular values of uPA and PAI-1 to carcinomas with an increase of uPA and/or PAI-1, there was lower rate of proliferation (average 8.5%) in the group with non-increased protein levels than in the group with increased protein level (average 13.9%); $p = 0.054$, Student's t-test (Fig. 1).

In a Spearman ranking correlation of the variables Ki67, uPA/PAI-1 PAI-1and RS OncotypeDX® there was a trend towards discernible correlations, presented in Table 3.

The differences in the RS became somewhat clearer in sub-group analysis taking into account the proliferation index (threshold 14%) and uPA/PAI-1 status (Fig. 2). With a proliferation of Ki67 > 14% and simultaneous elevation of uPA and/or PAI-1, an average and median RS was observed which already indicates an intermediate risk for a tumour relapse in 10 years (RS > 18). The differences were significant when compared with the group with Ki67 < 14% and non-increased uPA/PAI-1 ($p < 0.03$, Student's t-test).

Without taking into account proliferative activity, an intermediate risk of a tumour relapse (RS > 18) was even then to be observed when both uPA and PAI-1 are increased. If, however, only one of the two parameters was increased, the RS was below the numerical value of 18 as in cases with non-increased uPA/PAI-1 (Fig. 3), $p = 0.093$, Student's t-test.

With an isolated increase of PAI-1 a trend towards a more frequent high rate of proliferation (Ki67 > 14%) could be observed (Fig. 4).

Discussion

In this pilot study on a small collection of 25 patients from routine diagnostics, a complete set of tumour biology data, including a protein assay of uPA and PAI-1 and a multigene test (OncotypeDX®), was analysed. A primary expansion of the sample of patients was not achievable from the available resources, but even from the recent results valuable information could be obtained for a more comprehensive study to be planned in the future.

The study showed that with the help of a combination of the values of Ki67 and uPA/PAI-1 the general trend of the recurrence score (RS) to be expected from the

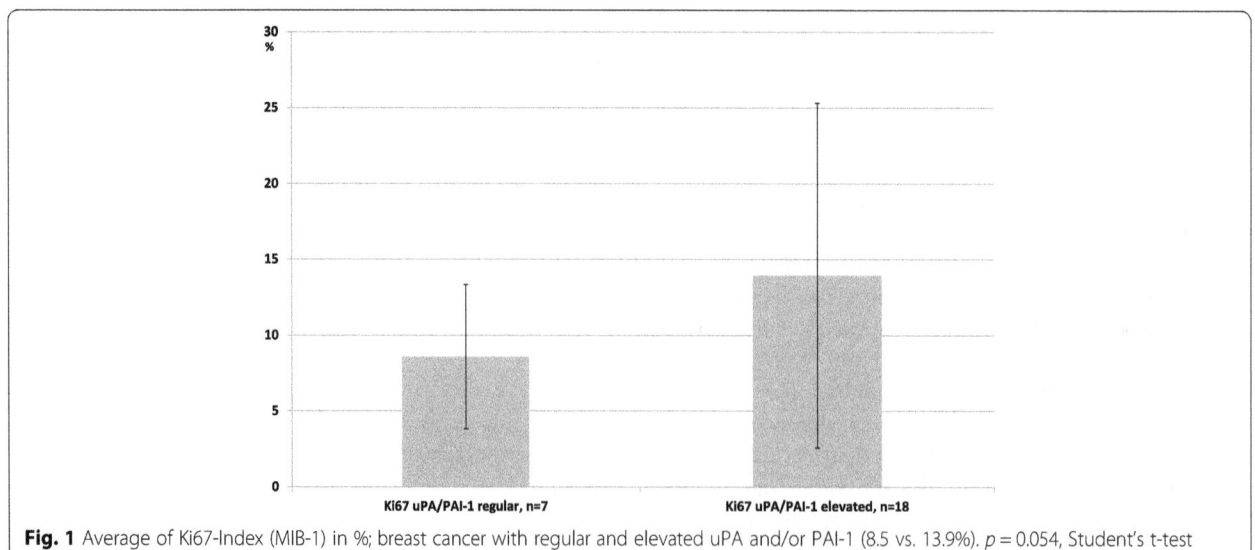

Fig. 1 Average of Ki67-Index (MIB-1) in %; breast cancer with regular and elevated uPA and/or PAI-1 (8.5 vs. 13.9%). $p = 0.054$, Student's t-test

Table 3 Positive correlations between different variables (Spearman correlation)

uPA/PAI-1 to RS OncotypeDX®	0.525
uPA/PAI-1 to proliferative index Ki67	0.460
Ki67 to RS OncotypeDX®	0.517

multigene test OncotypeDX® can be estimated. Particularly worth emphasising is the evidence of an already elevated recurrence score into the intermediate risk range if Ki67 was > 14% and the protein level of uPA and PAI-1 were increased, and of a RS consistently in the low risk range if both Ki67 and uPA/PAI-1 were not elevated. From this interaction the conclusion may be drawn that in clinical practice an appropriate analysis of this combination of parameters should be envisaged ahead of the multigene test. On the one hand, there are no doubts about the value of multigene tests. On the other hand, however, the costs for these tests are not assumed by some German health insurance schemes. The increasing cost pressure in routine care necessitates making the decision for a multigene test contingent on additional variables and to omit it if not essential in the case of an appropriate constellation of results (Ki67, uPA and PAI-1 all increased or Ki67 and uPA/PAI-1 all not increased). To our knowledge the interrelationships presented here have not yet been examined in the researchable literature. No indications can be derived from the available data as to whether a particular combination of parameters is also reliably associated with a high-risk recurrence score (e.g. by increasing the threshold of the critical Ki67 index from 14 to 20% or 25%). Therefore

a further study with a larger patient cohort should be planned. If the result of the pilot study can be confirmed, cost reduction by a factor of 10 could be achieved (according to verbal price information from involved laboratories) with a more targeted use of the multigene tests.

Links are known to exist between the Ki67 index and the values for uPA/PAI-1. Deluche et al. found lower Ki67 indices with negative uPA/PAI-1 than with increased values, with the threshold between low and high Ki67 being set at 20% [22]. They observed that when both parameters were taken into account in therapy planning, 9% fewer patients were received a recommendation for adjuvant chemotherapy than in cases where only the St. Gallen criteria were used. A qualifying comment to be made is that the ELISA (Enzyme-linked Immunosorbent Assay) for uPA/PAI-1 is only possible on fresh or frozen tumour tissue; ideally, a tumour sample of not less than 0.125 cm^3 must be available. The applicability of the procedure is thus limited by size of the tumour, because experience has shown that with tumour diameters of below 1.3 cm not enough tissue can be obtained without jeopardising the routine diagnostic procedures, especially with regard to the distance of the tumour from the resection margin. Although only an ELISA-based uPA/PAI-1 determination has been validated, efforts are being made to develop immunohistochemical assays for formalin-fixed paraffin-embedded tissue. A study has shown that the uPA/PAI values determined by means of immunohistochemical tests correlate significantly with the values of a validated ELISA [23].

The uPA/PAI-1 test is currently no longer recommended in the new version of the German S3 guideline

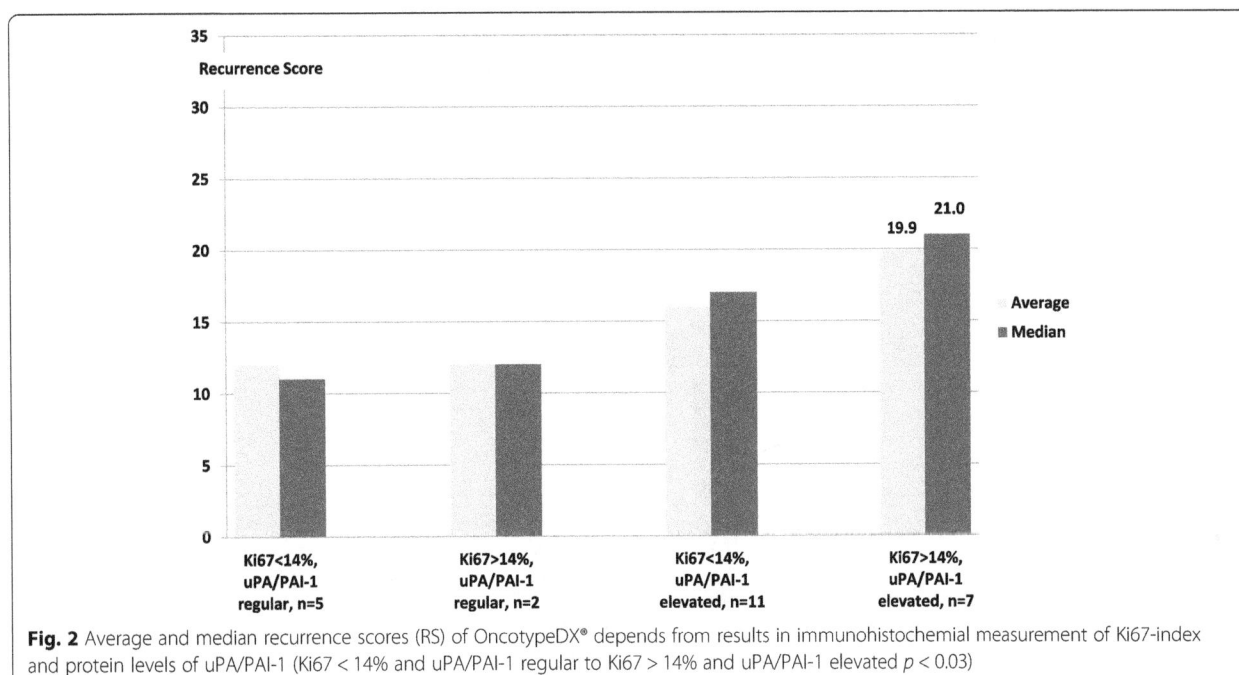

Fig. 2 Average and median recurrence scores (RS) of OncotypeDX® depends from results in immunohistochemial measurement of Ki67-index and protein levels of uPA/PAI-1 (Ki67 < 14% and uPA/PAI-1 regular to Ki67 > 14% and uPA/PAI-1 elevated $p < 0.03$)

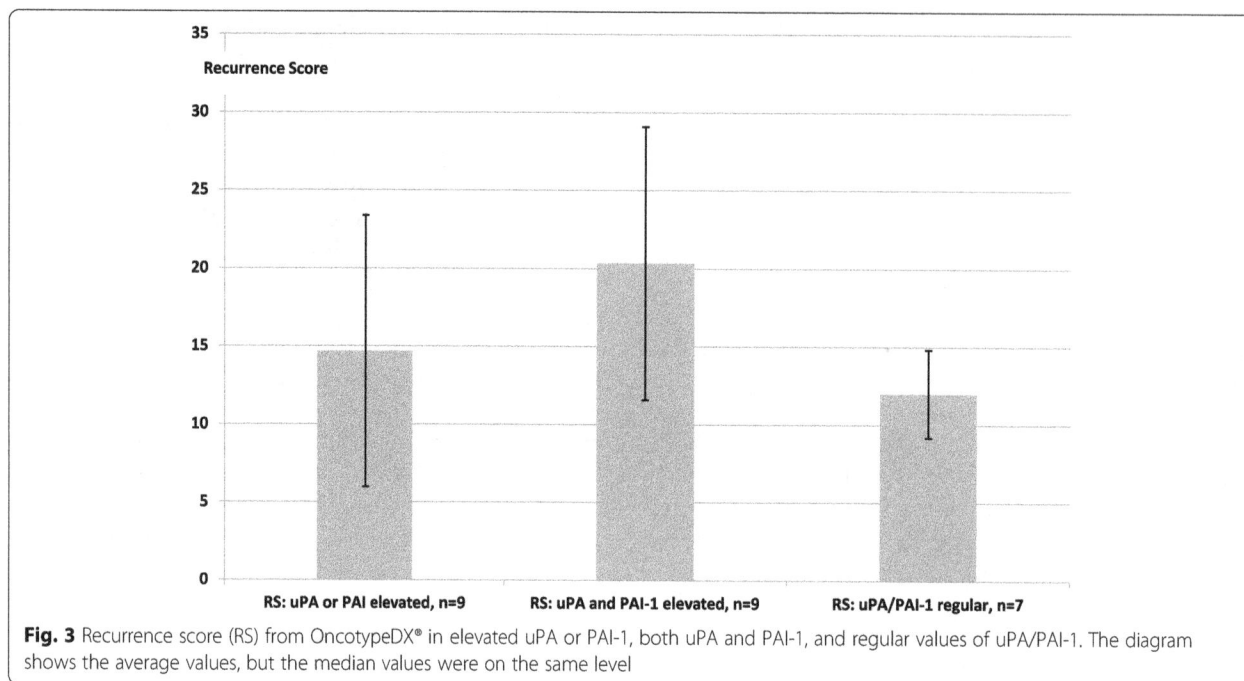

Fig. 3 Recurrence score (RS) from OncotypeDX® in elevated uPA or PAI-1, both uPA and PAI-1, and regular values of uPA/PAI-1. The diagram shows the average values, but the median values were on the same level

on breast cancer of 2017. The reason for this was the insufficient data situation for a prognostic assessment, because although the patients included in the older studies were given chemotherapy in the case of increased values, but no anti-hormonal therapy was administered when the values were not increased, so that no direct comparison of the prognosis of the two sample groups could be guaranteed on the basis of present therapeutic standards [24]. Furthermore, the Her2/neu status of the tumours was not known in previous studies. With regard to all breast carcinomas, however, there are indications that a link exists between uPA/PAI-1 and the known intrinsic subtypes. HER2-positive

or triple negative carcinomas are much more rarely uPA/PAI-1-negative than luminal-A type carcinomas [25].

According to the guidelines of the *American Society of Clinical Oncology* (ASCO), the levels of uPA and PAI-1 can be drawn upon for the decision for or against adjuvant chemotherapy; this is not recommended for Ki67 alone [26]. The analysis of uPA/PAI-1 can thus usefully supplement the information gained from conventional clinical-pathological parameters in the decision for or against adjuvant chemotherapy in cases of hormone-receptor-positive, Her2/neu-negative breast carcinomas [27], even before a multigene test has to be arranged. *A*

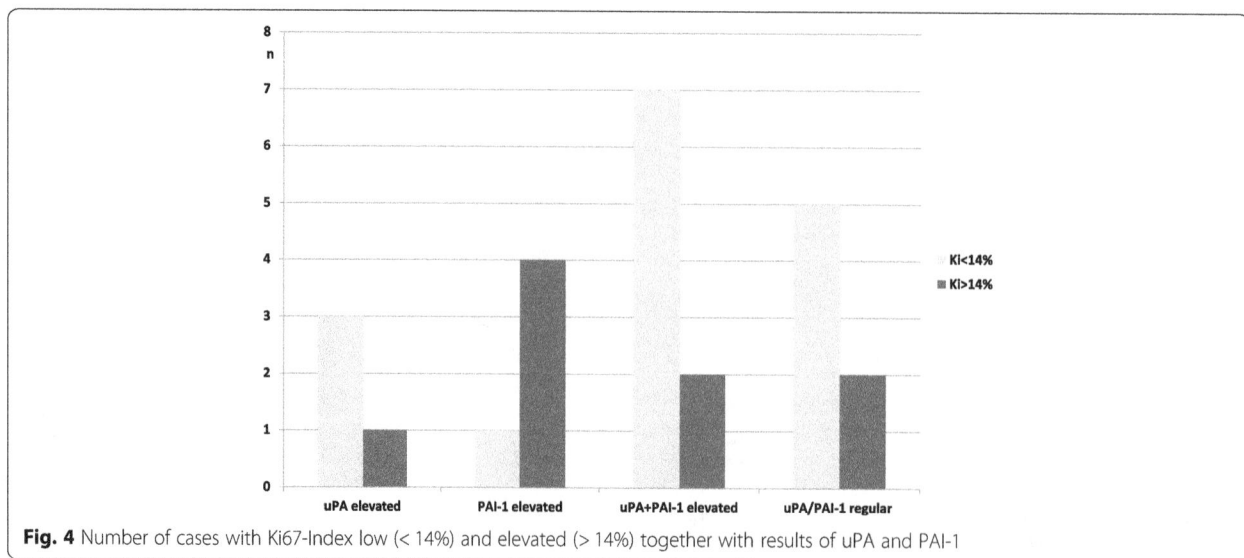

Fig. 4 Number of cases with Ki67-Index low (< 14%) and elevated (> 14%) together with results of uPA and PAI-1

further aspect is the difference in cost which can be seen as an additional argument in favour of uPA/PAI-1 testing. While this ELISA test tends to cost from 200 to 300 € (in Germany), the multigene array is much more expensive with around 4000 US$. If the uPA/PAI-1/Ki67 constellation points to low or higher risk this can be avoided in selected cases.

However, no conclusions concerning the success of chemotherapy may be drawn solely from increased values [28]. The risk stratification and therapy planning for a breast carcinoma never take place on the basis of an isolated parameter, not even if a multigene test is available, therefore the above assessment is not problematic.

Conclusions

The protein-based measurement of uPA/PAI from frozen tumour tissue and additional multigene tests enable a more differentiated risk assessment of the biological tumour behaviour than the sole evaluation of conventional criteria. The decision as to which test procedure is to be used can be made based on the evidence of clinical and methodical validation. In the overall context of the individual disease, extended analyses on tumour tissue must be critically weighed up in view of the benefit to be expected against the arising costs.

Acknowledgements
Acknowledgement to the technical staff of Pathology of Leopoldina Hospital Schweinfurt.

Funding
This publication was funded by the German Research Foundation (DFG) and the University of Wuerzburg in the funding programme Open Access Publishing.

Authors' contributions
HUV created the concept and execution of this study, MW interpreted the clinical data of uPA1/PAI-1 and multigene test, AS performed the data collection was responsible for approving the histomorphological/immunohistochemical characteristics of tumours. HUV and LF were major contributors in analysing and interpreting the data, statistical calculation, and writing the manuscript. All authors read and approved the final manuscript.

Competing interests
The authors declare that they have no competing interests.

Author details
[1]Pathology, Leopoldina Krankenhaus GmbH, Gustav-Adolf-Str 8, D-97422 Schweinfurt, Germany. [2]Department of Gynecology, Leopoldina Krankenhaus GmbH, Gustav-Adolf-Str 8, D-97422 Schweinfurt, Germany. [3]Institute for Pathology, University of Wuerzburg, Josef-Schneider-Str. 2, D-97080 Wuerzburg, Germany.

References
1. Lampelj M, Arko D, Cas-Sikosek N, Kavalar R, Ravnik M, Jezersek-Novakovic B, Dobnik S, Dovnik NF, Takac I. Urokinase plasminogen activator (uPA) and plasminogen activator inhibitor type-1 (PAI-1) in breast cancer - correlation with traditional prognostic factors. Radiol Oncol. 2015;49(4):357–64.
2. Binder BR, Mihaly J. The plasminogen activator inhibitor "paradox" in cancer. Immunol Lett. 2008;118(2):116–24.
3. Hildenbrand R, Schaaf A. The urokinase-system in tumor tissue stroma of the breast and breast cancer cell invasion. Int J Oncol. 2009;34(1):15–23.
4. Andreasen PA, Egelund R, Petersen HH. The plasminogen activation system in tumor growth, invasion, and metastasis. Cell Mol Life Sci. 2000;57(1):25–40.
5. Chen Y, Kelm RJ Jr, Budd RC, Sobel BE, Schneider DJ. Inhibition of apoptosis and caspase-3 in vascular smooth muscle cells by plasminogen activator inhibitor type-1. J Cell Biochem. 2004;92(1):178–88.
6. Ulisse S, Baldini E, Sorrenti S, D'Armiento M. The urokinase plasminogen activator system: a target for anti-cancer therapy. Curr Cancer Drug Targets. 2009;9(1):32–71.
7. Preissner KT, Kanse SM, May AE. Urokinase receptor: a molecular organizer in cellular communication. Curr Opin Cell Biol. 2000;12(5):621–8.
8. Rosenberg S. The urokinase-type plasminogen activator system in cancer and other pathological conditions: introduction and perspective. Curr Pharm Des. 2003;9(19):4.
9. Reuning U, Magdolen V, Wilhelm O, Fischer K, Lutz V, Graeff H, Schmitt M. Multifunctional potential of the plasminogen activation system in tumor invasion and metastasis (review). Int J Oncol. 1998;13(5):893–906.
10. Look MP, van Putten WL, Duffy MJ, Harbeck N, Christensen IJ, Thomssen C, Kates R, Spyratos F, Fernö M, Eppenberger-Castori S, Sweep CG, Ulm K, Peyrat JP, Martin PM, Magdelenat H, Brünner N, Duggan C, Lisboa BW, Bendahl PO, Quillien V, Daver A, Ricolleau G, Meijer-van Gelder ME, Manders P, Fiets WE, Blankenstein MA, Broët P, Romain S, Daxenbichler G, Windbichler G, Cufer T, Borstnar S, Kueng W, Beex LV, Klijn JG, O'Higgins N, Eppenberger U, Jänicke F, Schmitt M, Foekens JA. Pooled analysis of prognostic impact of urokinase-type plasminogen activator and its inhibitor PAI-1 in 8377 breast cancer patients. J Natl Cancer Inst. 2002;94(2):116–28.
11. Janicke F, Schmitt M, Pache L, Ulm K, Harbeck N, Hofler H, Graeff H. Urokinase (uPA) and its inhibitor PAI-1 are strong and independent prognostic factors in node-negative breast cancer. Breast Cancer Res Treat. 1993;24(3):195–208.
12. Rabi ZA, Todorovic-Rakovic N, Vujasinovic T, Milovanovic J, Nikolic-Vukosavljevic D. Markers of progression and invasion in short term follow up of untreated breast cancer patients. Cancer Biomark. 2015;15(6):745–54.
13. De Cremoux P, Grandin L, Dieras V, Savignoni A, Degeorges A, Salmon R, Bollet MA, Reyal F, Sigal-Zafrani B, Vincent-Salomon A, Sastre-Garau X, Magdelénat H, Mignot L, Fourquet A, Breast Cancer study Group of the Institut Curie. Urokinase-type plasminogen activator and plasminogen-activator-inhibitor type 1 predict metastases in good prognosis breast cancer patients. Anticancer Res. 2009;29(5):1475–82.
14. Meo S, Dittadi R, Peloso L, Gion M. The prognostic value of vascular endothelial growth factor, urokinase plasminogen activator and plasminogen activator inhibitor-1 in node-negative breast cancer. Int J Biol Markers. 2004;19(4):282–8.
15. Cronin M, Sangli C, Liu ML, Pho M, Dutta D, Nguyen A, Jeong J, Wu J, Langone KC, Watson D. Analytical validation of the Oncotype DX genomic diagnostic test for recurrence prognosis and therapeutic response prediction in node-negative, estrogen receptor-positive breast cancer. Clin Chem. 2007;53(6):1084–91.

16. Carlson JJ, Roth JA. The impact of the Oncotype DX breast cancer assay in clinical practice: a systematic review and meta-analysis. Breast Cancer Res Treat. 2013;141(1):13–22.

17. Goldstein LJ, Gray R, Badve S, Childs BH, Yoshizawa C, Rowley S, Shak S, Baehner FL, Ravdin PM, Davidson NE, Sledge GW Jr, Perez EA, Shulman LN, Martino S, Sparano JA. Prognostic utility of the 21-gene assay in hormone receptor-positive operable breast cancer compared with classical clinicopathologic features. J Clin Oncol. 2008;26(25):4063–71.

18. Albain KS, Barlow WE, Shak S, Hortobagyi GN, Livingston RB, Yeh IT, Ravdin P, Bugarini R, Baehner FL, Davidson NE, Sledge GW, Winer EP, Hudis C, Ingle JN, Perez EA, Pritchard KI, Shepherd L, Gralow JR, Yoshizawa C, Allred DC, Osborne CK, Hayes DF, Breast Cancer intergroup of North America. Prognostic and predictive value of the 21-gene recurrence score assay in postmenopausal women with node-positive, oestrogen-receptor-positive breast cancer on chemotherapy: a retrospective analysis of a randomised trial. Lancet Oncol. 2010;11(1):55–65.

19. Mamounas EP, Tang G, Fisher B, Paik S, Shak S, Costantino JP, Watson D, Geyer CE Jr, Wickerham DL, Wolmark N. Association between the 21-gene recurrence score assay and risk of locoregional recurrence in node-negative, estrogen receptor-positive breast cancer: results from NSABP B-14 and NSABP B-20. J Clin Oncol. 2010;28(10):1677–83.

20. Paik S, Tang G, Shak S, Kim C, Baker J, Kim W, Cronin M, Baehner FL, Watson D, Bryant J, Costantino JP, Geyer CE Jr, Wickerham DL, Wolmark N. Gene expression and benefit of chemotherapy in women with node-negative, estrogen receptor-positive breast cancer. J Clin Oncol. 2006;24(23):3726–34.

21. Wolff AC, Hammond MEH, Allison KH, Harvey BE, Mangu PB, Bartlett JMS, Bilous M, Ellis IO, Fitzgibbons P, Hanna W, Jenkins RB, Press MF, Spears PA, Vance GH, Viale G, McShane LM, Dowsett M. Human epidermal growth factor receptor 2 testing in breast Cancer: American Society of Clinical Oncology/College of American Pathologists Clinical Practice Guideline Focused Update. Arch Pathol Lab Med. 2018; https://doi.org/10.5858/arpa.2018-0902-SA.

22. Deluche E, Venat-Bouvet L, Leobon S, Fermeaux V, Mollard J, Saidi N, Jammet I, Aubard Y, Tubiana-Mathieu N. Assessment of Ki67 and uPA/PAI-1 expression in intermediate-risk early stage breast cancers. BMC Cancer. 2017;17(1):662.

23. Lang DS, Heilenkotter U, Schumm W, Behrens O, Simon R, Vollmer E, Goldmann T. Optimized immunohistochemistry in combination with image analysis: a reliable alternative to quantitative ELISA determination of uPA and PAI-1 for routine risk group discrimination in breast cancer. Breast. 2013;22(5):736–43.

24. Harbeck N, Schmitt M, Meisner C, Friedel C, Untch M, Schmidt M, Sweep CG, Lisboa BW, Lux MP, Beck T, Hasmüller S, Kiechle M, Jänicke F, Thomssen C, Chemo-N 0 Study Group. Ten-year analysis of the prospective multicentre chemo-N0 trial validates American Society of Clinical Oncology (ASCO)-recommended biomarkers uPA and PAI-1 for therapy decision making in node-negative breast cancer patients. Eur J Cancer. 2013;49(8):1825–35.

25. Witzel I, Milde-Langosch K, Schmidt M, Karn T, Becker S, Wirtz R, Rody A, Laakmann E, Schütze D, Jänicke F, Müller V. Role of urokinase plasminogen activator and plasminogen activator inhibitor mRNA expression as prognostic factors in molecular subtypes of breast cancer. Onco Targets Ther. 2014;28(7):2205–13.

26. Harris LN, Ismaila N, McShane LM, Andre F, Collyar DE, Gonzalez-Angulo AM, Hammond EH, Kuderer NM, Liu MC, Mennel RG, Van Poznak C, Bast RC, Hayes DF, American Society of Clinical Oncology. Use of biomarkers to guide decisions on adjuvant systemic therapy for women with early-stage invasive breast Cancer: American Society of Clinical Oncology clinical practice guideline. J Clin Oncol. 2016;34(10):1134–50.

27. Buta M, Džodić R, \DJurišić I, Marković I, Vujasinović T, Markićević M, Nikolić-Vukosavljević D. Potential clinical relevance of uPA and PAI-1 levels in node-negative, postmenopausal breast cancer patients bearing histological grade II tumors with ER/PR expression, during an early follow-up. Tumor Biol 2015; 36: 8193–8200.

28. Bellocq JP, Luporsi E, Barrière J, Bonastre J, Chetritt J, Le Corroller AG, de Crémoux P, Fina F, Gauchez AS, Kassab-Chahmi D, Lamy PJ, Martin PM, Mazouni C, Peyrat JP, Romieu G, Verdoni L, Mazeau-Woynar V. uPA/PAI-1, Oncotype DX™, MammaPrint(®). Prognosis and predictive values for clinical utility in breast cancer management. Ann Pathol. 2014;34(5):349–51.

23

Expression of DENDRIN in several glomerular diseases and correlation to pathological parameters and renal failure -preliminary study

Maja Mizdrak[1*], Katarina Vukojević[2], Natalija Filipović[2], Vesna Čapkun[3], Benjamin Benzon[4,5] and Merica Glavina Durdov[4,5]

Abstract

Background: In glomerular injury dendrin translocates from the slit diaphragm to the podocyte nucleus, inducing apoptosis. We analyzed dendrin expression in IgA glomerulonephritis and Henoch Schönlein purpura (IgAN/HSP) versus in podocytopathies minimal change disease (MCD) and focal segmental glomerulosclerosis (FSGS), and compared it to pathohistological findings and renal function at the time of biopsy and the last follow-up.

Methods: Twenty males and 13 females with median of age 35 years (min-max: 3–76) who underwent percutaneous renal biopsy and had diagnosis of glomerular disease (GD) were included in this retrospective study. Fifteen patients had IgAN/HSP and eighteen podocytopathy. Control group consisted of ten patients who underwent nephrectomy due to renal cancer. Dendrin expression pattern (membranous, dual, nuclear or negative), number of dendrin positive nuclei and proportion of dendrin negative glomeruli were analyzed.

Results: In GD and the control group significant differences in number of dendrin positive nuclei and proportion of dendrin negative glomeruli were found ($P = 0.004$ and $P = 0.003$, respectively). Number of dendrin positive nuclei was higher in podocytopathies than in IgAN/HSP, 3.90 versus 1.67 ($P = 0.028$). Proportion of dendrin negative glomeruli correlated to higher rates of interstitial fibrosis ($P = 0.038$), tubular atrophy ($P = 0.011$) and globally sclerotic glomeruli ($P = 0.008$). Dual and nuclear dendrin expression pattern were connected with lower rate of interstitial fibrosis and tubular atrophy than negative dendrin expression pattern ($P = 0.024$ and $P = 0.017$, respectively). Proportion of dendrin negative glomeruli correlated with lower creatinine clearance (CC) at the time of biopsy and the last follow-up ($P = 0.010$ and $P < 0.001$, respectively). Dendrin expression pattern correlated to CC at the last follow-up ($P = 0.009$), being lower in patients with negative than nuclear or dual dendrin expression ($P = 0.034$ and $P = 0.004$, respectively).

Conclusion: In this pilot study the number of dendrin positive nuclei was higher in podocytopathies than in inflammatory GD. Negative dendrin expression pattern correlated to chronic tubulointerstitial changes and lower CC, which needs to be confirmed in a larger series.

Keywords: Dendrin, IgA glomerulonephritis, Podocythopathies, Renal function, Immunohistochemistry

* Correspondence: mizdrakmaja@gmail.com
[1]Department of Nephrology and Hemodialysis, University Hospital Centre Split, Šoltanska 1, 21000 Split, Croatia
Full list of author information is available at the end of the article

Background

Dendrin is a proline - rich protein of still unclear function that was originally identified in telencephalic dendrites of sleep-deprived rats [1]. Apart from the brain, dendrin is found only in the kidneys, linearly expressed in podocytes along glomerular capillary loops [2]. As an integral part of the slit diaphragm (SD) complex, dendrin contributes to the regulation of podocyte function [3]. Dendrin has a possible role in the glomerular filtration, because it directly binds to nephrin and CD2-associated protein [2–5]. These proteins interact with p85 regulatory subunit of phosphatidylinositol 3-kinase, stimulating anti-apoptotic AKT signaling [3]. In response to glomerular injury and upregulated TGF-β, dendrin relocates from the membrane to the nucleus, thereby promoting apoptosis [3, 6]. Nuclear dendrin acts as a transcriptional factor of cytosolic enzyme cathepsin L, which proteolyzes CD2-associated protein, thereby increasing the apoptotic susceptibility to pro-apoptotic TGF-β [7]. On the other side, cathepsin L cleaves the regulatory GTP-ase dynamin and actin-associated adapter synaptopodin, causing a reorganization of the podocyte microfilament system, resulting in proteinuria [5, 7].

During fetal development of human kidney, dendrin is first detected at the *capillary loop stage* and it is never expressed in podocyte nuclei [2, 3, 8]. Due to this fact, nuclear relocation of dendrin in glomerular diseases (GD) is possible marker of disease [6]. The expression of dendrin in podocyte nuclei is found in small studies of different GD: FSGS, lupus nephritis (LN), membranous nephropathy (MN) and IgAN [6, 7]. Interestingly, significant proportion of dendrin positive nuclei was not found in MCD [2]. According to Kodama et al., large number of nuclear dendrin in IgAN could be an indicator of disease activity and its progression to glomerulosclerosis [7].

The aim of our pilot study was to evaluate possible difference in dendrin expression in inflammatory and non-inflammatory GD. We analyzed 11 IgAN, 4 HSP and 18 podocytopathies (11 primary FSGS and 7 MCD) and correlated with histological parameters and renal function at the time of the biopsy and the last follow-up.

Methods

Thirty-three patients whose percutaneous renal biopsy was performed from 1996 to 2015 in University Hospital Centre Split, Split, Croatia were enrolled in this study. Paraffin blocks of their biopsies were collected from the Department of Pathology and clinical data at the time of biopsy and the last follow-up in 2017 were collected from the hospital records. All biopsies were analyzed by light, immunofluorescence and electron microscopy making the diagnoses of IgAN, HSP, MCD or primary FSGS. Inclusion criteria were enough material in the paraffin block for immunohistochemical analysis and complete clinical data. The patients without adequate laboratory findings or paraffin blocks were excluded. In control group we analyzed glomeruli from ten patents with normal renal function, who underwent nephrectomy due to clear cell renal carcinoma. Five micrometer thin slides were cut from the paraffin blocks. Indirect immunohistochemistry was performed in Benchmark (Ventana Medical Systems, Inc. USA). The primary antibody was rabbit polyclonal anti-dendrin (Abcam, Cambridge, United Kingdom) diluted at 1:200 and incubated for 1 h. Secondary antibody was Optiview Detection kit (Ventana Medical Systems, Inc. USA) and incubation lasted 30 min. In immunofluorescence we used rabbit anti-dendrin (Abcam, Cambridge, United Kingdom), diluted at 1:200 and goat anti-nephrin antibody (G-20 Santa Cruse Biotechnology, Inc. Heidelberg, Germany), diluted at 1:300. They were applied simultaneously and left overnight in a humidified chamber at room temperature. The secondary antibodies were donkey anti-goat IgG (Alexa fluor 594 Molecular Probes Life Technologies, Oregon, USA), diluted at 1:300 and donkey polyclonal anti-rabbit IgG (Alexa fluor 488 Molecular Probes Life Technologies, Oregon, USA), diluted at 1:300. After washing in phosphate-buffered saline (PBS), DAPI (4′,6-diamidino-2-phenylindole) was applied and washed again. Stained sections were viewed and photographed, using a BX51 microscope (Olympus, Tokyo, Japan) equipped with a DP71 digital camera (Olympus), and processed with CellA Imaging Software for Life Sciences Microscopy (Olympus). Dendrin translocation to nuclei was presented by co-localization of dendrin, nephrin and DAPI in the same cell on immunofluorescence (Fig. 1).

Nuclear expression of dendrin was counted on immunohistochemical slide on the light microscope Olympus BX51, Olympus, Tokyo, Japan. Median was 6 glomeruli (min-max: 1–34) per slide. The same was done on immunofluorescence microscope. Since there was no statistical difference in number of dendrin positive nuclei between these two methods, only the results of the immunohistochemistry were presented in the further text. Number of dendrin positive nuclei was divided with the number of analyzed glomeruli and thus median (min-max) was calculated for each patient. Number of dendrin negative glomeruli was divided with number of analyzed glomeruli to get their proportion. Control slides were analyzed on one low magnification field (7 glomeruli in average) and analyzed on the same way. A pattern of dendrin expression in each glomerulus was assigned as membranous, dual, nuclear or negative. Only membranous staining was assigned as membranous, simultaneously positive membranous and nuclear staining as dual, only nuclear staining as nuclear and both negative membranous and nuclear staining with positive external control as negative (Fig. 2).

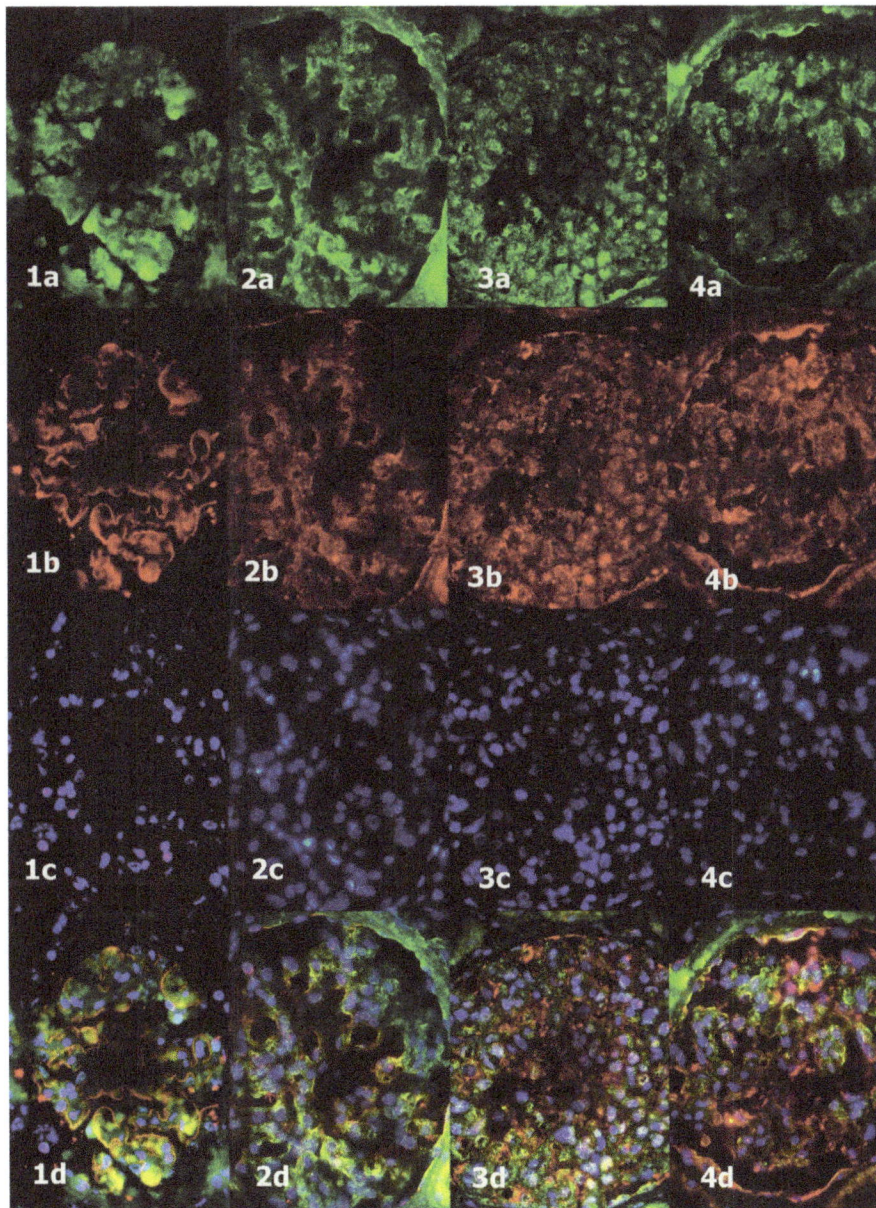

Fig. 1 Nuclear dendrin expression (arrows) in the control group (1) and glomerular diseases (2 - MCD, 3 - IgAN/HSP, 4 - FSGS); **a** - dendrin (green), **b** - nephrin (red), **c** - DAPI (blue), **d** - merge; fluorescence microscope, immunofluorescence staining, 400 x

Statistical analysis was performed using Statistical Package for the Social Sciences (SPSS) software (version 19 for Windows; SPSS Inc., Chicago, Illinois, USA). Statistical significance was set at $P < 0.05$, and all confidence intervals (CI) were at the 95% level. Spearman's correlation coefficient (Rho) was used to calculate degree of connection. Statistical significance of the difference in categorical characteristics of several independent variables was calculated by using χ^2 test. Fisher's exact test was used in the analysis of contingency tables when tested sample sizes were small. Analysis of statistical significance of differences in several numerical variables

was performed with the Kruskal-Wallis test and of differences between two groups with the Mann-Whitney test. The study was performed according to the Helsinki Declaration. Informed signed consent form was obtained from each patient (or parents if a child).

Results

In the study there were 20 (61%) males, with median of age 38.5 (min-max: 3–76 years) and 13 (39%) females, with median of age 35 (min-max: 4–62 years). Eleven (33.33%) patients had IgAN, four (12.12%) HSP, seven (21.21%) MCD and eleven (33.33%) FSGS. The distribution according to

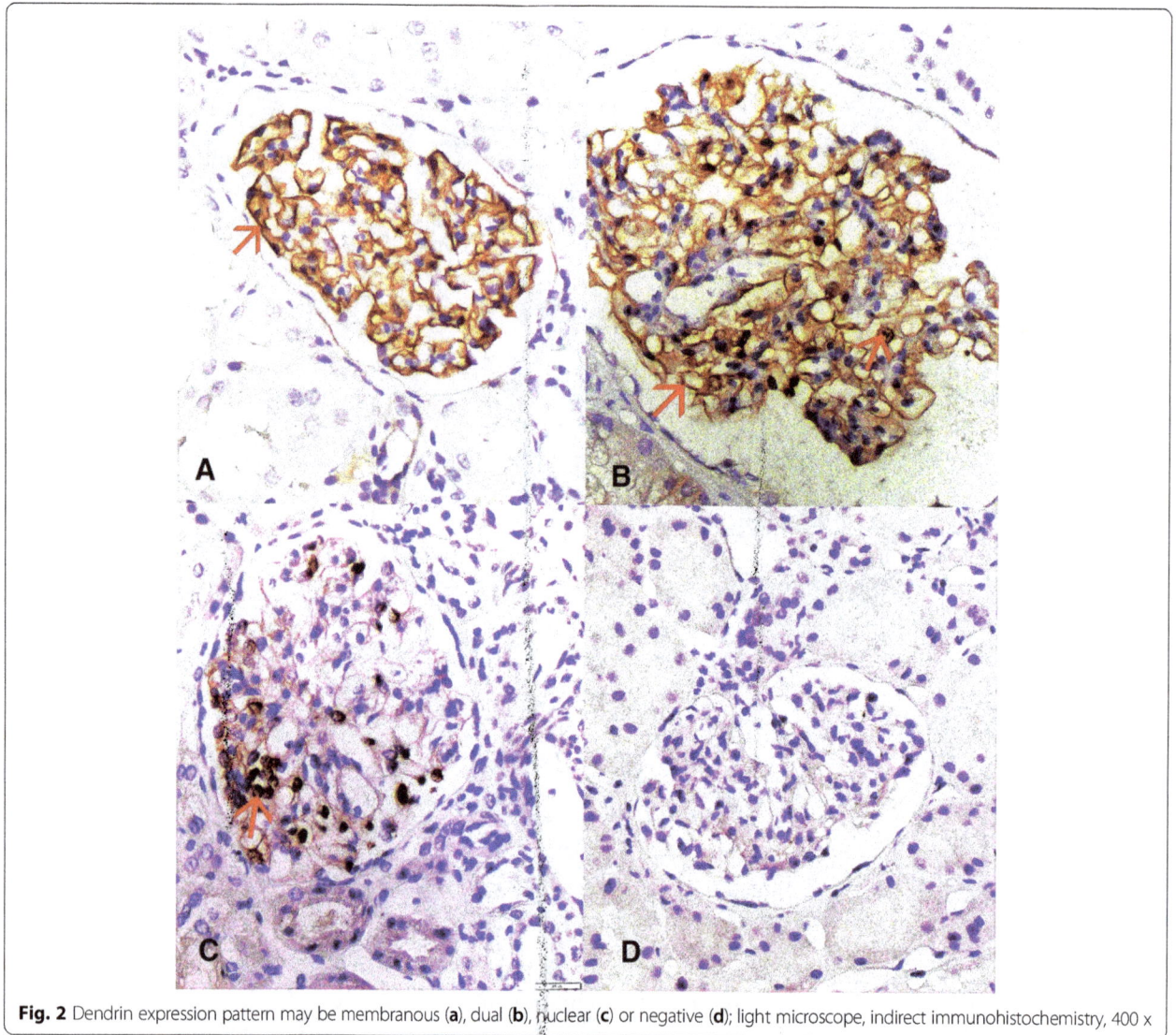

Fig. 2 Dendrin expression pattern may be membranous (**a**), dual (**b**), nuclear (**c**) or negative (**d**); light microscope, indirect immunohistochemistry, 400 x

the type of glomerular disease and clinical parameters is presented in Table 1. Due to small numbers, IgAN and HSP, and MCD and FSGS were analyzed together.

Patients with several GD were not significantly different in any clinical parameters. In further analysis types

of GD and the control group were analyzed according to median of number of nuclear dendrin expression and proportion of dendrin negative glomeruli (Table 2).

In IgAN/HSP median number of dendrin positive nuclei was 1.67 (min - max: 0.00–5.60) and in podocytopathies

Table 1 Distribution of 33 patients according to the type of glomerular disease and clinical parameters

Clinical parameter		Patients with glomerular disease				P
		Inflammatory		Non-inflammatory		
		IgAN (n = 11)	HSP (n = 4)	MCD (n = 7)	FSGS (n = 11)	
Hematuria	yes	4	4	1	4	0.169[a]
Hypertension	yes	7	1	5	9	0.163[a]
Proteinuria	≥ 3400 (mg/dU/24 h)	6	2	6	9	0.126[a]
Creatinine clearance (ml/min/1.73m^2) median value (min-max)	At the time of biopsy	96 (27–150)	84 (25–170)	89 (27–212)	62 (30–162)	0.800[b]
	At the last follow-up	59 (6–147)	75.5 (47–148)	103 (63–180)	51 (7–92)	0.942[b]

[a]Fisher's exact test
[b]Mann Whitney test

Table 2 Number of dendrin positive nuclei and proportion of dendrin negative glomeruli in glomerular diseases

| Dendrin expression | Glomerular disease ($N = 33$) | | | | |
| | Inflammatory ($n = 15$) | Non-inflammatory ($n = 18$) | | | |
	IgAN + HSP	MCD	FSGS	Control	P^a
Dendrin-positive nuclei[b]	1.67 (0.00–5.60)	5.90 (2.00–23.10)	2.80 (0.00–9.50)	0.50 (0.00–2.20)	0.004
Proportion of dendrin negative glomeruli[b]	0.50 (0.00–1.00)	0.00 (0.00–0.06)	0.27 (0.00–1.00)	0.00 (0.00–0.00)	0.003

[a]Kruskal Wallis test
[b]median (min-max)

3.90 (min – max: 0.00–23.10), ($P = 0.028$, $Z = 2.2$, $r = 0.38$, 95% CI 0.12–4.34). In further analysis MCD and FSGS were analyzed separately. Nuclear dendrin expression was different in IgAN/HSP, MCD, FSGS and control group ($\chi^2 = 13.10$; $P = 0.004$). Median nuclear dendrin expression was higher in MCD than IgAN/HSP ($P = 0.033$) and in MCD than the control group ($P = 0.003$). No difference was found between IgAN/HSP and FSGS ($P = 1.000$). Median of nuclear dendrin expression was not significantly different in MCD and FSGS ($P = 0.363$). Proportion of dendrin negative glomeruli was statistically different between GD ($\chi^2 = 13.60$; $P = 0.003$). In IgAN/HSP and FSGS proportions of dendrin negative glomeruli were higher than in the control group ($P = 0.015$ and $P = 0.035$, respectively). There was no difference between IgAN/HSP and FSGS ($P = 1.000$). Difference was not found between MCD and control group ($P = 1.000$).

CC at the time of biopsy did not significantly correlate to median of dendrin positive nuclei (Rho = 0.150, $P = 0.403$). According to Spearman's coefficient of correlation, CC at the time of biopsy and proportion of dendrin negative glomeruli showed negative correlation (Rho = – 0.444; $P = 0.010$). CC at the last follow-up significantly correlated to proportion of dendrin negative glomeruli (Rho = – 0.626; $P < 0.001$) and to median of dendrin positive nuclei (Rho = 0.433, $P = 0.012$). No difference was found in correlation between the level of proteinuria and median of dendrin positive nuclei (Rho = 0.324, $P = 0.066$), as well as proteinuria and proportion of dendrin negative glomeruli (Rho = – 0.284, $P = 0.109$).

Number of dendrin positive nuclei in IgAN/HSP was correlated to parameters of Oxford classification, but significant difference was not found (Table 3).

In eight IgAN samples with crescents median of dentrin positive nuclei was 1.58 (min – max: 0.00–3.85) and in seven IgAN samples without crescents 2.30 (min – max: 0.00–5.60) ($P = 0.479$). Proportion of dendrin negative glomeruli in the first group was 0.50 (min-max: 0.00–1.00), and in the former 0.33 (0.00–1.00) ($P = 0.668$). According to International Study of Kidney Disease in Children (ISKDC) classification, three patients with HSP were grade 3, and one grade 6.

Dendrin expression pattern was assigned to each patient according to predominate finding in whole slide, and it was nuclear in nine (27.27%), dual in sixteen

(48.48%) and negative in eight (24.24%) patiens. There was no difference between IgAN/HSP and podocytopathies in distribution of dual or nuclear dendrin expression pattern ($P = 0.299$). Also there was no difference in dual/nuclear versus negative expression pattern ($P = 0.418$). Dendrin expression pattern in 33 patients was correlated to pathohistological findings and clinical parameters of renal function (Table 4).

Dendrin expression pattern significantly correlated to median of CC at the last follow-up ($\chi^2 = 9.30$, $\eta^2 = 0.29$; $P = 0.009$). Mann-Whitney test in post-hoc analysis did not find any difference between the patients with nuclear or dual expression ($Z = 1.20$; $P = 0.234$). In patients with negative dendrin expression pattern, median of CC was significantly lower than in patients with nuclear expression pattern ($Z = 2.10$; $r = 0.52$; $P = 0.034$) and for 79.5 lower than in patients with dual expression pattern ($Z = 2.80$, $r = 0.59$, $P = 0.004$). CC at the time of biopsy and proteinuria were not significantly different between dendrin expression patterns ($\chi^2 = 5.20$; $P = 0.073$ and $\chi^2 = 3.1$, $P = 0.208$, respectively).

According to Spearman's coefficient of correlation, proportion of globally sclerotic glomeruli and number of dendrin positive nuclei showed negative correlation (Rho = – 0.409, $P = 0.018$). Significant correlations between number of dendrin positive nuclei and interstitial fibrosis (Rho = – 0.167, $P = 0.353$) or tubular atrophy (Rho = – 0.277, $P = 0.119$) were not found. Statistically significant positive Spearman's correlations were found in

Table 3 Number of dendrin positive nuclei according to Oxford classification of IgAN

Parameter	Number of cases	Dendrin positive nuclei median (min-max)	P^*
Mesangial hypercellularity (M)	M0 ($n = 2$)	1.50 (0.00–4.60)	0.941
	M1 ($n = 13$)	2.00 (0.00–5.60)	
Endocapillary proliferation (E)	E0 ($n = 11$)	1.50 (0.00–5.60)	0.549
	E1 ($n = 4$)	2.40 (0.00–3.85)	
Segmental sclerosis (S)	S0 ($n = 7$)	2.30 (0.00–5.60)	0.376
	S1 ($n = 8$)	1.50 (0.00–4.60)	
Tubular atrophy/interstitial fibrosis (T)	T0 ($n = 15$)	1.70 (0.00–5.60)	/
	T1 ($n = 0$)	/	
	T2 ($n = 0$)	/	

[*]Mann-Whitney test

Table 4 Dendrin expression pattern in relation to pathohistological and clinical parameters

Parameter	Pattern of dendrin expression in 33 patients with glomerular diseases			P^a
	Nuclear (N = 9)	Dual (N = 16)	Negative (N = 8)	
Interstitial fibrosis	0.05 (0.00–0.35)	0.01 (0.00–0.20)	0.10 (0.00–0.20)	0.024
Tubular atrophy	0.01 (0.00–0.35)	0.01 (0.00–0.20)	0.10 (0.01–0.25)	0.017
Globally sclerotic glomeruli	0.04 (0.00–0.35)	0.00 (0.00–0.21)	0.17 (0.00–0.50)	0.056
Creatinine clearance at the time of biopsy (ml/min/1.73m²)^b	53 (27–118)	108 (25–212)	58 (27–150)	0.073
Creatinine clearance at the last follow-up (ml/min/1.73m²)^b	68 (10–109)	91 (17–180)	11.5 (6–95)	0.009
Proteinuria (mg/dU/24 h)^b	6380 (1460–18,677)	5375 (100–28,254)	4150 (63–5250)	0.208

aKruskal-Wallis test
^{b}Median (min-max)

proportions of interstitial fibrosis (Rho = 0.363, P = 0.038), tubular atrophy (Rho = 0.437, P = 0.011) and globally sclerotic glomeruli (Rho = 0.451, P = 0.008) with proportion of dendrin negative glomeruli.

At last, dendrin expression pattern in all glomeruli was analyzed and different distribution according to type of GD was found (χ^2 = 52; P < 0.001) (Table 5, Fig. 3).

In IgAN nuclear pattern was found in 13% glomeruli and none in HSP (χ^2 = 9.60; P < 0.001). In MCD there was 3.9 times more glomeruli with nuclear dendrin expression pattern than in IgAN, but only one glomerulus with negative dendrin expression (χ^2 = 28; P < 0.001). IgAN had 3.1 times less glomeruli with nuclear dendrin expression than FSGS (χ^2 = 19.60; P < 0.001). Nuclear dendrin expression was found in MCD, in contrast to HSP (χ^2 = 28.20; P < 0.001). Dual pattern was 1.8 times more common in HSP than FSGS (χ^2 = 19.60; P < 0.001). In MCD one glomerulus had negative expression pattern and in FSGS 17% glomeruli (χ^2 = 12.10; P < 0.001).

Discussion

During glomerular injury, dendrin nuclear translocation promotes podocyte apoptosis, which is the main pathological mechanism of chronic kidney failure [9]. This pathway is strictly controlled by regulatory pro- and antiapoptotic molecules [10]. In an experimental model, the translocation from membrane to nucleus might be temporarily presented as a dual subcellular dendrin distribution [3]. In our immunohistochemical pilot study of human glomerular diseases, we have noticed not only dual, but also negative dendrin expression in several glomeruli. Dendrin expression pattern was different in analyzed types of glomerular diseases and higher proportion of dendrin negative glomeruli significantly correlated to lower creatinine clearance. We accentuate a term of *dendrin negative glomerulus* and suggest that dendrin expression might be irreversibly switched off in chronically damaged glomeruli. We assume that higher proportion of such glomeruli is possibly associated with podocyte loss and thereby is prognostically relevant to the kidney function. In our study, higher proportion of dendrin negative glomeruli has been significantly correlated to lower CC both at the time of biopsy and the follow-up, and for our best knowledge it is the first such data in the literature. Becherucci et al. explained the pathway of glomerulosclerosis in which dendrin has an important role. The limited podocyte death induced hypertrophy of survived podocytes; if podocyte loss had increased over a certain threshold, further step was the activation of parietal epithelial cells and their differentiation to podocytes, and if this compensatory mechanism was not efficient, induction of sclerosis followed [11]. In our study there were positive statistically significant Spearman's correlations between proportion of dendrin negative glomeruli and rate of interstitial fibrosis, tubular atrophy and globally sclerotic glomeruli. Higher proportion of globally sclerotic glomeruli was also correlated to lower number of dendrin positive nuclei what is in accordance with the literature. Kodama et al. found in the IgAN study that the number of dendrin positive nuclei was significantly higher in the renal biopsy specimens with only a few sclerotic glomeruli [7].

Table 5 Distribution of dendrin expression pattern in total number of glomeruli in analyzed glomerular diseases

Dendrin expression pattern	Total number of analyzed glomeruli in each type of glomerular diseases n (%)				P^*
	IgAN n = 52	HSP n = 34	MCD n = 75	FSGS n = 113	
Nuclear	7 (13)	0 (0)	38 (51)	42 (37)	< 0.001
Dual	29 (56)	27 (79)	34 (45)	51 (45)	
Negative	16 (31)	4 (12)	1 (1)	19 (17)	
Membranous	0 (0)	3 (9)	2 (3)	1 (1)	

*χ^2 test

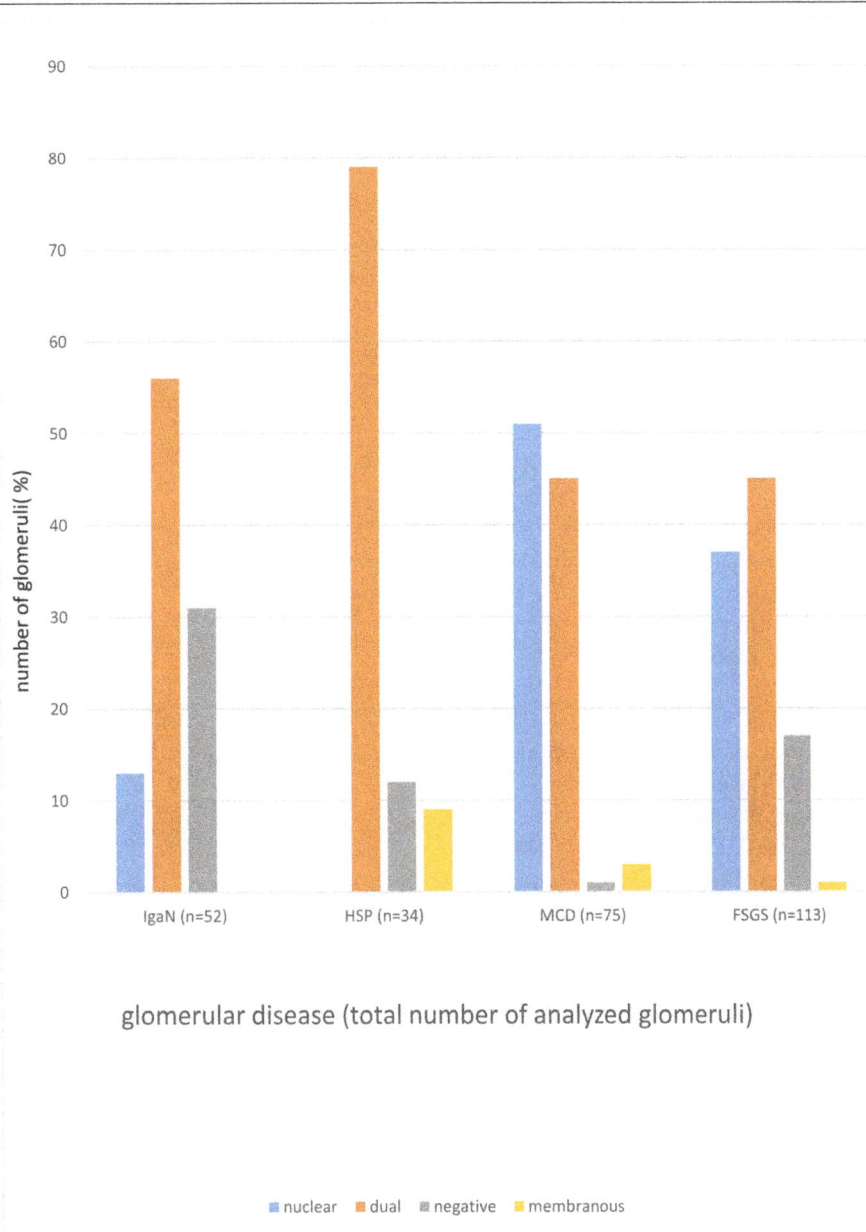

Fig. 3 Distribution of dendrin expression pattern in total number of glomeruli in analyzed types of glomerular diseases

According to previously reported small studies, nuclear dendrin relocation occurred in IgAN, FSGS, MN and LN [6, 7]. In the study of three cases of FSGS and MN and four cases of LN, Asunama et al. found significantly higher number of dendrin positive nuclei than in control (five cases) and MCD (three cases), in which a few dendrin-positive nuclei still were present [6]. Dunér et al. analyzed five patients with MCD and found cytoplasmic dendrin expression in areas with foot process effacement, but not in podocyte nuclei [2]. We used light and immunofluorescence microscopy and confirmed that number of dendrin positive nuclei was not significantly different between two

analyses. In our study clear nuclear relocation of dendrin in MCD was found. MCD is also podocytopathy caused by immunological factors despite regular light or immunofluorescence microscopy presentation [12]. Therefore, we assume that dendrin relocation is the response to glomerular injury, unrelated to type of the glomerular disease. In the future, a larger study would be necessary to examine dendrin nuclear expression in cohort of MCD patients of the same age.

Recent insights have defined the central role of the podocyte as both the regulator of glomerular development as well as the determinant of progression to glomerulosclerosis in podocytopathies [13]. In inflammatory GD - IgA nephropathy/HSP mesangial cell activation is an initial consequence of IgA deposition, but mesangial-podocyte crosstalk leads to indirect podocyte injury which has cytoskeletal and signaling consequences, ie. indirect podocyte injury also contributes to glomerular damage observed in IgAN [14].

We have examined dendrin expression pattern in all glomeruli of each type of glomerular diseases and have found the significant difference. In HSP, the disease with usually an acute clinical presentation, predominantly dual pattern of dendrin expression has been found, without nuclear expression and more membranous expression than in other GD. In IgAN dual and negative patterns were found and in podocytopathies predominantly nuclear and dual expression. Only one dendrin negative glomerulus was detected in MCD, in contrast to IgAN and FSGS (31 and 17%, respectively). These changes could be explained by the differences in the pathophysiological mechanisms, the clinical course and dynamics of a particular disease.

Conclusion

Relocation of dendrin from membrane to nucleus is a dynamic, gradual and multi-level process controlled and affected by numerous factors and signal pathways. We have found that dendrin translocation occurs in different types of glomerular diseases, including MCD, and dendrin expression presents in different patterns. The proportion of dendrin negative glomeruli could be a novel adverse prognostic factor of the kidney function. We propose that dendrin translocation and its correlation with kidney failure and pathological parameters should be interpreted in the context of dendrin expression pattern, not only as an absolute number of dendrin positive nuclei.

Abbreviations

CC: creatinine clearance; DAPI: 4',6-diamidino-2-phenylindole; FSGS: focal segmental glomerulosclerosis; GD: glomerular disease; GTP: hydrolyze guanosine triphosphate; HSP: Henoch-Schönlein purpura; IgAN: IgA nephropathy; LN: lupus nephritis; max: maximal; MCD: minimal change disease; min: minimal; MN: membranous nephropathy; PBS: phosphate-buffered saline; SD: slit diaphragm; TGB-β: transforming growth factor beta

Acknowledgements

Not applicable.

Funding

This paper received no specific grant from any funding source in the public, commercial, or not-for-profit sectors. This research was self-financed by the authors.

Authors' contributions

MM and MGD designed the study, analyzed histological slides, interpreted the results and drafted the manuscript. KV and NF performed immunofluorescence staining, analyzed histological slides and interpreted the results. VC and BB performed the statistical analysis and interpreted the results. BB made language corrections. All authors read and approved the final manuscript.

Competing interests

The authors declare that they have no competing interests.

Author details

[1]Department of Nephrology and Hemodialysis, University Hospital Centre Split, Šoltanska 1, 21000 Split, Croatia. [2]Department of Anatomy, Histology and Embryology, University of Split School of Medicine, Split, Croatia. [3]Department of Nuclear Medicine, University Hospital Centre Split, Split, Croatia. [4]Department of Pathology, Forensic medicine and Cytology, University Hospital Centre Split, Split, Croatia. [5]University of Split School of Medicine, Split, Croatia.

References

1. Neuner-Jehle M, Denizot JP, Borbély AA and Mallet J. Characterization and sleep deprivation-induced expression modulation of dendrin, a novel dendritic protein in rat brain neurons. J Neurosci Res 1996; 46: 138–151. [PubMed].
2. Dunér F, Patrakka J, Xiao Z, Larsson J, Vlamis-Gardikas A, Pettersson E, et al. Dendrin expression in glomerulogenesis and in human minimal change nephrotic syndrome. Nephrol Dial Transplant 2008; 23: 2504–2511. [PubMed].
3. Asanuma K, Campbell KN, Kim K, Faul C and Mundel P. Nuclear relocation of the nephrin and CD2AP-binding protein dendrin promotes apoptosis of podocytes. Proc Natl Acad Sci U S A 2007;104: 10134–10139. [PubMed].
4. Campbell KN, Wong JS, Gupta R, Asanuma K, Sudol M, He JC, et al. Yes-associated protein (YAP) promotes cell survival by inhibiting proapoptotic dendrin signaling. J Biol Chem. 2013;288:17057–62. PubMed.
5. Xiao Z, Rodriguez PQ, He L, Betsholtz C, Tryggvason K, Patrakka J. Wtip- and gadd45a-interacting protein dendrin is not crucial for the development or maintenance of the glomerular filtration barrier. PLoS One. 2013;8: e83133. PubMed.
6. Asanuma K, Akiba-Takagi M, Kodama F, Asao R, Nagai Y, Lydia A, et al. Dendrin location in podocytes is associated with disease progression in animal and human glomerulopathy. Am J Nephrol. 2011;537-49(PubMed):33.
7. Kodama F, Asanuma K, Takagi M, Hidaka T, Asanuma E, Fukuda H, et al. Translocation of dendrin to the podocyte nucleus in acute glomerular injury in patients with IgA nephropathy. Nephrol Dial Transplant 2013; 28: 1762–1772. [PubMed].
8. Takano K, Kawasaki Y, Imaizumi T, Matsuura H, Nozawa R, et al. Development of glomerular endothelial cells, podocytes and mesangial cells in the human fetus and infant. Tohoku J Exp Med 2007; 212: 81–90. [PubMed].
9. Huang Z, Zhang L, Chen Y, Zhang H, Yu C, Zhou F, et al. RhoA deficiency disrupts podocyte cytoskeleton and induces podocyte apoptosis by inhibiting YAP/dendrin signal. BMC Nephrol 2016; 17: 66. [PubMed].
10. Shirata N, Ihara K, Yamamoto-Nonaka K, Seki T, Makino S, Oliva Trejo AJ, et al. Glomerulosclerosis induced by deficiency of membrane-associated Gunylate kinase inverted 2 in kidney podocytes. J Am Soc Nephrol 2017; 28: 2654–2669. [PubMed].
11. Becherucci F, Lazzeri E and Romagnani P. A road to chronic kidney disease: toward glomerulosclerosis via dendrin.Am J Pathol 2015; 185: 2072–2075. [PubMed].
12. Alpers CE, Chang A. The Kidney. In: Kumar V, Abbas AK, Aster JC, editors. Robbins and Cotran Pathologic Basis of Diseases. Philadelphia: Elsevier; 2015. p. 917–8.
13. Wiggins RC. The spectrum of podocytopathies: a unifying view of glomerular diseases. Review article Kidney Int 2007. [PubMed].
14. Menon MC, Chuang PY, He JC. Role of podocyte injury in IgA nephropathy. Contrib Nephrol 2013; 181, 41–51. [PubMed].

24

Increased expression of claudin-17 promotes a malignant phenotype in hepatocyte via Tyk2/Stat3 signaling and is associated with poor prognosis in patients with hepatocellular carcinoma

Lemeng Sun[1], Liangshu Feng[2] and Jiuwei Cui[1*]

Abstract

Background: Hepatocellular carcinoma (HCC) is the second leading cause of cancer death in Asia; however, the molecular mechanism in its tumorigenesis remains unclear. Abnormal expression of claudins (CLDNs), a family of tight junction (TJ) proteins, plays an important role in the metastatic phenotype of epithelial-derived tumors by affecting tight junction structure, function and related cellular signaling pathways. In a previous study, we used a tissue chip assay to identify CLDN17 as an upregulated gene in HCC. Here we aimed to use molecular biology technology to explore the effect of CLDN17 on the malignant phenotype of HCC and the underlying molecular mechanism, with the objective of identifying a new target for HCC treatment and the control of HCC metastasis.

Method: The expression levels of CLDN17 in HCC tissues and histologically non-neoplastic hepatic tissues were explored by immunohistochemistry. Stable transfection of the hepatocyte line HL7702 with CLDN17 was detected by real-time polymerase chain reaction (PCR), western blotting and immunofluorescence. The impact of CLDN17 on the malignant phenotype of HL7702 cells in vitro was assessed by a Cell Counting Kit-8 (CCK8) assay, a Transwell assay and a wound-healing experiment. Western blotting was utilized to detect the activation state of Tyrosine kinase 2 (Tyk2) / signal transducer and activator of transcription3 (Stat3) pathway. A Tyk2 RNA interference (RNAi) was utilized to determine the impact of the Tyk2/Stat3 signaling pathway on the malignant phenotype of hepatocytes.

Results: In this work, our research group first found that CLDN17 was highly expressed in HCC tissues and was associated with poor prognosis. In addition, we demonstrated that CLDN17 affected the Stat3 signaling pathway via Tyk2 and ultimately enhanced the migration ability of hepatocytes.

Conclusion: In conclusion, we confirmed that the upregulated expression of CLDN17 significantly enhances the migration ability of hepatocytes in vitro and we found that the activation of the Stat3 pathway by Tyk2 may an important mechanism by which CLDN17 promotes aggressiveness in hepatocytes.

Keywords: Hepatocytes, Tight junction, Migration, CLDN17, Tyrosine kinase 2, Signal transducer and activator of transcription 3

* Correspondence: cjwjlu@126.com
[1]Stem Cell and Cancer Center, The First Bethune Hospital, Jilin University, Changchun, Jilin 130021, People's Republic of China
Full list of author information is available at the end of the article

Background

Previous studies have shown that the metastasis of epithelial-derived tumors is accompanied by abnormalities in tight junction (TJ) structure and function [1, 2]. Claudins (CLDNs) are the key proteins that form TJ, and accumulating evidence suggests that tumor cells frequently exhibit changes in the expression and localization of CLDNs [3]. For example, CLDN1 demonstrated to be overexpressed in colorectal cancer (CRC) compared with the level in the normal mucosa, and CLDN1 targeting with an anti-CLDN1 monoclonal antibody (mAb) resulted in decreased growth and survival of colorectal cancer (CRC) cells, suggesting that CLDN1 could be a new potential therapeutic target for CRC [4]. In addition, a database-augmented, exosome-based mass spectrometry approach identified circulating CLDN3 as a biomarker in patients with prostate cancer [5]. Moreover, high-level cytoplasmic CLDN3 expression is an independent predictor of poor survival in patients with breast cancer [6]. The TJ protein CLDN4 has been reported to be overexpressed in advanced ovarian cancer (OC) and Kaplan-Meier survival analyses and the log-rank test suggest that high expression of CLDN4 may have prognostic value in OC [7]. These observations revealed that the alterations in CLDNs expression may be related to tumorigenesis and cancer progression in various types of human carcinoma.

Additionally, CLDNs have been shown to participate in the transduction of intracellular/extracellular signals and may be related to tumorigenesis and cancer progression in human various carcinomas [8, 9]. For instance, genetic and pharmacological studies confirmed that the expression of CLDN3 was downregulated in colon cancer and that the loss of CLDN3 induced Wnt/β-catenin activation in a transducer and activator of transcription 3 (Stat3)-dependent manner to promote colon cancer malignancy [10]. Besides, a recent study revealed that enhanced CLDN18 expression activated ERK1/2 to contributed to the malignant potentials of bile duct cancer [11]. Our preliminary work showed that CLDN17 was strongly expressed in HCC tissues and cell lines and weakly expressed in non-neoplastic tissues and hepatocyte lines, which revealed that upregulated CLDN17 expression may play a role in the development of HCC. Furthermore, gene chip screening revealed that CLDN17 overexpression activated the tyrosine kinase 2 (Tyk2)/Stat3 pathway signaling pathway. To date, there has been no report on the impact of CLDN17 on the malignant phenotype of hepatocytes. In this study, we utilized molecular biology and other techniques to study the role and mechanisms of CLDN17 in malignant phenotype of hepatocytes and to identify novel targets for HCC treatment and the control of early metastasis.

Methods

Antibodies

Rabbit polyclonal antibodies against CLDN17 (cat. no. ab233333) and mouse anti-human β-actin (cat. no. ab8226) were purchased from Abcam (Massachusetts, US). Rabbit anti-human phospho-Stat1 (cat. no. #7649), rabbit anti-human phospho-Stat3 (cat. no. #9145, rabbit anti-human phospho-Tyk2 (cat. no. #68790), rabbit anti-human Stat1 (cat. no.#14,994), rabbit anti-human Stat3 (cat. no. #9139) and rabbit anti-human Tyk2 (cat. no. #13531) were purchased from Cell Signaling Technology (Boston, USA).

Cell culture

Human hepatocyte line (HL7702) and HCC cell lines (HepG2, Hep3B and Huh1) utilized in this study were purchased from Shanghai Cell Bank of the Chinese Academy of Sciences. These cell lines were cultured in Dulbecco's modified Eagle's medium supplemented with 10% fetal bovine serum (FBS) at 37 °C in a humidified incubator containing 5% CO_2.

Plasmid construction and transfection

The plasmid p-EGFP-C1/CLDN17 (NM_012131) was constructed and amplified by KeyGen BioTech Company. Two micrograms of plasmid DNA was transfected into cells using the SuperFect Transfection Reagent (TaKaRa, Japan) according to the manufacturer's protocol. A cell line stably expressing CLDN17 was selected in medium containing G418 (Thermo Fisher Scientific, Waltham, MA).

Real-time polymerase chain reaction (PCR)

Total RNA was extracted using a Perfect Pure RNA Cultured Cell Kit (Thermo Fisher Scientific, Waltham, MA) according to the manufacturer's protocol. Real-time PCR reactions was carried out as previously described [12]. The primer pairs used for CLDN17 and glyceraldehyde phosphate dehydrogenase (GAPDH) were as follows: CLDN17 forward (5′-ACCCAGCCATCCACATAG-3′) and reverse (5′- CCCTTGCTTCTTTCTGTTG-3′); and GAPDH forward (5′-AACGTGTCAGTCGTGGACCTG-3′) and reverse (5′-AGTGGGTGTCGCTGTFGAAGT-3′). The relative expression was based on the expression ratio of a target gene compared with that of GAPDH.

Western blotting

A bicinchoninic acid (BCA) Protein Assay Kit (Pierce Chemical Co., Rockford, Illinois, USA) was utilized to detect protein concentrations. Total protein (30 micrograms) was separated via 10% sodium dodecyl sulfate-polyacrylamide gel electrophoresis (SDS-PAGE) gel and then transferred onto a nitrocellulose membrane (Millipore, Temecula, California, USA). Next, the membrane was blocked and investigated with the following primary antibodies: rabbit anti-human phospho-Stat1, rabbit anti-human Stat1, rabbit anti-human phospho-Stat3, rabbit anti-human Stat3, rabbit anti-human phospho-Tyk2, rabbit anti-human Tyk2, rabbit anti-human CLDN17 and mouse anti-human β-actin. After 3 washes with phosphate-buffered saline (PBS), the membrane was incubated with horseradish peroxidase (HRP)-conjugated secondary antibody (Santa Cruz Biotechnologies, California, USA) at a 1:1000 dilution at 4 °C. Immunoreactive bands were detected using ECL western blot reagents (GE, Fairfield, Connecticut, USA) and analyzed with Image Lab 6.0.1 Software from Bio-Rad Laboratories.

Immunofluorescence method

The cells were fixed with 4% paraformaldehyde for 10 min at room temperature (RT) and then permeabilized with 0.1% Triton X-100 (Sigma-Aldrich, cat. no. 9002-93-1). Then, after blocking with 2% bovine serum albumin (Bote Biotechnological Corporation, Jilin, China) diluted in PBS for 30 min, the cells were probed with a primary rabbit anti-human CLDN17 antibody, which was diluted in blocking solution (1:1000 dilution) for 30 min at RT. The cells were incubated with Alexa Fluor®647-conjugated anti-rabbit IgG antibody (ab150093, Santa Cruz Biotechnologies, California, USA) at a 1:1000 dilution.

Cell counting Kit-8 assay

Cell proliferation curve generated by the colorimetric water-soluble tetrazolium salt assay using a Cell Counting Kit-8 (Dojindo, Kumamoto, Japan) as the protocol. The cells were seeded into 96-well plates in triplicate, and cell proliferation was recorded per 12 h for 4 days.

Wound-healing assay

The cells were maintained in a monolayer at 70% confluence on 24-well plastic dishes and the monolayer was scratched with a 100-μl pipette tip. The wounds were photographed light microscope (E100, Nikon Instruments Inc., Japan) (magnification × 200) at the same location at 0, 12 and 24 h.

Transwell chamber method

The cells were grown in a monolayer at 90% convergence and were maintained in FBS-free medium for 12 h. Matrigel (BD Biosciences, cat. no. 356234) was added to the upper Boyden chamber (Millipore, Bedford, MA) in 24-well plates and the plates were maintained in a cell incubator at 37 °C for 15 min. Then, medium containing chemotactic factors, which had been collected from the cell culture, was added to the 24-well plate. The cells were supplemented with Matrigel and cultured in a cell incubator at 37 °C for 6 h.

RNA interference (RNAi) method

Frozen glycerol bacterial stocks containing pGCSIL-scramble and pGCSIL-Tyk2-RNAi were purchased from Nanjing KeyGen Biotech Co., Ltd. The target was Tyk2-RNAi (29473), and the control insert sequence was pGCSIL-scramble. HEK 293 T cells (0.2×10^7) were seeded and maintained for 24 h to achieve 70–80% confluence in 6-well dishes (Costar, Cam- bridge, MA). Three plasmids, including of pGCSIL-Tyk2-RNAi or pGCSIL-scramble, 5 μg of the packaging vector pHelper 1.0 and 5 μg of a vesicular stomatitis virus glycoprotein (VSVG) expression plasmid vector, were added to Opti-MEM, with a final volume of 1.0 ml. Then, 50 μl of Lipofectamine was added to 950 μl of FBS-free medium. These two solutions were mixed and added to the cells. Lentiviral particles were harvested 48 h after transfection, and the viral titer was determined by counting green fluorescent protein (GFP)-expressing cells under a fluorescence microscopy (Nikon Diaphot 300®) with filters 96 h after transfection.

Patients and tissue samples

Biopsies were collected from 52 patients with pathologically confirmed the diagnoses of HCC who received treatment at The First Bethune Hospital of Jilin University between June 2007 and May 2012. The patients were carefully chosen based on the following criteria: no history of radiotherapy or chemotherapy and no prior malignant disease. The grade and classification of the HCC patients were based on the American Joint Committee on Cancer (AJCC) tumor node metastasis (TNM) staging system. Thirty cases of histologically non-neoplastic hepatic tissues and 10 cases of cirrhosis tissues were also obtained from hepatitis B virus infected patients who were treated at The First Bethune Hospital, Jilin University during the period between October 2006 and September 2011 that were identified to be histologically non-neoplastic. There were 16 men and 14 women with an average age of 49 years. The medical records of the patients were reviewed to determine the clinical and pathological characteristics.

Immunohistochemistry

An immunohistochemistry was utilized to explore the expression patterns of CLDN17 in 52 HCC tissues, 10 cirrhosis tissues and 30 non-neoplastic hepatic tissues. Of the 52 cases, 42 cases exhibited HBsAg infection, 17 cases exhibited occurrence and metastasis, and 34 cases were coupled with cirrhosis. The experimental method was described previously [13], and the antibody utilized was a rabbit anti-human CLDN17 antibody. The evaluation of protein expression levels was based on the percentage of positively stained tumor cells in combination with the staining intensity as previously described [14].

Follow-up

The patients with a pathologically confirmed diagnosis of HCC were followed-up for 60 months after diagnosis to assess occurrence and metastasis and to determine survival. The survival status of the patients was determined through a telephone interview or an outpatient visit before December 2017.

Statistical methods

All of the experiments were repeated 3 times, and all of the data are based on the mean ± SD of at least 3 experimental results. The experimental results were analyzed using Student's t-test, and the prognostic significance and value of CLDN17 expression was determined by the Chi-square test/Chi-square goodness-of-fit test. $P < 0.05$ was considered statistical significance.

Results

The expression of CLDN17 was upregulated in HCC cell lines and tissues

Real-time PCR and western blotting were utilized to detect the expression of CLDN17 in the human hepatocyte line and the HCC cell lines (Huh1, HepG2 and Hep3B). We found that the mRNA and protein expression levels of CLDN17 were low or absent in the human hepatocyte line HL7702 but high in HCC cell lines Huh1, HepG2 and Hep3B (Fig. 1a-c).

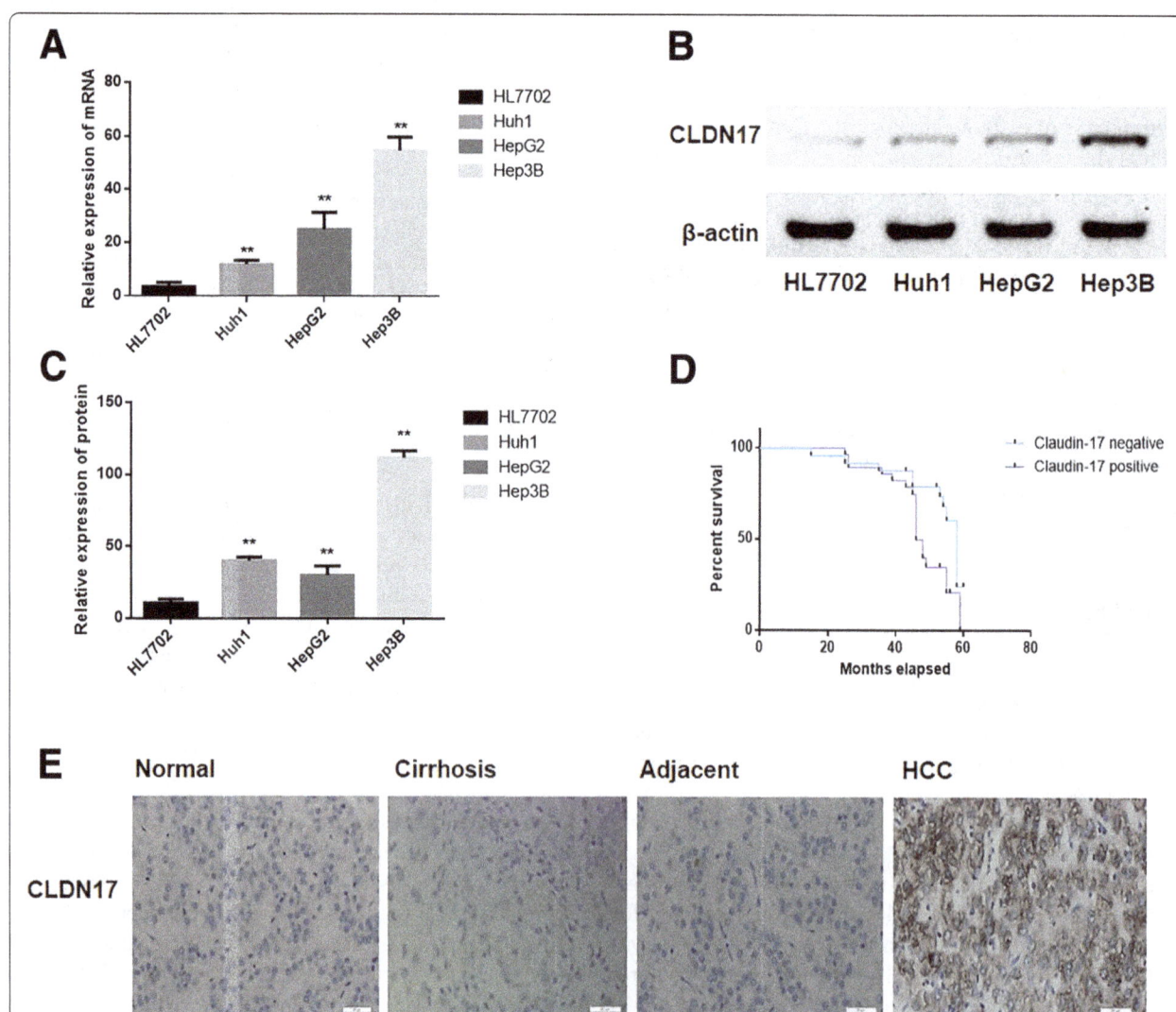

Fig. 1 The expression levels of CLDN17 in HCC cell lines and tissues. **a** The relative mRNA level of CLDN17 in the hepatocyte line and HCC cell lines; (**b**) The relative protein expression of CLDN17 in the hepatocyte line and HCC cell lines; (**c**) The corresponding statistical analysis of protein expression in the hepatocyte line and HCC cell lines; (**d**) The correlation between the expression of CLDN17 and survival in HCC patients; (**e**) The protein expression of CLDN17 in hepatocyte tissues, cirrhosis tissues, tissues adjacent to the tumors and HCC tissues. Note: * represents $P < 0.05$, ** represents $P < 0.01$, compared with the empty vector groups

CLDN17 expression was explored in 52 HCC tissues, 10 histologically non-neoplastic cirrhosis tissues, 10 histologically non-neoplastic tissues adjacent to the tumor and 30 histologically non-neoplastic hepatic tissues. As shown in Fig. 1e, the expression of CLDN17 in hepatic tissues and HCC tissues is located mainly in the cytoplasm and membrane. High expression of CLDN17 was observed in 53.8% (28/52) of HCC tissues 30.0% (3/10) of non-neoplastic cirrhosis tissues, 40.0% (4/10) of histologically non-neoplastic tissues adjacent to the tumor and in 40.0% (12/30) of hepatic tissues ($P = 0.0001 < 0.001$) (Table 1).

The log-rank test was utilized to analyze correlations between CLDN17 and clinical survival. As shown in Fig. 1d, patients with positive expression of the CLDN17 protein in tumors (median survival, 46.15 months) had a notably shorter survival than those with negative expression of the CLDN17 protein (median survival, 57.79 months).

Table 1 Expression of CLDN17 and the clinicopathological characteristics in HCC patients

Item	n	CLDN17 (+)	CLDN17 (−)	P
HCC tissues	52	28	24	< 0.01*
Hepatic tissues	30	12	18	
Age (years)				
≤ 60	21	11	10	1.000
> 60	31	17	14	
HbsAg				
+	42	23	19	1.000
-	10	5	5	
Cirrhosis				
+	34	18	16	1.000
-	18	10	8	
Occurrence and metastasis				
+	17	13	4	< 0.01*
-	35	15	20	
Serum AFP (ng/ml)				
< 400	22	13	9	0.637
> 400	30	15	15	
TNM stage (AJCC)				
I~II	27	17	10	< 0.01*
III~IV	25	11	14	
Histological grade				
Well-differentiated	24	15	9	< 0.01*
Moderately and poorly differentiated	28	13	15	

*Statistical significance was found with the Chi-square test/Chi-Square Goodness-of-Fit Test

The relationships between CLDN17 and clinical pathological indicators were also analyzed, and the expression of CLDN17 was not associated with age ($P = 1.000$), HBsAg absent status ($P = 1.000$), cirrhosis ($P = 1.000$), serum AFP level ($P = 0.637$) of HCC patients or clinical staging ($P = 1.000$) of HCC patients.

However, CLDN17 expression was associated with HCC occurrence and metastasis ($P = 0.001 < 0.01$), histological grade ($P = 0.001 < 0.01$) and TNM stage ($P = 0.001 < 0.01$) (Table 1).

Stable transfection of a hepatocyte line with CLDN17

The p-EGFP-C1/CLDN17 plasmid was utilized to transfect HL7702 cells. After G418 screening, a monoclonal strain of HL7702 cells was obtained, which was termed HL7702-CLDN17. Real-time PCR and western blotting were also utilized to detect the expression of CLDN17 in cultured cells. The results showed that the mRNA and protein expression levels of CLDN17 in the HL7702-CLDN17 group were notably higher than those in the empty vector groups ($P = 0.0001 < 0.01$; $P = 0.0001 < 0.01$, respectively) (Fig. 2a, b and d). Immunofluorescence was utilized to detect the localization of CLDN17 in HL7702-CLDN17 cells. The results showed that the expression of CLDN17 was primarily localized to the cell cytoplasm and membrane (Fig. 2c). These results demonstrated that clonal HL7702 cell line that stably expressed CLDN17 had been successfully established.

The impact of CLDN17 on the proliferation and migration of hepatocyte lines

The growth curve for the HL7702 cell line was generated by the CCK-8 method. The data revealed that the proliferation rates of HL7702-CLDN17 cells at 48 and 72 h were notably higher than those of the empty vector groups (Fig. 3a). A wound-healing experiment was utilized to detect the impact of CLDN17 on the migration ability of hepatocytes (Fig. 3b). The results showed that the migration distances of HL7702-CLDN17 cells were substantially greater than those of the empty vector groups at 12 and 24 h ($P = 0.0022$, < 0.01). The Transwell chamber method was also utilized to detect the migration ability of hepatocytes. Twelve hours after the cells were seeded, the cells that invaded through the membrane of the chamber were observed. The results showed that the number of invasive cells in the HL7702-CLDN17 group was notably higher than in the empty vector groups (Fig. 3c and d). These results suggested that CLDN17 clearly promoted the proliferation and migration ability of hepatocytes in vitro.

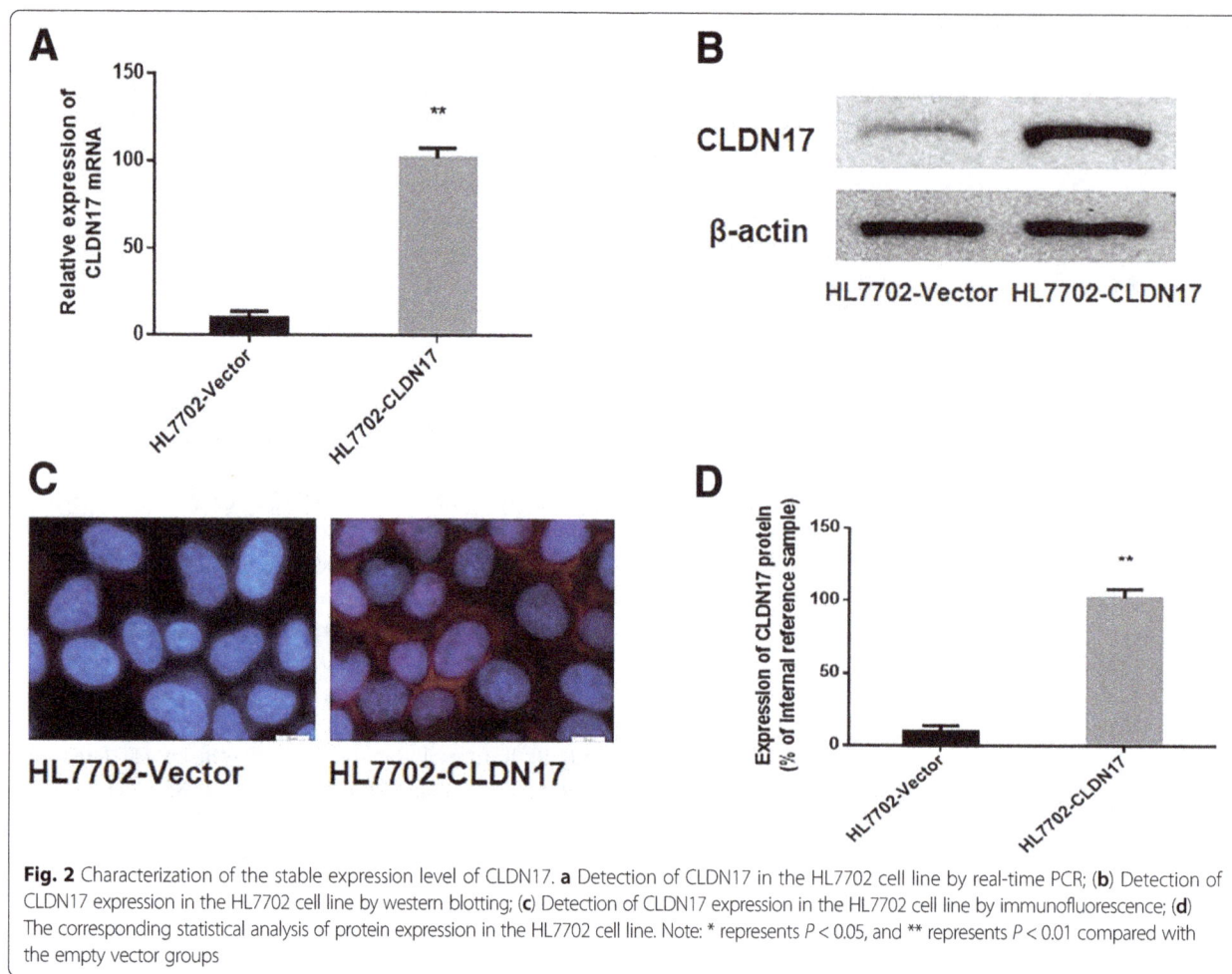

Fig. 2 Characterization of the stable expression level of CLDN17. **a** Detection of CLDN17 in the HL7702 cell line by real-time PCR; (**b**) Detection of CLDN17 expression in the HL7702 cell line by western blotting; (**c**) Detection of CLDN17 expression in the HL7702 cell line by immunofluorescence; (**d**) The corresponding statistical analysis of protein expression in the HL7702 cell line. Note: * represents $P < 0.05$, and ** represents $P < 0.01$ compared with the empty vector groups

The impact of CLDN17 on the Tyk2/Stat3 signaling pathway in hepatocytes

Western blotting was utilized to explore the activation state of the Tyk2/Stat3 pathway. The results showed that after the overexpression of CLDN17, the phosphorylation levels of Stat1, Stat3 and Tyk2 were substantially increased in the HL7702 cells (Fig. 4a and b). These data suggested that CLDN17 upregulation notably enhanced the activation of the Tyk2/Stat3 signaling pathway in the HL7702 cell line.

The impact of Tyk2/Stat3 signaling pathway activation on the invasion and migration ability of hepatocytes

To determine the impact of the Tyk2/Stat3 signaling pathway on the invasion and migration ability of hepatocytes, the pGCSIL-scramble plasmid and the pGCSIL-Tyk2-RNAi plasmid were utilized to transfect HL7702-CLDN17 cells. Western blotting was utilized to analyze Tyk2 expression and the phosphorylation level of Stat1 and Stat3 in these cells, and the results showed that the protein expression of Tyk2 was markedly downregulated in Tyk2-RNAi cells compared with the scramble group (Fig. 5a and b). The

data showed that after the knockdown of Tyk2, the phosphorylation level of Stat3 was notably downregulated while there was no significant change in the phosphorylation level of Stat1 in the HL7702 cell line that overexpressed CLDN17 (Fig. 5a).

A Transwell chamber assay and wound-healing assay were utilized to analyze the effect of Tyk2 on the invasive and migration ability of the examined cells. The results showed that the number of invasive HL7702 cells in the CLDN17-expressing cells was notably decreased following Tyk2 silencing in CLDN17-expressing cells (Fig. 5c and d). The migration distances of the Tyk2-RNAi cells were substantially shorter than those of the scramble group at 12 and 24 h (Fig. 5e).

Discussion

A number of studies have focused on the role of CLDNs in the tumorigenesis of HCC. For instance, CLDN1 has been described as a key factor in the entry of hepatitis C virus (HCV) into hepatocytes, and upregulated expression of CLDN1 was revealed to contribute to the promotion of epithelial mesenchymal transition (EMT) via the

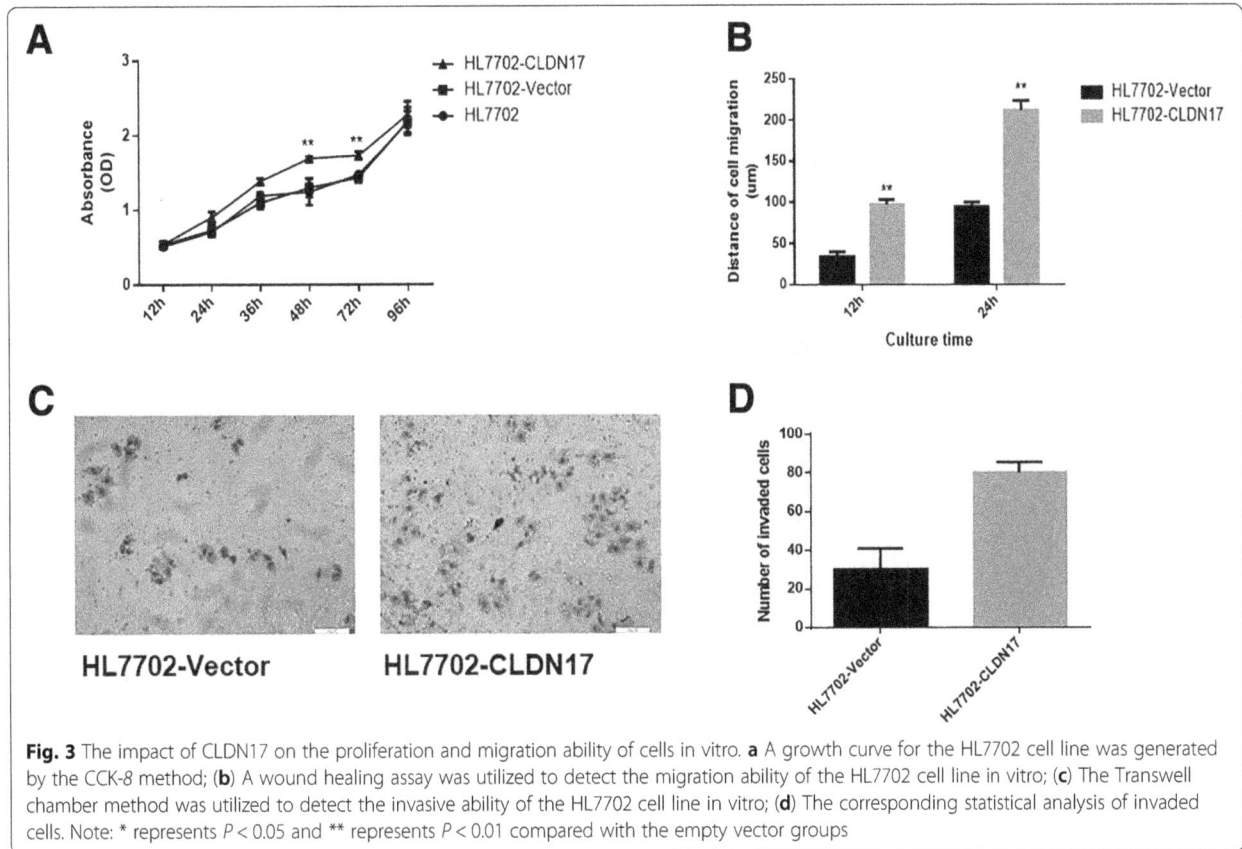

Fig. 3 The impact of CLDN17 on the proliferation and migration ability of cells in vitro. **a** A growth curve for the HL7702 cell line was generated by the CCK-8 method; (**b**) A wound healing assay was utilized to detect the migration ability of the HL7702 cell line in vitro; (**c**) The Transwell chamber method was utilized to detect the invasive ability of the HL7702 cell line in vitro; (**d**) The corresponding statistical analysis of invaded cells. Note: * represents $P < 0.05$ and ** represents $P < 0.01$ compared with the empty vector groups

c-Abl/Raf/Ras/ERK signaling pathway [15, 16]. Furthermore, it was demonstrated that CLDN3 is an epigenetically silenced tumor suppressor gene in HCC, and its overexpression notably inhibits metastasis by suppressing the EMT via the Wnt/β-catenin signaling pathway in HCC cells [13]. Besides, CLDN14 was epigenetically silenced via the trimethylation of lysine 27 on histone H3 (H3K27ME3) and was a novel prognostic biomarker in HCC [17]. Given the correlation between the expression levels of these CLDNs and the tumorigenesis of HCC, CLDNs represent potential novel therapeutic targets in patients with HCC.

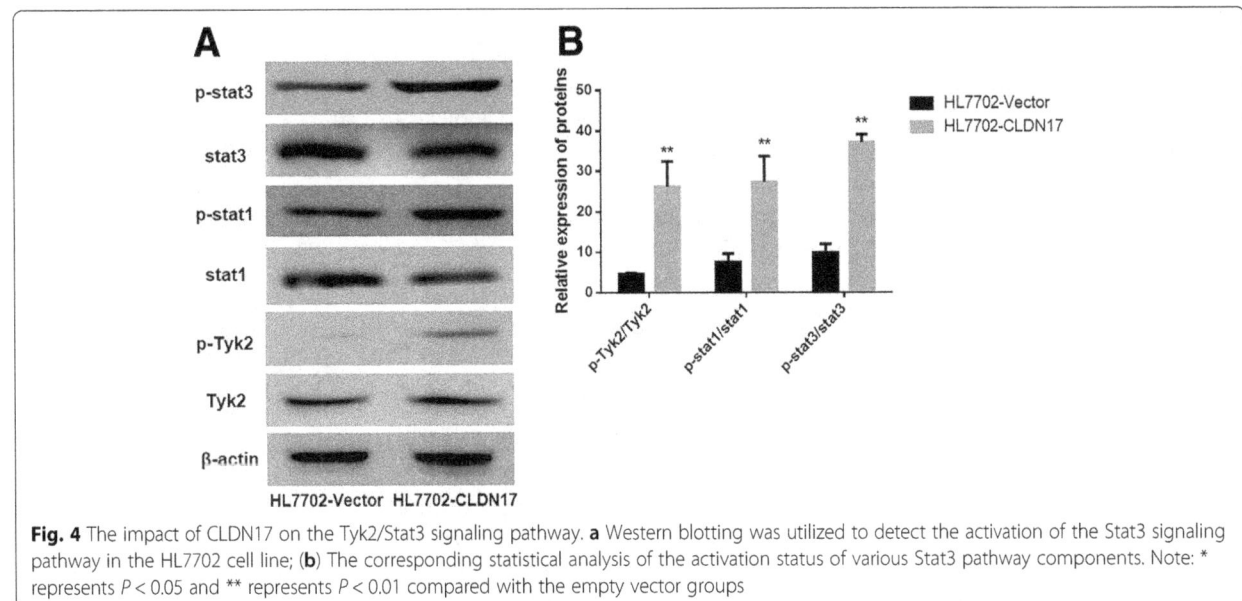

Fig. 4 The impact of CLDN17 on the Tyk2/Stat3 signaling pathway. **a** Western blotting was utilized to detect the activation of the Stat3 signaling pathway in the HL7702 cell line; (**b**) The corresponding statistical analysis of the activation status of various Stat3 pathway components. Note: * represents $P < 0.05$ and ** represents $P < 0.01$ compared with the empty vector groups

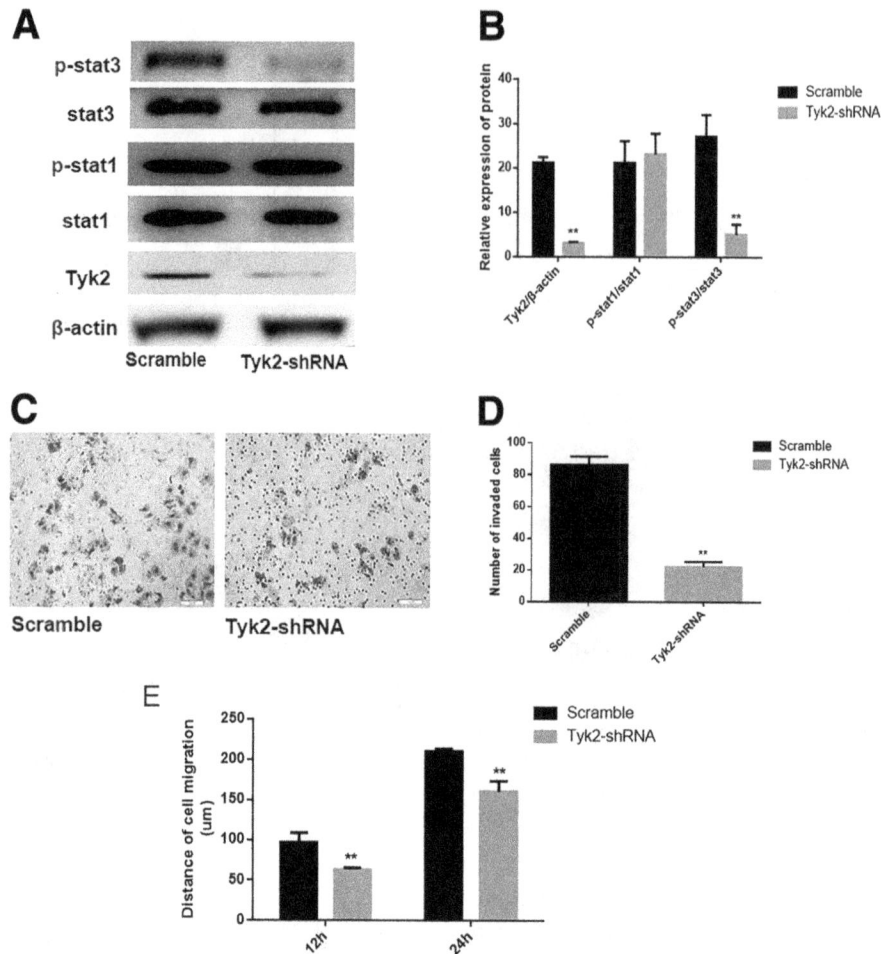

Fig. 5 RNAi was utilized to silence Tyk2 expression in CLDN17-expressing cells. **a** Western blotting was utilized to examine the effects of silencing Tyk2 and activating the Stat3 signaling pathway in the HL7702 cell line; (**b**) The corresponding statistical analysis of the activation of the Stat3 signaling pathway; (**c**) The Transwell chamber method was utilized to detect the impact of Tyk2 silencing on the invasive ability of the cells in vitro; (**d**) The corresponding statistical analysis of invaded cells; (**e**) A wound healing assay was utilized to detect the migration ability of the HL7702 cell line in vitro. Note: * represents $P < 0.05$ and ** represents $P < 0.01$ compared with the scramble group

CLDN17 is one of 27 members of the CLDN protein family, and our current understanding of the biological functions of CLDN17 is primarily limited to epithelial and epidermal permeability, barrier protection, and cell connections; reports on the relationship between CLDN17 and tumors are rare [18]. Our research group first found that CLDN17 expression was highly expressed in HCC tissues, and we speculated that the high expression of this gene may be involved with the tumorigenesis and progression in patients with HCC. Moreover, in the present study, we confirmed that CLDN17 markedly promotes the invasive ability of the hepatocyte line HL7702. Similar to our study, several studies have identified specific CLDNs as pro-oncogenes in human various cancers. For instance, previous work has shown that CLDN1 plays a key role in inflammation-induced growth and progression in patients with colorectal carcinoma [19]. Furthermore, Philip, R. et al. reported that CLDN7 expression in colorectal cancer

contributes to motility and invasion by promoting a shift towards EMT by recruiting EpCAM towards TACE/presenilin2 [20]. It was also revealed that CLDN7 is frequently overexpressed and promotes invasion in ovarian cancer [21]. However, in contrast to our results, other studies have shown that some CLDNs could be identified as tumor suppressor gene [22, 23]. For instance, the expression of CLDN1 was reduced in stage II and III rectal cancer and was established as a factor that correlates clearly with recurrence and poor prognosis [24]. In addition, the expression of CLDN6 was demonstrated to be silenced in cervical carcinoma tissues, and the restoration of CLDN6 expression suppressed cell proliferation and colony formation in cervical carcinoma cells in vitro, and tumor growth in vivo [25]. One potential reason for this difference is that the functions of CLDNs may be specific and dependent on different interacting molecules in different cells [26, 27]. In this manner, specific CLDNs may have specific impacts on the biological behavior of a given tumor [28–30].

At present, our results first indicated that the CLDN17 was overexpressed and highly associated with metastatic progression and prognosis in patients with HCC. Moreover, the overexpression of CLDN17 markedly promoted the invasion and migration abilities of the hepatocyte line HL7702. Furthermore, we also performed an initial exploration of the molecular mechanism associated with this effect, and we found that CLDN17 upregulation affected the Stat3 signaling pathway via Tyk2 and ultimately enhanced the migration ability of hepatocytes. Considering the limited therapeutic options for patients with HCC, the role of CLDN17 as a therapeutic target merits further exploration.

Conclusion

There have been few reports on the roles of CLDN17 in tumors, and many problems related to the specific molecular mechanisms must still be researched. In the present study, we confirmed that the overexpression of CLDN17 notably enhanced the malignant phenotype of the hepatocytes. In addition, the induction of Tyk2/Stat3 signaling may be one of the most important mechanisms by which CLDN17 promotes the migration ability in hepatocytes.

Abbreviations
AJCC: American Joint Committee on Cancer; CCK8: Cell Counting Kit-8; CLDNs: Claudins; FBS: Fetal bovine serum; GFP: Green fluorescent protein; H3K27ME3: Trimethylation of lysine 27 on histone H3; HCC: Hepatocellular carcinoma; HCV: Hepatitis C virus; Stat3: Signal transducer and activator of transcription3; TJ: Tight junction; TNM: Tumor node metastasis; Tyk2: Tyrosine kinase 2

Acknowledgements
We would like to thank American Journal Experts (AJE) for help with this manuscript.

Authors' contributions
Conceived and designed the experiments: JC. Performed the experiments: LS and LF. Analyzed the data: LF. Wrote the paper: JC. All authors read and approved the final manuscript.

Competing interests
The authors declare that they have no competing interests.

Author details
[1]Stem Cell and Cancer Center, The First Bethune Hospital, Jilin University, Changchun, Jilin 130021, People's Republic of China. [2]Department of Neurology and Neuroscience Center, First Hospital of Jilin University, Changchun, Jilin, China.

References
1. Escudero-Esparza A, Jiang WG, Martin TA. The Claudin family and its role in cancer and metastasis. Front Biosci (Landmark ed). 2010;16:1069–83.
2. Cunniffe C, Brankin B, Lambkin H, Ryan F. The role of Claudin-1 and Claudin-7 in cervical tumorigenesis. Anticancer Res. 2014;34:2851–7.
3. Turksen K, Troy TC. Junctions gone bad: claudins and loss of the barrier in cancer. Biochim Biophys Acta. 1816;2011:73–9.
4. Ouban A. Claudin-1 role in colon cancer: an update and a review. Histol Histopathol. 2018;11980. https://doi.org/10.14670/HH-11-980.
5. Worst TS, von Hardenberg J, Gross JC, Erben P, Schnolzer M, Hausser I, Bugert P, Michel MS, Boutros M. Database-augmented mass spectrometry analysis of exosomes identifies Claudin 3 as a putative prostate Cancer biomarker. Mol Cell Proteomics. 2017;16:998–1008.
6. Szasz MA. Claudins as prognostic factors of breast cancer. Magy Onkol. 2012;56:209–12.
7. Martin de la Fuente L, Malander S, Hartman L, Jonsson JM, Ebbesson A, Nilbert M, Masback A, Hedenfalk I. Claudin-4 Expression is Associated With Survival in Ovarian Cancer But Not With Chemotherapy Response. Int J Gynecol Pathol. 2018;37:101–9.
8. González-Mariscal L, Tapia R, Chamorro D. Crosstalk of tight junction components with signaling pathways. Biochim Biophys Acta Biomembr. 2008;1778:729–56.
9. Tsukita S, Furuse M, Itoh M. Structural and signalling molecules come together at tight junctions. Curr Opin Cell Biol. 1999;11:628–33.
10. Ahmad R, Kumar B, Chen Z, Chen X, Muller D, Lele SM, Washington MK, Batra SK, Dhawan P, Singh AB. Loss of claudin-3 expression induces IL6/gp130/Stat3 signaling to promote colon cancer malignancy by hyperactivating Wnt/beta-catenin signaling. Oncogene. 2017;36:6592–604.
11. Takasawa K, Takasawa A, Osanai M, Aoyama T, Ono Y, Kono T, Hirohashi Y, Murata M, Sawada N. Claudin-18 coupled with EGFR/ERK signaling contributes to the malignant potentials of bile duct cancer. Cancer Lett. 2017;403:66–73.
12. Livak KJ, Schmittgen TD. Analysis of relative gene expression data using real-time quantitative PCR and the 2(−Delta Delta C(T)) method. Methods. 2001;25:402–8.
13. Jiang L, Yang YD, Fu L, Xu W, Liu D, Liang Q, Zhang X, Xu L, Guan XY, Wu B, et al. CLDN3 inhibits cancer aggressiveness via Wnt-EMT signaling and is a potential prognostic biomarker for hepatocellular carcinoma. Oncotarget. 2014;5:7663–76.
14. Gao M, Li W, Wang H, Wang G. The distinct expression patterns of claudin-10, −14, −17 and E-cadherin between adjacent non-neoplastic tissues and gastric cancer tissues. Diagn Pathol. 2013;8:205.
15. Suh Y, Yoon CH, Kim RK, Lim EJ, Oh YS, Hwang SG, An S, Yoon G, Gye MC, Yi JM, et al. Claudin-1 induces epithelial-mesenchymal transition through activation of the c-Abl-ERK signaling pathway in human liver cells. Oncogene. 2013;32:4873–82.
16. Suh Y, Yoon CH, Kim RK, Lim EJ, Oh YS, Hwang SG, An S, Yoon G, Gye MC, Yi JM, et al. Claudin-1 induces epithelial-mesenchymal transition through activation of the c-Abl-ERK signaling pathway in human liver cells. Oncogene. 2017;36:1167–8.
17. Li CP, Cai MY, Jiang LJ, Mai SJ, Chen JW, Wang FW, Liao YJ, Chen WH, Jin XH, Pei XQ, et al. CLDN14 is epigenetically silenced by EZH2-mediated H3K27ME3 and is a novel prognostic biomarker in hepatocellular carcinoma. Carcinogenesis. 2016;37:557–66.
18. Koval M. Claudin heterogeneity and control of lung tight junctions. Annu Rev Physiol. 2013;75:551–67.
19. Cherradi S, Ayrolles-Torro A, Vezzo-Vie N, Gueguinou N, Denis V, Combes E, Boissiere F, Busson M, Canterel-Thouennon L, Mollevi C, et al. Antibody targeting of claudin-1 as a potential colorectal cancer therapy. J Exp Clin Cancer Res. 2017;36:89.

20. Philip R, Heiler S, Mu W, Buchler MW, Zoller M, Thuma F. Claudin-7 promotes the epithelial-mesenchymal transition in human colorectal cancer. Oncotarget. 2015;6:2046–63.

21. Dahiya N, Becker KG, Wood WH 3rd, Zhang Y, Morin PJ. Claudin-7 is frequently overexpressed in ovarian cancer and promotes invasion. PLoS One. 2011;6:e22119.

22. Ouban A, Ahmed A. Claudins in human cancer, a review. Histol Histopathol. 2010;25(1):83–90.

23. Zavala-Zendejas VE, Torres-Martinez AC, Salas-Morales B, Fortoul TI, Montano LF, Rendon-Huerta EP. Claudin-6, 7, or 9 overexpression in the human gastric adenocarcinoma cell line AGS increases its invasiveness, migration, and proliferation rate. Cancer Investig. 2011;29:1–11.

24. Yoshida T, Kinugasa T, Akagi Y, Kawahara A, Romeo K, Shiratsuchi I, Ryu Y, Gotanda Y, Shirouzu K. Decreased expression of claudin-1 in rectal cancer: a factor for recurrence and poor prognosis. Anticancer Res. 2011;31:2517–25.

25. Zhang X, Ruan Y, Li Y, Lin D, Quan C. Tight junction protein claudin-6 inhibits growth and induces the apoptosis of cervical carcinoma cells in vitro and in vivo. Med Oncol. 2015;32:148.

26. Lu Z: Functions of claudin-7 in human lung cancer. 2012.

27. Micke P, Mattsson JS, Edlund K, Lohr M, Jirstrom K, Berglund A, Botling J, Rahnenfuehrer J, Marincevic M, Ponten F, et al. Aberrantly activated claudin 6 and 18.2 as potential therapy targets in non-small-cell lung cancer. Int J Cancer. 2014;135:2206–14.

28. D'Souza T, Agarwal R, Morin PJ. Phosphorylation of claudin-3 at threonine 192 by cAMP-dependent protein kinase regulates tight junction barrier function in ovarian cancer cells. J Biol Chem. 2005;280:26233–40.

29. D'Souza T, Indig FE, Morin PJ. Phosphorylation of claudin-4 by PKCε regulates tight junction barrier function in ovarian cancer cells. Exp Cell Res. 2007;313:3364–75.

30. Li X, Li Y, Qiu H, Wang Y. Downregulation of claudin-7 potentiates cellular proliferation and invasion in endometrial cancer. Oncol Lett. 2013;6:101–5.

25

Molecular characterization of sessile serrated adenoma/polyps with dysplasia/carcinoma based on immunohistochemistry, next-generation sequencing, and microsatellite instability testing

Takashi Murakami[1,2]*, Yoichi Akazawa[1,2], Noboru Yatagai[1,2], Takafumi Hiromoto[1,2], Noriko Sasahara[2], Tsuyoshi Saito[2], Naoto Sakamoto[1], Akihito Nagahara[1] and Takashi Yao[2]

Abstract

Background: Colorectal sessile serrated adenoma/polyps (SSA/Ps) are considered early precursor lesions in the serrated neoplasia pathway. Recent studies have shown associations of SSA/Ps with lost MLH1 expression, a CpG island methylator phenotype, and *BRAF* mutations. However, the molecular biological features of SSA/Ps with early neoplastic progression have not yet been fully elucidated, owing to the rarity of cases of SSA/P with advanced histology such as cytologic dysplasia or invasive carcinoma. In this study, we aimed to elucidate the molecular biological features of SSA/Ps with dysplasia/carcinoma, representing relatively early stages of the serrated neoplasia pathway.

Methods: We performed immunostaining for β-catenin, MLH1, and mucins (e.g., MUC2, MUC5AC, MUC6, and CD10); targeted next-generation sequencing; and microsatellite instability (MSI) testing in 8 SSA/P lesions comprised of 4 SSA/Ps with high-grade dysplasia and 4 SSA/Ps with submucosal carcinoma.

Results: Lost MLH1 expression was found in 5 cases. All lesions studied were positive for nuclear β-catenin expression. Regarding phenotypic mucin expression, all lesions were positive for MUC2, but negative for CD10. MUC5AC and MUC6 positivity was observed in 7 cases. Genetically, the most frequently mutated gene was *BRAF* (7 cases), and other mutations were detected in *FBXW7* (3 cases); *TP53* (2 cases), and *KIT*, *PTEN*, *SMAD4*, and *SMARCB1* (1 case each). Furthermore, 4 of 8 lesions were MSI-high and the remaining 4 lesions were microsatellite-stable (MSS). Interestingly, all 4 MSI-high lesions displayed MLH1 loss, 3 of which harbored a *FBXW7* mutation, but not a *TP53* mutation. However, 2 MSS lesions harbored a *TP53* mutation, although none harbored a *FBXW7* mutation.

(Continued on next page)

* Correspondence: t-murakm@juntendo.ac.jp
[1]Department of Gastroenterology, Juntendo University School of Medicine, 2-1-1 Hongo, Bunkyo-ku, Tokyo 113-8421, Japan
[2]Department of Human Pathology, Juntendo University School of Medicine, Tokyo, Japan

(Continued from previous page)

Conclusions: SSA/Ps with dysplasia/carcinoma frequently harbored *BRAF* mutations. Activation of the WNT/β-catenin signaling pathway may facilitate the development of dysplasia in SSA/Ps and progression to carcinoma. Furthermore, our results suggested that these lesions might be associated with both MSI-high and MSS colorectal cancer, which might be distinguished by distinct molecular biological features such as lost MLH1 expression, *FBXW7* mutations, and *TP53* mutations.

Keywords: Sessile serrated adenoma/polyp, Colorectal carcinoma, MLH1, *FBXW7*, *TP53*, Microsatellite instability

Background

In 2003, Torlakovic et al. [1] reported evidence of abnormal proliferation in colorectal serrated polyps that superficially resembled hyperplastic polyps (but that could be distinguished histologically based on their abnormal architectural features) and introduced the terms "sessile serrated polyp" and "sessile serrated adenoma" to describe their observations. Currently, this category is designated as "sessile serrated adenoma/polyp (SSA/P)," as recommended by the World Health Organization [2]. SSA/P is considered as an early precursor lesion in the serrated neoplasia pathway, which largely results in colorectal carcinomas with high levels of microsatellite instability (MSI-high) [3–5]. Recent studies have shown associations of SSA/Ps and those with dysplasia/carcinoma with DNA methylation or lost protein expression of DNA-repair genes (i.e., *MLH1*) [1, 4, 6–9], a CpG island methylator phenotype [3, 4, 6, 7], and *BRAF* mutations [3, 4, 6–13]. This pathway is thought to be distinct from the conventional adenoma-carcinoma pathway, where adenomas progress to invasive colorectal carcinomas through the influence of several genetic alterations including adenomatous polyposis coli (*APC*) and *KRAS* mutations [4, 6, 10, 11, 14, 15].

Recently, targeted next-generation sequencing (NGS) has shown unprecedented potential for detecting underlying changes in the genetic architecture of cancer in a comprehensive and economically feasible manner, and the development of its platforms has enabled comprehensive analysis of genetic alterations in tumors [16, 17]. A comprehensive understanding of the genetic alterations associated with cancer could improve the molecular biological classifications of tumors and identify effective molecularly targeted therapies.

At present, the molecular biological features underlying the development of colorectal serrated neoplasia remain unclear. Hence, the aim of this study was to employ NGS to elucidate the molecular biological features of SSA/Ps with dysplasia/carcinoma, representing relatively early stages of the serrated neoplasia pathway.

Methods

Patients and materials

Eight colorectal lesions (from 8 different patients) were resected endoscopically or surgically at Juntendo University Hospital between 2014 and 2016, and used in this study. These lesions comprised 4 SSA/Ps with high-grade dysplasia and 4 SSA/Ps with submucosal carcinoma. The diagnosis of SSA/P was based on the following criteria described by Torlakovic et al. [1]: the presence of serration at the base of crypts, irregularly dilated crypts, irregularly branching crypts, and horizontally and/or laterally arranged basal crypts. The histologic features of the high-grade dysplasia were assessed as described previously [2, 12], as follows: a tubular, tubulovillous, or fused glandular pattern (mimicking conventional adenomatous high-grade dysplasia) or a serrated glandular pattern (preserving the serrated or saw-toothed structure with infolding of the crypt epithelium), which consisted of cuboidal and eosinophilic dysplastic cells with substantially larger nuclei and irregular thickening of the nuclear membrane (i.e. 'serrated-type' high-grade dysplasia). Submucosal carcinoma was defined as an obvious epithelial neoplasm histologically atypical enough to be diagnosed as at least high-grade dysplasia that was invading the muscularis mucosa into the submucosa. The inclusion criteria for SSA/P with high-grade dysplasia or with submucosal carcinoma included a component of ordinary SSA/P visible at the lesion edge that comprised at least 3 crypts, with an SSA/P-type histology required in 1 crypt. All samples were reviewed independently by 2 authors (TY and TM).

Typical morphologies in representative cases of SSA/P with submucosal carcinoma are shown in Fig. 1.

Clinicopathological analysis

For each patient, we recorded the age, sex, tumor location (proximal colon defined as proximal to the splenic flexure, remaining colon defined as distal), macroscopic type, whole tumor size (including both high-grade dysplasia or invasive carcinoma and in situ SSA/P), histological type (based on the World Health Organization's histological classification of tumors), depth of submucosal invasion, lymphovascular invasion, and lymph node metastasis.

Immunohistochemical analysis

Four-micrometer-thick serial tissue sections prepared from formalin-fixed and paraffin-embedded tissues were subjected to immunohistochemistry. Staining was performed using a Dako EnVision Kit with antibodies

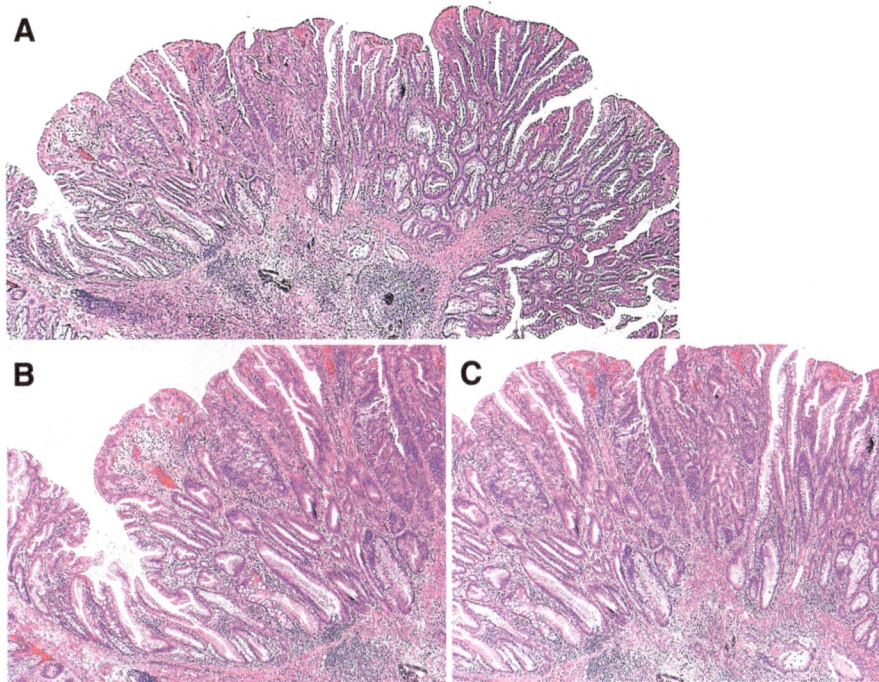

Fig. 1 Typical morphologies in a representative case of sessile serrated adenoma/polyp (SSA/P) with submucosal carcinoma (Case #6). **a** Dilated crypts with deep serration was seen on both sides of the lesion, and high-grade dysplasia with submucosal invasion was seen in the middle. **b** High-power field of (**a**) (the left side). Crypts with a serrated architecture included those that were irregularly dilated, irregularly branched, and horizontally arranged (basal), corresponding to SSA/P. **c** High-power field of (**a**) (the middle). Well-differentiated tubular adenocarcinoma was observed invading the submucosa. Adjacent SSA/P areas were observed towards both sides of the panel. An abrupt transition was evident between the 2 adjacent regions

against MLH1 (ab14206; 1:50 dilution; Abcam, CA, USA) and β-catenin (clone 14, 1:200 dilution; BD Bioscience, San Diego, CA, USA). Tumor phenotypes were evaluated by immunostaining with antibodies from Novocastra (Newcastle upon Tyne, UK; 1:100 dilution) against MUC2 (NCL-MUC-2), MUC5AC (NCL-MUC-5 AC), MUC6 (NCL-MUC-6), and CD10 (NCL-CD10–270). Appropriate positive and negative controls were used for each antibody.

Loss of MLH1 expression was noted when one or more clusters of tumor cells (minimal, focal, or multifocal) or all malignant cells showed no nuclear staining, compared with positive nuclear staining in normal epithelial cells and lymphocytes [1]. Expression of β-catenin, which generally showed an inverse relationship between membranous and nuclear (with cytoplasmic) reactivity, was only evaluated in terms of nuclear localization in this study. Nuclear β-catenin expression was considered as positive when distinct and strong nuclear staining was observed in over 5% of the tumor cells [9]. Membrane staining for CD10, and cytoplasmic staining for MUC2, MUC5AC, and MUC6 were judged as positive, when over 5% of tumor cells showed a positive reaction for each marker. The immunohistochemical staining results were evaluated by 2 authors (TY and TM).

DNA extraction

Genomic DNA was extracted from 5 formalin-fixed paraffin-embedded sections (10-mm-thick) using a QIAamp DNA FFPE Tissue Kit (Qiagen GmbH, Hilden, Germany), according to the manufacturer's instructions. Sections were stained lightly with hematoxylin, and only the dysplastic or carcinomatous areas in the lesions were microdissected with direct observation of the tissue under a light microscope. The DNA quality and integrity were checked spectrophotometrically.

Targeted NGS

The 50-gene Ion AmpliSeq Cancer Hotspot Panel v2 (Life Technologies) was used with the Ion-Torrent ™ Personal Genome Machine platform (Life Technologies, Foster city, CA, USA) in all experiments. This panel is designed to amplify 207 amplicons covering approximately 2800 mutations deposited in the COSMIC database from 50 oncogenes and tumor-suppressor genes commonly mutated in human cancers (*ABL1, AKT1, ALK, APC, ATM, BRAF, CDH1, CDKN2A, CSF1R, CTNNB1, EGFR, ERBB2, ERBB4, EZH2, FBXW7, FGFR1, FGFR2, FGFR3, FLT3, GNA11, GNAS, GNAQ, HNF1A, HRAS, IDH1, IDH2, JAK2, JAK3, KDR, KIT, KRAS, MET, MLH1, MPL, NOTCH1, NPM1, NRAS, PDGFRA, PIK3CA, PTEN, PTPN11, RB1, RET, SMAD4, SMARCB1, SMO, SRC, STK11, TP53,* and *VHL*).

The Ion AmpliSeq Library Kit, version 2.0 (Life Technologies) was used to amplify 10 ng of DNA according to the manufacturer's instructions. Sequencing beads were templated and enriched using the Hi-Q Template OT2 200 Kit, and sequencing was performed on 318v2 chips using the Hi-Q Sequencing Kit (Life Technologies) according to the manufacturer's protocols. Signal processing, mapping, and quality control were performed with Torrent Suite, v.5.0 (Life Technologies). Sequence variants were called using Ion Reporter, v5.2 using the AmpliSeq CHPv2 single-sample workflow and default settings. Variants were categorized according to whether they comprised a nonsynonymous or frameshift mutation, or stop codon in the exonic region. The limit of detection was a 5% mutational allelic frequency at $500 \times$ coverage or a 3% mutational allelic frequency at $1000 \times$ coverage for each tested region. The minimum coverage depth was $500 \times$.

MSI testing

DNA extracted from microdissected paraffin-embedded tumor sections and non-neoplastic tissues was analyzed by a polymerase chain reaction–based method, followed by capillary electrophoretic detection. MSI detection was performed using a panel of 5 mononucleotide microsatellite markers (BAT-25, BAT-26, NR-21, NR-24, and MONO-27). In accordance with National Cancer Institute guidelines, MSI at 2 loci or more was defined as MSI-high, instability at a single locus was defined as low levels of MSI (MSI-low), and no instability at any of the loci tested was defined as microsatellite-stable (MSS).

Results

Clinicopathological analysis

The detailed clinicopathological findings of the 8 SSA/P lesions are shown in Table 1. This study included 2 male and 6 female SSA/P patients, with ages ranging from 61 to 79 years (mean 69 years). Six lesions were within the proximal colon, and the remaining 2 lesions were in the distal colon. Macroscopically, sessile morphology was frequently observed among the studied SSA/P lesions. The mean tumor size was 18 mm (range: 10 to 31 mm).

Histologically, 4 lesions were high-grade dysplasias, and the other 4 lesions were well-to-moderately differentiated tubular adenocarcinomas invading into the submucosa, of which 1 lesion was accompanied with a mucinous component in the submucosa. Lymphatic invasion and lymph node metastasis were found in 1 case of SSA/P with carcinoma.

Immunohistochemical analysis

Loss of MLH1 expression was found in 5 cases. Without exception, all lesions were positive for nuclear β-catenin expression. Regarding phenotypic mucin expression, all lesions were positive for MUC2, but negative for CD10. MUC5AC and MUC6 were positive in 7 of 8 cases (88%). Immunohistochemical staining of these proteins in a representative case is illustrated in Fig. 2.

Mutation analysis

All SSA/P lesions had acceptable DNA integrity (the average RQ value was 0.18) and were subjected to NGS. The genetic alterations identified by NGS in 8 SSA/P lesions are summarized in Table 2. The most frequently mutated gene was *BRAF* (7 of 8; 88%), and the other detected mutations were in *FBXW7* (3 of 8; 38%), *TP53* (2 of 8; 25%), *KIT* (1 of 8; 13%), *PTEN* (1 of 8; 13%), *SMAD4* (1 of 8; 13%), and *SMARCB1* (1 of 8; 13%). The only *BRAF* mutation found was V600E (c.1799 T > A). The *FBXW7* mutations found were R278X (c.832 C > T), R479Q (c.1436 G >

Table 1 Summary of clinicopathological features in each case of sessile serrated adenoma/polyp (SSA/P) with dysplasia and invasive adenocarcinoma

Case No.	Age	Sex	Location	Macroscopic type	Size (mm)	Histological type	Depth of invasion (μm)	Mucinous component	Lymphatic invasion	Vascular invasion	Lymph node metastasis	Removal method
1	67	F	A	Sessile	10	HGD	Mucosa	–	–	–	–	EMR
2	69	M	S	Semipedunculated	10	HGD	Mucosa	–	–	–	–	EMR
3	79	F	C	Sessile	14	HGD	Mucosa	–	–	–	–	EMR
4	61	F	A	Sessile	18	HGD	Mucosa	–	–	–	–	ESD
5	61	M	D	Sessile	31	Well-ACA	Submucosa (400)	–	–	–	–	ESD + OPE
6	75	F	A	Sessile	15	Well-ACA	Submucosa (1100)	–	–	–	–	EMR + OPE
7	73	F	A	Sessile	25	Mod-ACA	Submucosa (2000)	–	+	–	+	OPE
8	65	F	T	Sessile	19	Mod-ACA	Submucosa (4000)	+	–	–	–	OPE

M Male, *F* Female, *C* Cecum, *A* Ascending colon, *T* Transverse colon, *D* Descending colon, *S* Sigmoid colon, *HGD* High-grade dysplasia, *Well-ACA* Well-differentiated adenocarcinoma, *Mod-ACA* Moderately-differentiated adenocarcinoma, *EMR* Endoscopic mucosal resection, *ESD* Endoscopic submucosal dissection, *OPE* Operation, + present; – absent

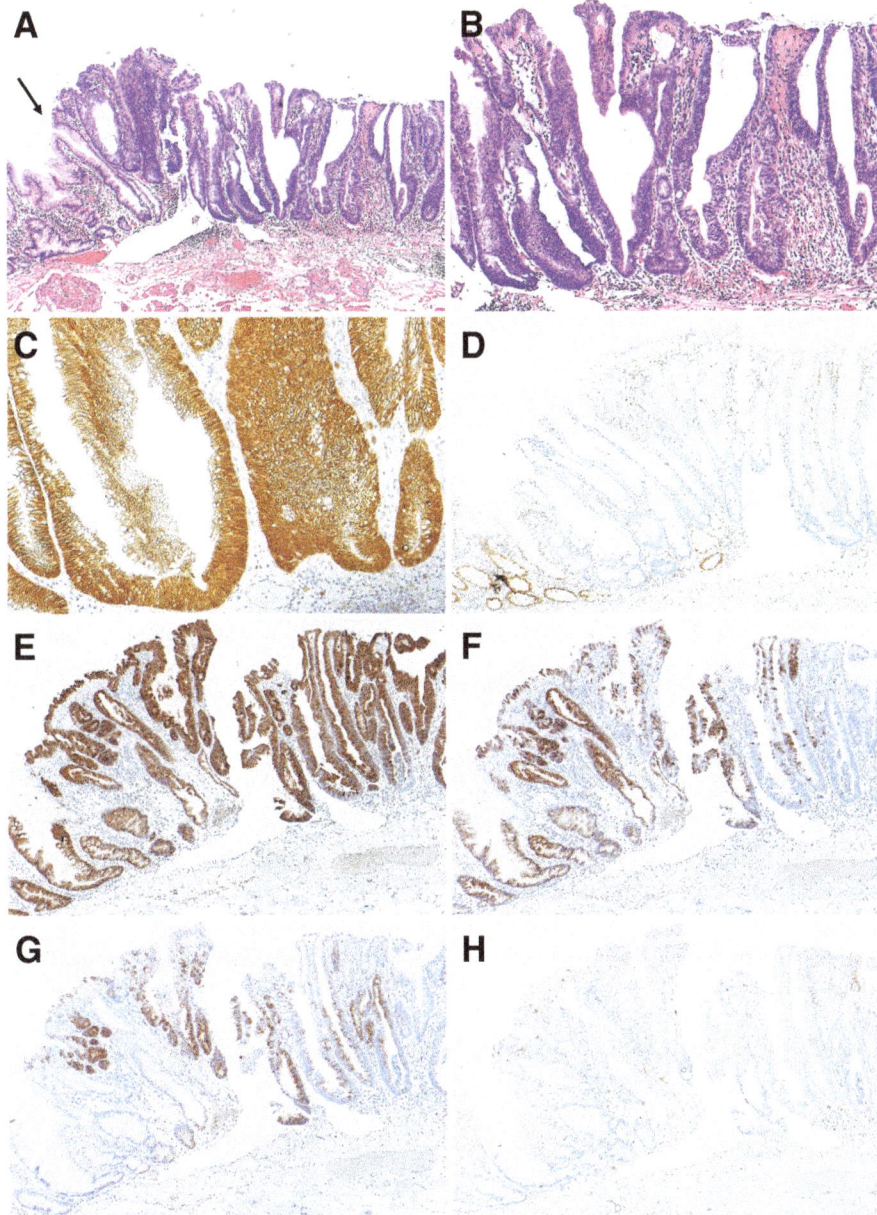

Fig. 2 Immunohistochemical staining in a representative case of sessile serrated adenoma/polyp (SSA/P) with dysplasia (Case #2). **a** Dilated crypts and deep serration, corresponding to SSA/P, were seen on the left side, and high-grade dysplasia without submucosal invasion was seen on the right side. An abrupt transition was seen between the 2 adjacent regions (arrow). **b** High-power field of (**a**) (the right side). A view shows high-grade dysplasia without submucosal invasion, which was pathologically consistent with SSA/P with cytologic dysplasia. The lesion showed nuclear β-catenin expression (**c**) and a loss of MLH1 expression (**d**). Regarding phenotypic mucin expression, the lesion was positive for MUC2 (**e**), MUC5AC (**f**), and MUC6 (**g**) expression, and negative for CD10 (**H**) expression

A), and Q508Q (c.1524 A > G). Examples of data analysis using the Integrative Genomics Viewer ™ software are shown in Fig. 3.

MSI testing
Of the 8 SSA/P lesions, 4 lesions (including 2 SSA/Ps with dysplasia and 2 SSA/Ps with carcinoma) were MSI-high and the remaining 4 lesions were MSS (Table 2).

Associations between immunohistochemistry, mutation analysis, and MSI
All 4 MSI-high SSA/P lesions showed a loss of MLH1 expression, and 3 of those lesions harbored an *FBXW7* mutation, but not a *TP53* mutation. In contrast, among the SSA/P lesion with MSS, only 1 showed loss of MLH1 expression, 2 cases harbored a *TP53* mutation, and no cases harbored an *FBXW7* mutation.

Table 2 Summary of molecular biological features in each case of sessile serrated adenoma/polyp (SSA/P) with dysplasia and invasive adenocarcinoma

Case No.	Group	Immunohistochemistry						Next generation sequencing analysis (Gene mutations)							MSI analysis
		MLH1 loss	β-catenin	MUC2	MUC5AC	MUC6	CD10	BRAF	FBXW7	KIT	PTEN	SMAD4	SMARCB1	TP53	
1	Dysplasia	−	+	+	+	+	−	+	−	−	−	−	−	+	MSS
2	Dysplasia	+	+	+	+	+	−	+	−	−	−	−	−	−	MSI-high
3	Dysplasia	+	+	+	+	+	−	+	+	+	−	+	−	−	MSI-high
4	Dysplasia	−	+	+	+	+	−	+	−	−	+	−	+	−	MSS
5	Carcinoma	+	+	+	+	+	−	+	−	−	−	−	−	−	MSS
6	Carcinoma	−	+	+	−	−	−	+	−	−	−	−	−	+	MSS
7	Carcinoma	+	+	+	+	+	−	−	+	−	−	−	−	−	MSI-high
8	Carcinoma	+	+	+	+	+	−	+	+	−	−	−	−	−	MSI-high

Dysplasia, SSA/P with high-grade dysplasia; Carcinoma, SSA/P with submucosal carcinoma; MSI-high, Microsatellite instability-high; MSS, Microsatellite-stable; +, present; −, absent

Discussion

Rare occurrences of *BRAF* mutations have been documented for conventional colorectal carcinomas, although they are frequent in dysplasia/carcinoma arising from SSA/Ps (50–90%) [3, 4, 9, 10, 12, 13]. In this study, *BRAF* mutations were detected in 7 of 8 SSA/P lesions, in accordance with previous reports [3, 4, 9, 10, 12, 13]. *BRAF* mutations result in activation of the RAS-RAF-MAPK pathway, and therefore our findings and previous reports [3, 4, 9, 10, 12, 13] suggest that those signaling pathways might be activated in serrated neoplasia.

We investigated the core protein-expression levels of MUC2, MUC5AC, MUC6, and CD10 because altered expressions of these proteins may be significantly correlated with the biological behavior of colorectal carcinoma and, possibly its prognosis. In this study, MUC2, MUC5AC, and MUC6 expression was frequently positive in the serrated lesions. MUC2 is a goblet cell-type mucin predominantly expressed in the colon. In contrast, MUC5AC and MUC6 are two gastric type mucins that are expressed in the surface foveolar epithelium and deep antral/pyloric glands, respectively, but not normally in colonic mucosa. MUC5AC and MUC6 expression have been strongly associated with tumorigenesis via the serrated neoplasia pathway [18–20], in agreement with our current findings.

The WNT signaling pathway involves β-catenin and plays a crucial role in the development of colorectal carcinomas through a conventional adenoma-carcinoma progression [21]. Several previous reports including our own [8, 9, 12, 13, 22] have also demonstrated that nuclear β-catenin accumulation is common in SSA/Ps with dysplasia and invasive carcinoma, but not in those without dysplasia. This observation implies that activation of the WNT/β-catenin signaling pathway is involved in the

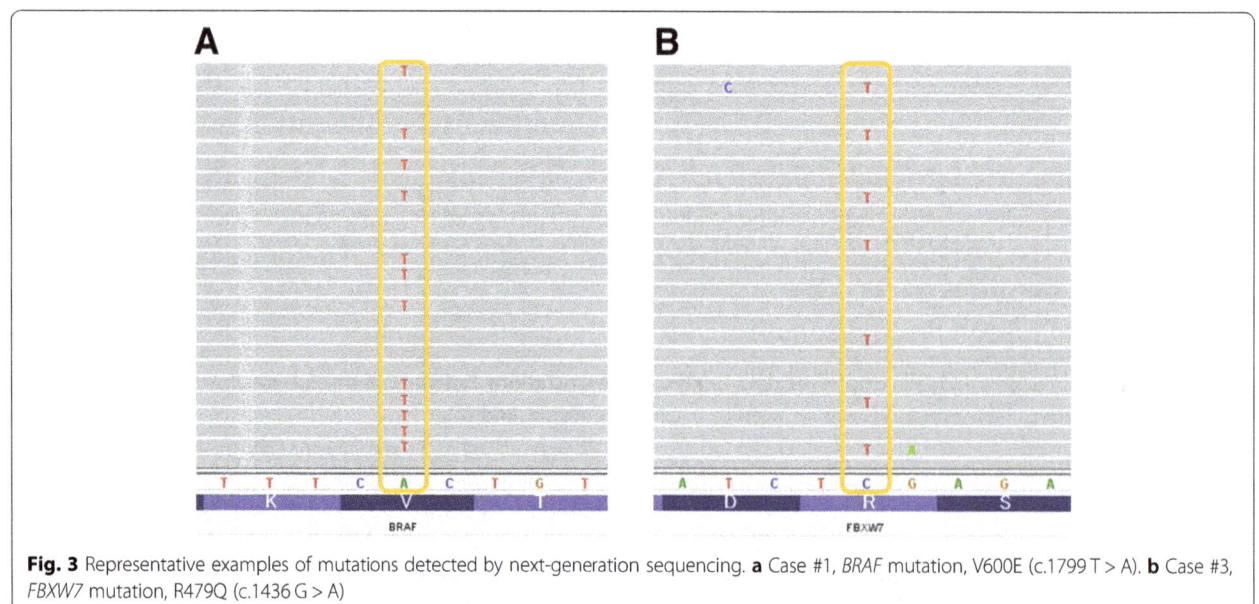

Fig. 3 Representative examples of mutations detected by next-generation sequencing. **a** Case #1, *BRAF* mutation, V600E (c.1799 T > A). **b** Case #3, *FBXW7* mutation, R479Q (c.1436 G > A)

development of dysplasia in SSA/Ps and progression to carcinoma. Although *APC* and *CTNNB1* mutations are major causes of WNT/β-catenin signaling activation in conventional-type adenomas, these genetic alterations are absent in SSA/Ps [13]. In this study, all serrated lesions examined also displayed nuclear β-catenin immunoreactivity, whereas no mutations in WNT/β-catenin signaling-associated genes (such as *APC* and *CTNNB1*) were found in the studied lesions. Previously, we reported that activation of the WNT/β-catenin signaling pathway might be associated with methylation of the associated genes, including *SFRP4*, *MCC*, and *AXIN2* [9]. This association could explain at least some of the discrepancies between β-catenin immunoreactivity and the lack of associated gene mutations.

The MSI phenotype has been regarded as a main subtype of colorectal cancers. Sporadic colorectal cancers with the MSI-high phenotype account for approximately 3–15% of all colorectal cancers [23]. MSI is a unique molecular alteration induced by deficiencies in the DNA-mismatch repair system and is characterized by unstable (variable length) microsatellites, a type of simple DNA sequence repeat. Some previous studies have shown that serrated neoplasia is associated with MSI-high colorectal carcinomas, which is accompanied with DNA methylation or loss of protein expression of DNA-repair genes such as *MLH1* [3–5]. In our study, all 4 MSI-high SSA/P lesions showed a loss of MLH1 expression, in accordance with previous reports [3–5].

A recent report by the Cancer Genome Atlas Project elucidated the molecular landscape of colorectal cancers and revealed that the hypermutated phenotype mainly overlaps with MSI status in colorectal cancers [24]. Many types of genetic mutations can occur in MSI-high colorectal cancers. Indeed, a previous report showed that mutations in various genes, including the tumor-suppressor gene *PTEN* and the oncogene *PIK3CA*, were caused by the instability of microsatellites in MSI-high colorectal cancers [25]. In this study, no MSI-high lesions harbored *PTEN* or *PIK3CA* mutations. However, it is interesting that 3 of 4 MSI-high lesions harbored an *FBXW7* mutation, whereas no MSS lesions harbored an *FBXW7* mutation. *FBXW7* is a tumor-suppressor gene located on human chromosome 4q that encodes a substrate-recognition component of SKP1–Cullin1–F-box protein-ubiquitin E3 ligase complexes [26]. These specific E3 ligase complexes negatively regulate the intracellular abundance of an expanding list of key oncogenic proteins such as cyclin E [27], c-JUN [28, 29], c-MYC [30, 31], MCL1 (myeloid cell leukemia 1) [32, 33], NOTCH [34–36], AURKA (aurora kinase A) [37, 38], KLF5 (Krüppel-like factor 5) [39], mTOR [40], and TGIF1 [41]. Therefore, the loss of FBXW7 function results in accumulation of its substrates, which leads to oncogenesis and progression of multiple cancers including colorectal cancers [42, 43]. A

study of over 500 primary tumors of diverse tissue origins suggested that *FBXW7* mutations occurred in approximately 6% of all evaluated tumors. Of these, the most commonly affected tumors were cholangiocarcinoma (35%), T-cell acute lymphocytic leukemia (31%), endometrial cancer (9%), and gastric cancer (6%) [43]. *FBXW7* has also consistently been identified as one of the most commonly mutated genes in colorectal cancer, being observed in 6 to 10% of all cases [43, 44]. Furthermore Chang et al. reported that *FBXW7*-mutant colorectal cancers had significant associations with MSI-high tumors in a large-scale study of 1519 cases [45]. Our findings and those previous reports indicated that *FBXW7* mutations might potentially be involved in the progression of MSI-high serrated lesions.

Activation of the second arm of the serrated neoplasia pathway, also driven by CpG island methylation of unspecified tumor-suppressor genes but not DNA-repair genes, may indicate progression to *BRAF*-mutant MSS carcinoma [46, 47]. Furthermore, as reported in earlier works [48–50], a strong inverse correlation was found between *TP53* alterations and the MSI phenotype. In this study, 2 of 4 lesions with MSS harbored a *TP53* mutation, whereas no MSI-high lesions harbored a *TP53* mutation, similar to previous observations [48–50]. The *TP53* gene encodes a tumor-suppressor protein containing transcriptional-activation, DNA-binding, and oligomerization domains. The encoded protein responds to diverse cellular stresses to regulate the expression of target genes, thereby inducing cell cycle arrest, apoptosis, senescence, DNA repair, or changes in metabolism [51]. Mutations in the *TP53* gene are reportedly associated with a variety of human cancers, including colon, breast, lung, and brain cancers [51]. Our findings and those previous reports indicated that *TP53* mutations are potentially involved in the progression of MSS serrated lesions. A schematic depiction of differences in the expression of key proteins and genetic alterations in the serrated neoplasia pathway is shown in Fig. 4.

Our study had a major limitation; the sample size was very small. A major impediment to investigating dysplasia/carcinoma arising in SSA/P is the rarity of this lesion. Additionally, a sufficient amount of specimen is necessary for NGS analysis, which limited the lesions that could be studied to those of 10 mm in diameter or more. These limitations lowered the statistical power of this study. Particularly, although the high rate of *FBXW7* or *TP53* mutations in the studied lesions is important, the possibility that this result was a chance occurrence cannot be denied, considering that only 2 or 3 cases of the studied lesions harbored *TP53* or *FBXW7* mutations, respectively.

To the best of our knowledge, few comprehensive genetic studies have been conducted in SSA/Ps with dysplasia and invasive carcinoma. Our results revealed mutations in *BRAF*, *FBXW7*, *TP53*, *KIT*, *PTEN*, *SMAD4*,

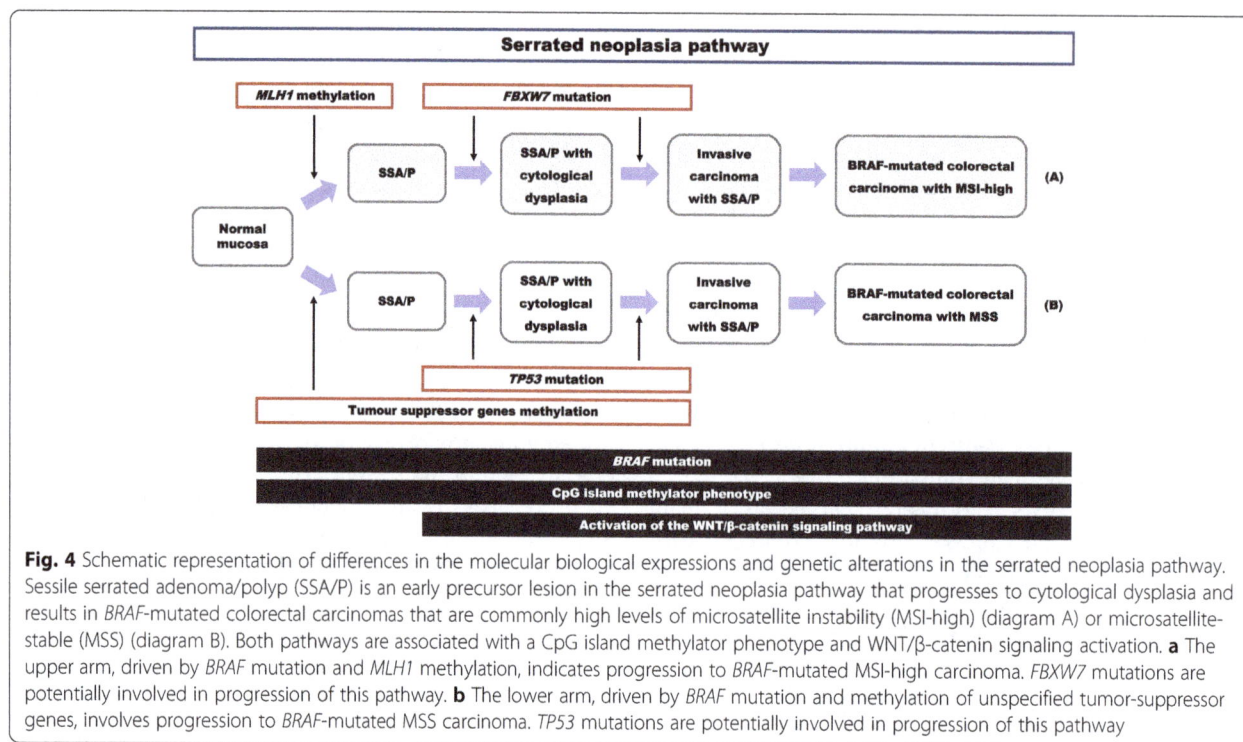

Fig. 4 Schematic representation of differences in the molecular biological expressions and genetic alterations in the serrated neoplasia pathway. Sessile serrated adenoma/polyp (SSA/P) is an early precursor lesion in the serrated neoplasia pathway that progresses to cytological dysplasia and results in *BRAF*-mutated colorectal carcinomas that are commonly high levels of microsatellite instability (MSI-high) (diagram A) or microsatellite-stable (MSS) (diagram B). Both pathways are associated with a CpG island methylator phenotype and WNT/β-catenin signaling activation. **a** The upper arm, driven by *BRAF* mutation and *MLH1* methylation, indicates progression to *BRAF*-mutated MSI-high carcinoma. *FBXW7* mutations are potentially involved in progression of this pathway. **b** The lower arm, driven by *BRAF* mutation and methylation of unspecified tumor-suppressor genes, involves progression to *BRAF*-mutated MSS carcinoma. *TP53* mutations are potentially involved in progression of this pathway

and *SMARCB1*. Furthermore, it is very interesting that all MSI-high lesions might be associated with MLH1 expression loss and mutation of *FBXW7*, but not *TP53*. Our results may help clarify the detailed mechanism of serrated neoplasia development. A comprehensive understanding of genetic alterations associated with the serrated neoplasia pathway could help identify effective molecularly targeted therapies.

Conclusions

In conclusion, colorectal SSA/Ps with dysplasia and invasive carcinoma frequently harbored *BRAF* mutations and showed nuclear β-catenin expression. Furthermore, these lesions might not only be associated with MSI-high colorectal cancer, but also MSS, and MSI-high and MSS serrated lesions might have distinct genetic features (such as *FBXW7* and *TP53* mutations). *BRAF*-mutant MSS colon carcinomas are particularly important because they have a dismal prognosis and an aggressive clinical course with adverse histologic features, such as lymphatic and perineural invasion and high tumor budding [52, 53]. Further investigations are required to elucidate molecular biological characteristics in the serrated neoplasia pathway in greater detail.

Abbreviations
APC: Adenomatous polyposis coli; MSI: Microsatellite instability; MSI-high: High levels of microsatellite instability; MSI-low: Low levels of MSI; MSS: Microsatellite-stable; NGS: Next-generation sequencing; SSA/P: Sessile serrated adenoma/polyp

Acknowledgements
The work was supported in part by a Grant-in-Aid from the Japan Society for the Promotion of Science (#18 K15796 to T. Murakami).

Competing interests
The authors declare that they have no competing interests.

Funding
No funds have been received for this study.

Authors' contributions
TM, YA, and TS designed the study; TM, YA, NY, TH, NS, TS, and NS performed technical procedures and acquired pathological and clinical data; TM, YA, AN, and TY analyzed and interpreted the data; TM drafted the manuscript; all authors reviewed and approved the final version of the manuscript. All individuals listed as co-authors of the manuscript have significantly contributed to this study.

References
1. Torlakovic E, Skovlund E, Snover DC, Torlakovic G, Nesland JM. Morphologic reappraisal of serrated colorectal polyps. Am J Surg Pathol. 2003;27:65–81.
2. Snover DC, Ahnen DJ, Burt RW, Odze RD. Serrated polyps of the colon and rectum and serrated polyposis. In: Bosman FT, Carneiro F, Hruban RH, Theise ND, editors. WHO classification of tumours of the digestive system. Lyon: IARC Press; 2010. p. 160–5.
3. Kambara T, Simms LA, Whitehall VL, Spring KJ, Wynter CV, Walsh MD, et al. BRAF mutation is associated with DNA methylation in serrated polyps and cancers of the colorectum. Gut. 2004;53:1137–44.
4. O'Brien MJ, Yang S, Mack C, Xu H, Huang CS, Mulcahy E, et al. Comparison of microsatellite instability, CpG island methylation phenotype, BRAF and KRAS status in serrated polyps and traditional adenomas indicates separate pathways to distinct colorectal carcinoma end points. Am J Surg Pathol. 2006;30:1491–501.
5. Patil DT, Shadrach BL, Rybicki LA, Leach BH, Pai RK. Proximal colon cancers and the serrated pathway: a systematic analysis of precursor histology and BRAF mutation status. Mod Pathol. 2012;25:1423–31.

6. Kim YH, Kakar S, Cun L, Deng G, Kim YS. Distinct CpG island methylation profiles and BRAF mutation status in serrated and adenomatous colorectal polyps. Int J Cancer. 2008;123:2587–93.

7. Kim KM, Lee EJ, Ha S, Kang SY, Jang KT, Park CK, et al. Molecular features of colorectal hyperplastic polyps and sessile serrated adenoma/polyps from Korea. Am J Surg Pathol. 2011;35:1274–86.

8. Dhir M, Yachida S, Van Neste L, Glöckner SC, Jeschke J, Pappou EP, et al. Sessile serrated adenomas and classical adenomas: an epigenetic perspective on premalignant neoplastic lesions of the gastrointestinal tract. Int J Cancer. 2011;129:1889–98.

9. Murakami T, Mitomi H, Saito T, Takahashi M, Sakamoto N, Fukui N, et al. Distinct WNT/β-catenin signaling activation in the serrated neoplasia pathway and the adenoma-carcinoma sequence of the colorectum. Mod Pathol. 2015;28:146–58.

10. Jass JR, Baker K, Zlobec I, Higuchi T, Barker M, Buchanan D, et al. Advanced colorectal polyps with the molecular and morphological features of serrated polyps and adenomas: concept of a 'fusion' pathway to colorectal cancer. Histopathology. 2006;49:121–31.

11. Spring KJ, Zhao ZZ, Karamatic R, Walsh MD, Whitehall VL, Pike T, et al. High prevalence of sessile serrated adenomas with BRAF mutations: a prospective study of patients undergoing colonoscopy. Gastroenterology. 2006;131:1400–7.

12. Fujita K, Yamamoto H, Matsumoto T, Hirahashi M, Gushima M, Kishimoto J, et al. Sessile serrated adenoma with early neoplastic progression: a clinicopathologic and molecular study. Am J Surg Pathol. 2011;35:295–304.

13. Yachida S, Mudali S, Martin SA, Montgomery EA, Iacobuzio-Donahue CA. Beta-catenin nuclear labeling is a common feature of sessile serrated adenomas and correlates with early neoplastic progression following BRAF activation. Am J Surg Pathol. 2009;33:1823–32.

14. Powell SM, Zilz N, Beazer-Barclay Y, Bryan TM, Hamilton SR, Thibodeau SN, et al. APC mutations occur early during colorectal tumorigenesis. Nature. 1992;359:235–7.

15. Miyoshi Y, Nagase H, Ando H, Horii A, Ichii S, Nakatsuru S, et al. Somatic mutations of the APC gene in colorectal tumors: mutation cluster region in the APC gene. Hum Mol Genet. 1992;1:229–33.

16. Meldrum C, Doyle MA, Tothill RW. Next-generation sequencing for cancer diagnostics: a practical perspective. Clin Biochem Rev. 2011;32:177–95.

17. Diaz Z, Aguilar-Mahecha A, Paquet ER, Basik M, Orain M, Camlioglu E, et al. Next-generation biobanking of metastases to enable multidimensional molecular profiling in personalized medicine. Mod Pathol. 2013;26:1413–24.

18. Walsh MD, Clendenning M, Williamson E, Pearson SA, Walters RJ, Nagler B, et al. Expression of MUC2, MUC5AC, MUC5B, and MUC6 mucins in colorectal cancers and their association with the CpG island methylator phenotype. Mod Pathol. 2013;26:1642–56.

19. Khaidakov M, Lai KK, Roudachevski D, Sargsyan J, Goyne HE, Pai RK, et al. Gastric proteins MUC5AC and TFF1 as potential diagnostic markers of colonic sessile serrated adenomas/polyps. Am J Clin Pathol. 2016;146:530–7.

20. Ban S, Mitomi H, Horiguchi H, Sato H, Shimizu M. Adenocarcinoma arising in small sessile serrated adenoma/polyp (SSA/P) of the colon: clinicopathological study of eight lesions. Pathol Int. 2014;64:123–32.

21. Morin PJ, Sparks AB, Korinek V, Barker N, Clevers H, Vogelstein B, et al. Activation of β-catenin-Tcf signaling in colon cancer by mutations in β-catenin or APC. Science. 1997;275:1787–90.

22. Bettington M, Walker N, Rosty C, Brown I, Clouston A, McKeone D, et al. Clinicopathological and molecular features of sessile serrated adenomas with dysplasia or carcinoma. Gut. 2017;66:97–106.

23. de la Chapelle A, Hampel H. Clinical relevance of microsatellite instability in colorectal cancer. J Clin Oncol. 2010;28:3380–7.

24. Cancer Genome Atlas Network. Comprehensive molecular characterization of human colon and rectal cancer. Nature. 2012;487:330–7.

25. Day FL, Jorissen RN, Lipton L, Mouradov D, Sakthianandeswaren A, Christie M, et al. PIK3CA and PTEN gene and exon mutation-specific clinicopathologic and molecular associations in colorectal cancer. Clin Cancer Res. 2013;19:3285 96.

26. Spruck CH, Strohmaier H, Sangfelt O, Müller HM, Hubalek M, Müller-Holzner E, et al. Hcdc4 gene mutations in endometrial cancer. Cancer Res. 2002;62:4535–9.

27. Koepp DM, Schaefer LK, Ye X, Keyomarsi K, Chu C, Harper JW, et al. Phosphorylation-dependent ubiquitination of cyclin E by the SCFFbw7 ubiquitin ligase. Science. 2001;294:173–7.

28. Nateri AS, Riera-sans L, Da Costa C, Behrens A. The ubiquitin ligase SCFFbw7 antagonizes apoptotic JNK signaling. Science. 2004;303:1374–8.

29. Wei W, Jin J, Schlisio S, Harper JW, Kaelin WG Jr. The v-Jun point mutation allows c-Jun to escape GSK3-dependent recognition and destruction by the Fbw7 ubiquitin ligase. Cancer Cell. 2005;8:25–33.

30. Welcker M, Orian A, Jin J, Grim JE, Harper JW, Eisenman RN, et al. The Fbw7 tumor suppressor regulates glycogen synthase kinase 3 phosphorylation-dependent c-Myc protein degradation. Proc Natl Acad Sci U S A. 2004;101:9085–90.

31. Yada M, Hatakeyama S, Kamura T, Nishiyama M, Tsunematsu R, Imaki H, et al. Phosphorylation-dependent degradation of c-Myc is mediated by the F-box protein Fbw7. EMBO J. 2004;23:2116–25.

32. Inuzuka H, Shaik S, Onoyama I, Gao D, Tseng A, Maser RS, et al. SCF (FBW7) regulates cellular apoptosis by targeting MCL1 for ubiquitylation and destruction. Nature. 2011;471:104–9.

33. Wertz IE, Kusam S, Lam C, Okamoto T, Sandoval W, Anderson DJ, et al. Sensitivity to antitubulin chemotherapeutics is regulated by MCL1 and FBW7. Nature. 2011;471:110–4.

34. Fryer CJ, White JB, Jones KA. Mastermind recruits CycC: CDK8 to phosphorylate the notch ICD and coordinate activation with turnover. Mol Cell. 2004;16:509–20.

35. Tetzlaff MT, Yu W, Li M, Zhang P, Finegold M, Mahon K, et al. Defective cardiovascular development and elevated cyclin e and notch proteins in mice lacking the fbw7 f-box protein. Proc Natl Acad Sci U S A. 2004;101:3338–45.

36. Tsunematsu R, Nakayama K, Oike Y, Nishiyama M, Ishida N, Hatakeyama S, et al. Mouse Fbw7/Sel-10/Cdc4 is required for notch degradation during vascular development. J Biol Chem. 2004;279:9417–23.

37. Mao JH, Perez-Losada J, Wu D, Delrosario R, Tsunematsu R, Nakayama KI, et al. Fbxw7/Cdc4 is a p53-dependent, haploinsufficient tumour suppressor gene. Nature. 2004;432:775–9.

38. Kwon YW, Kim IJ, Wu D, Lu J, Stock WA Jr, Liu Y, et al. Pten regulates Aurora-a and cooperates with Fbxw7 in modulating radiation-induced tumor development. Mol Cancer Res. 2012;10:834–44.

39. Wang R, Wang Y, Liu N, Ren C, Jiang C, Zhang K, et al. FBW7 regulates endothelial functions by targeting KLF2 for ubiquitination and degradation. Cell Res. 2013;23:803–19.

40. Mao JH, Kim IJ, Wu D, Climent J, Kang HC, DelRosario R, et al. FBXW7 targets mTOR for degradation and cooperates with PTEN in tumor suppression. Science. 2008;321:1499–502.

41. Bengoechea-Alonso MT, Ericsson J. Tumor suppressor Fbxw7 regulates TGFβ signaling by targeting TGIF1 for degradation. Oncogene. 2010;29:5322–8.

42. Cao J, Ge MH, Ling ZQ. Fbxw7 tumor suppressor: a vital regulator contributes to human tumorigenesis. Medicine (Baltimore). 2016;95:e2496.

43. Akhoondi S, Sun D, von der Lehr N, Apostolidou S, Klotz K, Maljukova A, et al. FBXW7/hCDC4 is a general tumor suppressor in human cancer. Cancer Res. 2007;67:9006–12.

44. Malapelle U, Pisapia P, Sgariglia R, Vigliar E, Biglietto M, Carlomagno C, et al. Less frequently mutated genes in colorectal cancer: evidences from next-generation sequencing of 653 routine cases. J Clin Pathol. 2016;69:767–71.

45. Chang CC, Lin HH, Lin JK, Lin CC, Lan YT, Wang HS, et al. FBXW7 mutation analysis and its correlation with clinicopathological features and prognosis in colorectal cancer patients. Int J Biol Markers. 2015;30:e88–95.

46. Leggett B, Whitehall V. Role of the serrated pathway in colorectal cancer pathogenesis. Gastroenterology. 2010;138:2088–100.

47. O'Brien MJ, Zhao Q, Yang S. Colorectal serrated pathway cancers and precursors. Histopathology. 2015;66:49–65.

48. Ionov Y, Peinado MA, Malkhosyan S, Shibata D, Perucho M. Ubiquitous somatic mutations in simple repeated sequences reveal a new mechanism for colonic carcinogenesis. Nature. 1993;363:558–61.

49. Kim H, Jen J, Vogelstein B, Hamilton SR. Clinical and pathological characteristics of sporadic colorectal carcinomas with DNA replication errors in microsatellite sequences. Am J Pathol. 1994;145:148–56.

50. Cottu PH, Muzeau F, Estreicher A, Fléjou JF, Iggo R, Thomas G, et al. Inverse correlation between RER+ status and p53 mutation in colorectal cancer cell lines. Oncogene. 1996;13:2727–30.

51. Rivlin N, Brosh R, Oren M, Rotter V. Mutations in the p53 tumor suppressor gene: important milestones at the various steps of tumorigenesis. Genes Cancer. 2011;2:466–74.

52. Pai RK, Jayachandran P, Koong AC, Chang DT, Kwok S, Ma L, et al. BRAF-mutated, microsatellite-stable adenocarcinoma of the proximal colon: an aggressive adenocarcinoma with poor survival, mucinous differentiation, and adverse morphologic features. Am J Surg Pathol. 2012;36:744–52.

53. Samowitz WS, Sweeney C, Herrick J, Albertsen H, Levin TR, Murtaugh MA, et al. Poor survival associated with the BRAF V600E mutation in microsatellite-stable colon cancers. Cancer Res. 2005;65:6063–9.

Permissions

All chapters in this book were first published in DP, by BioMed Central; hereby published with permission under the Creative Commons Attribution License or equivalent. Every chapter published in this book has been scrutinized by our experts. Their significance has been extensively debated. The topics covered herein carry significant findings which will fuel the growth of the discipline. They may even be implemented as practical applications or may be referred to as a beginning point for another development.

The contributors of this book come from diverse backgrounds, making this book a truly international effort. This book will bring forth new frontiers with its revolutionizing research information and detailed analysis of the nascent developments around the world.

We would like to thank all the contributing authors for lending their expertise to make the book truly unique. They have played a crucial role in the development of this book. Without their invaluable contributions this book wouldn't have been possible. They have made vital efforts to compile up to date information on the varied aspects of this subject to make this book a valuable addition to the collection of many professionals and students.

This book was conceptualized with the vision of imparting up-to-date information and advanced data in this field. To ensure the same, a matchless editorial board was set up. Every individual on the board went through rigorous rounds of assessment to prove their worth. After which they invested a large part of their time researching and compiling the most relevant data for our readers.

The editorial board has been involved in producing this book since its inception. They have spent rigorous hours researching and exploring the diverse topics which have resulted in the successful publishing of this book. They have passed on their knowledge of decades through this book. To expedite this challenging task, the publisher supported the team at every step. A small team of assistant editors was also appointed to further simplify the editing procedure and attain best results for the readers.

Apart from the editorial board, the designing team has also invested a significant amount of their time in understanding the subject and creating the most relevant covers. They scrutinized every image to scout for the most suitable representation of the subject and create an appropriate cover for the book.

The publishing team has been an ardent support to the editorial, designing and production team. Their endless efforts to recruit the best for this project, has resulted in the accomplishment of this book. They are a veteran in the field of academics and their pool of knowledge is as vast as their experience in printing. Their expertise and guidance has proved useful at every step. Their uncompromising quality standards have made this book an exceptional effort. Their encouragement from time to time has been an inspiration for everyone.

The publisher and the editorial board hope that this book will prove to be a valuable piece of knowledge for researchers, students, practitioners and scholars across the globe.

List of Contributors

Ming Zhao
Department of Pathology, Zhejiang Provincial People's Hospital, Hangzhou, China

Lixin Zhou, Li Sun, Dongfeng Niu, Zhongwu Li, Xiaozheng Huang, Qiang Kang and Lin Jia
Department of Pathology, Key Laboratory of Carcinogenesis and Translational Research (Ministry of Education), Peking University Cancer Hospital (Beijing Cancer Hospital), Beijing, China

Yan Song and Xun Zhang
Department of Pathology, Cancer Hospital of Chinese Academy of Medical Sciences, Beijing, China

Yunquan Guo and Feng Zhao
Department of Pathology, Xinjiang Medical University Affiliated Tumor Hospital, Urumqi, China

Peng Wang
Department of Pathology, Beijing Ditan Hospital, Beijing, China

Junqiu Yue
Department of Pathology, Hubei Cancer Hospital, Wuhan, China

Jinping Lai
Department of Pathology, Saint Louis University School of Medicine, Saint Louis, MO, USA

Dengfeng Cao
Department of Pathology and Immunology, Washington University School of Medicine, 660 S South Euclid Avenue Campus Saint Louis, MO 63110, USA

Bao-Hua Yu, Xiao-Yan Zhou, Da-Ren Shi and Wen-Tao Yang
Department of Pathology, Fudan University Shanghai Cancer Center, Dong-an Road 270, Xuhui District, Shanghai 200032, China
Department of Oncology, Shanghai Medical College, Fudan University, Shanghai, China

Bai-Zhou Li
Department of Pathology, the Second Affiliated Hospital of Zhejiang University, 88 Jiefang Road, Hangzhou 310009, China

Piotr Donizy and Agnieszka Halon
Department of Pathomorphology and Oncological Cytology, Wroclaw Medical University, ul. Borowska 213, 50-556 Wroclaw, Poland

Przemyslaw Biecek
Faculty of Mathematics and Information Science, Warsaw University of Technology, Koszykowa 75, 00-662 Warsaw, Poland

Adam Maciejczyk
Department of Oncology and Clinic of Radiation Oncology, Wroclaw Medical University, pl. Hirszfelda 12, 53-413 Wroclaw, Poland
Lower Silesian Oncology Centre, pl. Hirszfelda 12, 53-413 Wroclaw, Poland

Rafal Matkowski
Lower Silesian Oncology Centre, pl. Hirszfelda 12, 53-413 Wroclaw, Poland
Department of Oncology and Division of Surgical Oncology, Wroclaw Medical University, pl. Hirszfelda 12, 53-413 Wroclaw, Poland

Ana Paula Percicote and Gabriel Lazaretti Mardegan
Federal University of Paraná, Curitiba, Brazil

Elizabeth Schneider Gugelmim
Anatomic Pathology Service at the Pequeno Príncipe Hospital, Curitiba, Brazil

Sergio Ossamu Ioshii and Lúcia de Noronha
Department of Medical Pathology, Federal University of Paraná and School of Health of the Pontifical Catholic University of Paraná, Curitiba, Brazil

Ana Paula Kuczynski
Oncology Service at the Pequeno Príncipe Hospital, Curitiba, Brazil

Seigo Nagashima
School of Health of the Pontifical Catholic University of Paraná, Curitiba, Brazil

Peifeng Li, Jing Ma, Xiumin Zhang, Yong Guo, Yixiong Liu, Xia Li, Danhui Zhao and Zhe Wang
State Key Laboratory of Cancer Biology, Department of Pathology, Xijing Hospital and School of Basic Medicine, The Fourth Military Medical University, Changle West Road #169, Xi'an 710032, Shaan Xi Province, China

Kristen M. Plasseraud, Robert W. Cook and Federico A. Monzon
Castle Biosciences, Inc., 820 S. Friendswood Drive, Suite 201, Friendswood, TX 77546, USA

Jeff K. Wilkinson, Kristen M. Oelschlager, Trisha M. Poteet and John F. Stone
Castle Biosciences Laboratory, 3737 N. 7th St, Suite 160, Phoenix, AZ 85014, USA

Alia Albawardi and Saeeda Almarzooqi
Pathology Department, College of Medicine and Health Sciences, UAE University, Al Ain, United Arab Emirates

M. Ruhul Quddus
Department of Pathology, Women and Infants Hospital/Alpert Medical of Brown University, Providence, RI 02905, USA

Shamsa Al Awar
Obstetrics and Gynecology Department, College of Medicine and Health Sciences, UAE University, Al Ain, United Arab Emirates

Andreas H. Scheel
Institute of Pathology, University Hospital Cologne, Kerpener Str. 62, 50937 Cologne, Germany

Frédérique Penault-Llorca
Département de Pathologie, Centre Jean-Perrin, 58, rue Montalembert, 392, 63011 Clermont-Ferrand cedex 1, BP, France

Wedad Hanna
Department of Laboratory Medicine and Pathobiology, University of Toronto, Toronto, Canada

Gustavo Baretton
Institute of Pathology, University Hospital Dresden, Fetscherstr, 74, 01307 Dresden, Germany

Judith Burchhardt and Manfred Hofmann
Institute of Pathology Nordhessen, Germaniastraße 7, 34119 Kassel, Germany

Peter Middel
Institute of Pathology Nordhessen, Germaniastraße 7, 34119 Kassel, Germany
Institute of Pathology, University Hospital Göttingen, Robert-Koch-Str. 40, 37075 Göttingen, Germany

Josef Rüschoff
Institute of Pathology Nordhessen, Germaniastraße 7, 34119 Kassel, Germany
Targos Molecular Pathology GmbH, Germaniastraße 7, 34119 Kassel, Germany

Bharat Jasani
Targos Molecular Pathology GmbH, Germaniastraße 7, 34119 Kassel, Germany

Bo Zhu, Yichao Wang, Xiaolin Wang, Shiwu Wu, Lei Zhou, Xiaomeng Gong, Wenqing Song and Danna Wang
Department of Pathology, The First Affiliated Hospital of Bengbu Medical College, Bengbu, China
Department of Pathology, Bengbu Medical University, Bengbu, China

Xiaolong Liang, Jian Sun, Huanwen Wu, Yufeng Luo, Lili Wang, Junliang Lu, Zhiwen Zhang, Zhiyong Liang and Tonghua Liu
Department of Pathology, Peking Union Medical College Hospital, Peking Union Medical College and Chinese Academy of Medical Sciences, No. 1 Shuai Fu Yuan, Wangfujing, Beijing 100730, People's Republic of China

Junchao Guo
Department of General Surgery, Peking Union Medical College Hospital, Peking Union Medical College and Chinese Academy of Medical Sciences, No. 1 Shuai Fu Yuan, Wangfujing, Beijing 100730, People's Republic of China

Hyun-Jung Kim
Department of Pathology, Inje University Sanggye Paik Hospital, 1342, Dongilro, Nowon-gu, Seoul, South Korea

Ji Eun Kwon
Department of Pathology, Ajou University school of Medicine, Suwon, South Korea

Nam Hoon Cho
Department of Pathology, Yonsei Medical College of Medicine, Seoul, South Korea

Yeong-Jin Choi
Department of Pathology, Seoul St Mary's Hospital, The Catholic University, Seoul, South Korea

So Dug Lim
Department of Pathology, Konkuk University Medical center, Konkuk University School of Medicine, Seoul, South Korea

Yong Mee Cho
Department of Pathology, Asan Medical Center, Ulsan College of Medicine, Seoul, South Korea

Sun Young Jun
Department of Pathology, Inchun St. Mary's Hospital, The Catholic University, Incheon, South Korea

Sanghui Park
Department of Pathology, College of Medicine, Ewha Womens University, Seoul, South Korea

Young A. Kim
Department of Pathology, SMG-SNU Boramae Medical Center, Seoul, South Korea

Sung-Sun Kim
Departments of Pathology, Chonnam National University Medical school, Gwangju, South Korea

Mi Sun Choe
Department of Pathology, Keimyung University School of Medicine, Daegu, South Korea

Jung-dong Lee and Dae Yong Kang
Office of Biostatistics, Ajou University, School of Medicine, Suwon, South Korea

Jae Y. Ro
Department of Pathology, Houston Methodist Hospital, Weill Medical College of Cornell University, New York, USA

Paul Scorer, Marietta Scott, Nicola Lawson and Craig Barker
Precision Medicine Laboratories, Precision Medicine and Genomics, IMED Biotech Unit, AstraZeneca, HODGKIN, C/O B310 Cambridge Science Park, Milton Road, Cambridge CB4 0WG, UK

Marianne J. Ratcliffe and Jill Walker
Oncology Companion Diagnostics Unit, Precision Medicine and Genomics, IMED Biotech Unit, AstraZeneca, Cambridge, UK

Marlon C. Rebelatto
Translational Sciences, Research, MedImmune, Gaithersburg, MD, USA

Laura Fontana, Rossella Falcone and Anna Marzorati
Department of Pathophysiology and Transplantation, Università degli Studi di Milano, Via Francesco Sforza, 35 -20122 Milan, Italy

Eleonora Bonaparte, Chiara Pesenti, Leda Paganini, Silvia Tabano, Silvano Bosari and Monica Miozzo
Department of Pathophysiology and Transplantation, Università degli Studi di Milano, Via Francesco Sforza, 35 -20122 Milan, Italy
Division of Pathology, Fondazione IRCCS Ca' Granda Ospedale Maggiore Policlinico, Via Francesco Sforza, 35 -20122 Milan, Italy

Mario Nosotti
Department of Pathophysiology and Transplantation, Università degli Studi di Milano, Via Francesco Sforza, 35 -20122 Milan, Italy
Thoracic Surgery and Lung Transplantation Unit, Fondazione IRCCS Ca' Granda Ospedale Maggiore Policlinico, Via Francesco Sforza, 35 -20122 Milan, Italy

Stefano Ferrero
Division of Pathology, Fondazione IRCCS Ca' Granda Ospedale Maggiore Policlinico, Via Francesco Sforza, 35 -20122 Milan, Italy
Department of Biomedical, Surgical and Dental Sciences, Università degli Studi di Milano, Medical School, Via Francesco Sforza, 35 -20122 Milan, Italy

Paolo Mendogni
Thoracic Surgery and Lung Transplantation Unit, Fondazione IRCCS Ca' Granda Ospedale Maggiore Policlinico, Via Francesco Sforza, 35 -20122 Milan, Italy

Claudia Bareggi
Oncology Unit, Fondazione IRCCS Ca' Granda Ospedale Maggiore Policlinico, Via Francesco Sforza, 35 -20122 Milan, Italy

Silvia Maria Sirchia
Medical Genetics, Department of Health Sciences, Università degli Studi di Milano, via Antonio di Rudini, 8 -20142 Milan, Italy

Tomohisa Sakai, Yoshihiro Nishida, Shunsuke Hamada, Hiroshi Koike, Kunihiro Ikuta, Takehiro Ota and Naoki Ishiguro
Department of Orthopaedic Surgery, Nagoya University Graduate School and School of Medicine, 65 Tsurumai, Showa, Nagoya, Aichi 466-8550, Japan

Haiyue Wang, Zhongwu Li, Wei Sun, Xin Yang, Lixin Zhou, Xiaozheng Huang, Ling Jia and Dongmei Lin
Key Laboratory of Carcinogenesis and Translational Research (Ministry of Education), Department of Pathology, Peking University Cancer Hospital and Institute, No. 52 Fucheng Road, Haidian District, Beijing 100142, People's Republic of China

Bin Dong
Key Laboratory of Carcinogenesis and Translational Research (Ministry of Education), Department of Central Laboratory, Peking University Cancer Hospital and Institute, Beijing 100142, People's Republic of China

Ruping Liu
Beijing Institute of Graphic Communication, Beijing 102600, People's Republic of China

Mi-Jung Kim
Department of Pathology, Daehang hospital, 481-10 BangBae3-dong, Seocho-gu, 137-820 Seoul, Republic of Korea

Eun-Jung Lee, Do Sun Kim, Doo Han Lee and Eui Gon Youk
Department of Surgery, Daehang hospital, 481-10 Bang-Bae3-dong, Seocho-gu, 137-820 Seoul, Republic of Korea

Hyun-Jung Kim
Department of Pathology, University of Inje College of Medicine, Sanggye Paik hospital, Dongil-ro 1342, Nowon-gu, Seoul, Republic of Korea

Essam Ayad, Ahmed Soliman, Shady Elia Anis and Amira Ben Salem
Department of Pathology, Cairo University, Cairo, Egypt

Pengchao Hu and Youhong Dong
Department of Oncology, XiangYang No.1 People's Hospital Affiliated to Hubei University of Medicine, Xiangyang, Hubei 441000, People's Republic of China

Kerstin Hartmann, Kornelia Schlombs, Mark Laible and Claudia Gürtler
BioNTech Diagnostics GmbH, An der Goldgrube 12, 55131 Mainz, Germany

Marcus Schmidt
Department of Obstetrics and Gynecology, Johannes Gutenberg University, Langenbeckstraße 1, 55131 Mainz, Germany

Ugur Sahin
BioNTech AG, An der Goldgrube 12, 55131 Mainz, Germany

Hans-Anton Lehr
Institute of Pathology, Medizin Campus Bodensee, Röntgenstraße 2, 88048 Friedrichshafen, Germany

Cleo-Aron Weis, Hanaa Al-ahmdi and Timo Gaiser
Institute of Pathology, University Medical Centre Mannheim, University of Heidelberg, 68167 Mannheim, Germany

Jakob Nikolas Kather
Department of Medical Oncology and Internal Medicine VI, National Center for Tumor Diseases, University Hospital Heidelberg, Heidelberg University, Heidelberg, Germany

Susanne Melchers
Department of Dermatology, Venereology and Allergology, University Medical Center Mannheim, Heidelberg University, Mannheim, Germany

Marion J. Pollheimer and Cord Langner
Institute of Pathology, Medical University Graz, Graz, Austria

Miao Ruan, Tian Tian, Jia Rao, Xiaoli Xu, Baohua Yu, Wentao Yang and Ruohong Shui
Department of Pathology, Fudan University Shanghai Cancer Center, Shanghai, China

Department of Oncology, Shanghai Medical College, Fudan University, Shanghai, China

Keiko Segawa, Shintaro Sugita, Tomoyuki Aoyama, Hiroko Asanuma, Taro Sugawara, Yumika Ito, Mitsuhiro Tsujiwaki, Hiromi Fujita and Tadashi Hasegawa
Department of Surgical Pathology, Sapporo Medical University, School of Medicine, Sapporo, Hokkaido 060-8543, Japan

Terufumi Kubo
Department of Pathology, Sapporo Medical University, School of Medicine, Sapporo, Hokkaido 060-8556, Japan

Makoto Emori
Department of Orthopedic Surgery, Sapporo Medical University, School of Medicine, Sapporo, Hokkaido 060-8543, Japan

Hans-Ullrich Völker and Annette Strehl
Pathology, Leopoldina Krankenhaus GmbH, Gustav-Adolf-Str 8, D-97422 Schweinfurt, Germany

Michael Weigel
Department of Gynecology, Leopoldina Krankenhaus GmbH, Gustav-Adolf-Str 8, D-97422 Schweinfurt, Germany

Lea Frey
Institute for Pathology, University of Wuerzburg, Josef-Schneider-Str. 2, D-97080 Wuerzburg, Germany

Maja Mizdrak
Department of Nephrology and Hemodialysis, University Hospital Centre Split, Šoltanska 1, 21000 Split, Croatia

Katarina Vukojević and Natalija Filipović
Department of Anatomy, Histology and Embryology, University of Split School of Medicine, Split, Croatia

Vesna Čapkun
Department of Nuclear Medicine, University Hospital Centre Split, Split, Croatia

Benjamin Benzon and Merica Glavina Durdov
Department of Pathology, Forensic medicine and Cytology, University Hospital Centre Split, Split, Croatia
University of Split School of Medicine, Split, Croatia

Lemeng Sun and Jiuwei Cui
Stem Cell and Cancer Center, The First Bethune Hospital, Jilin University, Changchun, Jilin 130021, People's Republic of China

Liangshu Feng
Department of Neurology and Neuroscience Center, First Hospital of Jilin University, Changchun, Jilin, China

Naoto Sakamoto and Akihito Nagahara
Department of Gastroenterology, Juntendo University School of Medicine, 2-1-1 Hongo, Bunkyo-ku, Tokyo 113-8421, Japan

Takashi Murakami, Yoichi Akazawa, Noboru Yatagai and Takafumi Hiromoto
Department of Gastroenterology, Juntendo University School of Medicine, 2-1-1 Hongo, Bunkyo-ku, Tokyo 113-8421, Japan
Department of Human Pathology, Juntendo University School of Medicine, Tokyo, Japan

Noriko Sasahara, Tsuyoshi Saito and Takashi Yao
Department of Human Pathology, Juntendo University School of Medicine, Tokyo, Japan

Index